HEALING RESEARCH - VOLUME II

Popular Edition

HOW CAN I HEAL
WHAT HURTS?

Wholistic Healing
and
Bioenergies

Daniel J. Benor, M.D.

ISBN 0-9754248-3-1

This is the popular edition of Daniel J. Benor, M.D. *Consciousness,
Bioenergy and Healing*, Wholistic Healing Publications 2004. Parts of this
book appeared in a previous European version in *Healing Research: Holistic
Energy Medicine and Spirituality*, Copyright © 1992 Daniel J. Benor, M.D.

Wholistic Healing Publications
PO Box 502
Medford, NJ 08055, USA
(609) 714-1885   Fax (609) 714-3553
DB@WholisticHealingResearch.com

ACKNOWLEDGMENT OF PERMISSIONS TO REPRODUCE MATERIALS

I thank the many authors and publishers who have generously granted their permission to reproduce quotes in this book, in the spirit of healing.

I specifically acknowledge permissions for:
Benor, R. A holistic view to managing stress, In: Ronald A. Fisher & Pearl McDaid, *Palliative
Day Care,* London: Arnold/ Hodder Headline Group 1996, figure no. 12.1.

Besant, A and Leadbeater, CW, *Thought-Forms*, Wheaton, IL: Quest/ Theosophical 1971, Orig.
1925. Used by permission of The Theosophical Publishing House, The Theosophical Society,
Adyar, Madras 600 020, India

Reprinted from *J of Psychosomatic Research,* Volume 43, Miller, M. & Rahe, R H. Life
changes scaling for the 1990s, 279-292, © 1997 with permission of Elsevier Science

For paid permissions, I acknowledge:

The Atman Project by Ken Wilber. Quest Books, Wheaton, IL.

From: UNCOMMON THERAPY: The Psychiatric Techniques of Milton H. Erickson MD. By
Jay Haley. Copyright © 1986, 1973 by Jay Haley. Used by permission of W. W. Norton &
Company, Inc.

Swift, G. A contextual model for holistic nursing practice, from J. Holistic Nursing 1994,
12(3), 265-281, figures1 & 2, © 1994 by Sage Publications, Inc. Preprinted by Permission of
Sage Publications, Inc.

CONTENTS

INTRODUCTION   **1**

THE FOUR VOLUMES OF *HEALING RESEARCH*   **9**

CHAPTER 1: SELF-HEALING   **14**
Personality   19
Normality   33
Psychosomatic Disorders   34
The Body's Regulating Systems   35
Talking/Relational Psychotherapy   37
Physical Symptoms Addressed by Psychotherapy   40
Physical Symptoms Addressed by Bodywork Therapies   46
Psychological Conditioning (Reinforcement) and Behavior Therapy   47
Conditioning the Immune System   50
Body-Mind Therapies and Spiritual Healing   51
Psychological Conditioning, Feedback Loops, and Spiritual Healing   53
Suggestion   59
Hypnosis   74
Biofeedback   91
Unusual Human Abilities   95
Special Brain and Body Functions   100
Brain Hemispheric Functions   111
Self-Healing Programs   117
Spontaneous Remissions of Illness   129
A Few Words in Summary about Psychotherapies   132
The Mind and the Brain   133
Transpersonal Psychotherapy   135
Collective Consciousness and Spiritual Awareness   156
Preview of an Energy Healing Model   158

CHAPTER 2: WHOLISTIC ENERGY MEDICINE   **161**
Complementary/Alternative Medicine (CAM) Therapies   181
Bioenergies and CAM   183
CAM Modalities (from Acupuncture to Yoga)   185
Problems Addressed Effectively by CAM Modalities   354
CAM Issues   359

CHAPTER 3: THE HUMAN ENERGY FIELD 388
Auras 389
Kirlian Photography 404
Laboratory Measurements of Biological Energy Fields 411

CHAPTER 4: GEOBIOLOGICAL EFFECTS 439
Radiesthesia (Dowsing) and Radionics 439
Cosmobiology and Astrology 465

CHAPTER 5: SELF-HEALING APPROACHES AND EXERCISES: 476
Introduction 476
Background 477
Reasoning Your Way Through Stress 478
The Body: Index and Aid in Dealing with Stress 496
Feeling Your Way Through Stress 500
Unconscious Roots of Stress 506
Head Working with Heart 515
Varieties of Healings for Stress 533
Collective Consciousness 568
You're On Your Way to Self-Healing 569
CONCLUSION 570

Appendix A – Variations on the theme of psychotherapy 575

Notes 578

References 601

Glossary 619

Names Index 625

Subject Index 633

About the Author 648

TABLES

Chapter 1
Table II-1. Life-events inventory
Table II-2. Body terms and metaphors
Table II-3. Acceptance scales
Table II-4. Brain hemispheric functions
Table II-5. Status of four-year cancer
Table II-6. Two-year study of cancer patients treated by
           O. C. Simonton, M.D

Chapter 2
Table II-7. Chakras
Table II-8. CAM vs. Conventional Medicine

Chapter 3
Table II-9. Subjects' and experimenters' locations of pain
Table II-10. Various ways to define the world - Quantum physics vs.
           Newtonian physics

FIGURES

Chapter 1
Figure II-1. Jung polarities
Figure II-2. Angel
Figure II-3 Cartoon – placebo
Figure II-4. Balance
Figure II-5. The complete life cycle

Chapter 2
Figure II-6. Four aspects of health
Figure II-7. The interpenetrating process of healing
Figure II-8. Cartoon – Witch doctor?
Figure II-9. Movement and dance can be combined with healing
Figure II-10. The *Bagua*
Figure II-11. Healing works well with massage and aromatherapy
Figure II-12. Cartoon – Some of my instincts
Figure II-13. Cartoon – Meditation
Figure II-14. Cartoon – The memory of a happiness
Figure II-15. Stress management approaches

Chapter 3
Figure II-16. Kirlian fingertips disturbed balance
Figure II-17. Kirlian fingertip healthy
Figure II-18. Onion roots
Figure II-19. Relaxation circuit, one subject
Figure II-20. Classical diagram of polarities
Figure II-21. Relaxation circuit, two subjects

Chapter 5
Figure II-22. Ego states
Figure II-23 Cartoon – Why aren't you more grateful?
Figure II-24 Hexagrams of the I Ching
Figure II-25 The Norse Runes

DEDICATION

This book is dedicated to the many healers who have been my teachers – through the years of university, medical school, psychiatric training, and then through the countless workshops and classes with healers of a rainbow spectrum of wholistic approaches. This book is also dedicated to the careseekers who have been wonderful teachers themselves, helping me understand the wonders of the human condition.

This "baby" has been more than twenty years in gestation. I know it will continue to grow and mature, as my various teachers continue to bring me into ever deeper awarenesses of the spiritual truths that inform and quicken the adventure we call life.

I hope that a deeper wholistic awareness of our interconnection with each other and with the world around us will promote healings of societies and nations – not only of individuals - because our planet is in dire need of healing.

This book is also dedicated to the seekers who want to find deeper ways for helping themselves, as well as for helping others.

I wish you good healings!

FOREWORD

I have been exploring the realms of healing and parapsychology for more than forty-five years, and my interests have led me to perform extensive evaluations of clairvoyant diagnosis. The research I have conducted in this field has thoroughly convinced me of its validity and usefulness.

Dr. Benor's book goes well beyond anything that I have seen, in documen t-ing the abundance of work that has been done in the psychic-healing field. It would take several years to accumulate all of the information Dr. Benor provides, assuming one could locate all of the sources.

As in every such work, this outstanding presentation by Dr. Benor is not likely to sway or appeal to the mentally inflexible or to those with traditionally closed minds. But for the individual who is truly interested in exploring the information available, and who has a concept of that which is not "known" or is "uncontrolled," *Healing Research* provides an encyclopedic compilation of the material that has been made available up to this point in time. I am personally delighted to have had the opportunity to review the manuscript prior to its publication. Work such as this deserves wide dissemination.

– C. Norman Shealy, MD, PhD[1]

INTRODUCTION

*Real healing... must be "wholing," hence holy, if it is to be long
lasting – and worthy of mankind's unfolding potentials*
.   – Jeanne Pontius Rindge

In *HOW CAN I HEAL WHAT HURTS?* You will learn to understand your problems and heal yourself. You will also learn ways in which you may be helped to
heal through Complementary/Alternative Medicine (CAM).

CAM includes many self-healing approaches, such as relaxation, meditation,
imagery, journaling, fitness and proper diet. Self-healing can be boosted further
by CAM therapists who offer acupuncture, homeopathy, massage and other
methods that conventional medicine has largely ignored, but which the public are
embracing in a big way – because they are highly effective and have few side
effects.

If any of these therapies or terms is unfamiliar, the glossary at the end of the
book will be helpful.

How Can I Heal What Hurts is the popular version of *Healing Research,
Volume II.* The Professional Edition of this volume is generously supported with
research studies, notes and extensive references that are more detailed than the
average reader would want.

Volume I of *Healing Research* explores *wholistic spiritual healing*[2] - treatment
by the laying-on of hands and by mental intent, meditation, and prayer. There is a
massive body of research on spiritual healing. Two thirds of these studies show
significant effects of healing for a variety of problems in humans and animals.
There are also measurable effects on plants, bacteria, yeasts, cells in laboratory
culture, enzymes and DNA.

This evidence is surprising to most of my medical colleagues, who are largely
unfamiliar with CAM, and often very skeptical about spiritual healing. I don't
blame or fault doctors and scientists for their skepticism, because I, myself,
started out a strong disbeliever in healing. Being trained in psychology, medicine,
psychiatry and research, I knew all the conventional wisdom on why healing
couldn't possibly work. It was only in 1980, after nearly 20 years in the study and
practice of psychiatry, that I observed a physical change under a healer's hand
which completely convinced me this is a potent and valuable therapy.

Despite the research evidence, some skeptics continue to say that healing is no
more than a placebo ("sugar pill") effect, produced by healers' suggestions and

healees' expectations. This theory is clearly contradicted by the studies showing significant healing effects on animals, plants and other living things. The fact that healers can improve the health of animals and plants supports the healers' claims that healing is definitely more than a placebo.

The skeptics may not be entirely wrong, however. The placebo effect is actually a manifestation of the enormous self-healing abilities you have to alter your own states of health and illness. Self-healing can be activated intentionally or unconsciously by caregivers or by people working to heal themselves. Wise physicians who prescribe medicine know well that if they give their patients enthusiastic descriptions of anticipated benefits, they can make the effects of the pills much stronger. Self-healing can similarly contribute to treatments of any sort, including spiritual healing.

> *Are we so afraid to be wrong that we hide from the truth?*
> – John MacEnulty (9/13/03)

Improvements through the placebo effect show that you have enormous self-healing abilities. This book will help you to understand, activate and benefit from these highly effective and wonder-full approaches.

This second volume of *Healing Research* explores the following issues:

1. How can you heal yourself of serious physical diseases and psychological dis-eases?

There are two broad answers to this question.

The first is that everyone has vast mental and emotional resources which they can activate for effective self-healing. It is estimated that you are only aware of and using five percent of your brain capacity. Major portions of your brain are constantly monitoring and regulating body functions that you take completely for granted. You don't have to remind your body to breathe, circulate your blood or digest your food. Your unconscious mind, your hormones and your bioenergy fields handle these and many more body functions without your having to pay attention to them or even know about them.

Your brain also contains enormous stores of memories, mostly buried in your unconscious mind. Some of these memories may include traumas that can cause physical and emotional tensions – both of which can contribute to illness.

Your mind (conscious and unconscious) and body are intimately linked. In CAM therapies this is now acknowledged through the terms *mind-body* and *bodymind,* which are also coming into popular use. This book will explain how your bodymind can allow illness to occur and how you can learn to heal yourself by tapping into the enormous potentials of your mind-body awarenesses and connections. Chapter 1 of this book explains how you can heal yourself.

Varieties of CAM therapies teach how to use your mind to diagnose and treat your own psychological and physical conditions – to a far greater extent than was previously believed possible. Many of these self-healing therapies are explained in Chapter 2, and self-healing exercises that you can explore are suggested in Chapter 5.

The second answer to this question about self-healing is that the body consists of energy as well as matter. CAM therapists suggest that we can harmonize the biological energy patterns of the body and that this, in turn, harmonizes and heals the physical body itself. Chapters 3 and 4 of this book explain bioenergies.

Coming from the opposite direction, these same bodymind mechanisms may contribute to the original development of illnesses. Your mind-body stresses and traumas can express themselves as physical disease though mechanisms explained in Chapter 1. Prevention of illness through these same self-healing techniques is therefore another way you can benefit from CAM approaches.

2. How do biological energies (bioenergies) contribute to healing?

While Western medicine has focused primarily on the physical body, CAM therapists have long been aware that living creatures also possess *biological energy* bodies – which are composed of emotional, mental, relational, and spiritual levels of subtle energies. Each of these biofield levels is intimately interlinked with the others. Each level contributes to your states of health and illness. Each energy field may be addressed by healers, individually or in concert with the others, to improve your physical, psychological, and spiritual health, as well as your relationships with other people and with your environment.

We will consider numerous CAM therapies, many of which address biological energies in the body. Each therapy has its own traditions and understandings of how these bioenergies function, and how you can utilize them to promote health and treat illness: from ancient Chinese applications of *qi* to modern practices of acupressure and Applied Kinesiology; from Biblical healings by Christ and the apostles, and by countless healers in other ancient traditions around the world, to modern varieties of the laying-on of hands in Therapeutic Touch, Healing Touch, Reiki and other healing approaches now practiced in hospitals.

It is not yet clear whether the various CAM therapies are addressing different energies, or whether there is a single energy field that responds differently to different interventions. For instance, acupuncture treats symptoms and disorders by stimulating *meridians* (biological energy lines in the body) and *chakras* (major energy centers on the midline of the body). In spiritual healing (Reiki, Healing Touch), therapists use their hands to address the energy field that surrounds the entire body, as well as to assess states of health and intervene through the chakras. Homeopathy and flower essences offer vibrational remedies diluted in water and alcohol that are taken orally, to interact with the entire organism. We can begin to clarify how these energies function by studying all of these therapies with their various biological energies approaches.

Extensive experiences in these and many other CAM traditions suggest a variety of ways that energy fields in and around the body relate to your physical health and can be accessed in order to improve your health.

Western medicine has been slow to explore these therapies, and slower yet to accept and integrate them within its fold. Volume II of *Healing Research* describes mind-body medicine and spiritual healing as underlying elements that are common among to all therapies – in conventional medicine and CAM modalities.

Building on our clinical picture of bioenergies, we will then seek explanations for the mechanisms of action of biological energies.

Western (Newtonian) medicine meets bioenergy medicine

Modern research in quantum physics studies the behavior of particles and energies at the subatomic level. Quantum physics has proven two theories that challenge many of our conventional scientific concepts:

1. One theory is that matter and energy can be converted back and forth into each other. We address physical objects in our everyday world only as gross matter within Newtonian physics; but in quantum physics we can consider atomic and subatomic units of matter as either particles or as energies.

A chair you sit on feels pretty solid, and is constructed of materials such as wood, metal and cloth. It has a measurable size and weight. These are all properties that Newtonian physics has studied. Quantum physics tells you that the chair is composed of atoms and molecules that are held together by various energies, and there is a lot of space between the atoms and molecules. If we analyze these minute particles, we find that each embodies a certain amount (a *quantum*) of energy. Under certain conditions, we can interact with these particles as though they were just energy.

While quantum physics and conventional physics have been conceived conventionally as separate scientific domains, there is no reason not to assume that the realities of quantum physics cannot apply to a living organism.

2. The second theory is that the precise nature of some of the smallest units of matter are impossible to determine until they are actually observed. Only when an observer perceives their state do they take on the characteristics by which we define and identify them.

This indeterminacy suggests that objective reality as we conceptualize it is an illusion. In fact, at any given moment, we are surrounded by and composed of possibilities and probabilities rather than facts. The very act of scientific observation and measurement actually influences the outcome of the subject being observed.

Does this sound like science fiction? It certainly did to Newtonian physicists earlier in the 20th Century when Einstein first proposed this theory. However, through extensive, highly technical research, the quantum physicists have been able to prove that these theories are correct.

While these principles have been accepted as valid for inanimate matter, they have not been applied to living organisms by conventional science. These two principles fundamentally call into question our long-held Western belief in progressive, irreversible states of disease processes. Your physical conditions may vary according to the manners in which you perceive your own states, and may be altered as well by how caregivers perceive and address them. If the smallest units of subatomic matter can be seen as either particles or as waves of energy, then the function of *bioenergy* within the body takes on a new significance. Bioenergy of a disease process can be altered by how you perceive them, as well as by outside energies. They can offer you ways in which to heal yourself that have not been used in Western medicine.

Intuitives, healers and mystics have been making observations similar to those of quantum physicists over several millennia.[3] They report that they can address the bioenergy body to assess and enhance your health. This ancient wisdom of our ancestors is now being reconsidered in the light of a substantial body of research that is reviewed in the professional editions of *Healing Research, Volumes I and II*.[4] After centuries of independent development, these two seemingly separate paths – modern medicine and traditional medicine – are converging.

As we progress toward the fullest understanding of our bodies and how they function in the world, we will benefit from both of these healing traditions. Quantum physics has not supplanted Newtonian physics. Each still has its place. It is the same with Newtonian medicine and wholistic, bioenergy medicine. This book considers the best of both, to offer a unified theory to guide and inspire the future of healing practice.

Healing in practice

"Linda," a pretty but frail woman looking ten years older than her age of thirty-six, consulted me for a series of severely disabling chronic problems. She had been suffering for eight years from fatigue, headaches, stomachaches, diarrhea, generalized muscle aches, weakness, fitful sleep and sometimes even sleepless nights, extreme tiredness, mental fuzziness ("brain fog") and multiple food allergies.

Her family doctor had initially treated her headaches and stomachaches with a variety of medications. While these partially alleviated her pains, they further diminished the quality of her life – which was already seriously limited by her multiple symptoms. Side effects of the medications included worse mental fog, constipation and stomach cramps, weight gain, increased irritability, and a generalized allergic reaction to one medicine that required other medicines to deal with it.

Prior to her illness, she worked long hours as a broker in an investment firm. As she began having difficulties maintaining the wearing pace of work her job demanded, her employer was less than sympathetic. This added stress was the straw that forced her to seek leave on medical disability – a difficult challenge when her doctor could not find a specific medical diagnosis to explain her multiple symptoms. Her boyfriend of three years left her, not finding the emotional resources to support her through her ordeals. He, like her employer, accused her of being lazy and of making up her symptoms to avoid the stresses of her demanding job.

With the help of a wholistic physician, we established that Linda was suffering from chronic fatigue syndrome, fibromyalgia and candidiasis – all diagnoses that conventional medicine does not even acknowledge, much less treat. Over a period of two years, her multiple symptoms required a series of dietary changes, nutritional supplements, lifestyle adjustments and counseling. Spiritual healing, acupuncture and self-healing techniques helped her to deal with her pain and to regain her normal sleep patterns. Gradually, she was able to return to working (at a less stressful job), and to resume a normal life – after coming to appreciate that her body demanded appropriate attention and coddling, which was actually an expression of her inner emotional needs for the same.[5]

Linda's case is not unusual. There are many problems for which conventional medicine can offer only limited, symptomatic relief. CAM therapies often are much more helpful with these symptoms and illnesses.

The content and style of this book will help you appreciate that Complementary/ Alternative Medicine has its own ways of perceiving, understanding and addressing health and illness. While different in many ways from conventional, Western ways of addressing health issues, CAM is a valid scientific system in and of itself.

In the domains of energy medicine that we will explore, the portal of logic and linear analysis represents only one of several doorways to understanding and interacting with our world. There are additional approaches to these explorations that are equally valid – through emotion, intuition, imagery, metaphor, bioenergies and spiritual awareness.

In conventional science and medical care, logic and linear reasoning are seen as the only valid methods for analyzing and understanding the world of matter, including the human body. Even if this view is valid, it clearly is not comprehensive enough to explain or to guide you in effectively navigating the complex realms of your inner experiences. Your inner worlds are vital to your wellbeing. They include emotions of love, anger, anxiety, depression and hate, and personal contexts of relationships, collective culture, and spiritual awareness. All of these impact your experiences of both health and illness in numerous ways – yet they are beyond the realm of direct examination or objective measurement. These are sorely ignored and neglected in most of conventional Western medical care.

Conventional science dismisses these immeasurably important elements as inaccurate, subjective, imaginary or mystical – in short, as a lot of nonsense. This is a bias of conventional beliefs and thinking that is illustrated in the very word "nonsense." Many aspects of dis-ease and disease addressed by CAM approaches are not directly available to your outer senses, and not measurable by "objective" instruments. The assumption in Western medicine is, therefore, that they cannot be valid or relevant factors for treatment, which in fact they are not – within those frames of reference that are restricted to conventional medicine's linear system of assessment and physical methods of treatment.

Many aspects of the approaches used in CAM therapies are not cut from the fabric of the physical, measurable world of our outer senses. They are woven instead of the inner threads of feelings and intuition, and often include spiritual awarenesses. All of these are just as valid as our outer senses. To dismiss love or anger as irrelevant aspects of your whole self is to ignore the greater portions of your life experience.

The reasonable man adapts himself to the world. The unreasonable one persists in trying to adapt the world to himself. Therefore, all progress depends on the unreasonable man.

– George Bernard Shaw

The worlds of inner knowing are inclusive rather than exclusive. They are better understood with *both/and* approach rather than through *either/or* subdivisions. Inner knowing allows you to see the outer, physical world as one part of the structure of reality – which is connected and interwoven with your inner worlds. You have been given a left brain that specializes in linear awareness and processes, as well as a right brain that specializes in intuitive, patterned awarenesses.

If you disregard the potential of the intuitive, you are ignoring at least half of the images that your brain is capable of projecting on the screen of your consciousness, not to mention the vast and incredibly rich variety of information that is available through much of your unconscious mind. And your intuitive mind has a vast, rich potential for extending your health awareness and healing abilities.

Extensive research in parapsychology[6] shows that your mind can reach outside the limits of your physical body, and can also connect with events from the past and the future. These awarenesses may extend beyond space and time, into spiritual dimensions. This *transcendent consciousness* can be enormously helpful to you in improving your health.

Because such concepts are at variance with Western scientific ways of thinking, many conventional caregivers still reject wholistic concepts. Others, more open to the both/and approach, are able to see these contradictions as reasons to re-examine and expand the basic assumptions of conventional science and medicine. This book makes a strong case for the proposition that it is time to bring Western medical science into the world of a broader reality – or, more accurately, of broader realit*ies*.

Wholistic Integrative Care

Modern Western (Newtonian) medicine is excellent for dealing with infections and physical trauma, and it is currently exploring genetic engineering – which holds both wonderful promises and potential disasters of unknown magnitude.[7]

Wholistic medicine is much more useful in many cases than Newtonian medicine for dealing with chronic illnesses and psychological problems, as we see in countless clinical examples – like in Linda's story, above.

Wholistic care is also a challenge to CAM therapists. Many CAM practitioners make the opposite error of not applying linear analyses to their therapies. CAM therapists may rely entirely on their inner awarenesses to guide their assessments and treatments. They may neglect scientific evaluations of their clinical assessments and treatments, and experimental validations of theories to explain their "unusual" results. This can lead to the error of accepting approaches that are no more than placebos, born of theories that have no validity outside the imaginations of those who propose them. Suggestion is an aspect of every healthcare intervention. There may be remedies in homeopathy, flower essence therapy and aromatherapy, or manipulations in chiropractic and craniosacral therapy, or rituals recommended in spiritual healing which are of no more value than a sugar pill. Linear analyses that explore whether therapies actually accomplish what they claim to do are ethically necessary, in order to assure that we are not charging for services that are, in effect, variations on the theme of suggestion.

Many CAM practitioners are now acknowledging the need for objective linear studies to confirm that their approaches are potent and effective. Chapter 2 of the professional edition of this volume reviews extensive research that does precisely that, with growing numbers of studies of CAM therapies published by conventional caregivers in medical journals. There is a considerable body of evidence confirming that acupuncture, massage, biofeedback, spiritual healing, creative arts therapies, and other CAM approaches offer significant benefits.

Despite their differences, there is every reason to suggest that CAM and conventional therapies can and should be used in combination with each other. *Integrative* or *blended* systems of care provide the best of all possible therapeutic worlds.

> **It is important to note that using conventional linear language to describe non-linear treatments will distort the analysis of these interventions to a greater or lesser extent. To provide a truer taste of the essence of wholistic and bioenergy interventions, this volume includes numerous counterpoint quotations that are matched to the linear text. Through metaphor, imagery, poetry, humor and linear contrasts, we can open ourselves toward the wider, feeling and intuitive nature of these interventions. These draw upon and resonate with the gestaltic, intuitive and spiritual aspects of our consciousness for healing on multiple levels.**

Knowing with the heart is a complement to knowing with the head;
knowing with the head is a balance to knowing with the heart.
                                                        – D.B.

Technical notes
A glossary at the end of the book explains technical terms.

The professional edition, *Consciousness, Bioenergy and Healing*, contains about 1,500 references. This, the popular version of *Healing Research, Volume II*, is designed for easy reading. Only a few, selected references are included in this edition, other than quoted text references.

Similarly, the professional edition includes many more endnotes.

In summary to this Introduction
The complexities of relationships between body, emotions, mind, relationships and spirit make it difficult to analyze these elements and their interconnections separately. There will therefore be overlaps and cross-references in various sections of the analysis of wholistic healing in this book. It is somewhat like exploring the patterns of threads in a multi-colored carpet, where some hues will be more visible because they are on the surface and more densely threaded in some places, while other colors may still be present but more subtly contributing their hue in that section, and yet other tints may be present but only visible beneath the surface after some probing.

THE FOUR VOLUMES OF
HEALING RESEARCH

Though Volume II of this series is complete in itself, it also serves as an extension of the material covered in Volume I, and creates a basis for understanding materials presented in Volumes III and IV. Taken as a whole, the four volume series presents a thorough exploration of the theories and processes of spiritual healing and bioenergy medicine, as well as a broad examination of the related scientific research.

Volume I: *Scientific Validation of a Healing Revolution*
The first volume in the series summarizes an extensive body of research confirming claims by spiritual healers that they can effect improvements in the health of the healees who flock to them, suffering from all the ailments known to humankind.

Volume I defines *spiritual healing* (abbreviated to *healing*) as any purposeful intervention by one or more persons wishing to help another living being to change for the better, using processes of focused intention, or light manual contact or hand movements near the subject of the healing. Healers may also invoke outside agents such as God, Christ, or other individual "higher powers," as well as spirits and universal or cosmic forces or energies. They may call upon special healing energies or forces residing within themselves, apply various techniques of psychokinesis (mind over matter), or activate self-healing powers or energies that are latently present in the healees.

Volume I also reviews anecdotal reports, and an impressive body of research which demonstrates significant healing effects on people, animals, plants, bacteria, yeasts, cells in laboratory culture, enzymes, and DNA. Out of 191 controlled studies of healing, 124 demonstrate significant effects. If we select from these the 50 most rigorous studies, 25 show effects that could occur only one time in 100 and another 12 at a level of 2 to 5 times in 100.

This volume further discusses how spiritual healing may be seen as part of the spectrum of parapsychological, or *psi* phenomena.[8] The term *psi* is derived from the Greek letter Ψ (pronounced *sigh*), used in parapsychology to include telepathy, clairsentience, psychokinesis (PK), and pre- or retro-cognition.[9]

Based on the evidence from the controlled studies presented in Volume I, supported further by many less rigorous studies and anecdotal reports, I take it as a given that spiritual healing does exist, beyond any reasonable doubt.

Volume I address es the question, "Is there adequate research to confirm that spiritual healing is effective?" or more simply, "Does spiritual healing work?" and answers with a resounding "Yes!" Volume I also supplies a wealth of clues to the mystery of *how* healing works.

Volume I, Popular Edition, reviews how healers from around the world describe their work; summarizes in layman's terms the extensive research in healing; surveys the research in parapsychology as a context for understanding spiritual healing.

Volume I, Professional Supplement, reviews only the controlled studies and pilot studies of spiritual healing, in much great detail than the popular edition.

Volume II (Popular Edition): *How Can I Heal What Hurts?*
Volume II continues where Volume I left off, to further address the question: "How does healing work?" This volume deals with therapies involving subtle energies that healers can sense with their hands, and that some can visually perceive as auras of color around living beings. These energies have been reported for thousands of years, yet mainstream modern science has been slow to acknowledge, much less examine them.

Biological energies appear to interact in turn with environmental energies. Research is explored on the effects of earth energies, sunspots, and other influences of heavenly bodies as suggested by astrology, and their relevance to spiritual healing is considered.

Environmental energies interact with the bodymind and with the bioenergy body. We commonly acknowledge this by noting that some places have positive energies or "vibes" – such as a church or a special place in nature. Similarly, we may feel negative vibrations in other places, without apparent reason. These can be so distinctly unpleasant that we avoid being in that space.

We are beginning to appreciate that these perceptions may actually relate to healing energies and harmful energies, as they impact our own biofield and bodymind.

Throughout this volume, wherever possible, I suggest self-healing approaches you can use to explore, understand and heal your problems, bringing greater harmony, healing and happiness into your life. These self-healing exercises are detailed in Chapter 5.

To conclude, I summarize the observations and research discussed in each of the chapters of volume II, and point toward several pathways into a future of integrated care. The separate themes of each chapter are interwoven throughout the fabric of this volume, and the threads are so intricately intertwined and the patterns so complex that it is impossible to separate them entirely from one another. Together they form an over-arching pattern that is as yet beyond our full understanding. The entire tapestry of existence is contained in the complexity of the grand design.

The professional version of Volume II, *Consciousness, Bioenergy and Healing,* reviews and discusses the controlled studies and pilot studies of self-healing, CAM and bioenergy therapies in greater detail. It is extensively referenced for further reading and research. It does not contain Chapter 5 of the Popular Edition, which has a collection of self-healing exercises.

Volume III: Science, Spirit, and the Eternal Soul

After centuries of ignoring spiritual aspects of healing, Western science is now applying its own methodology to explore and confirm an inner nature of Nature that does not conform to common, linear logic.

Volume III explores studies of consciousness extending beyond the body, as in out-of-body and near-death experiences.

Volume III also reviews research from quantum physics that observers actually shape what they perceive, and therefore that there is no way to define an *objective* reality, as Western science has presumed. The processes and phenomena observed by scientists may be altered by their theoretical assumptions, through the methods and instruments used for their observations, and the interpretations and explanations they impose on their data. Ever so subtly, the so-called "impartial" scientific observers influence that which they observe, in the very process of observing it.

> What appears to be an objective statement is actually *a statement of collective agreement* among observers concerning the commonality of their subjective experience. Thus, the so-called 'objective' stance, championed so enthusiastically by traditional scientific medicine, is really just a cover-up for a "subjective" stance, a stance which attempts to separate and dissect things which cannot ultimately be separated or dissected. Furthermore, in spite of the fact that the subject-object division is an untenable proposition, modern medicine persists in choosing to invalidate subjective experience in favour of what it conceives as an objective – with disastrous results.
> – *Michael Greenwood and Peter Nunn (p.29)*

Volume III further explores extensive research on the mystical and spiritual aspects of healing, including fascinating evidence for the survival of the spirit after death. Though this kind of spirituality was the exclusive reserve of religion in Western society during recent centuries, other societies have traditionally used spirituality in practical ways for diagnosing and healing illness.

Amazingly, the findings from research in spiritual dimensions that has been published from laboratories on six continents presents a coherent picture of spiritual dimensions of reality.

In Volume III, I invite you to explore with me these realms of healing that are paradoxically distant yet very near at hand. They are far from the *material* universe that conventional Western society has proposed as the only real and valid one. Yet they are as near as they can possibly be, for they reside within each of us and can be explored quite readily if we are willing to examine our inner awarenesses and to explore our relationships to our surroundings with open minds and hearts.

Volume IV: *Compendium of Theories and Practices in Spiritual Healing*

Volume IV synthesizes the materials from the three preceding volumes, and presents a range of theories to explain the processes of spiritual healing. It also includes my personal experiences with healing as a medical doctor, psychotherapist, healer and researcher.

Spiritual healing and many of the complementary therapies address the energy aspects of the body. Volume IV explores the broader and deeper implications of this ancient yet new view of our existence, and the healing approaches which are opened through a wholistic understanding of our place in the cosmos.

The overall goal of the series is to promote non-linear ways of seeing and learning about healing energies and processes, to complement our conventional, linear analyses. Both approaches are needed for a full understanding of healing.

Does all of this stretch your credulity to the point of discomfort? Have I exceeded your *boggle threshold*? Your skepticism is clearly warranted, because until recently many of the claims referred to above were made without the benefit of validation through modern scientific investigation. Today we are beginning to comprehend these subjects through more systematic research, and through better understanding of the underlying assumptions – both on the side of conventional medicine and of CAM therapies. Conversely, we are also beginning to legitimize our own individual, personal explorations of these realms through our inner, intuitive senses.

The length of these volumes is a reflection of the complex structure of the house of our human existence. Our linear methods of examining and analyzing this edifice lead us to shine a spotlight into each of its windows one at a time. But we must not forget that while we are examining any one room, myriads of vital activities are proceeding in all of the other rooms simultaneously. In fact, the "windows" and "walls" we perceive are largely of our own creation, produced by the very process of investigation through our physical rather than our intuitive senses. The metaphor of the house better suits the study of physical aspects of health. For CAM and bioenergy medicine, the image of a complex web of interpenetrating energy fields is more appropriate.

The *Healing Research* series considers the healing powers of our body, mind, emotions, relationships (with each other and with our environment) and spirit as a tightly interwoven and unified system. The benefits of the wholistic approach is well illustrated in a story related by a woman patient to Bernie Siegel, a wholistic surgeon. This patient complained to him that during exploratory surgery her previous surgeon had discovered that she was suffering from inoperable cancer. As she awoke from the anesthesia, her surgeon had told her that all that she could do was to hope and pray. "How do I do that?" she asked. He replied, "That's not my department." She therefore sought out Dr. Siegel, a surgeon who is comfortable in helping people deal with spiritual as well as physical issues.

This series is intended to help us respond to such pleas with our hearts and our spirits, and not only with our minds. I suggest that you skim the chapters in each book before reading them, or read each volume with the expectation that you will re-read it in the future. The complexity, integrity and beauty of the web of our existence cannot be appreciated fully by examining its infinite strands individually.

This study, in all its complexity, is not simply an intellectual exercise. Understanding our intimate relationships with each other and with the world around us is essential to our healing of this planet and of our relationships with it.

Man did not weave the web of life,
He is merely a strand in it.
Whatever he does to the web,
He does to himself.

— Chief Seattle

CHAPTER 1

Self-Healing

This need to dissect and examine each separate component of life may have originally led to specialization. The specialization... has become increasingly specific, so that today we find the absurd situation of a specialty mechanic polishing his small part to a high degree of efficiency without caring whether the whole functions...

– Paul Solomon

This book is about wholistic healing – the healing of the whole person, on all levels of being. In western medicine, experts are trained to address limited subsections of people. This is more efficient, and is virtually necessary in this age of information overload. Rarely, however, is there an expert who can help you address your problems on all of their levels – to include body, emotions, mind, relationships and spirit.

You will see how you can play a major role in maintaining your own health as well as in preventing and dealing with any illness you may develop. This chapter invites you to explore your mind-body and bodymind connections and many wholistic approaches for dealing with physical and psychological problems. Spiritual issues will be mentioned frequently, but not discussed here in detail.[10]

Poor health is not a thing that exists separately from a sick person – a thing to hand over to a specialist whose manipulations will make *it* better. The first step in a wholistic approach is to understand the meaning of the illness. "What is going wrong?" should be the initial question, and this should be asked not only about the *physical* aspects of the illness, but also about the larger context of a person's life.

First, there are mechanical factors to consider – for example, if you suffer from backaches you may be straining your back by lifting incorrectly or by sitting for long periods in a chair that is not well matched to the height of your work. But we should look beyond these physical mechanics and ask, "Why are you allowing yourself to lift things incorrectly? Could the pain in your back partially result from tensions contributed by emotional factors? Could you be holding back emotions, for instance, which is putting tension into muscles that go into spasm? "Is there a part of you that might welcome the attention and sympathy which the pain invites from those around you?"

More subtle and complex still are the connections between emotional factors and ailments caused by known external and internal physical problems. For example, although everyone is exposed to viruses and bacteria, only some get sick. In addition to physical factors, such as poor diet or impaired immune functions, and psychological issues may also contribute to your vulnerability to infection. For instance, research shows that we are much more vulnerable to all sorts of illnesses during times of bereavement or other emotional stresses. Pains from known physical problems, such as trauma, arthritis or neurological disorders, may be markedly worsened if you are emotionally upset. To clarify whether such factors might be present in your illness you must ask, "What might my body be telling me through this symptom?"

This link between emotion and illness has even been formalized into a *Life-Events Scale*. (See Table II-1.) The death of a family member, loss of a job, or retirement would be obvious sources of stress in your life. More surprising contributors on the stress list are *positive* events, such as marriage, the birth of a child and relocation. In fact, any factor that involves change or increases tension can apparently predispose you to illness. A score of more than 200 life change units (LCU) on this Inventory indicates that you are in serious risk of becoming ill, and scores of 300 or higher are commonly found in people with major illnesses (Miller/ Rahe).

Emotional stresses can predispose people not only to infections, but also to metabolic, cardiovascular and degenerative diseases, and even to cancer. Strong emotions can make the body susceptible to illness due to sheer exhaustion, or through alterations in the level of muscle tension, hormones, antibodies, or white blood cells, and probably also through variations in several levels of biological energies that are as yet poorly defined.

Personality and stress
How you respond to stress may depend on your personality – the traits you inherited in your genes and developed as you learned how to navigate your way through life.

For instance, one well-studied aspect of the mind-body relationship is the link between Type A personality and heart disease. People with this personality type are extremely driven to achieve personal goals that often are poorly defined. They are intensely competitive; hotly pursue advancement and recognition; tend to push themselves to complete tasks rapidly; and over-schedule activities that have strict deadlines. Type A personality can contribute to elevated cholesterol, early development of heart disease, risk of angina (heart pains) and heart attacks, and death from heart disease. Hostility seemed to be the primary factor in predicting Type A susceptibility to risk from heart disease.

A common denominator in Type A behaviors is the poor management of aggression. In an excellent review of this (and other, related mind-body) research,

Table II-1.   Life Events Questionnaire

Life change event	LCU
Health	
An Injury or illness which kept you in bed a week or more or sent you to the hospital	74
An injury or illness which was less serious than above	44
Major dental work	26
Major change in eating habits	27
Major change in sleeping habits	26
Major change in your usual type and/ or amount of recreation	28
Work	
Change to a new type of work	51
Change in your work hours or conditions	35
Change in your responsibility at work	
More responsibility	29
Fewer responsibility	21
Promotion	31
Demotion	42
Transfer	32
Troubles at work	
With your boss	29
With coworkers	35
With person under your supervision	35
Other work troubles	28
Major Business adjustment	60
Retirement	52
Loss of job	
Laid off from work	68
Fired from work	79
Correspondence course to help you in your work	18
Home and Family	
Major change in living conditions	42
Change in residence	
Move within the same town	25
Move to a different town, city, or state	47
Change in family get-togethers	25
Major change in health or behavior of family member	55
Marriage	50
Pregnancy	67
Miscarriage or abortion	65
Gain of a new family member	
Birth of a child	66
Adoption of a child	65
A relative moving in with you	59
Spouse beginning or ending work	46
Child leaving home	

To attend college	41
Due to marriage	41
For other reasons	45
Change in arguments with spouse	50
In-law problems	38
Change in the marital status of your parents	
Divorce	59
Remarriage	50
Separation from spouse	
Due to marital problems	76
Due to work	53
Divorce	96
Birth of a grandchild	43
Death of spouse	119
Death of other family member	
Child	123
Brother or sister	102
Parent	100
Personal or social	
Change in personal habits	26
Change of school of college	35
Change in political beliefs	24
Change in religious beliefs	29
Change in social activities	27
Vacation	24
New, close, personal relationships	37
Engagement to marry	45
Girlfriend or boyfriend problems	39
Sexual difficulties	44
"Falling out" of a close personal relationship	47
An accident	48
Minor violation of the law	20
Being held on jail	75
Major decision regarding your immediate future	51
Death of a close friend	70
Major personal achievement	36
Financial	
Major change in finances	
Increased income	38
Decreased income	60
Investment and/ or credit difficulties	56
Loss or damage of personal property	43
Moderate purchase	20
Major purchase	37
Foreclosure on a mortgage or loan	58

From Miller/ Rahe

Harris Dienstfrey (1991) points out that aggression is not a uniform characteristic in all people:

> ... Some people are aggressively competitive because it is a sport-like activity that gives them pleasure. Some people are aggressively competitive because they are filled with envy. Some people are aggressively competitive because they want to prove their superiority over other people. (p. 23)

People with Type B personality are not driven by ambition or competitiveness, and are not worried by deadlines.

It is therefore important to explore beneath the presence of aggression, to learn what is causing it and then how to deal with it. These psychological variables have not been taken into account by most investigators, who tend to lump all aggression under the same generic label. In my clinical practice I find that the concept of the Type A personality is readily appreciated by people who have difficulty relaxing, and who are constantly on the go. Cardiac counseling regarding healthy diet and other life habits, combined with focused counseling to address Type A behaviors, can reduce the risk of recurrent heart attacks by half.

Reduction of tensions can decrease the incidence and severity of many other illnesses as well. This may be one of the most important ways in which doctors, therapists and healers can help you. The mere presence of a caregiver, inviting you to share your anxieties, may alleviate much of your distress and initiate self-healing. The drift of medical practice into more time-efficient and cost-effective practice, with briefer visits and less time to talk with you, may be one of the reasons you are reading this book or seeking CAM therapies.

Your powers for healing are enormous. Even with a serious illness, you might have a spontaneous remission without the intervention of professional therapists or healers. We all have enormous innate potentials for self-healing that are largely unexplained, unexplored, and even unacknowledged by conventional medicine.

We can learn from the growing wholistic health movement how the role of healthcare providers can shift from taking on responsibility for curing patients to advising careseekers on ways in which they can care for themselves – through their own choices and actions, such as with proper diet, exercise and other forms of self-care.

Wholistic or *whole person care* acknowledges the intimate connection between mind, emotions and body. You may play a role in the development of the illness in varieties of obvious and subtle ways. Conversely, with healing awarenesses, attitudes and practices you can prevent illnesses, and can deal with them effectively if they do develop. This chapter explores many of the ways in which you can develop these sorts of sensitivities and skills.

Wholistic health practitioners also encourage integration of treatments that are less familiar to conventional caregivers, such as homeopathy and acupuncture. These CAM therapies help to maintain health and to deal with the roots of illnesses when they appear, rather than simply treating the *symptoms* of ill health.

Let me invite you now to look through some of the helpful windows and doorways I have found in the house of healing, to explore how people can make themselves ill or make themselves better.

I start with basic explanations of how your bodymind develops, evolves and functions.

PERSONALITY

The neurotic builds dream castles in the air.
The psychotic lives in them.
The psychiatrist collects the rent.
— Anonymous

Personality development

The person you are today is an accumulation of a lifetime of experiences. Your biological regulators all act like a computer – including your genetic programs, nervous and immune systems, and hormones, your biological energy fields, and your enormous files of stored memories of experiences. Your biocommputer is infinitely more complex than any hardware or software that has yet been developed by modern technology. You are endowed with physical and psychological characteristics that are uniquely yours, and your body has a range of capabilities to perceive and respond to your environment. You have strengths that may help you to resist environmental stresses and weaknesses that may leave you vulnerable to challenges – such as physical and emotional fatigue, substances in foods and airborne particles that may cause allergies, assaults on your immune system from bacteria and viruses, severe changes in temperature, and the like. Your personality, expressed in your physical and psychological makeup, is a unique combination of these and multitudes of other factors.

The psychological characteristics that make up your personality can be analyzed and described according to many perspectives. I share a few here that I have found particularly helpful.

Personality factors

A series of personality traits were evident in babies at the age of one month, and will persist as predispositions with minimal changes throughout life (Thomas, et al). These include:

1. Activity levels – high or low in general, being more awake in the morning or in the evening;
2. Rhythmicities in eating, sleeping and other activities – preferences for regular periodicity or for irregular schedules;
3. Adaptability – flexible and going with the flow, or unbending and easily rattled by changes;
4. Approach/ withdrawal – extroverted and reaching out spontaneously, or quiet, introverted and passive;
5. Threshold for response – sensitive and quick to respond, or unbothered and slow to respond to noise, intrusive touch and other environmental stimuli;
6. Intensity – preferring soft, gentle and quiet exchanges, or rough and tumble interactions;

7. Moods – even, with a narrow range, or punctuated with wide-ranging ups and downs;

8. Distractibility – shifting gears easily or with difficulty from one awareness or activity to another;

9. Persistence – remaining focused on tasks with greater or lesser intensity.

Understanding these factors may help you adjust your life to achieve greater harmony in many ways.

For instance, imagine to yourself that you are a person who prefers regular rhythms to your life, with breakfast, lunch and dinner at the same time each day. Imagine that you marry and have a baby who is totally irregular in eating and sleeping schedules. Or, vice-versa, that you eat and sleep when hungry or tired, and have a baby who is happiest when fed every four hours and unhappy if her sleep schedule is disrupted. Simply understanding your mutual differences in preferences on the rhythmicity and adaptability factors may help you work out the compromises that promote harmony rather than conflict.

Knowing where you are on factors such as adaptability, intensity, distractibility and persistence may help you in deciding how compatible you are with a partner in work or your personal life, and may help you work out differences that otherwise could cause dissonance and. friction.

Coming from the opposite direction, when there is a tension between you and others in your life, you might ask, "Are there personality variables here that are abrasive and irritating?"

Simply identifying and discussing these differences can open up ways to compromise and greater harmony.[11]

Jungian personality types
Another typology of human characteristics was devised by Carl Jung. Jung pointed out that everyone has a personality type that is dominant in the area of one or two of four parameters, which are paired in polar opposites. These are the polarities of *thinking* ←→ *feeling*, and *intuition* (inner senses) ←→ *sensation* (outer senses). He also noted that there are introverted and extraverted styles of relating to the world. (See Figure II-1.)

Figure II-1. Jungian polarities

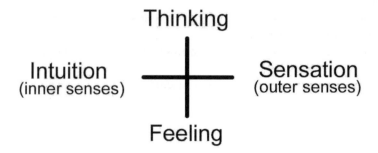

Thinking type people organize their perceptions of the world and their responses to it through logical analysis and planning. They usually do not pay much attention to their feelings, and may even label feelings as *illogical, unreasonable,* and *unreliable.* (Our society overvalues this mode of relating to the world, as witnessed by the pejorative connotations of these terms.) A scheduled, predictable world is most comfortable for the thinking types.

> *Discipline and letting go, the two paths as one, guide me always.*
> *Work and trust, another way of saying it.*
> *Knowing takes us to its limit, its edge. We go beyond.*
> *We learn, come to understanding, let go of our understanding and pass into the unknowable, the highest knowledge.*
> *Without discipline we increase our ignorance.*
> *Without letting go we build a prison of information.*
> *The two paths merge as one, breathing in, breathing out.*
> – John MacEnulty (8/29/2003)

Feeling types are described by Jung in terms of *values*, but my own view is that these types of people may also be described in terms of *emotionality*. They experience life as a montage of emotions and values. Experiences that are emotionally charged feel real and alive, interesting and exciting, and are highly valued. Thoughts alone are colorless. Plans are acted upon if one is in the right mood, and communication is engaged through the tones and nuances of interaction more than through their content. The feeling types respond most to activities and experiences that excite and stimulate, be it with attraction or withdrawal.

> *The heart has reasons that reason knows nothing of.*
> – Blaise Pascal

Intuitive types grasp information in broad patterns and mental maps. They intuit their way through situations, often without even conceptualizing to themselves the process by which they make their decisions. Intuitive perceptions come in wholes – and any individual part that they might analyze represents less than the truth. They instinctively know the right things to do in familiar situations. With new challenges, intuitives may simply know successful ways through a morass rather than deducing solutions, using specific details and leaps of inspiration rather than step-by-step reasoning. I've been amazed and amused to see intuitive people who come up with the accurate answers to challenging problems in mathematics or the sciences but can't even begin to explain how they arrived at their answers. Many intuitives suffer in school when they come up with correct answers on their exams but are unable to explain how they arrived at them, and may even be unfairly accused of cheating.

> *The intuitive mind is a sacred gift and the rational mind is a faithful servant. We have created a society that honors the servant and has forgotten the gift.*
> – Albert Einstein

Sensation types notice every detail in the world around them – form, color, and sound are the threads with which they weave the fabric of their reality. Everything has its place. Shaping, organizing and moving bodies and objects around is important and satisfying. Every incident has its cause and effect, and if these are not apparent in the present, it is merely because insufficient efforts have been applied to fitting things into their proper order.[12]

> *Nothing is more indisputable than the existence of our senses.*
> – Jean Le Rond d'Alembert

Each of these polarities may be expressed through an *introverted* (inner directed) or *extroverted* (outer directed) style of relating to the world.

Introverted people are guided by inner awareness, heeding their feelings and intentions to direct their actions and responses to the world around them. The expectations and demands of the outer environment will not influence them as strongly as their inner worlds of thought, intuitions and emotions. Such people will appear thoughtful, introspective and quiet, if they are of moderately introverted. They are their own worst critics, setting their inner barometers for behavior and response according to their own opinion of themselves, and not readily influenced by external pressures. Extremes of introversion are seen as deviant from psychological and social norms, and may include excessive shyness, social isolation, depressed withdrawal, disregard for expectations of friends and family, and the like.

In contrast, *extroverts* are outgoing and highly responsive to social situations. They seek interactions with others, pay a lot of attention to others' expectations, and want to conform in order to be accepted. At the extremes of the scale, extroverts are unhappy unless others join with them in their exuberance. Some may seem to have no opinions of their own, structuring their world around others' views and norms. Another pattern of extroversion may be seen in hypomanic or manic personalities, who push their views upon others and may experience their emotions to a great extent through the reactions of others, having great difficulty in perceiving their own roles in creating the responses set up by their own behaviors.

Within each of these polarities there are degrees of insightfulness and wide ranges of behavior, so the basic polarities explain some but not all aspects of people's various ways of being in the world.

Extroverts focus on objects/ people external to themselves, and experience the world as a series of interactions with these *outside* objects. *Introverts* are focused on their inner awarenesses, living their conscious lives under the influence of whichever of the four polarities are dominant in them, without becoming too tightly bound to the outer world.

> *The Science Graduate asks "How does it work ?"*
> *The Economics Graduate asks "How much does it cost ?"*
> *The Engineering Graduate asks "How can we make it ?"*
> *The Liberal Arts Graduate asks "Do you want fries with that ?"*
> – Jesse N. Schell

Shadow aspects of personality

While each person may readily acknowledge their own primary traits, they may not be aware that their polar opposites are also alive and active in the *shadow* aspects of their being – those parts of themselves that exist outside of their conscious awareness. We tend to block these awarenesses because we would rather not acknowledge them, to ourselves or others.

Until recently, we have been encouraged to maintain cultural stereotypes of men as thinking/ sensation primaries, and women as feeling/ intuitive primaries. Women's Liberation has been a transforming force in helping to acknowledge our neglected polar opposites, giving women permission and encouragement to develop their *thinking* and *sensation* aspects, while men's groups encourage men to acknowledge their *feeling* and *intuitive* sides.

Unconsciously, people may choose a friend or mate with opposite polar preferences because they find this stimulating and balancing, but also because they can let the other express the aspects of themselves that they would rather not acknowledge or deal with. For example, a husband (with primary introverted, thinking/sensation functions) may be happy to see his wife (with primary extroverted, intuitive/feeling functions) handle the decorating and entertainment at home. The wife may likewise leave the finances and mechanical repairs to her husband – thus each avoids engagement with their shadow or *inferior* polarities. This kind of partnership of polarities can work in the opposite direction as well. The feeling partner can help the thinking partner to be more aware of their own feelings, and vice-versa.

> *If my heart could do my thinking would my brain begin to feel?*
> – Van Morrison

The *shadow* aspect of our unconscious mind also shuts away those parts of our being that make us uncomfortable, and that we would rather not acknowledge to ourselves and to others. This shadow carries all of our forgotten, unacknowledged, deeply buried old hurts with their accompanying angers and resentments; all the little and great envies and desires that parents and religious institutions teach us we ought not to have, though we invariably do – and more besides.[13]

In addition to managing *shadow* aspects of our emotions and personalities, our unconscious mind also serves as a vast storehouse for factual memories. But while the unconscious is very much a part of us, it is extremely challenging to perceive and comprehend how it functions.

> *It is difficult to become consciously aware of the unconscious! This way of thinking is, for most of us, a vast unknown that we visit each night in our dreams, but usually find irrelevant to daily life. Since it is unfamiliar, some people think of it as strange, even frightening, and therefore necessary to keep under control.*
>
> *If you think of the stars in the night sky as separate points of light, the circling mind connects them to the constellations. It joins apparently disparate things with bonds of analogy, metaphor, and possibility. It spins an infinity of choices. It is where your words exist before you speak them. It is*

> *the "you" that has no face. It is the source of ritual, mystery, and magic,*
> *the sacred space within you, where prayer originates.*
>
> — Dawna Markova (p. 26)

These *shadow* parts of our psychological makeup are every bit as much a part of ourselves as the other aspects that are within our conscious awareness. As such, they influence our beliefs, perceptions, feelings and actions – often completely without our conscious awareness. These are our irrational desires and fears, our un*reason*able reactions – precisely because they abide and function deep below the level of our reasoning mind. They operate outside of our *persona* – the part of our selves that we construct and groom in order to present the best possible face to ourselves and to those around us. We may become aware of our *shadow* parts when we catch ourselves in excessively strong outbursts of hurt or angry feelings, when we examine our dreams, or when others point out that they feel our behaviors are inappropriate.

Similarly, the shadow aspects of our personalities seek expression just as much as our conscious polarities do. For instance, a *thinking* primary person will also have feelings that want and need to be expressed. If the feelings are held in, they tend to build up until they find some outlet, often under conditions of pressure or stress, when the dominant polarity loses some of its control. When these repressed feelings finally do come to expression, it is often through interactions with other people that stir the *shadow* to strong responses, and many times the eruption into consciousness and expression in words or actions occurs in ways that are counter-productive. Explosions of emotion, in turn, often generate negative reactions. Such experiences discourage people from giving vent to their shadow sides.

There are many ways that shadow feelings can influence a person's life. They may lead to depression, anger, negative beliefs about one's ability to succeed, or poor interpersonal relationships.

Case: "Todd" was a highly successful businessman who had been married for 14 years to "Julie," a music teacher. Over the years, Todd found himself developing an increasing irritation with Julie's emotionality. She was completely up-front in saying what she felt, when she felt it, and had no hesitation in expressing laughter, tears or anger. Whenever they argued, which was becoming more and more frequent, Todd was upset as much by how she expressed her feelings as by whatever it was they were arguing about. Julie, for her part, felt that he was increasingly cold and distant, less and less interested in spending time with her. She was increasingly enraged when they disagreed, which was highly out of character for her.

A marriage counselor suggested that each might do well to sort out some of their feelings in individual therapy. Todd reluctantly accepted this suggestion, overcoming his unhappiness with the referral because the counselor came very highly recommended and he truly wanted to save their marriage, as much for the children's sake as for his own. Over a period of several months, Todd was surprised to discover that a lot of the anger he was venting on his wife was actually excess anger that came from a deep well of negative feelings that he was carrying inside himself from his childhood. Julie's emotionality had stirred these buried feelings, but before he was conscious of them, he simply vented them at the source of their arousal, rather than at their original sources – his own parents, who had argued and fought each other bitterly for many years, sometimes getting into physical fights which had terrified him.

Both of Todd's parents had had to work long hours to earn enough to support their four children. While they said that they loved Todd, he never felt sure they really meant it because they were rarely there to help him when he was upset or feeling needy. Being a bright student, Todd sought approval and gratification by earning good grades.

Todd stuffed his feelings of hurt and anger in what I call *the emotional trash bucket* of his unconscious mind. As a child, this was the best he could do. He couldn't change his parents, couldn't fire or replace them and couldn't leave. Had he not stuffed these feelings away, he would have suffered the constant emotional distress and pain of feeling unloved and unwanted by his parents.

Case (continued): Early in their relationship, Julie's emotionality had appealed to Todd because he could enjoy seeing her releasing feelings that he himself would never have expressed. Indeed, he rarely would have acknowledged harboring such feelings himself. Over the years of living together, however, his unconscious mind gradually absorbed (through the freedom exhibited by Julie in expressing her feelings) that it did not have to keep the lid on his emotional trash bucket shut so tightly. So when Julie stirred his feelings, they started to leak out.

As Todd was able to recall and release in counseling the feelings from his emotional trash bucket that had been stored away in his childhood, they no longer spilled out when his wife became emotional.

In her own individual counseling, Julie learned as well about feelings she had been carrying from her childhood. She had always felt frustrated that her father was cold and distant most of the time, but highly volatile and explosive when he was drunk – at which point she was frightened of him. While Todd had not been withdrawn when they married (and never had a drinking problem), his increasing discomfort with Julie's feelings had led him to withdraw emotionally in their relationship as their arguments became increasingly heated. This stirred her childhood fears and angers, which were vented initially on Todd. She, too, was able to sort through her childhood feelings in counseling so that they no longer intruded inappropriately in her marriage.

The computer model of mental functions

Have you ever stopped to realize that the basic programs running in your personal bio-computers were written by a child? When you were just starting to explore the world, you learned from experience how to respond to the world around you. To the degree that you were raised in a nurturing and trustworthy environment, had a tolerable amount of stress and adequate support to deal with distress, you learned to trust. If your family was loving, you learned to form emotionally satisfying intimate relationships with others. If your early environment was one of misunderstanding, mistrust, painful relationships or abuse, and if you didn't have adequate support to deal with the pressures and upsets in your life, you had to learn to protect yourself, as Todd did.

As an infant, you had a restricted understanding of your environment, and limited abilities to cope with it. Very basic and important parts of your learning occurred before you even had the chance to develop language or reasoning capacities. The coping programs you developed in childhood were mostly unconscious, and are stored in the shadow parts of your mind that exist below your conscious awareness. They are so basic to your overall personality structure that they have become second nature, and their influence seems self-evident – "That's just the way I am."

The basic functional structures of your personality are the skeleton programs upon which the flesh of your life is sculpted – both systematically, by family, school, religious and other societal institutions, and coincidentally, through your uniquely personal life experiences.

Such personality factors are certainly relevant to how people respond to health challenges. If you shut the lid tightly on your inner emotional bucket, your body may be one of the ways that your unconscious mind seeks to alert you to the burden it is carrying – and ever so eager to let go of. If you are open to letting your unconscious mind speak its needs, you may deal more successfully with stressful challenges.

Such factors may similarly explain many of the differences between those who respond and those who remain indifferent to healing interventions.

Personality disorders and psychoses
Consider the agony of Tonia, an infant who yearns for warmth and closeness but receives only harshness and indifference from her parent(s). Unable to conceive of time in the future (because her unprogrammed computer has yet to learn that concept), she is aware only that she is miserable, and likely to remain so forever.

Rather than allowing her to suffer, Tonia's unconscious mind may intervene to help in several ways. It may bury some of her hurts in forgetfulness, keeping them isolated from her conscious mind so that she will suffer less. It may, for instance, shut away the hurt of being unloved, and allow a facade of indifference to develop, to hide this fundamental insecurity so that she suffers less. Unfortunately, this protection is provided at the cost of the shutting off (*repression*) portions of her being from her own conscious awareness. It reduces the immediate pain of rejection, but it does so by sweeping the hurt feelings under the carpet of her unconscious mind, where they remain stored in all their intensity. Thus neglected, they can fester like a boil, subtly influencing or sometimes grossly poisoning her future relationships through her unresolved hurts from the buried past.

Tonia's unconscious mind may redefine reality for her so that horrendous, unbearable truths are softened to tolerable miseries. Rather than accepting that her parents do not want *her,* her child mind may create fantasies that *she has done something for which she is being punished.* As a result, she may develop a negative self-image, anticipating hurt and rejection from anyone close to her.

Emotions play an enormous part in our lives. Much of our understanding of psychology comes from analyzing observable behaviors. However, much of our behavior is based on our underlying feelings, both conscious and unconscious.

Daniel Goleman, in his best-selling book, *Emotional Intelligence*, shows that emotional awarenesses and interactions are not simply second-rate experiences that are somehow inferior to our thinking ways of engaging with the world. Emotions are not logical, in the sense that they are not built upon consciously reasoned patterns and plans. In our Western culture, we are conditioned to believe that anything that is not *logical* is not *reasonable*. But our emotions have reasons for existing, even though we may not be consciously aware of them. Furthermore, our emotional reactions may guide us with greater accuracy and deeper truth – since they are not as easily misled by superficial appearances or prejudiced by logical expectations.

As children, many of us convince ourselves that showing our feelings is the wrong thing to do because this can upset our parents, teachers and friends. Due to such pressures our unconscious mind may be programmed to avoid showing feelings from the time we are old enough to respond to social pressures – which can even start before we can speak.

> *The subconscious, like the earth, knows only to reproduce what is planted in it.*
>
> – Alice Steadman

These unconscious programs tend to be self-validating. Mistrustful people see their interactions with others through mistrusting eyes, and therefore respond to others with defensive behavior. They will generally steer clear of close relationships, to avoid what they anticipate will be an inevitable disappointment. Other people will tend to react in a complementary manner, not seeking relationships with those who send out signals that they do not want others close to them. This in turn confirms what the mistrustful people already believed – that they are unwanted. They may even view any trusting approaches by others with suspicion.

This process may be influenced by factors such as the age and developmental stage at which traumas or lack of adequate emotional support are experienced, by the availability or absence of emotionally nourishing alternatives for the suffering person and by inherited genetic personality factors. The complex interplay of multiple factors produces a great diversity of symptoms, and sometimes leads to disagreements even among experienced therapists about possible causes and diagnoses of emotional disorders.

Problems of a moderate nature in this category may lead to what we term *personality disorders*, an example of which could be a person who is excessively shy. More serious imbalances may lead to inward withdrawal and social isolation. The opposite, of extremely volatile and stormy relationships, may occur in a borderline personality disorder. The borderline craves closeness but strongly fears rejection, and is constantly struggling with those who are close to them – over issues of trust, mutual responsibilities for problems in the relationship and major fears of rejection.

The most severe disturbances of this kind may precipitate (or contribute to) psychoses, particularly in those who are genetically susceptible. Psychotics are individuals who have retreated so far from interaction with others that they have difficulty differentiating between their inner and outer worlds. Their emotional responses may be inappropriate and out of place in the outer world. Anyone may become psychotic if they are exposed to sufficiently severe stress. Those who are chronically psychotic are called *schizophrenic*.

Problematic personality disorders may require prolonged psychotherapy for change to occur. The most reliable treatment for psychoses is with tranquilizers. Properly prescribed, they can greatly reduce psychotic symptomatology, and allow people to live a reasonably normal life. However, if the major tranquilizers are used alone, without accompanying therapeutic treatment, they are very often unsatisfactory as a long-term solution. For one thing, they can produce unpleasant and debilitating side effects. Furthermore, they do not alter patterns of behavior deriving from complex, psychological processes and family interactions that maintain and perpetuate severely dysfunctional modes of relating. These may require psychotherapy for effective treatment.

> *Removing symptoms is like taking the lid off the pot, so it is no longer boiling over. Finding the emotional causes is like taking the pot off the stove.*
>
> – James Gordon

Neuroses
Discrete traumatic experiences, milder cases of unsatisfied emotional needs, and successful defense in a person of stronger genetic constitution may result in less severe protective responses on the part of the unconscious mind.

The trauma precipitating a neurotic crystallization into a lifelong crippling habit need not be a major one. It may simply be an insult that is poorly tolerated by the incompletely programmed computer of a child's unconscious mind, which may then convince the child to suppress certain aspects of their being. Typically, children will have an encounter with a parent in which they feel that they cannot be themselves and still be loved.

Case: Two-year-old Tommy presented his mother with a picture. Previously she had praised him for his drawings, but this time she furiously scolded him, "You bad child! How could you do something like that? Go to your room!" Because Tommy's mother didn't tell him she was only upset this time because he drew the picture on the wall, and he was overwhelmed by the intensity of her anger and the words "You bad child" (which he had heard many times before), he imprinted a negative image of himself on his mental hard drive.

Minor painful experiences of this sort can be emotionally crippling in little ways. Tommy might simply avoid drawing in the future. More serious emotional injuries could lead to more debilitating consequences. Tommy might hold off from sharing any spontaneous aspects of his feelings, believing that he is bad and that people will get angry with him and reject him if he reveals his inner feelings. Again, uncounted multitudes of factors could contribute to a child's responses, including their threshold for dealing with intense stimuli, how often their parents scold them in ways that are belittling, whether they have emotional support from anyone else, and so on.

Processes of this kind are usually repressed from the child's conscious mind by that part of him which protects him from emotional distress – his unconscious mind.

However, in order to censor emotional material effectively, the unconscious has to be aware of what it is protecting the child from. It must plant a sign on the spot in the carpet under which it has swept the discomforts, identifying what is hidden there. Then it has to stand vigilant guard by that spot, to keep the dirt from being stirred up into conscious awareness by future life events. All of this effort requires emotional energies, and creates tensions in the unconscious mind, which constantly maneuvers to screen out potentially distressing facts and feelings in order to prevent emotional pains from reaching the conscious mind.

If it is particularly vigilant, the unconscious may go a step further. It may continue to distance Tom from other, somewhat similar situations that threaten to stir up the repressed emotions which he felt as a child. In later life, a person like Tom may find himself avoiding women, for instance, as a result of the accumulated minor and major painful experiences he had with his mother.

Anxiety is the warning signal from the unconscious to the conscious that some external or internal threat is perceived or anticipated, or that the habitual rules for safe and acceptable behavior are being disobeyed. When the unconscious succeeds in masking from our awareness the origin of our anxiety that we run into difficulty. It is when Tom becomes uncomfortable with his pattern of avoiding women for no logical reason that he may become aware of the workings of his unconscious mind.[14] Tom can then become aware of the factors that are causing the anxiety and he can deal with the cause, whereupon the anxiety will usually dissipate.

See Chapter 5 for a variety of self-healing approaches that can help with problems of these sorts.

Mental defense mechanisms

Each of us has mental constructs of our self in our mind. These are complex edifices that we build as we grow, drawing on our experiences of personhood – as individuals and as members of family and society. The frame for the house we build is provided in our genetic makeup. The bricks and mortar are given to us by our family and culture. The ways in which we lay them down, and the appearance of the facade (*persona*) that we design to protect ourselves and present ourselves to the world, will be determined by our personal reactions to our life experiences. We may also build fences or even walls around this house of self for protection from real or imagined possible attacks.

Our defenses are not constructed only to protect us against the outer world. We also build dark closets and cellars where we can dump unpleasant experiences and feelings that we do not wish to deal with, or which we feel are beyond our capacities to master through less drastic measures. If these experiences were sufficiently traumatic, we may need massive doors behind which to barricade them from our conscious awareness.

In general, we tend to feel that the walls we have constructed around ourselves *are* our selves. We defend them valiantly against confrontations with others, whose outer fortifications are inevitably different from our own. We become uncomfortable when questioned about our choices of materials, or the shape we give to our walls. It is easier to maintain the fantasy that these walls are genetic inheritances, or the products of our childhood training, rather than admitting that they are the products of our own choices. We usually have many options for introducing new colors or undertaking extensive remodeling. Whether we choose to add defenses or remove our boundary defenses may influence our openness or resistance to healing of dis-ease or disease.

We have many ways of defending the boundaries of what we experience as our selves. If we are very firm in our defenses and our walls are thick, we may simply ignore the differences between ourselves and others.

> The neurotic builds dream-castles. The psychotic lives in them. The psychiatrist collects the rent.
>
> – Anonymous

Anna Freud, the daughter of Sigmund Freud, is the clearest writer on defense mechanisms. She detailed a series of ways in which we respond to stress. Her focus is primarily on how we handle anxiety in adaptive or maladaptive ways.

The most obvious form of anxiety is based on reality factors, such as fears of going out at night in an unsafe neighborhood. This is best handled by avoiding the dangerous situation or by taking appropriate precautions to assure our safety.

Unrealistic anxieties[15] arise from internal conflicts between our natural impulses and the ways we are inclined to respond to these – shaped by our personality, upbringing and societal expectations.

Defense mechanisms help us to deal with anxieties. They are automatic, usually unconscious responses. They are based on internal interpretations of reality, distorted through our individual perceptions and ways of responding to the anxieties. The defense mechanisms change how we perceive the problems and our responses to them.

Repression is the most common defense. By burying the issues in the unconscious mind, we don't feel the anxiety as strongly. Furthermore, it remains outside of our awareness so we aren't plagued by memories of the anxiety. Repression can be selective, with only the distressing parts of a memory being buried. You might remember that you visited your parents, but conveniently forget about the unpleasant interactions you had with them.

Denial is a more complete form of repression, in which you might completely forget you visited your parents. Denial is more common in childhood, when your reasoning powers are not as mature and you can more easily create and accept fantasies as being real. In adulthood, denial is common as an initial reaction to a severe loss or threat of one, as in bereavement. Initially, it is helpful in softening the blow of a loss. Prolonged, it can become problematic. Denial is also common in addictions. Others may clearly see that a person is addicted to alcohol or drugs, while she may completely deny she has any problem.

Everyone uses repression and denial to some degree. The more you use these defenses, however, the more psychological energies you have to keep investing in maintaining your unawareness of wheat you have shut away in the closets and caves of your unconscious mind.

Projection allows you to reduce your anxieties by saying that someone else has the thoughts that make you uncomfortable. This process is entirely unconscious. You might be angry with someone. Having been raised to believe that feeling or letting out your anger is wrong, you could project your anger onto them, accusing them of being angry with you.

Intellectualization allows you to separate yourself from uncomfortable feelings, by focusing only on the facts of an experience. If someone in your family is diagnosed with an illness, you might spend lots of time studying everything you can about the disease and avoid feeling the anxiety, disappointment or fear about the possible consequences of the disease.

Regression may be activated under severe stress. When adult defenses aren't adequate to deal with a very high level of anxiety, the unconscious mind may revert to defense mechanisms that worked in earlier years. For a child, sucking a nipple, a pacifier or a thumb may have been comforting. When stressed, adults often revert to comfort eating or smoking – oral activities which worked in childhood.

Displacement shifts the target of one's feelings from one that might be dangerous to a safer target. Letting your anger out at your boss when he treats you unfairly might jeopardize your job, so you are likely to swallow down your feelings rather than giving him a piece of your mind – or worse. Having swallowed down these feelings at work, you might find yourself venting the excess angers at your wife or children.

Reaction formation transforms your negative feelings into positive ones. Having been hurt or neglected in childhood by your family, you might choose to work a in a caregiving profession. By helping others, you vicariously enjoy their receiving the care that you never had.

Rationalization is a defense mechanism whereby you reorganize your understanding of a problem after is occurs. If you're not invited by a friend to his party, you could convince yourself that you really didn't want to go, anyway. This helps to maintain your self-esteem.

In our western society, where thinking is emphasized so much over feelings, this is a defense that is very popular – in national as well as individual defense mechanisms. We often rationalize that others have constructed their walls based on mistaken beliefs, from plans that were given to them by ignorant designers (i.e. different from our own). If we are charitable, we may excuse others for their ignorance in misinterpreting the Master's plans. If we need targets for displaced angers, we may elevate ourselves by denigrating others, claiming that our architects descended from traditions that are closer to God or that our designers remain truer to the Ultimate Design – which then justifies us in exploiting, mistreating or abusing these "others."

If our defenses are not as massive, our unconscious mind may eventually hint to us that we might be needlessly hiding behind our ramparts, or going about in suits of armor that might in reality be unnecessary burdens. These inner voices are most likely to emerge as we mature, and especially when we feel safe and are not operating under overwhelming stresses. If we are uncomfortable with such inner suggestions that we may not have to defend ourselves so strongly, we may repress them, sometimes without ever letting them reach our conscious awareness. It is really easier to let old habits continue, rather than to challenge or dismantle them. If we do allow such criticisms of our defenses to surface to awareness, or if circumstances confront us with our disproportionate responses to what others handle better, we may deny that such questions have arisen within us. We may project our doubts onto others, blaming *them* for making us uncomfortable.

For instance, people commonly remark, "He made me angry when he said that..." But in reality, no one can *make* us feel something that is alien to ourselves. More often we resonate with something the other person does or says, and we don't wish to acknowledge that the feelings aroused in us are related to the *shadows* in our dark closets. Such encounters with repressed materials challenge our beliefs, and often we are more comfortable hiding behind our carefully constructed defenses. Rather than acknowledge our inner discomforts, we project blame for them upon others (Benor 2003).

To put this in a more concrete example, if Gerry calls me a jerk, my response could be anger if I feel insecure and she rattled the door on the closet behind which I hid my past hurts that led me to be insecure and angry. Gerry offers me the lovely opportunity to dump some of my anger on her. It is easier for me to be angry than to examine what lies behind that door which makes me vulnerable to be upset by such a taunt. If I'm not insecure, I don't have to bite on the bait. I might ask myself questions such as, "What did I say or do to offend Gerry?" or "Why is Gerry in a bad mood today?"

Our fears keep us locked into our defenses – fears of being hurt by imagined or perceived attackers, and fears of failing or otherwise disappointing ourselves and others. Our defenses in turn hold our earliest fears locked inside of us, and the secondary fear of being re-traumatized keeps us from releasing the earlier fears. We are often tied into knots of fears, as Ronald Laing has so brilliantly pointed out:

> I don't respect myself
> I can't respect anyone who respects me.
> I can only respect someone who does not respect me.
> I respect Jack
> *Because* he does not respect me.
>
> I despise Tom
> *Because* he does not despise me.
>
> Only a despicable person
> can respect someone as despicable as me.
>
> I cannot love someone I despise.
>
> Since I love Jack
> I cannot believe he loves me.
>
> What proof can he give?
> – Ronald Laing 1970 (p. 18)

Among healers and wholistic therapists, involvement in spiritual development may actually be a form of defense against awareness of their own emotional tensions. Blaming our misfortunes on bad *karma* or getting deeply involved in spiritual practices may sometimes be *spiritual bypasses* around psychological problems.

There are many other ways in which we may defend ourselves from uncomfortable awarenesses and we cannot explore all of these here. The examples above should suffice to explain the principles behind our habits and methods of hiding our own feelings from ourselves.

NORMALITY

> *Mental health doesn't mean always being happy - if it did,*
> *nobody would qualify.*
>
> – Ashleigh Brilliant

Now that we have reviewed some types of psychological problems, you may well ask, "So, how do you get to be a normal person?"

The answer is that there is no general agreement on a definition of psychological normality. Everyone has some measure of defensiveness, some unresolved hurts, and some quirks of personality that make her or him uniquely different from everyone else. On the positive side, most would agree that normal people have a flexibility to behave and respond adaptively to various challenges and stresses in their lives.

The concept of psychological normality encompasses a general range of individuality that is considered reasonable within a given society. The acceptability of differing beliefs and behaviors varies between countries and cultures, and even in different communities within the same culture.

Everyone also has their unique emotional thresholds for feeling stress, for becoming distressed, and their breaking points – intense situations and stresses that will prove intolerable, and will result in psychological decompensation. At what point, then, can we say that a person is psychologically abnormal? We all have general concepts of normality, and can readily agree when presented with an example of a person whose behaviors or beliefs deviate in major ways from our accepted norms, but we may still have difficulty judging for ourselves and agreeing with others when confronted with individuals who deviate mildly or moderately from our shared idea of normality. Conversely, while others may not feel that a certain person is abnormal, this person may herself believe that she is not normal. In other cases, people may lack any awareness that they are abnormal.

A second factor in determining the line between normality and abnormality relies upon the opinions of those assessing whether people are normal or not.

> *Who I really am is one of those difficult questions I prefer to leave to the*
> *experts.*
>
> – Ashleigh Brilliant

In the end, we must simply live with complex personal and generally accepted standards for distinguishing between psychological normality and abnormality, between sanity and insanity. And there will always be broad gray areas in which a person's normality may be disputed.

 Some of the above may appear to be rather nit picking, and the reader may be wondering why this is relevant. The assessment of psychological disorders and of their severity is of major importance in deciding whether various treatments are helpful for people with those disorders. The variability in human nature challenges the researcher to develop valid and reliable ways of assessing deviations from normality.

 Standardized psychological questionnaires are often used for such purposes. When these are given to thousands of subjects, norms for responses can be calculated. These then become helpful tools for clinicians and researchers in assessing psychological abnormalities and changes that may be the result of a given treatment.

> *Anybody who behaved normally all of the time would not be completely normal.*
> – Ashleigh Brilliant

PSYCHOSOMATIC DISORDERS

> *What a man thinks of himself, that is which determines, or rather, indicates, his fate.*
> – Henry David Thoreau (1854)

The body can become a series of battlegrounds in the unconscious mind's maneuvers to protect us from unpleasant experiences.

 When danger is perceived, either consciously or unconsciously, the body becomes tense. This is an automatic reflex reaction involving the nervous system and hormones. The body is preparing to respond to the perceived threat by fleeing or fighting. When we fight or flee the tension is discharged, and our bodies can again relax.

 When either circumstances or the own defenses (often unconsciously) prevent us from dealing with the sources of our tension, there can be a chronic buildup of stress without an appropriate release. Our bodies then suffer the consequences of prolonged tension. Blood pressure rises, muscles remain taught and may spasm and stress hormones continue to circulate. People frequently are unaware that emotional tensions lie behind their symptoms, because these processes are managed by the unconscious mind.

 Tense muscles will ultimately start to complain by hurting. Backaches and headaches are common results of stress, but other muscles can also spasm and ache. Once we feel the pain, a vicious circle is initiated: Pain → Anxiety → Muscle tension → Spasm → Pain increases, and so on.

 Similar muscle spasms in our lungs can produce a narrowing of the airways in the bronchioles, bringing on asthmatic attacks; tension in arteries throughout our body resulting in elevated blood pressure; spasms in cardiac arteries causing angina (heart pain from insufficient blood supply) and in muscles along the skull producing migraines; excessive gastric acid secretion leading to heartburn and ulcers; spasm in the gut, and other such disorders.

Subtle and insidious changes in the immune system may also occur due to chronic tensions. White cells and antibodies are less effective in protecting the health of people who are under stress. This may contribute to their developing infections, and may increase their susceptibility to serious illnesses such as AIDS and cancer.

Secondary gain is another psychological mechanism which can initiate cycles that maintain and perpetuate pain and other symptoms. Pain may be useful in some situations, despite the fact that it causes us discomfort and we consciously wish to be rid of it. For example, pain can provide an acceptable excuse for not attending a social event that might be stressful, for avoiding unwanted sexual relations, for not going to work, or for sidestepping other unpleasant obligations or demands. Conversely, a symptom may gain us caring responses from family and friends, and greater closeness – in relationships where we might hesitate to ask for such attention, or where others hesitate to offer it.

> *The sick man is more than half a rascal. He may only be sick because he hasn't the courage to clean house.*
> – Sherwood Anderson

The unconscious mind, searching for the most immediate way to relieve our anxieties, might thus help us avoid facing stressful situations by aggravating and perpetuating pains that are present due to any cause. A chronic headache may flare up "conveniently" (though unconsciously) when an unfavorite aunt or mother in law phones to invite a person to dinner. Secondary gain may then reinforce the pain-tension-spasm cycle when this pattern recurs in other situations as well.

Subtle energy blocks and imbalances that occur as a result of tension and stress may also produce a variety of symptoms. I will discuss this further in subsequent sections.

THE BODY'S REGULATING SYSTEMS

The deeper levels of the brain concern themselves with monitoring and regulating the vital, routine functions of the body, such as breathing, temperature control, heartbeat and blood pressure. They also maintain a suitable chemical balance in the bloodstream to provide an optimal environment for the various tissues and organs.

These functions are controlled via a diffuse network of nerves that run from the brain, along the spinal cord and out through various nerves to reach every part of the body. This network is called the *autonomic nervous system (ANS)*. The ANS tenses skeletal muscles via the *sympathetic nervous system (SNS),* and relaxing them via the *parasympathetic nervous system (PNS).*

The SNS is activated when we prepare for fight or flight. It increases the heart rate and blood pressure, and stimulates the adrenal glands to produce adrenaline and steroids that enhance body functions. It constricts the arteries in the extremities in order to increase the amount of blood available to the larger muscles and internal organs. It heightens our anxiety and our alertness to potential dangers. All of these factors serve us well in emergencies, as they increase our awareness of what is going on around us, and enhance our strength and stamina for immediate physical response to danger. However, when the SNS is chronically activated, as in conditions of long-term, low-grade stress, it can be harmful to our health, as discussed in the section above, on vicious circles.

The PNS also activates the digestive tract and other organs. Again, these functions are beneficial as long as the organ activities remain within a normal range. But when chronically over-activated, various problems, such as ulcers, can result.

Hormones are chemical regulators in the body. They act as catalysts in chemical reactions, facilitating and regulating the biochemical activity of the body to make it more efficient. Hormones prepare us for action, assist in initiating digestive processes, regulate blood sugar levels, respond when allergens intrude in the body, prepare the uterus for pregnancy, bring on lactation, and more.

The *pituitary* and *pineal glands*, located at the base of the brain, are centers for regulating hormone production in endocrine glands around the body. These crucial regulating organs are also influenced by our states of mind and emotions. Stress can therefore produce over-activity of the endocrine glands, as in the condition of hyperthyroidism.

The *immune system,* consisting of white cells and antibodies, protects the body against invading organisms that cause disease. Over-activity of this system can cause problems such as allergies, and may also contribute to chronic illnesses such as arthritis, asthma, and other disorders.

While the correlation between chronic stress and immune system disorders was known for many years, there was no known mechanism to explain how stress could cause these changes. In recent years it was discovered that there are several dozens of *neuropeptides* (chemical messengers) that are produced by nerve cells in the brain to communicate with each other. These same neuropeptides are also found in white cells. We are just beginning to appreciate that the immune system is so closely knit together with the nervous system that they may in fact function together as a single system. Receptors for neuropeptides are also found in the spinal cord, intestines, kidneys, gonads and other organs. This suggests yet another mechanism whereby the brain/mind and body may act in concert.

With chronic stress producing chronic over-activity of the nervous, endocrine and immune systems, these systems can become exhausted and depleted. They will then be unable to provide us with optimal protection, and we may develop chronic fatigue syndrome, fibromyalgia or other stress-related illnesses.

Since our states of mind can influence the levels of activity in all of these systems, they also offer us access to self-corrective measures for alleviating our own physical problems. Direct access to our unconscious control mechanisms can be achieved through hypnosis, biofeedback, imagery, focused relaxation therapy and other techniques, while indirect access is available through any of the various stress reduction techniques.[16]

While direct interventions to alter our maladaptive body functions are available, we often find that the unconscious mind resists changes in its habitual patterns of response to stress. Psychotherapy may be needed along with these techniques in order to deal with psychological defenses.

TALKING/ RELATIONAL PSYCHOTHERAPY

A person who diagnoses and prescribes for his own afflictions has a fool for a physician and often a corpse for a patient.
— Anonymous

How can we find our way out of difficult habits and self-destructive patterns of perceiving, responding and relating to the world? While it is possible to learn from life experiences, to learn to activate an enormous spectrum of self-healing approaches, and to reprogram our own unconscious mind, the process of doing this may be difficult and sometimes challenging in the extreme when we undertake it on our own, without help.[17]

We may dig such deep ruts for ourselves that we cannot even see out of them to find other paths which might be easier to travel. It is extremely hard for people in the thick of emotional difficulties to see alternatives to their unhelpful or maladaptive behaviors, much less get to the roots of their own problems and deal with them. We may also persist in maladaptive behavior patterns from habit. We tend to try harder in ways we already know rather than seeking new ways to cope, even if the old approaches have not succeeded and may actually have contributed to our problems. In effect, we only dig our ruts ever deeper. For instance, if we habitually withdraw from stressful situations, we may completely isolate ourselves when we are under severe stress. This can lead to a state of depression that leaves us with less energy to cope – and thus another vicious circle is established.

But he that hides a dark soul, and foul thoughts
Benighted walks under the midday sun,
Himself is his own dungeon.
— John Milton

Another common problem is that the unconscious mind, programmed in childhood to protect us against emotional dangers and distresses, is quite resistant to change. We may be far removed from the original hurts that initiated our defensive habits, but we still tend to avoid similar psychological discomforts as though the original dangers were still present. Without any conscious awareness that we are doing so, we resist all logical arguments for change.

Resistance is about standing on yourself and saying you can't move...
— Jessica Macbeth

CASE: Sid's father shouted at him a lot when he was young, and would spank him severely if he talked back. Sid learned to protect himself by clamming up and do-

ing his best to not stir his father's wrath. In later life, Sid was unable to assert himself with his boss at work, even when he knew he was in the right. He would cringe if his boss raised his voice, and was constantly afraid of criticism – even though he was very knowledgeable and skilled in his job. He sought counseling after his friends at work repeatedly challenged him over why he didn't stand up to his boss.

The very act of consulting a health care professional may in itself reduce tension, since it gives us someone who can provide support, and we can then hope for some relief. Many methods of psychotherapy approaches are available, involving an enormous variety of therapist-client interactions. These range from supportive relationships to introspective, reflective processes (such as psychoanalysis and psychodynamic therapy), to more action-oriented therapies (such as cognitive behavior modification). They may include techniques such as hypnosis, relaxation, and meditation, as well as therapeutic family and group interactions, and they may also involve attention to mind-body relationships.[18]

CASE (continued): Sid chose a gestalt therapist, whose way of working with people is to have them hold a dialogue between various aspects of their problem. Sid held a discussion between the part of himself that wanted to have it out with his boss and the part that was afraid to do so. Over a series of therapy session, this led to explorations of other times when Sid had had conflicts like this, particularly in his childhood.

How does psychotherapy work? Jean Shinoda Bolen (1979, p. 69 - 70) discusses how psychoanalysis, one of the many forms of psychotherapy, can help.

> [D]oing analysis is analogous to gardening. The relationship between analyst and patient, with its rules of confidentiality and its quality of sanctuary where it is safe to bring up anything, serves as a container for the process of growth. Removing weeds and rocks, and tilling and watering the soil are preliminary tasks in gardening and are like the psychotherapy phase of analysis. The hindrances to growth, the weeds and rocks – whether in one's early family life or in one's current situation – need to be eliminated. Whatever has crowded out the individual's growth needs to be recognized and removed. Water, that is like feeling, must be brought to the situation in order to allow the defenses to soften and be penetrated. In this way, feelings from others can get through to provide nourishment, like water gets through to the roots of a plant that have been in parched, thick, clayey soil. In analysis, growth occurs underground or deep in the unconscious; later, it manifests itself in what shows above ground.
>
> What comes into being depends on the nature of the seed. A good gardener helps each plant to grow fully and produce whatever it was meant to: whether fruit or vegetable or flower, to be fully whatever it was meant to be – oak, redwood, geranium or cactus.
>
> Often an analyst is a supporting pole for a period of time in another person's life. Most growing things become sturdy enough to eventually

continue on their own, absorbing the water and sunshine of the environment, taking nourishment from the soil in which they are now deeply rooted, in a life of significant soil.

The therapist provides a safe environment in which to explore what is hurting or emotionally unsettled. She helps to sharpen the focus on where the problems lie and how they developed. As we develop greater trust, the therapist gives support so that we don't have to be afraid that releasing our feelings will overwhelm us. She can point out ways in which we might over- or under-estimate our participation, responsibilities or guilt in creating, maintaining or deepening our own problems. Our feelings toward the therapist and our beliefs about what she feels toward us will often be similar to feelings and beliefs we have with regard to other people, but in therapy we can discuss them openly. The therapist can provide feedback as to where we may be distorting or exaggerating our reactions to her, and can thereby help us to correct our erroneous beliefs and maladaptive responses.

Being in the presence of a person who is unconditionally accepting and who gives us reliably objective feedback provides a corrective emotional experience. We may learn to trust that another person can really be there for us – in ways that our parents and mentors may not have been able to

Analysis of our dreams and fantasies can be enormously productive in revealing our unconscious patterns of belief and responses to challenges in our lives. Dreams may also be keys to some of the doors behind which we locked our feelings when they were too painful for us to deal with.

CASE (continued): Sid released intense feelings in several of the hypnotherapy sessions. These stimulated dreams, which opened into earlier and earlier layers of memories of traumatic experiences. The turning point in the therapy came when he recalled a minor experience, but to four year-old Sid a very traumatic one. Sid was all dressed up for Easter services. He loved going to church because this was a time his family was together in a relaxed atmosphere – in contrast to the frequent tensions at home. His mother was often exhausted from being both a homemaker and working as a saleswoman in a department store, and his father was often short-tempered after working long hours as a taxi driver. In the middle of the Easter service, Sid needed to go to the bathroom. His father shushed him several times when he tried to ask to be taken to the restroom. Unable to hold it in any longer, he wet himself. His father, obviously embarrassed (and probably feeling some guilt for having ignored Sid's needs), shamed Sid publicly when he saw he had wet his pants.

Sid felt doubly betrayed by his father, first for not having been sensitive to his feelings and for not responding to his needs and second, for shaming him in front of several other children in the church.

We may learn as much from the *hows* of our interactions as we do from the *whats*. Analyzing our thought processes, our feelings and our interpersonal interactions may more quickly reveal how our unconscious mind works than addressing the content of our thoughts and beliefs.

CASE (continued): Sid's healing in therapy came as much from the acceptance extended by his therapist as it did from the release of the buried memories and feelings. This corrective experience was a balm for the wounds he had carried from this and other painful interactions with his father.

All of these aspects of psychotherapy can help us let go of the childhood programming that may be exerting a negative influence in our adult lives.

CASE (continued): Coming to trust his therapist, Sid began to shed his distrust and fear of authority figures – a distrust generalized by his unconscious mind in its attempts to protect him from further anticipated betrayals, as he had experienced with his father. Gradually, Sid became more assertive at work and was eventually able to stand up for himself with his boss.

The processes of positive change involved in psychotherapy also have great bearing on our understanding of how self-healing and healer-healing work. The unconditionally acceptance of the caregiver for the careseeker is a major element in every therapeutic interaction, whether the therapy focuses on talking, prescribing remedies, manipulating the body or any other therapeutic exchange.

There is also a caution here, however, in interpreting reports of positive effects of healing interventions. Because people may respond to the therapeutic relationship alone, any treatment modality – whether through talking therapies, bioenergies, physical manipulation of the body, prescription of medications or taking herbal remedies – must take into account the possibility that the presence of the caregiver may have been an important, or possibly even the essential element in the success of the treatment.

Beyond the caring attention of the therapist, there are many theories and clinical approaches to helping through psychotherapy. Several of these are discussed below and many others are detailed in the next chapter. Appendix A provides a brief description of a range of psychotherapies.

PHYSICAL SYMPTOMS ADDRESSED BY PSYCHOTHERAPY

> *The body is a vehicle for the soul and spirit, and a metaphor for wheat is transpiring in the whole person.*
> – DB

We often experience various physical sensations when repressed feelings are activated unconsciously under stress. As discussed above, these may range from muscle tension and tightness to spasms and pain. Such reactions may simply be conditioned responses of tension in our bodies, which became associated with early traumas or with the expression of particular unpleasant emotions. Alternatively, the actual memory of the emotion may have been stored in some way within the complaining muscles and tendons, or in another aspect of our body functions. Let us consider, for illustration, at some healing experiences of a person with a psychosomatic problem.

CASE: Susan, a 23-year-old university student, came for psychotherapy because she was lonely and depressed. Susan's father had been killed in an auto accident when she was eight years old. She felt deeply hurt, and also furious with him for "abandoning" her. The unconscious does not differentiate between loss through deliberate abandonment, divorce, death or illness. The unavailability of a parent to meet the child's needs creates a justifiable rage.

Eight-year-old Susan told her mother she was angry, but her mother was grieving the loss of her husband and became upset by her daughter's words. Susan then felt guilty for adding to her mother's burden of pain. In the unfolding of this drama, Susan learned not to express her emotions. One of her ways of holding them in was to clench her jaw tight, literally biting off the words and keeping her mouth tightly shut in order to keep her feelings from spilling out.

Susan's unconscious mind then stepped in to protect her from feeling her unpleasant emotions, which were also partially unacceptable to her own conscience. Her unconscious helped her by keeping these feelings buried so that they were no longer consciously experienced as a source of anguish.

This worked well as a temporary solution, but it eventually had unfortunate consequences. Susan's unconscious mind, in its attempts to protect her from feeling hurt, began to work overtime. Any experience that might potentially remind Susan of the unpleasant memories locked away in her dark mental closets had to be prevented from disturbing her. This constant awareness of what to keep away from was manifested in Susan's conscious mind as a sense of uneasiness and irritability in any related situations that she encountered later in life. Although she had a pleasant personality and was good-looking, she had no real friends. She also suffered from tension headaches at the sides of her head.

Whenever she started to get close to someone, she would get into silly arguments with him, and soon ended the relationship. Susan's unconscious was trying to protect her, first from the unresolved childhood grief over her father's death with the pain and anger of being abandoned, and second, from the possibility of suffering the same feelings of rejection and hurt if she allowed anyone else to get close to her emotionally.

Susan's psychotherapist helped her to search her unconscious memories and feelings in order to understand her current irrational behavior. He explained how the muscles that tighten her jaw are attached at the one end to the jawbone and at the other end to the sides of her head. Muscle relaxation exercises provided substantial relief from the headaches. Her therapist also taught her to pay attention to her headaches – as red flags to alert Susan to situations in which she was clenching her jaw to hold in her feelings.

Once the roots of the problem were identified, Susan experienced, with considerable intensity, many of the repressed memories with all their attached sadness and anger. There were several therapy sessions during which she raged and cried as though her father had just recently died. These emotions were released from her unconscious at this point in her life because she could now cope with them more competently. Furthermore, she trusted in her therapist's support to help her to deal with these emotions and to find more constructive ways of handling rejections – both actual and anticipated ones which never actually materialized but which still were a source of agony to her. Although the feelings of anger and hurt were still painful, Susan now had many more alternatives for coping with them as an adult.

After working through the pent-up anger she felt toward her father, Susan found she no longer needed to distance herself from her friends. She also stopped having headaches.

The intensity of such emotional releases (*abreactions*) testifies to how well the unconscious represses these feelings. They remain in their dark closets, carefully guarded from scrutiny but intact in all their raw power. This is especially common with grief, which is one of the most painful experiences in life.

Cues that can alert us to seek psychotherapy often take the form of somatic complaints. We may have headaches or other symptoms for which our doctor cannot identify a physical cause. Sometimes it is enough for the doctor simply to ask us what might be making us feel tense, and we realize what is making us up tight. In other instances we might need to speak with a counselor or therapist to discover the sources of the tension underlying our physical problems. The psychotherapist can help us work out what is triggering the symptoms and why. Often the symptom turns out to be a learned (*conditioned*) response, which became associated with tension in the context of an original emotional trauma. Thereafter, we may experience the same response in similarly tense situations.[19] A case of this kind was presented to me when a young man sought my help with an awkward problem.

CASE: Peter, aged 22, would become nauseous whenever he faced the prospect of dating a girl. If he forced himself to take the girl out, he sometimes even vomited. He had avoided dealing with the problem for several years by burying himself in his studies. Now that he was out of school and working, he was becoming increasingly frustrated and angry with himself.

Peter was successful in his work as a nurse, seemed otherwise free of emotional problems, and could not see any logical reason for his difficulties. I decided that behavioral therapy promised to provide the most direct relief, and I taught Peter some relaxation techniques. I then asked him to fantasize, while in a relaxed state, that he was approaching women to talk with them, or that they were approaching him. This taught him to remain relaxed when getting close to women. After three weeks of practice, Peter reported that his feeling of nausea in the actual presence of women was much reduced.

During the following session, Peter spontaneously recalled an important event from his senior year in high school. He had been in the school cafeteria where his best friend's girlfriend worked. As she dished a portion of peas onto his plate, she hinted that she would like him to ask her out. He was very upset, feeling attracted to her, but also reluctant to betray his best friend. He declined politely, but felt nauseous and could not finish his meal. That was when his nausea had begun.

Once Peter's unconscious mind released these memories with their attached emotions, he no longer felt any nausea in the presence of women. Peter's unconscious had kept him away from women in his adult life because of conflicts that had been buried deep in his psyche some years earlier. His headaches and nausea cleared up when his emotional conflict was sorted out.

While insights into the origins of a problem may surface during behavioral thera-pies, this is not a requirement for cures of chronic symptoms. People may relinquish their physical problems without any awareness of the original traumas or ongoing causes behind them.

Psychotherapy has contributed significantly to our understanding of healing. It uncovers processes by which the unconscious protects the conscious mind. The unconscious behaves in a very literal, mechanistic, computer-like fashion. Its re-actions are involuntary, reflexive, and frequently simplistic to the point of childish irrationality. Situations that make us uncomfortable are dealt with to *im-mediately* reduce the tension, even though it may not actually resolve the problem. In fact, the long-term effects of the automatic, unconscious response may be to worsen the problem. The unconscious mind, in its childish way, does not consider the long-range implications of such protectiveness over the whole person. Psychological conflicts are rapidly repressed and unpleasant tensions are reduced. However, muscle tensions and other symptoms that frequently accom-pany emotional stress may then accumulate, with no apparent cause to explain their presence.

This is most clearly and dramatically seen in *conversion* reactions (sometimes called *hysterical* reactions). In these cases, drastic changes such as paralyses or sensory deficits may appear quite suddenly, with no apparent physical cause. Here is a clinical example of how this might occur.

CASE: John was a church-going, well-mannered, 32-year-old clerk, and a good husband and father to two lovely children. Under stress from company problems that threatened his job, combined with some unexpected financial burdens at home, he exploded one day in anger at his wife. He even raised his fist, but did not strike her. This was very uncharacteristic of him, and he was immediately apologetic and remorseful. The next morning he awoke with a feeling of weakness in his right arm. This developed over the next two days into total paralysis of the arm and hand

Neurological evaluation showed no physical disease, but revealed a pattern of paralysis typical of a conversion reaction. In psychotherapy John proved to be a good hypnotic subject. Under trance he revealed that he had been so angry at his wife that he was ready to strike her. This was clearly very much out of character, and contrary to the dictates of his conscience. It was apparent that John's uncon-scious mind had punished him through this paralysis for feeling the extreme anger, and at the same time had prevented him from expressing this dangerous emotion. John made a very rapid recovery as his anger was uncovered and re-leased during hypnotic trance. This process of repressing his feelings and hiding them from his own awareness was explained to him, and with the help of further the psychotherapy he no longer had to repress his anger or punish himself for it.

Since all of these processes occur in the unconscious mind, people are initially unaware of the causes of their conversion symptoms. When a person uncovers the roots of his symptoms under hypnosis, the strong emotions that were repressed may be released. Upon coming out of the hypnotic trance, he can be instructed to recall the information he had repressed. In many cases this process will relieve his symptoms permanently. Hypnosis is particularly effective in treating conversion reactions, and with appropriate therapy they may be cleared up very quickly.

The process is the same, whether it leads to conversion reactions or simply to feelings that are buried in the unconscious without external symptoms. The pain of sexual, physical, or emotional abuse, for instance, may be repressed in this way, when the trauma is still fresh and overwhelming. However, the buried hurts may later produce disabling psychological symptoms. With the support of a therapist, the pain can be released, and the symptoms will then resolve.

> *Though this be madness, yet there is method in it.*
> – William Shakespeare (*Hamlet*)

Arthur Janov vividly describes how headaches, ulcers, constipation, asthma, hypertension, muscle tensions, epilepsy and many other problems have been alleviated as a result of his method of therapy, which prescribes screaming to enable the release of pent-up emotions. Janov's descriptions are amongst the clearest I have found on releasing tensions, as well as other symptoms associated with emotional blocks, through psychotherapy.[20]

Other avenues for uncovering the meanings in the many and varied ways the body speaks – through gestures, sensations and symptoms - and for releasing symptoms have been developed in several mind-body psychotherapies.

Gestalt therapy invites people to imagine themselves as the part of their body that has made an idiosyncratic unconscious movement, as in a nervous tic (Perls).

CASE (continued): In the example of Sid (mentioned above), the therapist noticed that his hands were clenched into fists. When Sid was asked about this gesture, he had no clue what his body might be saying. He was instructed to speak for his fists – that is, to put words to the gesture. In this way he was able to identify and verbalize anger his unconscious anger, which he then realized had been provoked not only by his boss, but also through chronic, unexpressed frustrations in his marriage. His unconscious mind had been expressing this anger through his fists in nonverbal communication in the therapy session, as well as through the paralysis which initially brought him to the therapy.

Physical symptoms such as pain may also clear up when their meaning is perceived through gestalt therapy, as a person puts words to the tensions behind the symptom and as emotions locked within the body are released.

Relaxation techniques such as muscle relaxation, meditation, and breathing exercises can help to relieve many aspects of emotional and physical stresses. Most of these techniques are easily learned and profoundly effective.

If you would like to take a brief break from reading to explore one or more of these exercises, you can go to the Appendix and explore *muscle relaxations*.

Another bodymind therapist, a psychiatrist named Wilhelm Reich, was one of Freud's disciples He believed that a life force, which he called *orgone energy,* permeates all things in the universe. . Reich felt that health depends on maintaining an adequate flow of this energy throughout the body. He taught that for various defensive reasons, people with mental disturbances develop muscular rigidity (*armoring*), which is often associated with sexual inhibitions. This tension could block the natural flow of body energy. Reich developed a variety of breathing and muscle exercises to help release these energy blocks.

Reich's disciples subsequently branched out and developed variations on his methods. *Bioenergetics*, developed by Alexander Lowen, uses exercises and stress postures to achieve similar results. *Core-energetics therapy* is another related approach, developed by John Pierrakos. *Rolfing* is a related form of therapy in which very deep massage and pressure are applied to the muscles, tendons and fascia (connective tissues) in order to heighten body sensations related to underlying psychological tensions, sometimes to the point of inducing pain. Unconscious memories and feelings locked within the tissues may be released through this method.

The *Feldenkrais, Alexander, and Hellerwork methods* are gentler forms of body-based psychotherapy. They aim to build posture and correct habits of movement so that people feel better within their bodies. They focus on improving positive behaviors, in addition to addressing pathological patterns.

Rubenfeld Synergy Therapy extends this type of bodywork to focus on the emotions underlying body tensions and other symptoms, helping to release habitual defensive patterns along with whatever energy has been locked into the body in a maladaptive way.

Massage, in its many variations may release muscle tensions.

Working with the body through any of these or other approaches may help to release such defensive patterns much more quickly than talking therapy alone.

Initially, however, this kind of work may raise anxieties and confused feelings because the unconscious mind believes that the defensive patterns it has employed for many years, programmed in childhood, are needed for protection. On the positive side, Ilana Rubenfeld explains how such confusion could actually facilitate change.

> "Fusion" means "union." "Con" can mean either "with" or "opposed to."
> Thus the word "confusing" means both a pulling apart *and* a joining, both
> of which are vital to the process of change. I encourage clients to feel con-
> fused, because you have to be willing to be disorganized in order to get
> reorganized. If you are in a dysfunctional habit pattern, it cannot be
> changed unless it is interrupted, and interruption means confusion. We get
> anxious and hate it; it's often bewildering. But we cannot experiment with
> new, *non*habitual behavior unless we experience the discomfort of our old
> ways breaking apart. We cannot change without first falling into what I
> have called "the fertile void." (p. 20)

These therapies all release tensions and their associated memories from the mind and body. They demonstrate that the unconscious mind will frequently lock up conflicting emotions, complex problems, and uncomfortable memories inside the muscles and tissues of our bodies. In the practice of these and other related therapies, chronic pains and other symptoms are frequently relieved when physical and emotional tensions, and the associated memories and emotions, are finally released.

With these therapies we begin to see that body and mind are so intimately re-lated that the terms, *bodymind therapy* and *mind-body therapy* may be appropriate and helpful concepts.

Spiritual healing is another therapy that can relieve many symptoms in similar ways. Aspects of psychotherapy will always be involved in healing – through suggestion on the part of therapists and through expectations of healees. This does not mean that healing is merely a form of suggestion. The controlled studies re-viewed in Volume 1 show that healing is another bodymind therapy, a potent intervention which is significantly more than just a placebo effect.

Meditation produces many benefits for physical and psychological wellbeing. Meditation may bring about spontaneous emotional releases, sometimes accom-panied by marked improvements in physical symptoms. It appears that when we calm ourselves through meditation, the unconscious mind realizes it does not have to protect us any more from feeling the hurts of old traumas that it buried at the time we experienced them. Meditators who are unprepared for such releases may be surprised, distressed or even dismayed – feeling that these are negative effects of meditation. They are usually only negative if the meditator responds with fear. If such emotional releases are recognized and accepted as part of the healing process, they can be enormously helpful.

These therapies provide many avenues for addressing psychological and physi-cal problems. Pain is particularly responsive, even when it is caused by known physical causes such as trauma, arthritis or other disease processes.

PHYSICAL SYMPTOMS ADDRESSED BY BODYWORK THERAPIES

And your body is the harp of your soul,
It is yours to bring forth sweet music from it or confused sounds.
                                        – Kahlil Gibran

Massage in its numerous variations can alleviate many symptoms, including pain and anxiety. By manually kneading the muscles, massage releases chronic physi-cal tensions. Emotional tensions, stored in the muscles, tendons and ligaments, may be released at the same time. As with meditation, such releases may be un-expected.

Spiritual healing can have similar effects. Skeptics might suspect that spiritual healing is no more than a mechanical laying-on of hands, a kind of massage that uses simple physiological methods to relieve tension through muscular relaxation. In practice, the laying-on of hands usually involves only light touch at the most, and frequently includes hand-movements that are made around the healee's body without actually touching. The application of pressure to release symptoms is not used in spiritual healing.

Spiritual healing also has a broad range of overlaps with various forms of psy-chotherapy, as it can bring about releases of old psychological traumas. Another of the common suspicions of skeptics (and it certainly was one of my own initial impressions) is that reports of spiritual healings must involve hysterical symp-toms that are cured through suggestion, or through the healer's soothing presence or counseling. While this may be true in a few cases, there are many more instances of confirmed problems of physical origins that have responded to spiritual healing.

Healing is really much more than a form of body therapy. It reduces anxieties and seems to directly relax the muscles, or to activate mechanisms within the healee's body to release tensions in the muscles, without physical pressure.

Healing may in fact be a helpful adjunct to enhance massage and other body therapies. My own clinical experience is that healing facilitates these releases considerably more than the physical interventions alone. Several therapy approaches have been developed that include healing, such as Network Spinal Analysis and the Bowen technique.

Many complementary therapists may even be healers without knowing it – especially those involved in manual therapies. Growing numbers of these therapists are consciously including healing in their ministrations, finding that the combination of the two is more potent than either of the practices used alone.

PSYCHOLOGICAL CONDITIONING (REINFORCEMENT) AND BEHAVIOR THERAPY

> *A dog will salivate out of habit when a bell is rung. What bells do you respond to in your life?*
>
> – DB

Ivan Pavlov's study is a classic in the area of psychological conditioning (also called *reinforcement*). He demonstrated that if a bell is rung whenever food is presented to a dog, the dog will learn to associate the sound of the bell with the food. He will start to salivate whenever he hears the bell, even if he does not receive food at that time. In other words, the dog has become conditioned to the bell as a stimulus producing salivation.

Such conditioning can occur in humans without our conscious awareness. If psychologists smile (or in any other manner provide *reinforcements*) whenever their clients behave in a particular way, such as reporting dreams or discussing their feelings, the clients will be conditioned by such reinforcements to repeat the behaviors with a greater frequency. This is one of the reasons why Freudian clients come to have Freudian dreams, while Jungian clients have Jungian dreams. They are simply fulfilling their therapists' expectations, responding to reinforcements provided by their respective therapists. This may occur without the conscious awareness of either therapists or clients.

The examples presented above are from the controlled context of the psychologist's office. However, the same principles apply in the less structured settings of everyday life. Anyone may have a sudden sensation of physical tension (such as tightness in muscles or stomach cramps) when they experience an emotional event. This may then lead to conditioning of the body to become tense (or to cramp up) whenever that emotion is felt or the event is recalled or repeated. Such randomly reinforced connections between bodily conditions and environmental stimuli or emotional reactions may be totally unconscious. We may suffer a number of physical symptoms, believing them to be purely related to malfunctions of our body. We may have no awareness of any connection with the original chain of events that reinforces and maintains those symptoms. Remember that Peter, who felt nausea associated with dating women, at first had no idea how this symptom had developed.

Psychotherapists have learned to relieve symptoms using these same processes of reinforcement, in what is called *behavior therapy*. Therapists repattern their clients' responses to stimuli, so that the clients will no longer suffer from physical discomfort. The natural conditioning or reinforcing circumstances are first identified, and the clients are then taught to relax or to respond in some other, more adaptive manner to the same stimuli. The case of Peter, described earlier, illustrates this process of corrective conditioning.

A popular version of this technique is *cognitive behavioral therapy*, in which the therapist confront clients with the illogical nature of their fears and then helps them to sort out logical approaches for dealing with them.

CASE: Harry was terrified of dogs. He readily admitted that although he had been bitten by a dog as a child, this was no reason to cringe every time he passed a little dog on a leash while walking down the street – as much as twenty or thirty years later. The avoidance of dogs may have been a good survival technique in childhood but it was totally unnecessary, inconvenient, and sometimes embarrassing to him a quarter of a century later, at age 32.

Prior to therapeutic interventions, clients tend to hold onto such symptoms quite tenaciously.

CASE (continued): Harry's cognitive behavior therapist suggested a pattern of exercises that paired positive images with the fearful feelings which arose whenever Harry even thought of a dog. Every time he mentally pictured a dog and felt he wanted to cringe, the therapist directed him to imagine himself on a beach on a warm, relaxing holiday. Harry would then relax, basking in the sun of his mental beach imagery. By repeatedly alternating this process of imagining a dog, then imagining a relaxing scene, Harry was able to reprogram his unconscious, automatic dog alarm so that it no longer went off whenever he saw a harmless dog.

It may not be necessary to achieve *conscious awareness* of the original causes of tensions in order to be rid of them. We may let go of old patterns of behavior when new and better ones serve us better – but too often our habit patterns are firmly engrained, and do not change, even if they are maladaptive and causing us considerable discomfort or even distress and pain. A fear of heights or of flying, which might have developed from negative experiences that we may not even recall, can keep us from hiking up a lovely mountain or from flying off on a refreshing holiday, or even from emptying leaves out of the drain spout, if this simple task requires us to climb a ladder.

Sometimes our unconscious habits can be quite complex in their origin and their expression.

CASE: Gina's fear of her verbally abusive father had generalized over her 25 years of life into a fear of any authority figure, a hesitant manner of relating to anyone with a loud voice, and anxieties about dating men. Since there was no single image that she could use for conditioning herself to let go of all of these fears and defensive habits, her therapist helped her to partialize her problems. Gina made a list of all of her fears, and then chose which one she wanted to work on first. She was able to shape her behaviors one at a time, to overcome the entire complex of her fears, and to eliminate the residues of real pain that she had experienced in childhood because of her abusive father.

Richard Bandler and John Grinder have taken the concept of conditioning several steps further. They use related techniques to establish more adaptive responses, or even chains of responses, of an emotional and cognitive nature. Their approach is called *Neurolinguistic Programming (NLP)*. They touch the client at a randomly chosen part of his body, as a means of *anchoring* (conditioning) the response that they are teaching.

CASE: George was so nervous about speaking in public that he would forget his materials, fumble helplessly with notes he had prepared and stuttered – despite the fact that he was an excellent teacher in a one-to-one situation. The therapist told him to picture himself in a lecture situation where he would be highly anxious. The therapist then touched George on one of his knuckles while he was imaging himself in that situation. Next, the therapist instructed George to picture himself feeling competent, relaxed and comfortable in giving a lecture to a large audience – while the therapist touched him on the next knuckle, near the first "anchor." On touching each spot again, the feeling that had been anchored there was elicited. (This is an important observation, in and of itself – as discussed below.) The therapist then touched the two spots simultaneously, and the positive anchor neutralized the negative one. This conditioned George to relinquish his chronic, distressing patterns and to feel confident and comfortable when lecturing in public.

You might wish to explore this technique for yourself, following suggestions outlined in Chapter 5, which also describes several variations and elaborations of NLP techniques.

NLP clearly demonstrates how easily and quickly the body may become linked through conditioning to respond to various stimuli. We saw in the case of George that once an image and its related feelings were anchored in a body location by a touch, the same image and feelings would be elicited on repeatedly touching the same spot. If a person happens to have a body sensation at a time when she has a negative experience, the memory of that experience may become linked to the sensation. At any time in the future that the same body sensation occurs, the memory of the negative experience may be invoked again. This may explain how traumatic experiences produce some physical symptoms, as discussed below.

Behavioral techniques can be highly effective in treating discrete problems such as phobias and focused anxieties, as in fear of heights or fear of speaking in public. Recent research also confirms that these techniques can be potently effective in treating depression, particularly when combined with antidepressant medication.

CONDITIONING THE IMMUNE SYSTEM

Our cells are constantly eavesdropping on our thoughts and being changed by them. A bout of depression can wreak havoc with the immune system; falling in love can boost it... Joy and fulfillment keep us healthy and extend life. This means that the line between biology and psychology can't really be drawn with any certainty...

– Deepak Chopra

Research shows that conditioning (psychological reinforcement) can influence biochemical processes within the body. The most startling discovery in this area has been that our immune responses can also be psychologically conditioned.

Experiments by Robert Ader and Nicholas Cohen have demonstrated that the immune systems of mice can be conditioned to respond to chemical stimuli. When experimenters gave mice saccharine mixed with cyclophosphamide (a chemical that produces severe abdominal pains), they found that the mice could be conditioned to respond to the saccharine alone as though they were receiving both chemicals. Some of the mice that received only saccharine after undergoing the conditioning process even died. In their search to understand why this happened, Ader and Cohen found that cyclophosphamide suppresses the immune system. They then deduced that the saccharine alone was having the same effect on the conditioned mice, to the point that they were succumbing to infections. Subsequent experiments confirmed this conjecture. .

This breakthrough has generated an enormous number and variety of studies and has led to further insight into how the mind and the immune system interact.

Until recently, science had no explanation for how the immune system could *remember* an antigen, even many years after an initial exposure to it. People who have had measles or other diseases, or who have been immunized against these diseases in childhood, will be able to fight off similar viruses for many years, sometimes throughout the rest of their lives.

One possible explanation involves the white blood cells, which form a major component of the immune system. In the past few years it has been discovered that white cells contain many of the identical chemicals that nerve cells produce at their junctures (neuropeptides). These neuropeptides provide a chemical modality for communications between nerve cells. The fact that the very same series of neuropeptides are also found in white cells suggests that the white cells may pass information on to the brain for storage. It also suggests that the mind may communicate with and influence the immune system through these same neuropeptides. In effect, the white blood cells appear to be able to act as an extension of the *central nervous system*.

In many of the same ways that the mind can influence the immune system, it appears that it can also affect the cardiovascular system. Dean Ornish has shown that a combination of relaxation, meditation and imagery therapy, together with regular exercise and a healthy diet, can bring about dramatic improvements in the condition of people with cardiac disease, even if they are very seriously ill and in need of cardiac surgery. The Ornish approach is finding increasing acceptance as a technique for dealing with cardiovascular disease.

While the precise mechanisms for mind-heart communications have yet to be elaborated, it is clear that they are present. The interactions of the mind with the immune system have been called *psychoneuroimmunology* (*PNI*), and some are starting to use the term *Psychoneurocardiology.*

BODY-MIND THERAPIES AND SPIRITUAL HEALING

Many of the levels on which spiritual healing may occur overlap with the fields of practice of both conventional and unconventional psychotherapies.

Therapists who treat body tensions are directly addressing the deeper interactions of people with their own bodies. Understanding how the mind and body interact can help them to formulate physical exercises to facilitate therapy. Reich, Lowen, Pierrakos, Feldenkrais and others who have explored body-focused therapies have developed astonishing shortcuts to reaching, releasing, analyzing and clearing repressed emotional traumas.

How can these sorts of body-mind communication occur? I believe three principal factors are at play here. First, the body is able to store memories, especially intense ones. Second, when the therapist is comfortable with touch and with intense emotional expressions, then clients will be more likely to benefit from therapies that promote rapid releases of buried hurts. Third, bioenergies provide links between consciousness and the body. Healers may apply many of these same methods intuitively, without deliberately planning these interventions.

Conventional Freudian and psychodynamic psychotherapies have emphasized the analysis of thoughts and the cautious verbal exploration of repressed emotions. They have often ignored the mind-body connection, or worse – avoided it. Thirty years ago I was warned by several of my psychiatry instructors about the dangers of touching clients – a convention that today has actually been written into law in some American states. This blanket caveat becomes a feedback loop that is often initiated by the therapist, leading to unfortunate self-fulfilling prophecies. If therapists are not comfortable with touching, then they will surely convey their anxieties to their clients by their verbal tone and non-verbal communications. They will then cue clients to believe that it might be dangerous if they are touched by their therapists (or by extension, if they are touched by anyone else). This can lead either to repression of feelings and avoidance of touch, or to anxieties if they do allow themselves such interactions. At the same time, therapists will feel that their caution is validated by their clients' anxious responses. This type of negative feedback loop is comparable to the apocryphal story of the mental patient who snapped his fingers loudly and frequently "to scare away the tigers." When someone pointed out that there were no tigers around, he replied, "See! It works!" In the same way, a client's fears and a therapist's anxieties can be woven into a vicious circle that will certainly not benefit the clients, though it may benefit the therapist by slowing the progress of treatment.[21]

The issue of the avoidance of touch during psychotherapy has been complicated by cases of therapists who have sexually abused their clients. This has increased the professional pressure on therapists to avoid touching, lest their caring touch be misinterpreted as a sexual advance.

In contrast, most spiritual healers are comfortable with touching healees, and this may actually facilitate self-healing in all of the many ways that touch is comforting, enhances bonding and promotes relaxation.

Reinforcement theories and practices demonstrate how tensions can become linked to environmental or internal cues. In the example of George, who was treated with Neurolinguistic Programming, we saw that through structured use of touch one can weaken an old perception and anchor a new one. Not only does this demonstrate ways in which initial tensions may get caught within the body, but it also provides a means for the therapist to introduce new emotional responses to old anxiety-triggering cues. In this instance, as in many others we will consider throughout this book, we can appreciate that including the bodymind in therapy represents a major advance beyond basic conditioning techniques.

As we saw in the example of the laboratory mice, more recent research indicates that immune responses can also become conditioned. It is therefore highly probable that behavior therapy and other psychotherapies can also contribute to the treatment of illness through enhancement of immune functions. Psychoneuroimmunology (PNI), discussed later in this chapter, is a therapy built on this understanding.

These observations suggest bases for understanding the ways in which the body internalizes stresses, and then develops the disease patterns of malfunction. Similarly, these mechanisms point to ways in which healers may evoke more constructive and healthy patterns of behavior and bodily function without needing to activate psi powers.

A healer can provide relief from emotional problems in several other ways as well. For instance, healers usually take time to listen to their clients' problems. This is something that conventional doctors and nurses are doing less and less, as pressures from limited budgets and "efficient" medical management limit the time they spend with patients.

Healers may also be helpful when people become stuck in vicious circles of anxiety and tension associated with pain and illness. Simply offering hope may be enough to reduce anxiety, and may thus relieve tensions and reduce the discomforts of the entire vicious circle. The very suggestion that people may be getting help from spiritual healing may produce relief through placebo effects (considered below). Healers may also discuss ways for healees to relax and avoid stressors, and this can have similar results.

Some healers are adept at psychological counseling. They might be able to help people deal with secondary gains, by confronting healees about their needs for attention which their symptoms and illnesses may generate, and by suggesting ways to approach difficult situations that they are avoiding. Healers may thus be able to help their clients through a variety of clinical interventions, even if they have no special spiritual healing abilities.

Conversely, there may often be elements of psi and healing in conventional psychotherapy – unbidden and perhaps even without the conscious awareness of the therapists or clients. Some therapists can intuit their clients' tensions, inner conflicts and needs; some have a healing *presence* that clients warm to. This may seem speculative, but is supported in research. Many studies confirm that most people have *psi* (psychic) abilities.[1] Similarly, several healing studies demonstrate that many people who make no claim to healing abilities can produce healing effects. It does not require a great leap of faith to believe that therapists of all varieties may introduce aspects of psi and healing in their therapy.

PSYCHOLOGICAL CONDITIONING, FEEDBACK LOOPS, AND SPIRITUAL HEALING

There are many possible connections between conditioning and spiritual healing, especially touch-healing.

During a laying-on of hands, a healer may reprogram a healee's responses to a stressful situation without even being aware of doing so, as we have seen is possible in Neurolinguistic Programming.

My experience with NLP and my observations of spiritual healings lead me to believe that in most cases, far more occurs in healing sessions than a mere reconditioning of responses to given stimuli. Conditioning is inevitably a part but not all of what may occur in spiritual healing.

Psychoneuroimmunology introduces a new understanding of the potential control that the mind can exercise over the body. The mind's influence over the immune system is another clue to mechanisms whereby the body might "spontaneously" rid itself of diseases, including cancer, with the help of imagery techniques, suggestion, or spiritual healing. The mechanisms involved may reside within the healee, who can activate them when encouraged by the therapist.

There are loops of connections between the body and the unconscious mind which can have positive and negative effects. On the positive side, body functions such as blood pressure and temperature are kept within limits that are optimal for survival. If our blood pressure falls, our nervous system sends signals to raise it. If the ambient temperature rises, we sweat in order to lower our body temperature. These automatic reactions help to keep body processes functioning within physical and chemical ranges that are conducive to life.[2]

On the negative side, such feedback loops may become stuck in *vicious circles.* For instance, we have already considered how anxiety can produce muscle tension. If this becomes a chronic condition, it may eventually lead to muscular spasms → pain → anxiety → tension, → worse spasms → etc., in a cycle that can become difficult to interrupt.

Feedback loops function on psychological and social levels as well. In relating to other people, we all tend to adopt certain patterns. These are determined partly by the personality we develop from birth, but to an even greater extent they are influenced by feedback that we receive in the course of our social interactions. Having adopted a particular set of patterns, we usually continue to follow them without much thought. If three-year-old Sally knows she can obtain a favorable response from her parents by whining, then she will be likely to whine automatically when she asks for something. In turn, her parents will become accustomed to her behaving as a whiner, although they may still complain about it. It is easier for them to respond automatically to her whining behavior than to encourage her to act in new ways, which would require them to think before reacting to her new approach. The rebellious teenager invites stricter controls, which stimulate further rebellion. The nagging wife sets off the drinking husband, who goes out and drinks because she nags, which only brings more nagging... and so on.

> *My, how you've changed since I've changed.*
> – Ashleigh Brilliant

Such relational patterns may be experienced as positive rather than negative, but they may still be maladaptive. A husband may be better at math than his wife, and may therefore take on the responsibilities of handling all of the bills and other finances in a marriage, while his wife may take on all the responsibilities for so-cial arrangements. While such tacit, complementary partnerships may be convenient, they also leave each partner without the challenges that could develop their skills in the reciprocal areas of responsibility. In the Jungian framework, we would observe that this mutual complementarity leaves people less likely to ex-plore their weaker polarities. In a more problematic variation on this theme, a child may be helped by parents (in homework, tasks of daily living or making decisions) to the extent that the child never develops the skills or confidence to care for herself. The parents feel needed in being helpful, the child feels nurtured in being cared for. We call these relationships *co-dependent*.

An understanding of these types of feedback loops is important to the practice of psychotherapy and healing. First, persons who are ill relate to the world as *peo-ple-with-symptoms*. Even though these symptoms may be troublesome or even devastating in their effects, people caught up in vicious circles may have diffi-culty in relinquishing the maladaptive behaviors that perpetuate their own suffering. An example of this sort was described to me many years ago.

CASE: Morris, a young man in his early twenties had scarred corneas from in-fancy. When corneal transplants were first developed he was a prime candidate for this procedure, which promised to restore full vision. Upon the removal of his bandages, his family and the doctors were all tremendously excited to see his re-sponse to his newly acquired ability to see.

After adapting to his new perceptions, Morris was absolutely delighted. Over a period of a few months, however, he became seriously depressed and finally committed suicide.

A psychological post-mortem revealed that it had been too difficult for him to adjust to life as a seeing person. He had been used to receiving extra help be-cause of his blindness, and when he could see, he was expected to cope more independently. Unfortunately, he could not adapt to the new expectations.

This is an extreme example, but it illustrates the difficulty of adjusting to life after the symptoms to which a person may have become completely accustomed are finally eliminated.

In many instances people *consciously* wish to be cured of their symptoms, but *unconsciously* have numerous reasons for retaining them (secondary gains), and may therefore unconsciously resist improving.

Relatives of people who experience this kind of dramatic healing may similarly find it difficult to adjust to their recovery. The sick person may have been satisfying many needs of other family members through their illness, such as permitting or encouraging more open displays of affection or caring; providing an excuse for avoiding uncomfortable situations, such as traveling or work; or keeping a spouse or other relative from leaving the relationship. Their symptoms may also have become entangled in various power struggles for dominance or competition.

> *The chicken is the egg's way of getting more eggs.*
> – Alan Watts

Relatives often subtly encourage family members to remain ill, or at least not to improve too rapidly or too completely. In the illustration presented above of the drinking husband and the nagging wife, even if the husband were to stop drinking, he might encounter responses such as: "Well! So you forgot to stop at the bar on the way home today, did you?" or "I wonder how long this bout of sobriety can last!" Once we get ourselves into chronic vicious circles, it is difficult to extricate ourselves, and to differentiate between cause and effect.

Figure II-2 Positive transformation

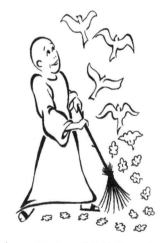

Image courtesy of Keith Chopping

Psychotherapy may be able to break vicious circles of negative interactions, partly through elements of suggestion and gradual symptom relief. In addition, a positive seed may be planted in the minds of the participants, and the opposite of a vicious circle may be established. For lack of an appropriate phrase, I have coined the term, *sweetening spiral*. With healing we may feel better → be less tense → have less pain → feel better → etc. Similar sweetening spirals can develop in our social interactions as we progress through the healing process.

There are other subtle therapist-client feedback loops that can develop in the course of treatment. In conventional psychotherapies, and especially in psycho-analysis, the therapist is frequently cautioned against delving into psychologically sensitive areas too quickly, lest the client be overwhelmed by anxiety and possibly even decompensate into psychosis.

My personal experience in for people with a variety of emotional problems in America, England and Israel contradicts these caveats. If a therapist is comfortable with (and not afraid of) his clients' intense emotions, and if the clients have confidence in the therapist, then there is very little danger that clients will be frightened unduly by their own feelings, even when these are quite intense.

Similar observations about handling intense emotions have been made by therapists practicing *Gestalt Therapy*, *Transactional Analysis* and *Primal Scream Therapy*.

Doctors, patients and researchers frequently get stuck in self-validating feedback loops. For instance, conventional doctors may enjoy feeling competent and needed. They may relate to their patients in authoritarian manners, heightening their sense of superiority. Many patients are pleased to come to a specialist who can identify, explain and treat their problems, and are often comforted by being given a diagnosis and a prescription. By keeping the focus at the level of symptoms and physical illnesses, these doctors and patients avoid dealing with underlying emotional issues that may be causing and perpetuating the problems. This avoidance loop is reinforced by their relief at not having to deal with unpleasant feelings that could be upsetting to both caregiver and careseeker. This avoidance comes with a cost, however. Rather like an abscess that is neglected because it would be painful to lance it to drain the pus, when emotional pus is not released it continues to fester and may lead to toxic conditions.

Similarly, healers and healees may also develop feedback loops of beliefs and practices.

A healer's reputation for bringing about rapid improvements in people's health might predispose healees to relinquish their illnesses more readily. Part of the success reported by healers may also be due to self-selection of healees who are emotionally ready to get better. Healees' high expectations when they come for spiritual healing may facilitate more rapid change, as compared with the expectations they might bring to other health care professionals whose methods are more familiar and predictable. Healees may need only the "permission" of the healer to abandon old habit patterns and adopt new ones. Being successful will then further enhance the healers' confidence.

In another sweetening spiral, healers who are not afraid of their healees' emotional intensity may facilitate releases of long-repressed conflicts and feelings, merely through their own acceptance that this is safe for the client to do.

Not all such feedback loops are positive, however. Healers' egos may become inflated when they are successful in helping people. They may push healees to improve when healees are not yet emotionally ready – because the healers want the aggrandizement of dramatic results and adulation from healees and other observers. Healees may choose healers of this sort when they are not ready to explore their psychological issues that are behind their symptoms. They may relinquish their presenting symptoms, avoiding having to deal with their underlying problems and satisfying the healers, but may find the symptoms returning later or may develop other symptoms.

Feedback loops can act to slow the acceptance of healing within conventional medicine. Many in the scientific community have tended toward skepticism and disbelief in psi and spiritual healing because they find that the related phenomena are too alien to their everyday experiences and customary belief systems. (To put it more colloquially, healing exceeds their *boggle threshold.*) People who are uncomfortable with information that contradicts their worldview are more likely to turn to others who share their disbelief for confirmation of the views they already hold, rather than to re-examine (much less relinquish) their cherished and well-defended perspectives.

Let me share a response I received in my search for surgeons to participate in a research project on healing:

> *Benor:* Here are some experiments on animals, plants, enzymes and humans, which show that healing works.
>
> *Surgeon.* Why are you giving me references from such weird sources? Aren't there articles in reputable journals?
>
> *Benor:* Reputable journals have been prejudiced against publishing such articles.
>
> *Surgeon.* How can I believe, then, that these are reputable studies? Why wouldn't better journals publish these results?
>
> *Benor:* It seems they aren't comfortable with this sort of thing.
>
> *Surgeon.* Well, what you tell me looks promising, but what will my colleagues think? What about my patients? They'll probably think I'm losing it!
>
> *Benor:* We can explain that we're doing this study to explore whether such forms of healing are effective. It may be that it's all due to the effects of suggestion. If that's true, the study will also be useful.
>
> *Surgeon:* I'll have to think it over...
>
> *Surgeon* (at a later date): You know, if this stuff about healing were actually true, I'd have to change my whole belief system. It can't be true!

Such attitudes have nourished the prejudice against research on spiritual healing, and against the publication of related studies. There is a clear social resistance to change, and this is reinforced by feedback loops of social disapproval of any deviation from the norm.

> *[I]gnorance of ignorance... is the fundamental limit of our knowledge.*
> – Francis Jeffrey

To examine spiritual healing we must be willing to rise above these defensive feedback loops, and change our established patterns of belief.

Healers who work in research settings anecdotally confirm many of the above speculations. They tell me that people referred to them by doctors have significantly different expectations from people who are self-referred for healing. There is often less readiness to change in the doctor-referred patients, who may have various emotional reasons for holding onto their illnesses. The referring doctor may actually want these patients to get well more than the patients do themselves.

Returning to positive feedback loops in spiritual healing, we often find that healing seems to require a strong belief on the part of healers in their own ability to heal successfully. To some degree, the greater their confidence, the greater the healers' effectiveness may be.

The healees' confidence in the healer is likewise an important factor in the relative success or failure of healing. Healers may function best when they can successfully establish an atmosphere of confidence in and enthusiasm for spiritual healing. The belief and encouragement of those around them may strengthen their own belief and confidence, and thus enhance their healing effectiveness.

Conversely, disbelief on the part of observers or participants may inject uncertainty into healers' minds, which then interferes with their healing. This situation has been frequently observed in psi and healing research. Gifted subjects almost uniformly report that they feel inhibited by skeptical observers. Disbelievers and skeptics have viewed this as a *hedge* on the part of healers. They regard it as an excuse for evasion of scrutiny by investigators who might expose the healers (or psi subjects) as fakes or charlatans. While this may be so in some instances, I find this an unlikely hypothesis when I consider the many gifted, sincerely dedicated and highly successful healers who practice with great honesty and integrity.

We will consider some of these issues further at the end of this chapter, under the headings of *transpersonal psychotherapy* and *psi and psychotherapy.*

Theoretical consideration of feedback loops
Cognitive feedback loops function on many levels. Gary Schwartz (1984) is a biofeedback specialist and researcher of bioenergies. He hypothesizes that there are nine principal levels of processes. They link imagery and physiology in a hierarchical system that ranges from cellular homeostasis to social interaction:

Schwartz proposes that the various levels, from the physical levels of self-regulation, through various psychological levels.

> 9. Social interactions
> 8. Motivation and belief
> 7. Education and insight
> 6. Cognitive-emotional-behavioral-environmental self-control
> 5. Discrimination training
> 4. Motor skills learning
> 3. Operant conditioning
> 2. Classical conditioning
> 1. Homeostatic-cybernetic self-regulation (p. 36)

Through links of imagery connecting various levels of feedback loops, Schwartz suggests that the mind may influence the body's regulating (*homeostatic*) mechanisms at many levels. Therapists may intervene at any of these levels to help their clients alter unhealthy patterns of body, mind, emotion and relational problems.

Schwartz's list is actually simplified. For instance, there are more levels in the physical system. Regulative functions of level (1) include atomic, molecular, cellular, tissue, organ, neurological, hormonal, energy field and organismic levels. His observations are also relevant to visualizations used in therapy. At the opposite end of the spectrum, we may add various dimensions of spirit.[24]

Schwartz further observes that systems tend to assume autonomous purposes and to persist in the course set by their original purpose until new imagery initiates new connections within and between levels – in effect, "replacing the worn or outmoded gears," "resetting the thermostat," or redefining the programming.

More relevant to our discussion of therapies, there is the hierarchy of conventional medicine:

5. Spirit
4. Relationships
3. Mind
2. Emotions
1. Body

Each level has elements that influence the levels above and below it, and each is influenced by those levels in return. Conventional medicine views the body as the base of the pyramid, upon which all the others stand. Emotions, mind and spirit are seen as the products of the brain's electrochemical and hormonal processes.

Wholistic healing may reverse this hierarchy, viewing spirit as the base of the pyramid. Other models may equally apply, as discussed in the next chapter.

SUGGESTION

> *Notoriously, throughout the ages, warts are likely to respond to any method other than the orthodox treatment of the time. Orthodox suggestion with or without hypnosis in the hospital or consulting room is less likely to result in the disappearance of a wart than, for example, the burying of half a potato in the light of a full moon. It may be of significance that many forms of treatment which are successful while the rationale is accepted by the therapist begin to fail when new information casts doubt on this acceptance. The sword of logic pierces the shield of conviction, and treatment technique is no longer successful, one of the main factors in the 'suggestion' situation having been eliminated. Too much, but still not enough, knowledge may thus be a handicap in therapeutics.[25]*
> – Louis Rose

Suggestion is a most effective way of bringing about changes in numerous physical and psychological conditions. Most people will respond favorably to verbal and non-verbal suggestions that their condition will improve – when these are given by a therapist or other authority figure. Pains will decrease, anxieties will melt away, blood pressure will go down, and the potency of other therapies may be markedly enhanced. For instance, post-surgical pain can be reduced by telling people that after surgery they may feel some pain, but the anesthetic will last for a number of hours, and they can then receive pain medicine if they need it. The patients are thus mentally prepared to deal with pain, so they don't get anxious when they experience it. Because they are not nervously anticipating the pain, their stress hormones and muscle tensions will be lower, and they will deal more calmly with the pain when it comes. The experience of the pain will therefore not be as intense or distressing. This can markedly reduce the severity of the pain that they experience and significantly reduce the need for pain medicine.

Suggestions may be given directly, as described above, or they may subtly accompany other therapeutic interventions. A pill handed to you by a nurse with the comment, "Here, this will take your headache away," will have a more potent effect than a pill left at your bedside with the comment, "Take this if you need something for pain."

Suggestions can be profoundly effective when given by a strong authority figure and when applied deliberately, as will be discussed below.

Scope for the skeptics who doubt that spiritual healing is real

Sadly, suggestion is often viewed in Western medicine as a less legitimate intervention or a treatment of lesser value than other forms of therapy, rather than being seen as beneficial in and of itself, or as a form of self-healing that can and should be actively promoted.

For a variety of reasons, our society has come to discount the self-healing aspect of getting well. Doctors emphasize the contributions that they can offer toward healing illnesses, such as prescribing medications and surgical interventions, but they largely ignore the contribution that healees bring to their own healing.

Doctors label self-healing as a *sugar-pill* or *placebo reaction,* with a negative connotation. To a doctor seeking scientific evidence for the efficacy of a new treatment, the placebo effect is a nuisance because it makes it difficult to judge whether patients are responding to the treatment itself or simply to the suggestion that they are receiving something that will help them.

Let me illustrate this with a rather extreme example of components of suggestion in spiritual healing,. The following excerpt is a typical specimen of the skeptic's point of view. With a clearly disparaging attitude, journalist George Bishop describes first-hand encounters with several healers, including Dr. Harold Plume and his mediumistic guide Hoo Fang, and the well-known charismatic healers, *Kathryn Kuhlman, Oral Roberts,* and others.

Bishop draws parallels between patients going to healers and patients being treated with placebos by physicians. He feels that both healers and physicians can alleviate symptoms but that there is an added danger with spiritual healing. The healer does not have the education to know when medical treatment is required, in addition to or in place of suggestion or emotional release. Bishop believes that because healing treatments are not derived from logical, linear reasoning, they are simply not to be trusted. He discounts the value of medical intuition.

Bishop is especially thorough in his portrayal of the intense emotional atmosphere of a revival meeting (often termed *faith healing*, or *spiritual healing* in the US), and in his discussion of how this might contribute to the healings by heightening suggestibility. He himself attended such a gathering with specific instructions from the program director of his radio station to expose the healer's (presumably) fraudulent operation. His personal experience as a skeptic struggling with effects of suggestion illustrates well the challenges generated by unconventional healings. It is often difficult to move beyond the boundaries of the perceived limits of our world!

> ... I stationed myself in the healing line and was soon in the glare of the floodlit stage shuffling toward an evangelist who appeared to be healing all comers.
>
> ... I felt myself caught up in the general excitement. The lights glaring down from the tent poles, the crowd chanting prayers and punctuating them with great shouts of thanks to the Lord when a healing was announced, the organ hitting inspirational chords... I found myself getting anxious to do my part, to do what was expected of me. I craned my neck to one side to see what the procedure was so that, when my turn came, I wouldn't foul the whole thing up... By the time I was two people away from the evangelist I regretted being there most heartily – I was not afraid of what would happen to me as much as I feared disappointing the crowd...

The healer merely gave Bishop a quick blessing and passed him along the line. Bishop was relieved that he had not given a poor performance.

> ... The feeling of participation, even though one... may be, as in the writer's case, specifically opposed to it, is fairly common to anyone not used to the glare of a public spotlight before a large, enthusiastic crowd... This eagerness to go along, tacked onto a basic emotional instability and honed by a team of shrewd, experienced selection assistants, makes for a successful, inspiring healing revival that has the audience reaching appreciatively for purse and wallet.

Bishop's views are typical of people who have only a superficial understanding of healing and related phenomena. Unfortunately, with preconceived biases many valuable observations, especially when they are still in their infancy, may be thrown out along with the bath water of rejected beliefs. We tend to automatically discredit whatever is unfamiliar, if it jars with our conventional belief systems.[26]

The value of suggestion
Spiritual healing can teach us much about the power of suggestion.

> *A healer's greatest magic lies in a patient's willingness to believe. Imagine a miracle and you're half way there.*
> – Dana Scully (Gillian Anderson, *The X-Files*)

Some researchers believe that suggestion and placebo effects are a nuisance, because they interfere with their evaluations of various treatments. This has given suggestion a bad name in the medical community.

Many researchers consider suggestion to be a worthwhile, legitimate and important part of various forms of healing. For example, Jerome Frank (1961), a psychiatrist at Johns Hopkins University, presents a classic discussions on the value of suggestion in many contexts. Though this material was written 25 years ago, much of Frank's wisdom remains valid today.

Frank begins with the complex skein of interactions between people and their environments. He emphasizes that illness, especially when chronic, reduces self-esteem, restricts their interactions with their environment, and eventually can lead to despair. In turn, this can cause family and friends to withdraw, since they feel that the patients' illnesses threaten their own security. The result is a vicious circle of increasing frustration and withdrawal on the part of all participants.

Frank feels that modern medicine focuses mainly on the illness itself and its social ramifications, rather than on the whole patient and the greater context in which he lives. Non-medical healers regard illness "as a disorder of the total person, involving not only his body but his image of himself and his relations to his group; instead of emphasizing conquest of the disease, they focus on stimulating or strengthening the patient's natural healing powers" (p. 47). Frank adds that people's relationship with their world, including their spiritual world, is included in the scope of the healer's ministrations. Illness is viewed as a manifestation of the dysfunction of a person within their total environment. Although purely physical causes are recognized as contributing to disease, the healer does not concentrate on these exclusively. The function of the healer is usually far broader than that of the Western doctor.

The patient's background provides the healer with a wider range of *handles* for intervention than are usually appreciated or employed in Western medicine. Frank points out that patients come to a healer with a set of expectations about how the healer will conduct the treatment. The patient feels that the healer is endowed with either powerful personal abilities or the skill to channel potent forces from higher sources such as spirits, cosmic energies, Christ or God. With this mind-set, the patient is primed to respond to the healer's suggestions.

Healers act in ways that enhance these pre-existing expectations. They will usually first invoke the aid of potent outside sources of healing power – through prayers, channeling of spirit guides or explanations of the cosmic energies that they feel they are transmitting. This also will allow them to disclaim personal responsibility for any potential failures. If the healing either occurs slowly or does not materialize at all, the fault can be attributed to the external agencies, whose ways are inscrutable to human beings. Healers may also refer those patients whom they suspect they cannot help to other practitioners. These attitudes and maneuvers maintain the image of the healer's power and thus preserve a high expectation of success in the patients.

Healers may act to enhance expectations even further. A group of patients whose hopes have been collectively raised through prayers, hymns, sermons or other invocations of higher powers will encourage the individual patient's anticipation of success. Such is the atmosphere of waiting rooms, prayer-halls, and American faith healers' mass rallies. The expectation is further strengthened when patients see the healer appear to, or actually succeed in healing other patients.

Frank also reviews the literature on persuasion from the point of view of experimental psychology. He cites particularly the work of Robert Rosenthal on experimenters in psychological laboratories who give a wide variety of subtle cues to experimental subjects, thereby inducing them to conform to the investigators' expectations. Experimenters may often be unaware that they are subtly guiding their subjects in such ways to respond in particular manners.

The following is a classic example of unwitting effects of suggestion that were caused by experimenters' own expectations.

CASE: An experimenter gave several assistants a series of photographs to show to the experimental subjects, who were asked to rate the photographs according to the degree of success or failure demonstrated in the faces of the people in the photographs. Half of the assistants were told that previous experience had shown that the photos were rated successful, while the other half were advised the opposite – while the photographs were actually selected because they actually were rated independently as being neutral as regards to a successful appearance. The assistants repeatedly obtained results that confirmed their expectations! They were not told that they themselves were the subjects of the investigation and were totally unaware that they had biased the results of the photograph evaluations.

Analysis of tapes of these interviews revealed multiple, subtle verbal cues given by the assistants to the subjects. Many of these cues were transmitted very rapidly, and thus were able to influence the subjects' first response.

This phenomenon of experimenter bias has been labeled the *experimenter effect* or the *Rosenthal effect*. Similar results have been noted in numerous learning experiments. For instance, when laboratory assistants were told that a group of rats were more intelligent than average, they found that those rats performed better on maze tests, and the reverse occurred when they were told that the rats were less intelligent than average. When teachers were told that certain students were bright (though actually they were no brighter than average), these students improved on their intelligence test scores, while others in the same class did not.

Frank also discusses the effects of suggestion in medical settings, where it is usually called the placebo effect. Doctors cue their patients to expect particular results from their treatments. Patients can even be led to expect physiological effects that are opposite to the known pharmacological properties of a drug. For instance, a woman with nausea and vomiting was given ipecac, which causes vomiting, but she was told that this medicine would calm her stomach. In this case, the drug had the suggested effect rather than its known pharmacological result of stimulating vomiting.

> *Our remedies in ourselves do lie,*
> *Which we ascribe to heaven.*
> – William Shakespeare

Frank considers numerous other factors in therapist-patient interactions that lead to psychotherapeutic change, and his book provides an excellent review of suggestion as an essential part of all forms of healing.

Lessons from medical anthropology

Emilio Servadio studied folk healers in the Italian countryside, focusing on unconscious and paranormal factors. He noted that patients' concepts of what disease means may vary enormously according to their cultural background. He found that "There is a whole range of pathological or psychopathological phenomena that are evidently, though quite unconsciously, lived from inside as an 'ill' more in a moral than in a universal medical sense."

Ills such as these may be blamed on numerous factors, including the *evil eye*, witchcraft, evil spirits, or punishments for evil thoughts or forbidden deeds. Within these cultural beliefs, patients may appropriately anticipate that the required healing will come from a magician or healer with magical powers, rather than from a modern doctor. The magician interacts with the patient in a manner that is consonant with the patient's beliefs and expectations, and in this way provides a form of basic psychotherapy that is culture-specific. The magician addresses factors that are of vital importance to the patient under the patient's own belief system. Such factors would not even be considered by the modern doctor. Therefore, in these cases the doctor often has less success than the magician or healer.

A large number of studies have been published on culture-specific illnesses and their treatments. It is extremely rare, however, for any of these studies to seriously addresses the spiritual healing aspect of medical anthropology. Even among experts in the area of healing practices in other cultures, many are unaware of the spiritual healing components in shamanistic healings. Western scientists tend to carry the beliefs of their own cultures into their studies, explaining away effects of spiritual healing because (within the scientists' belief systems) these simply do not and cannot exist.

Placebo effects

Placebo effects are responses by patients to inactive medication or treatment, and they clearly represent reactions to suggestion. Approximately one-third of all patients with almost any ailment who receive any form of treatment will report some improvement. This is true even if the treatment is only a chemically inactive sugar pill. The placebo effect, sometimes termed the *sugar-pill reaction*, has been thoroughly researched and has obvious relevance to healing research.

> *Belief is a potent medicine.*
> – Steven E. Locke and Douglas Colligan

The term *placebo* derives from the Latin, "I shall please" and "placate."

Placebo effects were recognized as early as the Sixteenth Century. In 1572, Michel de Montaigne observed that "There are men on whom the mere sight of medicine is operative." He gave the following example:

> [There was] a man who was sickly and subject to [kidney] stone, who often resorted to enemas, which he had made up for him by physicians, and none of the usual formalities was omitted... Imagine him then, lying on his stomach, with all the motions gone through except that no application has been made [no active ingredient was used]! This ceremonial over, the apothecary would retire, and the patient would be treated just as if he had taken the enema; the effect was the same as if he actually had... When, to

save the expense, the patient's wife tried sometimes to make do with warm water, the result betrayed the fraud; this method was found useless and they had to return to the first. (Cogprints)

There are many variations on the theme of placebo reactions.

- People may have a stronger reaction to an experimental drug when they know that the comparison drug they may be given is also an active medication, rather than an inert substance.

- Experimental subjects have a stronger response to either placebos or aspirins when these are identified by a well-known brand name than when they are given blank tablets.

- When subjects were given either chloral hydrate (a strong sedative) or amphetamine (a stimulant) without receiving any clues as to which they were getting, they were unable to tell the differences between the effects of the two medications.

The placebo reaction is not restricted to medicinal therapies, and may occur with any form of treatment. This forces ethical therapists to examine which of their ministrations, or what proportion of them, may stimulate placebo reactions. The subtlety and pervasiveness of such problems in evaluating medical treatments is demonstrated by Beecher's research on a type of cardiac surgery called *internal mammary artery ligation.*

The procedure consisted of tying off certain inessential arteries that appeared to divert blood unnecessarily away from the heart. Patients with angina (heart pains experienced upon exertion) who underwent this surgery reported definite improvement as a result of this surgical intervention. Measurable positive changes were even noted on their electrocardiograms (EKGs) and on tests of ability to cope with physical exertion. The ligation involved major surgery, with all the attendant risks of hospitalization, exposure to anesthesia and invasion of the body. However, the benefits appeared to outweigh the risks and costs.

Beecher conducted a study in which patients in one group were told they would receive internal mammary ligation surgery, but in fact were given only a superficial surgical skin wound, while another group actually underwent the full surgical procedure. The findings of the study showed that those who had the sham surgery improved just as much as those who had the actual procedure. This was true even in regard to the objective measures by cardiograms and tests of physical stress.

> *Our body is a machine for living. It is organized for that. It is its nature.*
> *Let life go on in it unhindered and let it defend itself, it will do more than if*
> *you paralyze it by encumbering it with remedies.*
> – Leo Tolstoy

Modern medicine has generally viewed suggestion and placebo effects with disdain and disparagement, complaining that susceptible patients waste doctors' valuable time with imagined problems that clear up without real treatment. What these doctors are actually saying is that people don't always bring them the medical problems which they were trained to treat. Many complementary therapists and spiritual healers know the wisdom of providing emotional support and appropriate healing suggestions, so that people can gather the energies they need to heal themselves.

Figure II-3.

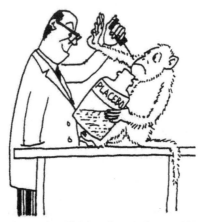

Cartoon by Bill Sykes, from *Caduceus,* 1988,
Issue No. 3, with permission of the publishers

Placebo reactions are forms of self-healing. Though neglected and even denigrated by our mechanistic Western society, they are well recognized and widely used by shamans and other effective healers to help people deal with their diseases and dis-eases.

The mechanisms by which placebos work are complex and still a matter of considerable speculation. The unconscious mind is prone to being imprinted with messages given by authority figures, as well as by a person himself. Emphatic or authoritative statements or even simple repetitions of words may impact people deeply, programming their unconscious mind to respond to particular stimuli. Expectations of therapists and careseekers may predispose to placebo reactions.

There is ample evidence that we ourselves program our own bodies to develop symptoms and illnesses through negative suggestions. Metaphors relating to body parts and functions abound. See Table II-2 for a sampling of these. If a person repeatedly says, "What a pain in the neck this is!" or "My blood pressure is rising!" it is not a surprise that their body may develop neck pain or hypertension. While this is not a researched observation, I have seen this occur many times in my practice of psychotherapy.

Negative placebo effects (*nocebo effects*) may also occur in clinical practice. A common way for grim negative suggestions to be implanted is when a doctor tells patients they have only so many months to live. In effect, this is as bad as placing a curse on a person, whose unconscious mind may respond literally, conforming to the expectations of this authority figure by bringing an end to life at the predicted time.

Table II-2. Body terms and metaphors

BODY: disembodied; em--

HEAD: ache, big, brainy; bursting, cool, dense; fat; foggy; fuzzy; good; have -- examined; like a hole in the --; hot; -- in a good space; into your --; light; migraine; numbskull; pig; poor -- for; reaching a --; shit--; splitting; stuffed; swelled/ swollen; thick (head; skull)

MIND: blew; brainless; closed; deep; dreaming; drifting; --ful; fuzzy; --less; losing one's-; muzzy; nervous (wreck); of two --; open; out of one's --; shallow; sleeping on decision; sticks in my --; thinker; thinking straight; thoughtful; thoughtless

NERVES: found; high strung; lost; nerveless; -- of steel; nervous; nervy; rattled; raw; shaken; shattered; shot; some --; taut; tense; up tight; unnerving; wound up; wracked

EYES: black; blank; bleary; blinded; bright; burning with desire; clouded; cried my -- out; crinkled; cross-eyed (with tiredness or overwork); don't want to see; empty; clear; cross-eyed; scathing glance (look); keen; nobody home; red-eyed; sad; can't see straight; sharp; shot lightning from --; shut--; sight for sore --; tearful; tearjerker; twinkling; weeping -- out

NOSE: bent out of shape; big; blocked; bloody; brown --; cut off to spite face; gets up my -; nosy; Pinocchio; sniffs out; snooty; snotty; sticking -- into someone's business

EARS: cloth; deaf; don't want to hear that; --ful; keen; musical; sensitive; sharp

MOUTH: big; bigger than stomach; bite (has a -- to it; lip; -- off more than can chew; tongue); biting remark; chew (lip; on; up); fat lip; foot in --; chew on that; get chops around a situation; keep your -- shut; lip(s) (giving a bunch of --); loose tongue; sharp tongue; well, shut my --; shut up; slip of the tongue; smile; sour taste; speak (clearly; up); speechless; spit it out; stiff upper lip; tastes (bad, bitter, good, sharp, sour, sweet); teeth on edge; tight lipped; tongue in cheek; tongue tied; toothless; voice (cool; crooning; grating; piercing; warm)

NECK: full up to my --; pain in the --; sticking -- out; stiff

THROAT: can't swallow down; choking on--; choked up; cough up; craw full; full up to--; sticks in my --; (can't; hard to) swallow that; swallow down (feelings; insults; pride; sorrow)

CHEST: get it off --; puffed out

BREASTS: generous; giving; milk of human kindness; nurturing; weaning

LUNGS: breathe easy; blow (cool; gasket; hot and cold; it; off steam; stack; temper); blown away; can't breathe; catch one's breath; cough up; froze; holding one's breath; puffing; take a breather; take a deep breath; wheezing along

HEART: ache; attack; big; bleeding; blood boiling; blood pressure up; break; cold; cross your -- and hope to die; cruel; eating my -- out; empty; -- felt; frozen; full; --less; good; lonely; open; palpitated; pierced; pressured; --rending; sticks in my --; shaken to the core of my --; shut down; skipped a beat; sticks in my --; stopped; swelled; warm; warmed; weighing on --; -- went out to

BLOOD: bad; bloody; -- brother/ sister; cold --; -- froze; hot --; in my --; thin --; warm --

STOMACH: bellyaching; belly full; belly laugh; burns; can't --; digest; eaten up with (anger; jealousy); eating (away at; heart out; words); full (of it; up to); gut feeling; hungry for... ; indigestion; in knots; lies heavy in gut; like a rock; rumbling; sick to --; sensitive; soured; spill guts; hard to stomach; stuffed; swollen; tears one's guts apart; want to (could) vomit

SPLEEN: --ful; splenetic; venting --

LIVER: bilious; jaundiced; liverish

KIDNEYS/ BLADDER: holding back; big/ little pisher/ pisser; pissed drunk; pissed/ peed off; wet knickers/ pants;

WOMB/ OVARIES: birthing (idea; project); broody; good flow; knocked up; menstrual (pre-, post); pregnant (expectation, pause)

PENIS/ TESTES: balls (has, no); balled/ balls-up; big balls; cock- (around; half; up); dick (around; face: head); jerk-off; prick; schmuck; wanker

VAGINA: cunt; loose; pussy, putz
SEX: coming on; fuck (--er; --ed up; off); loose; orgasmic; oversexed; pimp; sexy; sleazy; sowing (and reaping) wild oats; turned on; undersexed; whore
ANUS/ BUTTOCKS: ass; asshole; bum; butt (in, out); constipated; fart; fat; holding (back; in, tight); pain in--; shit (head, hot, face; in pants); soft as a baby's bottom; tight ass
BACK: -- against the wall; --breaking; --up; backed into it; bent (over backwards, all out of shape); get one's -- up; --off; pat on --; pain in --; sit up and pay attention; stiff
ARMS/ HANDS: black/ brown thumb; cold hands/ warm heart; pain in the elbow; even handed; fighting tooth and nail; fumbling; giving the finger; green thumb; ham fisted; heavy handed; lend/ lift a hand; light fingered; limp wrist; nimble fingers; raise a fist/ hand; rule of thumb; sharp elbows; sticky fingers; stiff arm; strong arm; all thumbs; thumbs up; tight fisted; two left hands
LEGS/ FEET: Achilles' heel; best foot forward; cold feet; dipping a toe in the water; down at the heels; earthed; flat footed; footing bills; foot in (grave, it; mouth); foot loose; grounded; kicking (the bucket; habit; myself; up a fuss); knees (turned to jelly; weak); on the ground; shot self in foot; stand (can't--; last--; make a--; -- firm; --tall); stepping out; sticking a foot out; stood up; stumblefoot; stand (alone; firm; proud; take a --; tall; together; --up; --up and be counted); two left feet; walking a (narrow; straight) line; well heeled
MUSCLES: aching; bearing up; can't bear; burdened; carrying a burden/ load/ weight; flexible; frozen; hang loose; overburdened; pull self together; rigid (with fear); rooted to the spot; (having) shakes; stiff; in stitches; up tight; (sick and) tired; weighed down; wobblies; wound up
SPINE/ SKELETON: being straight; burdened; can't bear it; carrying (a load; too much); chill went up my --; crooked; feel it in my bones; rigid; pointing the bone; shivers up --; shoulder up; spine chilling; --less; can't stand --; stand tall; stand up and be counted; stooped over; stooping to; stretched (too far; to breaking point); all twisted up; unsupported
SKIN: allergic to... ; blanched; blushed; breaking out; burning up; made my -- creep; flaky; flushed; itching to; pale; picking (at; on); pimply; red faced; thick; thin; ticklish; tore my -- out
HAIR: bad hair day; bristled; hackles rose; hair turned grey; pulling my hair out; stood on end
TOUCH: aching to--; easy touch; smooth touch; tickled; touched; touching; touchy; untouchable
FEEL: bad; calm; emotional (overcome); feelings (bury, frenzied, good, hide, hurts to... ; uplifting), smooth; like square peg in round hole; tied up;
BALANCE: balanced; on an even keel; flipped out; im--; lost --; pushover; set me back; un--; upset
DEATH: cry oneself to --; dead (end; heat; on my feet; on target; roll over and play); --of me; (nearly) died of (embarrassment; fright; shame); doing me in; dying to; end of me; ending up; finished me off; killing me; nearly died; scared to --; sick to --; slays me; wish I was dead

In traditional cultures, shamans may deliberately curse or put a hex on a person, causing illness and even death. While this may appear medically unethical, one must realize that the shaman in many cultures serves the multiple functions of doctor, counselor, arbitrator of interpersonal and inter-tribal conflicts, and mediator between man and nature and between man and the spirit worlds. In these cultures, there are no police, no courts, and no jails. The shaman therefore uses nocebo hexes to enforce social justice – placing a curse on a person who is accused of a transgression and removing it when restitution has been made.

It is not surprising to learn that in different cultures there may be different distributions of common psychosomatic problems. For instance, placebos have been enormously helpful to German people suffering from stomach ulcers (60 percent rates of healing), while far fewer respond in Brazil (7 percent). On the other hand, placebos administered in the treatment of hypertension are relatively ineffective in Germany, compared to responses in other countries. While this has yet to be confirmed in research, I would speculate that some of these differences relate to body metaphors that may be more common in one language than another, leading to more nocebo effects for those particular organs in one culture than in another.

What is clear is that placebos can be potent activators for self-healing. Research is now confirming that placebo reactions produce changes in the brains of people who are suffering from depression or anticipating they will receive nicotine, and one would expect similar findings with other placebo responses.

Suggestion, placebo effects and the need for formal research in healing

Most skeptics, like George Bishop, regard spiritual healing as nothing more than a placebo. They tend to take an element of the whole to be the whole. The metaphor I use to describe this is a set of weighing balances, like the ones used for fruit in country markets. Suppose we put a ten-pound weight of stress in one pan, and in the other we put all of the efforts and therapies used to combat the stress, adding measures of relaxation, proper diet, hope, will, love and spiritual healing to cope with the burden. Finally, when we add suggestion to the pan, the balance tips, and healing occurs. A casual observer might thus assume that suggestion is the one factor that tipped the balance. But we should also be aware of the hope, will, love, healing, and other measures that have likewise contributed to the healing. (See Figure II-4.)

Figure II-4. A variety of factors counter stress

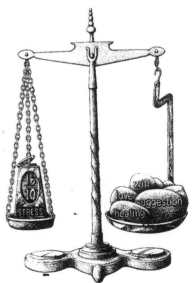

In spiritual healing, it is even more confusing and difficult to discern the causal factors. As yet we have no reliable measures to tell us whether various healers' contributions have the effect of adding a grape, a watermelon, or nothing at all to the balance of health and illness. The skeptics may in fact be entirely right in the case of some healers. I have observed some whose efforts seem to involve little more than a good bedside manner. But I have met other healers who have brought about striking improvements in severe medical problems, when medicine had nothing more to offer.

The difficulty is that in any particular case it may be impossible to identify which problems are responding to placebo effects and which, if any, are responding to something else. It is for this reason that careful, controlled studies of healing (and all other forms of treatment) are advisable.

Acceptance
Acceptance is one contributor to healing that is vastly under-rated clinically, and sorely neglected in research. Randall Mason et al. noted that the rates of recovery for patients undergoing retinal detachment surgery varied widely. They studied psychological elements in the speed of wound-healing following this surgery, identifying a critical factor that they called *acceptance*. This is the ability to take in stride the stress of having to undergo surgery. Patients with a high degree of acceptance appreciate the difficulties involved in their illness, but do not overreact or excessively fear the effects of surgery on their future. Although they may fear the procedures involved and may feel pain, they are able to remember that their discomforts will be temporary. A high degree of optimism is maintained, even if these patients are warned that possible negative effects such as blindness may result from the surgery. By contrast, patients with low acceptance seem to lose perspective. They become overly concerned about the possible negative results of surgery, to the point that this may become emotionally overwhelming. (See Table II-3.)

> *Acceptance of reality is the beginning of taking responsibility for your life. Often you can control events, but just as often you must adapt to circumstances beyond your control. How you adapt – the thoughts you think, the words you speak, and the attitude you take – determines your state of health and your chance for recovery...*
> – Barbara Hoberman Levine (p. 40)

In this study, the authors found that the rate of physical healing correlated very significantly with the presence of high (versus low) acceptance. When the study was repeated by the same authors, their initial findings were confirmed. This factor has not been studied by others, but it seems likely that this contributes to the variability of responses to healing and other therapies. It may also be related to meta-anxiety, discussed later.

> *The Lord gave, and the Lord took away.*
> *Blessed be the name of the Lord.*
> – Job

The will to live

A last aspect in this discussion of our control over our lives through suggestion is our expectation of how long we will live.

Curt Richter of Johns Hopkins University experimented on this important factor in healing – the will to live (Watson 1975). He arranged for rats to swim in a container of water that was roiled constantly so that the rats could not rest. He kept them in the water until they died of exhaustion. In this experiment, Richter found that wild rats died more quickly than domesticated ones. However, if the wild rats were removed from the water just prior to death, they quickly recovered. When subsequently returned to the tank, they continued swimming much longer than previously. The experience of being removed once from the tank had apparently given them hope. Thereafter they were willing to exert themselves for much longer periods than they had been before, prior to the hope-instilling experience.[27]

Lyall Watson, commenting on Richter's experiment, speculates that the rats' initial behavior may be similar to that of humans who have been *hexed* or cursed with a death-sentence. Such people can become ill, though they suffer from no recognizable medical problems. They may languish and die within a few weeks or days, despite all medical efforts to help them. Watson surmises that they die from loss of hope.

The potentially fatal nature of the feeling of hopelessness was demonstrated in German concentration camps in the *musselman phenomenon*. Some prisoners survived for months under grueling conditions, but then gave up the struggle to live, perhaps because of despair that they would ever be free. They simply gave up and died, even though no additional stress was applied. No physical explanations for their deaths were apparent. They appeared to have lost the will to live.

Others have shown the opposite: the ability put off death. It is not rare to find people with terminal illnesses lingering past the medically predicted date of their death – when they have a specific reason to stay alive. They may wait for the arrival of a relative from afar, for the celebration of a date of particular importance (such as a family birthday, graduation or holiday).

Conversely, there are those who are ready to let go of their anchors to physical life but linger and linger – until a member of the family or significant other comes to a point where they can let go of the relationship. The decision to let go may occur without any direct communication between the relative who is holding on and the person who is waiting to die. The release to break the link to life appears to be communicated telepathically or in some other, spiritual dimension.

Suggestion, in summary

A major portion of the change that transpires following any treatment may be the product of suggestion or placebo effects. This is commonly taken to indicate that the complaints of patients who improve due to suggestion are imaginary or caused by emotional or physical tensions, and are therefore susceptible to self-healing by suggestion that helps them to relax emotionally and physically. In fact, the opposite appears more likely: suggestion can alter many body processes, for illness or health.

Spiritual healing, combined with an element of suggestion, may inject a will to live and to fight for health, and/or may encourage an attitude of acceptance. Few

Table II-3. Acceptance scales

REACTION SCALES	Accepts totally	Accepts cautiously	Accepts with reservations	Accepts w/ resignation	Rejects
1. Reaction to Detachment	Confronts directly	Shaken but goes on	Advances fearfully	Bogged down	Trapped, back-to-wall
2. Reaction to Surgeon	Trusts	Praises hopefully	Seeks reassurance	Submits	Suspects
3. Reaction to Surgery	Optimistic about results	Hopefully certain about success	Vacillates in expectation	Unwilling to hope	Pessimistic
4. Reaction to Chaplain	Companionship in interpreting life	Seeks agreement for positive philosophy	Seeks consolation avoids discussion of inner conflict	Seeks respect for virtue and wisdom of compliance	Perceives as alien force or expects him to mourn
5. Reaction to Others	Meets on equal terms	Acts as host	Is not sure how to react	Expects sympathy and concern	Gives sense that no response to him is adequate

	Confident he can cope	Hopefully he can cope	Ambivalent about coping ability	Doubtful he can cope	Convinced he cannot cope
6. Coping Ability	Confident he can cope	Hopefully he can cope	Ambivalent about coping ability	Doubtful he can cope	Convinced he cannot cope
7. Self Care Ability	Able to do things for self and be helpful	Tries to do things for self and cooperate	Torn between desire to do and inability to do	Helpless and makes obvious displays of it	Acts as if entitled to services
8. Self-Image	Accepts self and situation (without special concern)	Displays positive image (embarrassed by dependence)	Keeps things in check (ambivalent about dependence)	Self-pitying (recognizes dependence with pity)	Sulking or detachment (angry over dependence)
9. Conversation	Willing to converse in depth	Pursues pleasant conversation	Caught between response and preoccupation	Talks mostly about affliction of self	Avoids open contacts with others
10. Philosophy of evil	Accepts bad with good	Wonders how the bad fits	Seeks assurance 'this is not all bad'	What can you 'do'? (It's Gods will)	'It's a dirty trick'

* From Mason, et al.

healers have considered these factors. Any of the organ systems that respond to suggestion could conceivably be responding to healers' interventions through the healers' suggestions, rather than through spiritual healing. The same is true for every other CAM intervention.

Alternatively, it is possible that some healers have a psychic gift of eliciting or stimulating self-healing, which is similar to the processes elucidated in studies of suggestion, but more powerful than suggestion alone (perhaps operating through telepathy, as reported by C. M. Barrows – in the section on hypnotic suggestion below). Well-structured, research could probably tease out the more likely among these alternatives. With this hypothesis I do not mean to indicate that all placebo reactions are examples of spiritual healing. Clearly, many placebo effects are caused by socially induced suggestion, relaxation or other self-healing processes that are familiar to Western medicine.

Let us now continue our exploration of the mechanisms of suggestion in greater depth.

HYPNOSIS

From a psychobiological perspective... so-called resistance is a problem in accessing state bound information and transducing it into a form in which it can be utilized for problem-solving.
— Ernest Rossi (1986, p. 87)

Historical Notes

In the mid-nineteenth century, Franz Anton Mesmer popularized a treatment he called *animal magnetism,* which was the forerunner of hypnosis. In his induction technique he performed what he called *magnetic passes* around the body of the subject. Initially he did this with iron magnets but later he used only his hands. Part of the process appears to have involved elements common to laying-on of hands healing. Today, hypnosis is a widely practiced form of psychotherapy, practiced without passes of the hypnotists' hands around the body.

Hypnosis is a special, extremely powerful method of harnessing the power of suggestion. In some instances it seems to involve direct activation of unconscious portions of the mind.

Profound awareness of an amazing spectrum of bodily functions and alterations in these functions may be brought about through hypnosis. Pains resulting from many different causes can be markedly reduced or eliminated using this technique. This discovery has led to a better understanding of pain, by demonstrating that it is more than a series of messages transmitted from a part of the body that is experiencing stress or damage. The subjective experience of pain is much more complex than the stimulation of nerve endings that transmit impulses to the brain, which in turn interprets them as physical pain.

Under hypnosis, people may be told that they have no pain, and their pain can simply stop. This may be pain from an injury to the skin such as a burn, from a deeper injury like surgery, from cancer or from other causes. In some cases, people will report that their pain has completely disappeared. At other times they report that it is still there, but they don't have to attend to it or worry about it, and it no longer bothers them. People under hypnosis can also be induced to alter their memory of chronic *intermittent* pain, so that they are not left with the hopeless feeling that they have nothing to anticipate but more pain throughout the rest of their lives. This is a true blessing, because the anticipation of more pain may produce as much misery as the experience of pain itself.

From the mid-nineteenth century, hypnotic suggestion has even enabled surgeons to operate without anesthesia. The effectiveness of hypnotic anesthesia for major surgical procedures has been confirmed in the scientific literature in recent decades, in cases of hemorrhoid and cardiac surgery, vein stripping, and caesarian section.

When patients' limbs are placed in plaster casts and their joints are immobilized for several weeks, the joints typically "freeze" and are very stiff and painful upon removal of the casts. If the limbs are immobilized under hypnosis, even for weeks at a time, they may not freeze up or hurt when movement is resumed.

The skin is especially responsive to hypnotic suggestion. If a deeply hypnotized subject is told that she is being touched with a hot iron, she may develop redness and even blistering on her skin – although in actuality she has only been prodded by the finger of the hypnotist. Herpetic blisters (shingles) may also be brought out under hypnosis. Several cases of *fish-skin disease*,[28] which is normally unresponsive to medical treatment, showed dramatic improvement under hypnosis. Burns heal more rapidly with hypnosis, and warts may be eliminated, even under a very light trance. The hypnotist simply suggests that after several days (commonly two weeks) the warts will fall off – and in a high percentage of cases they actually do. It should be noted that numerous forms of suggestion other than hypnosis may be just as effective in removing warts (e.g. painting the wart with food coloring). A recent variation on this theme is to cover them with duct tape for two weeks. They will often come off when the tape is removed.

Hypertension (high blood pressure) responds well to hypnosis, as does asthma. Bone fractures can also heal more quickly under hypnotic suggestion. In isolated cases, it has even been shown that traumatic bleeding may be halted through hypnosis. Patients who are prepared for surgery with hypnotic suggestions bleed very little during their operations.

Another form of bleeding that hypnosis has been helpful in controlling is hemophilia. Persons suffering from this condition lack particular biochemical clotting factors, due to genetic defects. This causes them to bleed profusely from even the slightest cut, often for days. They may even die from a minor cut if they are not treated. Yet with hypnosis hemophiliacs can undergo dental extractions, a procedure that normally could be fatal to them. In one investigation, the need for blood transfusions in a group of child hemophiliacs was decreased by a factor of 10 over the period of a year, through the application of self-hypnosis.

Hormonal changes can also be induced under hypnosis. Favorable responses have been recorded with diabetes, menstrual problems, and breast development.

There are four styles of hypnotic induction that are commonly employed. The first utilizes monotonous, rhythmic stimulation such as focusing on a swinging pendulum or other object, while the hypnotist suggests that the subject will relinquish control over their own behavior to the hypnotist. The second method solicits the active cooperation of the subject, and uses more direct suggestions without elaborate inductions. The third is a more coercive technique, in which hypnotists forcefully assert their authority, and subjects instantly relinquish their will to the hypnotist. And last, there is self-hypnosis, in which subjects give themselves instructions to enter a hypnotic state.

Most people are able to enter some levels of the hypnotic state, ranging from slight relaxation to very deep trance. Estimates vary, but a commonly accepted standard for conventional approaches is that one in five can enter a clinically useful trance state for deep work, while two out of three can do light suggestive work under hypnosis. Practitioners of NLP estimate that the percentages are actually much higher. Herbert Spiegel and David Spiegel developed a screening test for hypnotic susceptibility. They instruct the prospective subject to roll their eyes upward as far as they can. The less the iris is visible below the margin of the upper eyelid, the greater the susceptibility to hypnotic induction. Close to three-quarters of those who are rated susceptible using this test are able to enter a clinically productive trance state.

In deeper hypnotic states, a person's unconscious mind appears to be open to interventions by the hypnotist. Vast stores of memory that are normally inaccessible to the subject's conscious mind may thus be explored. For example, hypnotic subjects may connect with long-forgotten memories from very early childhood. This is called *hypnotic regression.* Some even claim to recall memories from their own birth, and from within their mother's womb.

Taking this a big step further, there are practitioners who report successes in resolving clients' current-life problems by accessing memories of past-life traumas that have persisted into the present, and are causing current difficulties.[29]

When subjects relinquish control of their conscious mind, the hypnotist is able to suggest alternative behaviors that the subjects' unconscious mind may accept. To some extent, the hypnotist is able to reprogram perceptions and conceptualizations held by the subject.

Some hypnotherapists suggest that people experiencing severe trauma may commonly enter a state that is equivalent to a trance. This makes them particularly open to helpful suggestions from those who are caring for them – for example, to minimize their acute suffering from pain.

With deeper trance, the subject may also have amnesia for what occurs under hypnosis.

Hallucinations suggested by the hypnotist may be fully experienced by subjects in all sensory modalities as though they are real experiences. For example, if a person in hypnotic trance is told that there is a cute animal or a dangerous one present in the room, they will behave exactly as if they can perceive that animal in the room. Conversely, sensory blocks may also be inserted under hypnosis. Subjects may report negative hallucinations, meaning that they are unable see something that is actually present, because the hypnotist has told them that it is not there. When commanded by the hypnotist, subjects may develop amnesia for particular events or thoughts.

The response of the unconscious mind under hypnosis is extremely concrete and literal, so hypnotherapists learn to state suggestions very precisely and sequence them with care. An apocryphal story tells of a hypnotherapist who lost contact with his subject when he gave the instruction: "You will hear nothing but the sound of my voice." The subject stopped responding entirely, and it was only hours later that she wakened on her own. She had apparently taken the first four words of his instruction literally, and had simply tuned out all sounds, so that she could not accept any further suggestions.

Lessons from hypnosis have been helpful in other areas of therapy. The unconscious mind can respond quite literally to suggestions that are given without hypnosis, in a concrete manner which is similar to that observed under hypnosis. Psychotherapists often find that their patients have absorbed parental injunctions or scoldings during their childhood, which have remained imprinted in their unconscious minds. Words said forcefully in anger, such as "You stupid fool!" or "You clumsy oaf!" can have devastating consequences for the rest of a person's life, if the unconscious mind is deeply imprinted with that negative self-image.

Subjects may also be induced to do strange and ludicrous things by stage hypnotists for the amusement of an audience. For example, when told that they are chickens, they may cluck, flap their arms, and make other bird-like motions. Such casual and frivolous use of hypnosis is deplorable, and sometimes dangerous. People may accept hypnotic suggestions in such a setting that can open up serious conflicts that were previously repressed. In one such case, the subject did not come out of a stage trance for several days.

Usually, subjects will not cooperate with suggestions that go against their moral or ethical beliefs. If told to do something that would compromise their normal standards, subjects are likely to simply refuse, or even to waken from the trance. However, a crafty hypnotist may trick subjects into believing that they are acting under circumstances which accord with their morals, when in fact they do not.

Explaining hypnosis
Despite centuries of study, experts do not agree on what actually occurs during hypnosis, much less on the mechanisms that could explain it.

Leslie LeCron, an expert hypnotist, suggests that the trance state achieved by mesmerists of the last century may have been different from the hypnotic states commonly invoked today. For one thing, the early mesmerists' inductions lasted four or five hours. The passes of hands around the body performed during these inductions may also have produced effects not often observed today, and this may account for some variations between early and modern reports. For example, the mesmerists refer to a very deep stage of hypnosis called *plenary trance*, which was achieved through inductions that lasted several hours, and which is rarely seen today. In this state, physiological processes such as heartbeat and breathing were markedly reduced. Subjects were reportedly able to remain in plenary trance for up to two weeks, not requiring food or drink. These deep trances may also account for some of the early reports of successful induction of psi abilities under hypnosis.

Theodore X. Barber, who researched hypnotic phenomena for many years, found that many of the results achieved with hypnosis can be equaled by subjects who apply their own willpower, enhanced with suggestion, to physical tasks – *without hypnotic induction*. Barber maintains that what is commonly assumed to be a special mental state that is induced under hypnosis does not actually represent an altered state of consciousness or trance. Critics of his views propose that all subjects who follow suggestions are, in effect, in a state of hypnosis. Barber counters with the criticism that studies of hypnotic phenomena rarely include a control group that is given suggestion without hypnotic induction. When Barber studied both modalities, he actually found that suggestion without induction was superior in producing many effects.

Sheryl Wilson and Theodore Barber identify a personality type that they find in about four percent of the population. This is an individual who has the ability to visualize mental images extremely vividly, is able to enter trance states quite easily, and is prone to experiencing psi phenomena. (Psi abilities were found in 92 percent of the specially gifted individuals studied). The authors suggest that psi does not correlate with hypnosis per se, but rather with people who have this special personality type, who are excellent candidates for hypnosis.

At the turn of the century, C. M. Barrows reported numerous cases in which he telepathically suggested away the pains of toothaches, facial spasms and other disorders. He was able to achieve these results even when his subjects were unaware that he was attempting telepathic hypnotic anesthesia. He carefully experimented with the states of mind that he experienced during the treatments, and found that focusing on the desired condition in the patient was successful, but that intentionally attempting to transmit the instructions was not.

In the mid-nineteenth century, a number of scientists explored the use of remote hypnotic inductions in treating selected subjects. Under carefully controlled conditions, they were repeatedly able to induce trance from a distance, and in some cases even to transmit orders that were executed by the subjects.

Leonid Vasiliev, a (then) Soviet researcher, also found that he could induce hypnotic trances telepathically with selected subjects, and he was able to demonstrate this repeatedly in controlled laboratory conditions. Under hypnosis, some of his subjects' muscles could be made to contract when the hypnotist pointed his finger at the muscle or at its nerves. Under hypnosis, some of Vasiliev's subjects could also locate the position of the hypnotist's hand when their eyes were closed and the hypnotist's hand was not touching their body.

Vladimir L. Raikov another (then) Soviet researcher, claimed that he could suggest to hypnotized subjects that they were reincarnated artists, thereby enhancing their artistic talents. This technique was effective only in subjects who were able to achieve deep trance states

Another case of possible relevance to the subject of hypnosis is the legendary Indian rope trick, performed by fakirs in the East. Typically a performer throws a rope into the air, where it hangs apparently suspended without visible support. The fakir then sends his assistant (usually a young boy) up the rope, and the boy disappears at the top. When the fakir orders him down, there is no response. The fakir, seemingly enraged, grabs a sword and climbs the rope, also disappearing at its nether end. Sounds of a struggle are heard, and the dismembered body of the boy comes tumbling piecemeal down to the ground. The fakir then climbs down the rope with his bloody sword, and covers the bodily remains of the boy with a cloth. A moment later he removes the cloth and the boy rises, unharmed.

A lawyer named Mordecai Merker presents a case for *mass telepathic hypnosis* as an explanation of the Indian rope trick. His evidence, which he feels would stand up in any court, consists of eyewitness accounts from a variety of apparently reliable people who claim that they have photographed performances of the rope trick, but found that the photographs did not correspond with their recollections of the events. The pictures showed the fakir and his assistant throwing the rope up into the air, but the rope merely fell to the ground and the fakir and his helper simply stood motionless for the duration of the performance.

On the basis of the evidence, my impression is that mass hypnosis seems a possible explanation for the Indian rope trick.

Skeptics propose that some cases of apparent healings, especially *psychic surgery,* could likewise be the result of mass hypnosis. In psychic surgery, developed separately in the Philippines and South America, healers perform surgical operations without anesthesia or sterile technique. Healees experience no pain, no bleeding and no infections. Their wounds heal very rapidly, sometimes instantly. Some psychic surgeons use knives, others insert their bare hands into the body. Here, the mass of evidence reviewed in *Healing Research, Volume III* appears to contradict the hypnosis hypothesis and support the legitimacy of the psychic surgery.[30]

Possible mechanisms for physical effects experienced under hypnosis

One hypothesis commonly adduced to explain many of the above-mentioned physical phenomena is that people have a natural ability to control the muscles surrounding their blood vessels. This is normally a function of the autonomic nervous system, and as such it usually is not under conscious control. However, biofeedback clearly demonstrates that it is possible to bring such processes under intentional control.

For instance, reddening of the skin under hypnosis is caused by dilation of blood vessels, and sophisticated laboratory instruments have been used to confirm capillary dilation and accelerated capillary blood flow in the skin under hypnotic suggestion. Bleeding can be halted by the reverse process, i.e. by a constriction of blood vessels. It has been suggested that warts may disappear because they are deprived of nutrition due to constriction of blood vessels, which can lead to their "starvation" so that they dry out and drop off. It is hypothesized that cancers might similarly be deprived of sustenance by restriction of blood flow. Blistering under hypnosis is harder to explain. By extending known mechanisms, one could imagine blood vessels dilating sufficiently to allow exudation of serum into the tissues.

In the treatment of asthma, the primary effect of hypnosis is probably a relaxation of muscle spasm in the bronchioles (tubes leading to the lungs). There may also be allergen-specific antibodies or other blood components that respond to hypnosis, through mind-body connections discussed elsewhere in this chapter.

Many hypnotic effects may derive in part from psychological relaxation, for example in cases of hypertension, asthma, irritable bowel syndrome, hormonal disorders and other conditions. Emotional relaxation could interrupt the vicious circle of stress → anxiety → tension → physical symptoms → more anxiety → more tension → etc.

No one has yet proposed adequate hypotheses to explain cases in which ichthyosis and hemophilia improve under hypnosis. Though we cannot as yet completely explain these cases and others, it is evident from studies of hypnosis that a vast potential resides within each of us for self-healing, which can be released through the power of suggestion.

Hypnosis and psychotherapy

Hypnosis has been used extensively in psychotherapy (hypnotherapy) to explore the unconscious foundations of patients' symptoms and conflicts. With hypnotic treatment, memory may be remarkably improved, and patients may achieve extremely accurate recall of minute details from earlier years. During this form of therapy, psychological defenses are often bypassed. Even memories that were repressed following severe traumatic experiences may be retrieved. Details that otherwise might require many weeks or months to extract from the patient's memory can be recovered rapidly - in a few sessions or sometimes even in a few minutes. Emotional blocks can also be lifted under hypnosis, either temporarily or permanently. Unconscious causes underlying neurotic conflicts may be more rapidly revealed in a hypnotic trance, while they might not otherwise be recognized by patients in their conscious state. [31]

The following is another composite example.

CASE: Fourteen-year-old Linda was raped by a boyfriend. She felt utterly betrayed and devastated. She dared not tell her parents or friends because she knew they would blame her rather than offer understanding or support. Within days, she "forgot" about the incident – that is, she pushed it out of her conscious mind.

Being a bright student, Linda buried herself in her studies. She went on to a successful career in nursing, which provided much satisfaction. It also gave her the excuse to avoid romantic involvement with men, because when she was not working evening shifts she was sleeping off her exhaustion from overwork.

But when the initial bloom of satisfactions in her professional advancements faded, Linda became depressed. A hypnotherapist suggested that she go back to the past under trance to discover the reasons for her unhappiness, and the rape came to light in the first session. Working through the emotional trauma associated with this experience took many months. Linda had to get in touch with and resolve her buried feelings of fear, outrage, anger, betrayal, guilt, sadness, and deep hurt. Eventually she was able to do all of this, and she came to a healing place of forgiveness for herself and for the rapist. Linda then stopped running away from relationships, and was happily married several years later.

Posthypnotic suggestions are another potential benefit of hypnotherapy. These are instructions given by hypnotherapists to subjects who are in hypnotic trance, with the injunction that they should be acted upon at some point after the subjects come out of the trance, and without memory of the hypnotic instructions. Subjects will usually carry out these suggestions very literally, as though their unconscious mind has been specifically programmed for the task. This can be helpful in strengthening patients' resolve, and in reminding them to change unhealthy habits such as overeating and smoking. For instance, suggestions may be implanted to make people recall the consequences of smoking or eating every time they reach for a cigarette or a snack.

One classical use of hypnosis, developed by Freud and others, is to explore the repressed conflicts that can lead to *hysterical* (today called *conversion*) symptoms. These are symptoms of psychogenic origin, typically a paralysis (as in the case of John, described earlier in this chapter) or sensory malfunction, which derive from unconscious psychological conflicts. Sufferers may experience intense anger, inappropriate sexual arousal or other unacceptable feelings. In order to protect them, their unconscious mind can completely isolate these emotions from their conscious awareness. In some cases it might even go further – causing the body to develop physical symptoms – in order to prevent them from taking any action based on the forbidden emotions, and simultaneously to punish them for harboring these feelings. Such physical symptoms can influence a very wide range of sensory and motor systems throughout the body. They may include muteness, deafness, blindness, various paralyses, and many types of altered sensations, ranging from lack of dermal sensitivity to severe pains.

Multiple personality disorder (MPD), also called d*issociative disorder*, is another syndrome for which hypnosis can be an effective therapy. People suffering from MPD have unconsciously split off and isolated the aspects of themselves that they find difficult to integrate within their primary personality. Sexual feelings are commonly isolated in this way, when the superego (conscience) cannot tolerate them. This rather extreme method of coping with uncomfortable feelings is usually found only in cases of very severe abuse in childhood. The helpless child may use this drastic form of psychological self-defense to isolate intensely painful experiences and feelings that would otherwise be overwhelming. Once the pattern of personality splitting under stress is established, it may be repeated in later life in reaction to further traumas.

Under hypnosis, the various personality "multiples" can be contacted and addressed by the hypnotist. With long-term hypnotherapy it is possible to help people reintegrate the divided aspects of their personality.[32]

While multiple personality is an extreme and rare disorder, all of us have functional personality splits in varying degrees. You may behave differently toward your wife than you behave toward your children, and in yet another manner with your neighbor, your doctor, and so on. There are facets of yourself that come forward and other facets that are reticent to express themselves to each person with whom you interact. At various times you may be more or less open to the characteristics in yourself that you consider to be faults or shortcomings. In effect, you may appear to be a different person under different circumstances, in different moods, in different surroundings and in the context of different relationships

A caution is in order here. It must be stressed that only competent therapists should use these hypnotherapy techniques. Injudicious probing of unconscious conflict by untrained hypnotists can produce anxiety and can even worsen existing psychiatric conditions. Furthermore, posing leading questions during hypnosis can produce false responses and false memories if subjects compliantly respond to direct or implied suggestions.

Hypnosis does not necessarily require the repeated intervention of a therapist. Some people can learn to hypnotize themselves. The actual mechanisms of self-hypnosis remain unclear, inasmuch as subjects are giving the instructions to themselves, while simultaneously receiving and responding to them. It has been hypothesized that people may be able to "split" their consciousness in order to achieve this. Self-hypnosis can aid relaxation and reinforce posthypnotic suggestions.

Hypnosis and spiritual healing

Hysterical symptoms (conversion reactions) usually develop in people with a type of personality that responds well to hypnosis and other sorts of suggestions. This means that almost any authoritative figure can initiate healing if they suggest a behavioral improvement while the patient is in a supportive setting, or conversely, if they command the hysteric to change in the context of a highly charged, emotional environment. Such atmospheres are deliberately created by some American faith healers. Although no studies have been conducted in this area, it seems entirely within the realm of probability that interventions by religious leaders, appropriate prayers, visits to shrines such as Lourdes, and other suggestive curative agents could produce relief of conversion symptoms. This is especially likely in the case of revival meetings, where the contagious enthusiasm and emotionality of audience participation could further heighten the effects of suggestion. Because of this possibility, medical professionals have suspected that many reports of the more dramatic spiritual healings are considerably less miraculous than naive lay people might take them to be. Such cures are presumed by many knowledgeable health practitioners to be no more than remission of hysterical symptoms.

My own impression is that this conclusion is too exclusive. Some alleged healings undoubtedly are due to such processes but I seriously doubt that all of them are. The clearest evidence showing that healings in revival meeting settings are far more than conversion reactions comes from a remarkable book by Richard Casdorph. Investigating a series of healings by the late Kathryn Kuhlman, who gave healings in these sorts of settings, Casdorph provides detailed case presentations, including confirmation of organic disease by examining physicians, with laboratory and X-ray reports (reproduced in the book) prior to and following healing treatments, and personal reports by the healed and their families. Casdorph describes cured cases that include bone cancer, malignant brain tumor, disabling arthritis and multiple sclerosis. When supported by laboratory studies, none of these could be due to conversion reactions.

Explorations of Multiple Personality Disorder point to some possible explanations for healing. Remarkable studies show that when one "member" of a multiple personality is allergic, diabetic, cross-eyed, exhausted, or in other ways physically debilitated, other personalities in that same individual may not exhibit these physical conditions at all, or not to the same degree. Furthermore, EEGs and brain blood flow patterns may differ when different personalities are present. These findings seem to indicate that the body is an extension of the mind, and that with a change of mind the body can be dramatically transformed. From this we can speculate that spiritual healing may in some cases entail the relinquishing of unhealthy templates for mental/emotional personality or self-image. Conversely, spiritual healing may in other cases manifest as the acceptance of healthy templates.

In cases of MPD, a fragment of the self may be identified that has access to knowledge about all of the separate personalities. This inner "individual" may become an ally of the therapist in integrating all of the parts into a coherent whole.

Within the cast of MPD characters there may be yet another personality that is so much more aware and emotionally centered as to be an enormous resource to the therapist in helping the client sort out the other, emotionally troubled personalities. Ralph Allison and Gretchen Sliker, each writing about MPD and related phenomena, call this the *Inner Self-Helper*. At times this fragment of the MPD patient's self appears to possess wisdom and knowledge far exceeding what would be expected in a person suffering from this syndrome, and this may indicate access to something in the realms of transpersonal dimensions, such as a collective consciousness or *higher* consciousness.

Healers often suggest that healees call upon their *higher selves* to find the causes and cures for their illnesses. Such suggestions may allow us to access aspects of our unconscious minds that we otherwise would not exercise. In my own practice I have found that some people indeed possess this hidden ability. We have only to call upon our inner self-helper to discover the reasons for our woes and problems, and to learn the steps we may take to alleviate and correct them.

Other healers suggest that spirits of departed people, nature spirits and angels may help in these ways.

A more conventional explanation of this phenomenon is also possible. It may be that we clothe our unconscious mind or spirit in the raiment of a wise advisor, who interprets the messages we receive from our own deeper selves or from transpersonal awareness. Each of us could endow our inner helper with the personality and garments we imagine she or he merits, much as each of us molds our picture of the Deity worshipped in our culture to resonate with our own expectations.

> *God created man in His image and man returned the compliment.*
> – Jerome Lawrence/ Robert E. Lee

Suggestive and hypnotic influences without formal induction

Helpful responses to suggestion may also occur in cases other than psychosomatic illness. People with emotional problems or physical, ailments of organic origins may benefit from suggestion as well. Here I have deliberately used the word "suggestion" rather than "hypnosis," although this distinction is in itself a gray area.

The late Milton Erickson was one of the world's greatest hypnotists. He was especially skillful in using methods of suggestion in clinical situations without invoking the classical hypnotic trance (Haley 1973), as in the following incident involving his son.

> Three-year-old Robert fell down the back stairs, split his lip, and knocked an upper tooth back into the maxilla. He was bleeding profusely and

screaming loudly with pain and fright. His mother and I went to his aid. A single glance at him lying on the ground screaming, his mouth bleeding profusely and blood spattered on the pavement, revealed this was an emergency requiring prompt and adequate measures.

No effort was made to pick him up. Instead, as he paused for breath for fresh screaming, I told him quickly, simply, sympathetically and emphatically, "That hurts awful, Robert. That hurts terrible."

Right then, without any doubt, my son knew that I knew what I was talking about. He could agree with me and he knew that I was agreeing completely with him. Therefore he could listen respectfully to me, because I had demonstrated that I understood the situation fully. In pediatric hypnotherapy, there is no more important problem than so speaking to the patient that he can agree with you and respect your intelligent grasp of the situation as he judges it in terms of his own understanding.

Then I told Robert, "And it will keep right on hurting." In this simple statement, I named his own fear, confirmed his own judgment of the situation, demonstrated my good intelligent grasp of the entire matter and my entire agreement with him, since right then he could foresee only a lifetime of anguish and pain for himself.

The next step for him and for me was to declare, as he took another breath, "And you really wish it would stop hurting." Again, we were in full agreement and he was ratified and even encouraged in this wish. And it was his wish, deriving entirely from within him and constituting his own urgent need. With the situation so defined, I could then offer a suggestion with some certainty of acceptance. This suggestion was, "Maybe it will stop hurting in a little while, in just a minute or two." This was a suggestion in full accord with his own needs and wishes, and, because it was qualified by a "maybe it will," it was not a contradiction to his own understanding of the situation. Thus he could accept the idea and initiate his responses to it.

As he did this, a shift was made to another important matter, important to him as a suffering person, and important in the total psychological significance of the entire occurrence - a shift that in itself was important as a primary measure in changing and altering the situation.

The next procedure... was a recognition of the meaning of the injury to Robert himself – pain, loss of blood, body damage, a loss of the wholeness of his normal narcissistic self-esteem, of his sense of physical goodness so vital in human living.

Robert knew that he hurt, that he was a damaged person; he could see his blood upon the pavement, taste it in his mouth, and see it on his hands. And yet, like all other human beings, he too could desire narcissistic distinction in his misfortune, along with the desire even more for narcissistic comfort. Nobody wants a picayune headache; if a headache must be endured, let it be so colossal that only the sufferer could endure it. Human pride is so curiously good and comforting! Therefore Robert's attention was doubly directed to two vital issues of comprehensible importance to him by the simple statements, "That's an awful lot of blood on the pavement. Is it good, red, strong blood? Look carefully, Mother, and see. I think it is, but I want you to be sure."

Thus there was an open and unafraid recognition in another way of values important to Robert. He needed to know that his misfortune was catastrophic in the eyes of others as well as his own, and he needed tangible proof that he himself could appreciate. By my declaring it to be "an awful lot of blood," Robert could again recognize the intelligent and competent appraisal of the situation in accord with his own actually unformulated, but nevertheless real, needs.

By this time Robert had ceased crying, and his pain and fright were no longer dominant factors. Instead, he was interested and absorbed in the important problem of the quality of his blood.

His mother picked him up and carried him to the bathroom, where water was poured over his face to see if the blood "mixed properly with water" and gave it a "proper pink color." Then the redness was carefully checked and reconfirmed, following which the "pinkness" was reconfirmed by washing him adequately, to Robert's intense satisfaction, since his blood was good, red, and strong and made water rightly pink.

Then came the question of whether or not his mouth was "bleeding right" and "swelling right." Close inspection, to Robert's complete satisfaction and relief, again disclosed that, all developments were good and right and indicative of his essential and pleasing soundness in every way.

Next came the question of suturing the lip. Since this could easily evoke a negative response, it was broached in a negative fashion to him, *thereby precluding an initial negation by him,* and at the same time raising a new and important issue. This was done by stating regretfully that, while he would have to have stitches taken in his lip, it was most doubtful if he could have as many stitches as he could count. In fact, it looked as if he could not even have ten stitches, and he could count to twenty. Regret was expressed that he could not have seventeen stitches, like his sister, Betty Alice, or twelve, like his brother, Allan; but comfort was offered in the statement that he would have more stitches than his siblings, Bert, Lance, or Carol. Thus the entire situation became transformed into one in which he could share with his older siblings a common experience with a comforting sense of equality and even superiority. In this way he was enabled to face the question of surgery without fear or anxiety, but with hope of high accomplishment in cooperation with the surgeon and imbued with the desire to do well the task assigned him, namely, to "be sure to count the stitches." In this manner, no reassurances were needed, nor was there any need to offer further suggestions regarding freedom from pain.

Only seven stitches were required to Robert's disappointment, but the surgeon pointed out that the suture material was of a newer and better kind than any that his siblings had ever had, and that the scar would be an unusual "W" shape, like the letter of his Daddy's college. Thus the fewness of the stitches was well compensated.

The question may well be asked at what point hypnosis was employed. Actually, hypnosis began with the first statement to him and became apparent when he gave his full and undivided, interested and pleased attention to each of the succeeding events that constituted the medical handling of his problem.

At no time was he given a false statement, nor was he forcibly reassured in a manner contradictory to his understandings. A community of understanding was first established with him and then, one by one, items of vital interest to him in his situation were thoughtfully considered and decided, either to his satisfaction or sufficiently agreeable to merit his acceptance. His role in the entire situation was that of an interested participant, and adequate response was made to each idea suggested.

This vignette illustrates how dramatic changes can be brought about in the experiences and attitudes of people with serious physical problems, applying the principles of hypnosis. Erickson's suggestions to his son were highly effective on many levels. First the child's *meta-anxiety* (anxiety about being anxious, leading to panic) was reduced. His attention was then redirected to aspects of the situation that his parents got him to consider in a new light, demonstrating not only their understanding of the situation but also their control over it. The child's pain was either reduced via his altered perception, or forgotten when his attention was redirected.

Another clinical report shows how hypnotists may also be able to dramatically influence people's *self-perceptions* and *self-image*. Erickson was asked to help a fourteen year-old girl who had developed the idea that her feet were much too large. Over a period of three months she became increasingly withdrawn, not wanting to go to school or church, or even to be seen in the street. She would not allow the subject of her feet to be discussed, and would not go to a doctor. In the role of a physician, Erickson visited the girl's mother, who happened to be sick at the time.

> Studying the girl, I wondered what I could do to get her over this problem. Finally I hit upon a plan. As I finished my examination of the mother, I maneuvered the girl into a position directly behind me. I was sitting on the bed talking to the mother, and I got up slowly and carefully and then stepped back awkwardly. I put my heel down squarely on the girl's toes. The girl, of course, squawked with pain. I turned on her and in a tone of absolute fury said, "If you would grow those things large enough for a man to see, I wouldn't be in this sort of a situation!" The girl looked at me, puzzled, while I wrote out a prescription and called the drugstore. That day the girl asked her mother if she could go out to a show, which she hadn't done in months. She went to school and church, and that was the end of a pattern of three months' seclusiveness. I checked later on how things were going, and the girl was friendly and agreeable.

This interaction demonstrates how extensive changes in a person's attitudes and behaviors may be introduced through subtle but powerful clinical suggestions. My training and experience as a psychiatrist would suggest that the girl was suffering a severe phobic or obsessive disorder, or even a psychotic decompensation.

She seemed to be withdrawing from reality into an inner, autistic world created out of her own fears. I would have predicted that prolonged psychotherapy, possibly involving the prescription of tranquilizers, would be required. Yet Erickson brought about dramatic improvements in this girl's perceptions of herself and in her behavior through a single meeting with her.

It is difficult to know, from the meager details provided, whether this was a very limited, focal phobia or whether other psychopathology was present. While it is difficult to generalize from a single case report, such a dramatic improvement in a teenager with such severe symptoms suggests that others with similar problems might benefit from these sorts of interventions. In other cases, however, more generalized or more severe pathology in the child or in the family might prevent such brief interventions from having as dramatic results as reported in this case.

Explaining hypnosis

Authorities on the subject disagree about the nature and even the substance of hypnosis. Furthermore, numerous experiments demonstrate that merely through an exertion of their own willpower, people can accomplish much that is currently thought to be possible only under hypnotic trance. Bandler and Grinder, following in the footsteps of Erickson and other gifted therapists, have developed hypnotic techniques that do not require elaborate trance induction processes (such as monotonous repetition of instructions or focusing the eyes on a pendulum). In their systems of therapy, NLP, hypnotic induction is achieved very rapidly by the therapist simply giving instructions to the subject. This supports Barber's contention that hypnosis may be no more than a mutual agreement between hypnotist and subject that each will behave in particular ways, since people can perform most of the feats ascribed to hypnotic trance when they are not hypnotized, merely by exerting maximum effort.

Although opinions differ on what hypnosis is, several common denominators appear in the classical descriptions of this type of phenomenon:

1. focusing of attention on limited sensory cues and thought processes;
2. exclusion of extraneous sensory cues and thought processes;
3. instructions given in a repetitive, even monotonous manner by oneself or another person, usually in a rhythmic pattern, or instructions given in an authoritative manner by another person, as in NLP;
4. a particular mind-set, with a series of culturally determined expectations for behavior conducive to hypnotic trance;
5. enhanced access to unconscious memories and repressed emotions;
6. improved abilities to imprint new information in memory;
7. increased control over bodily functions;
8. enhanced ability or even an internal compulsion to apply oneself to specific goals, once these goals have been impressed upon the mind under hypnosis;
9. behavior throughout the hypnotic and posthypnotic states resembling everyday conduct as governed by the unconscious mind, e.g. using literal, concrete, simplistic logic and thought processes (such as taking the hypnotist's suggestions literally, and repressing awareness of parts or all of the hypnotic experience after waking from the trance state);

10. ability to suspend belief and judgment in accordance with suggestions given, even when they contradict everyday reality;

11. ability to isolate and compartmentalize mental and emotional aspects of the self.

Experts disagree about the psychological mechanisms that are involved in hypnotic trance. Hypnotists also differ in their criteria for depth of trance. Moreover, no commonly accepted method of objectively identifying the presence or depth of a trance state has yet been developed. Some feel that suggestions given to subjects in light trance may ultimately (although perhaps not immediately) be as effective as those given in deep trance.

The mechanisms by which people are able to greatly enhance their control over mind and body while they are in the hypnotic trance state is not clear. One hypothesis is that under hypnosis, greater concentration allows them to apply their mental energies more effectively. This can be compared to learning disciplines that allow maximal use of physical force, such as karate. Merely by concentrating, without apparent hypnotic induction, practitioners can achieve feats of unusual strength, such as stretching the body rigidly between two chairs with only head and heels supported. The question remains whether they may be practicing the equivalent of self-hypnosis (whatever that is).

Another theory is that unconscious portions of the brain and/or mind are accessed under hypnosis, which would explain the greater range of stored information available and the enhanced control over physiological functions.

If we take this a step further, we encounter the further possibility that vast potentials for self-healing exist within us, but they are blocked by cultural disbeliefs that hypnosis is able to bypass. Given permission, encouragement and support, we are able to activate our self-healing capacities.

Underlying the effectiveness of suggestion and hypnosis is the ability to alter our perceptions and beliefs about ourselves. Our emotional and physical pains may not change in their intensity, but our beliefs about them may shift, so that they do not make us as anxious, afraid, depressed or bitter.

> *[T]he belief system that possesses perception is not just abstract in nature. It is fuelled by imaginative, creative power. It is an active, dynamic shaping of the meaning and impact of the world by the mind. And so to rethink the world in the act of seeing it means putting out a deep re-appraisal of what we see. Then we start to experience the world as being different...*
> – John Heron

Metaphors and imagery in suggestion and hypnosis
Metaphors and imagery may form another basis for suggestion. For example, Milton Erickson would talk at length with a patient about planting and growing tomatoes. Embedded within his discussion would be imagery with subtle metaphoric messages relevant to the patient's problems. "*Planting tomato seeds*" could suggest planting seeds of inspiration or change in the person's life. "*Preparing the soil, watering plants, and applying fertilizer*" could suggest giving attention to details that might help to bring the patient's projects to fruition.

In our everyday use of language, body-related words are frequently used metaphorically to describe our relationships, and body parts are used in metaphors that describe our emotional reactions. For example, a particular weakness may be called someone's *Achilles' heel*. An annoying person or situation may become *a pain in the butt* or *a headache*. I might *have a hard time swallowing* something that *I don't want to hear*. Someone who complains may be *bellyaching*, or speaking in other metaphoric body language, as summarized earlier in Table II-2.

If we say such phrases emphatically or repeat them often to ourselves, or if others say them to us, we may begin to tense up the part of our body that is addressed in the metaphor. Chronically tense muscles can eventually go into spasm, with serious pain. Through such mechanisms we develop an enormous range of somatic symptoms, such as tension headaches and bellyaches.

More serious illnesses can develop when chronic tensions activate the autonomic nervous system and neurohormonal mechanisms. Psychosomatic theory recognizes that there are particular illnesses that can be strongly correlated with chronic stress, including asthma, hypertension, thyroid dysfunction, peptic ulcers, irritable bowel syndromes, migraines, and more.

Chronic stress can also affect the immune system, leading to the development of other illnesses and syndromes. These include allergies (particularly those that are manifested in the skin – our boundary with the world around us), chronic fatigue syndrome, fibromyalgia and cancer.

When we delve even further into the physiological mechanisms of disease and healing, we find that there is an energetic aspect to the body that can play a crucial role in these regards. As discussed in greater depth in Chapter 3, the mind can shape our *biological energy fields*, which in turn will influence the physical body. The contributions of biofields to health and illness add another dimension to *mind-body* (or *bodymind*) medicine.

Many doctors, nurses and other conventional caregivers focus exclusively on the physical body and are completely unaware of any of these additional mechanisms for developing symptoms and illnesses. They treat the symptoms of these illnesses but ignore underlying stresses that may be contributing to, or actually causing and maintaining the problems. This is like tightening the lid on a pot of soup that is boiling over, rather than turning down the heat or removing the pot from the stove.

By exploring the meanings of symptoms and helping patients to vocalize what their bodies are saying, we can decipher the physiological metaphors for dis-ease in people's lives that often manifest as disease. This is one of the main contributions of wholistic medicine.

Yet another benefit of healing metaphor can be found in the generalization of imagery that can be internalized in very personal ways, thus influencing many related problems that may be present in numerous nuances and variations.

CASE: Jeremy came to therapy for help to overcome a fear of speaking in public. Though he was a successful bank manager, he found himself panicking when he had to speak to any group of people and therefore giving a poor impression at public and corporate meetings. This was hindering his career. As he began work in psychotherapy, he found that this was actually only one of many anxieties – all relating to lessons learned in growing up with very strict and critical parents. He was afraid to explore new situations, anxious when faced with several choices, browbeaten by his wife, and still unable to contradict his parents when they made unreasonable suggestions and demands.

By working with imagery of a monster that was always critical, he was able through this one root of his problems to reach many of the branches on the tree of anxieties grew out of his childhood experiences.

Such generalizations of an initial problem may escape notice and may not be dealt with through more direct approaches that focus on cognitive awareness and that may miss some of the emotional and other branches of problems. Metaphors and imagery reach into a person's unconscious and help to heal whatever problems resonate with them.

It is quite probable that Erickson's stepping on the girl's foot dealt metaphorically with many more branches and roots of problems than were apparent in the chief complaint of her feet being too big.

More on suggestion and spiritual healing

Reports reviewed above have demonstrated that good hypnotic subjects also often have psi abilities. The nature and reasons for this correlation are as yet unclear.

Vasiliev's observation that under hypnosis subjects' muscles contracted when the hypnotist pointed at them or at their innervating nerve may be explained in several ways. Telepathic control may be involved, although this seems unlikely, since Vasiliev arranged for anatomically naive experimenters to point to where the nerves are located (without knowing they were doing so), and the appropriate muscles still contracted. Perhaps subjects were able to read the minds of the experimenters. The existence of this sort of *super-ESP* would be stretching accepted psi explanations a little, but it is not beyond the realm of the psychologically conceivable.[33] Another possibility is that the hypnotic state produces greater receptivity in the subject to a field or emanation originating in the experimenter. This might or might not be related to healing energies.

The receptors for psi impressions in the brain have yet to be identified. The correlation of hypnosis with psi suggests that identical or overlapping sections of the brain might be involved in both phenomena. This would appear a fertile subject for research with brain imaging.[34]

Wilson's and Barber's observations on the power of simple suggestion and maximal investment of efforts may be relevant to healing in several ways. Some healings may partially or totally owe their success to suggestions of the hypnotic type. Subtle but potent suggestions, perhaps even given without conscious intent by healers, may produce some of the improvements attributed to healings. A few healers use hypnotic suggestions deliberately for relaxation and hypnotherapy, in addition to giving spiritual healing., They report that each of these approaches enhances the effects of the other.

Healers may also release blocks to innate self-healing abilities, either through spiritual healing or through suggestion. Many healers claim that they do no more than catalyze or activate healees' own healing powers. Healees may then heal their own body/mind.

Some studies have demonstrated that hypnotic trance and other alternative states of consciousness enhance people's abilities to use their psi faculties. I do not know of any study on the effects of hypnosis per se on healers' abilities. But since healing gifts often appear in persons who are gifted with other psi faculties, there is every reason to believe that hypnosis might be a helpful adjunct in teaching student healers, or enhancing already developed healing abilities.

Further observations have supported this theory:

1. Meditation has been recommended as a path to developing healing abilities. Meditational and hypnotic states of mind appear to overlap in many ways.
2. Most healers report that they enter a meditative state when they are performing healings.
3. Healers who invoke the aid of spirits often use variants of hypnosis to enter the mediumistic (channeling)[35] state, in which they diagnose and heal.

The compartmentalizing of aspects of the self under self-hypnosis resembles in a loose way what occurs in Multiple Personality Disorder. One portion of the self gives hypnotic instructions and another portion accepts them. Such splittings of the self indicate that the mind can isolate modules of consciousness or of the personality, which then appear to function independently of each other. Consciousness of the *self* as an entity may alternate between the modules, or may coexist within separate modules.

When a split in consciousness occurs, it may appear to the self and to others that an alien personality is *possessing* the individual. Some healers claim they can help by eliminating "possessing entities," and it may be that in some such cases they are actually healing unconscious mental splits.[36]

The complexities of these issues can only lead one to agree with William James: "Our science is a drop, our ignorance a sea."

BIOFEEDBACK

> *O Lord, there are tubes in the body which should be opened and tubes in the body which should be closed. If it be thy will, let those which should be open remain open and those which should be closed remain closed.*
> – Jewish prayer

Biofeedback is something we all use without being aware of it. A child learns to aim the spoon into her mouth through visual biofeedback. She sees her hand moving and learns to adjust the movements of her hand and arm muscles so that the food lands where she wants it to.

Electronic and mechanical devices may provide people with information about their internal body states, of which they are otherwise unaware. Many of these states are highly correlated with emotional tensions, and this is why they form the basis for lie detector tests, for example. These technologies can also be helpful learning tools to help people control their own internal reactions to stress. An electrode may be placed on the body to measure the surface *electrical skin resis-*

tance (*ESR*) or underlying muscle tension. The measurements are displayed on a dial or translated into a tone that varies with the amount of tension. People can use this feedback to alter their internal states because they can immediately tell when they are doing something that either increases or decreases their tension. Biofeedback can thus enable people to gain control over many body processes.

Through biofeedback we can learn to influence many other physical functions on a conscious basis, even those that are normally controlled by unconscious, automatic regulating mechanisms. This control is not achieved spontaneously because under normal conditions there is no sensory feedback available. For example, you are usually unaware of your heart rate, or blood pressure and therefore have no way of either increasing or decreasing either. With biofeedback you can learn to alter your heart rate and blood pressure voluntarily.

In biofeedback therapy, subjects are told to alter the level shown on the dial or to change the tone that represents a given physiological measurement. Instructions are not provided on how to do this, since no effective descriptions for this process have yet been found. In fact, subjects will usually do best if they do not force themselves to relax. Elmer Green (1972) observes:

> In active volition that you use for operating the normal muscles, the harder you try presumably the better it works, but when you're trying to control the involuntary nervous system the harder you try the worse it works. You have to learn how to talk to the body, tell it what you want it to do, have confidence in it, allow it to do it and detach yourself from the results. If you don't do that it won't work. If you keep worrying about it or thinking about it won't do it. It's like forcing yourself to go to sleep, which doesn't work very well either. And about the time you give up trying to force yourself to go to sleep then you go to sleep.

Through trial and error a subject can learn to control these functions, just as infants learn to control their hands from visual, tactile and kinesthetic feedback, by trial and error.

It was once thought that certain muscles in the body are not susceptible to voluntary control. The apparent reason for this was that people had not received adequate feedback to know when these "involuntary" muscles were contracting or relaxing. A simple example, which you can test yourself with a little patience, involves the iris muscle of the eye. By providing feedback with a mirror, many people can learn to contract or dilate that muscle voluntarily. Average learning time is about an hour.

Self-regulation may provide control over tensions in the following areas: voluntary muscles throughout the body (I learned to wiggle my ears with feedback from a mirror); portions of the bowel; blood pressure; heart rate; selective blood vessels (as in your hands to make them hands warmer or cooler, or in your head to relieve migraines); brain waves; skin resistance, and more.

Mechanisms for self-regulation

Biofeedback is helpful for treating the pain component of many diseases. Pain is usually associated with tension. It may result from the primary disease process, as with inflammation of joints in arthritis, or from inadequate blood supply caused by spasm in the arteries with migraines or blockage of blood vessels, as in atherosclerotic heart disease. Pain can also lead to the vicious circles of anxiety → tension → muscle spasms → pain → more anxiety → etc. For example, with tension one may get headaches caused by spasms of muscles attached to the skull.

Relaxation may also help with breathing problems. Asthmatics may also find themselves in vicious circles: wheezing → anxiety → tension in the body → constriction of airways → more wheezing → more anxiety → etc.

In these situations, a twofold healing process may be activated through relaxation. First, relaxation breaks the vicious circles detailed above. Second, releasing tension in various muscles may interrupt the primary disease processes. When bronchioles relax, we breathe easier, literally and metaphorically. If arteriospasm is reduced by relaxation, more blood will reach the affected tissues, and the pain will ease. Other mechanisms that have not been so well studied may also be involved at the primary level, such as reduced inflammation due to hormonal, immune, or other biochemical alterations that are enhanced through relaxation.

Implications for self-healing

Illnesses may be initiated when people are sensitized in particular organ systems. Some seem to have skin, bowels or other parts that are more sensitive than usual. In such cases, these parts of the body respond first to tension. They may have had spontaneous internal feedback learning (unassisted by external feedback loops) via sensations of bowel tension, skin sweating, rashes or other subtle cues. Some people may become sensitized cognitively (by the examples of relatives with organic or psychosomatic illnesses) to pay attention especially to these parts of their body. Their use of language may program their unconscious minds to tense up particular parts.

Initially, control is initiated through anxieties and tensions that produce pain or other problems. In therapy, improvement of these same conditions is facilitated under hypnotic or other suggestion - which reverse the direction of previously learned controls, producing relaxation rather than tension.

One psychologist provided an exotic example of this sort of self-control, teaching himself to beat his heart in any desired rhythm (*Brain/Mind* 1983a). Another unusual example is the practice of *tumo* in Tibet, in which meditators develop the ability to stay warm in sub-zero weather, and can raise the temperature of their extremities at will to above-normal levels.

Yoga adepts, after years of practice, have been known to demonstrate highly unusual levels of control over many aspects of their bodies. Other people may practice yoga or other forms of meditation for these purposes or may spontaneously develop unusual control over body functions in the course of meditation. These unusual feats are not the ultimate goals, per se, of the meditative practices. They do, however, serve for some people as ways of motivating and demonstrating mental focus, which is a landmark of meditation. They also provide feedback to those meditating, proving that they are advancing in their spiritual practices.

The unconscious mind appears capable of taking control and regulating various body functions, given the proper mind-sets. If self-regulation can be learned with biofeedback, the body can potentially also be induced by suggestion to make the same changes, even without such training. Hypnosis can elicit unusual control over the body, without preliminary practice. We must be cautious, therefore, in assessing any therapy that addresses problems which are subject to self-regulation.

Biofeedback and spiritual healing
There are several ways in which biofeedback may be associated with spiritual healing.

Control over body functions similar to that achieved in biofeedback may be a part of spiritual healing. A variety of illnesses associated with the physiological mechanisms discussed above could be alleviated by patients developing their abilities to control their own bodies. Many people clearly have the potential to learn self-regulation, but we are far from clear on the mechanisms that might activate these self-healing potentials. We must therefore be cautious in crediting spiritual healing with changes that could be the result of self-regulation, activated by suggestion, self-hypnosis, etc. This does not rule out the possibility that spiritual healing directly activates some of the mechanisms that suggestion alone does not. Spiritual healing and suggestion may complement each other, with the two in concert being more effective than either alone.

A special case of biofeedback is that of electroencephalogram (EEG) biofeedback. Numerous studies have confirmed that it is possible to enhance relaxation by increasing the level of alpha brain waves. Deeper relaxation and meditative states may be achieved with increases in the slower delta and theta waves.

The *mind mirror* of C. Maxwell Cade and Geoffrey Blundell is a device that displays on a panel of lights the amount of brain-wave activity at various frequencies as it occurs simultaneously in both brain hemispheres. Cade found that the more effective healers have symmetrical activity in the two brain hemispheres. This provides a potential mode of biofeedback that might help people to develop their healing abilities through a visual display of their EEGs.

Brain-wave patterns of healer and healee become synchronized during healings. Bruce MacManaway (1983) observed that this effect is strengthened when several healers work on one subject simultaneously. While this has not been used yet as biofeedback, it appears to suggest another piece of supporting evidence, or possibly another pathway for spiritual healing to occur.

Demonstrations of *allobiofeedback* provide scientific proof that one person can remotely influence the body of another. The researchers measured the skin resistance (GSR) of a subject, displaying this on a meter that was placed in front of a healer in a distant room. Using this feedback, the healer was able to alter the subject's GSR through distant healing. This series of experiment was repeated with different healers and subjects, and produced highly significant results – that could occur by chance less than one time in a billion.[37] This mechanism provides another potential model for teaching healing – giving healers immediate feedback on a physiological effect of their healng.

Deena Spear has used mental influence over violins as feedback to confirm to students that they can also learn distant healing.

Biofeedback as taught by Elmer and Alyce Green may also lead to marked transformations in consciousness and spirituality.

UNUSUAL HUMAN ABILITIES

God's miracles belong to those who can concentrate on one thing and limit themselves.

– Baal Shem Tov

There are many well authenticated reports of physical feats that are beyond normal human abilities. These reports demonstrate that the human body may be able to accomplish unaided some of the same effects that are achieved through spiritual healing. They may also shed some light on the processes that are involved in self-healing. Vladimir Kuznetsov proposes the term *anthropomaximology* for the study of unusual physical powers.

An example is Jack Schwarz, who has an unusual degree of control over some of his bodily functions. He was carefully scrutinized in the act of piercing his flesh with large needles by Elmer Green. Not only did he report that he felt no pain, but no bleeding was noted upon withdrawal of the needles, the wound closed within minutes, and healing occurred within a day or two without infection or scarring. This control was apparently only possible when he anticipated the injury. He said:

> Now if you would take the needle and you would sneak behind me and put it in my buttocks or anywhere else I would jump up too and scream out, but if you told me you were going to do that, then I already knew that I had to be alert to control it, so no pain would be felt because I was aware that disharmony would take place that the skin would be destroyed and that therefore blood might come forth. Then I have to start to work right away on it. I detach myself from this physical body and from the outside. I get the image that the blood will keep flowing and that in a way you make it flow so fast that it hardly actually can even get out of your vein.

Others have developed such abilities in contexts of religious practices.

The Parmann Project has reported on a group of Sufis in Jordan who pierce their bodies with spikes, swords and knives as an act of religious faith. They report no pain, bleeding, injuries to internal organs or subsequent infections, and claim that healing occurs within minutes. Some may only pierce the flesh of their arm or cheek, while others may pierce their abdomen through and through. They claim that this ability is conferred with 100% success by masters who transfer the self-healing ability through a blessing and a ritual handshake. I have seen photographs and videotapes of these piercings, and I met a western psychologist, Professor Howard Hall of Case Western University, who observed them and videotaped them first hand and confirmed that these are not magicians' stage tricks.

Alfred Stelter mentions two individuals with unusual abilities to control body processes associated with wounds. The first is Therese Neumann, a devout countrywoman who demonstrated stigmata (wounds on the body that appear spontaneously at places where Christ's body was wounded during crucifixion). Many similar cases have been reported over several centuries. What was unusual in Neumann's case was that she apparently could survive without more than a token intake of food and water over many years.

The second person described by Stelter was a Dutchman, Mirin Dajo, who was able to let people pierce his body completely through with swords without suffering any pain, and with immediate closure of the wound upon withdrawal of the blade. He too was scrutinized by scientists, and even X-rayed. All examinations confirmed that no tricks were involved. A similar adept, Daskalos, is described by Kyriakos Markides.

Rustum Roy describes a type of Qigong practice called *bigu*, with which people are able to live for periods of months and years with an intake of less than 300 calories daily.

Max Freedom Long relates how South Sea islanders are able to walk on hot lava without being harmed. He also describes in detail a person who handled fire and very hot objects, but suffered no burns. This man could even touch a red-hot iron poker with his tongue. He claimed that he was able to do this by "becoming one with the fire," and added that he could do it only if knew he had not injured anyone in any way or caused sorrow to anyone.

Firewalking was also a fad in the US during the 1980's. Many thousands of ordinary people (including myself) learned to enter an alternative state of consciousness (ASC) in a brief workshop and then walked on coals as hot as 800-1,200°F with no pain or damage to our feet. Only a handful of people have ever been burned in the process.

The practice of *trial by fire* is used in some cultures as a form of popular justice. The accused are required to touch a very hot object with some part of their body, to place a hand in boiling water, or some other variant on this theme. The belief is that if they are innocent, they will remain unharmed.

Berthold Schwarz describes a Pentecostal church in the U.S. where members pass burning acetylene torches over their skin (and also handle poisonous snakes and ingest strychnine) with no ill effects. These activities are meant to demonstrate their religious faith. Several of Schwarz's observations may provide clues to the mystery of firewalking. He reports that the hair and clothes of the faithful are not scorched when their limbs or faces are exposed to flames. One member held his hand, dripping with fuel oil, in flames for ten seconds and the oil did not catch fire – while an iron poker dipped in the same oil caught fire immediately. The faithful reported that concentration and faith are required for them to perform these feats.

Max Freedom Long describes a woman who could walk on sword blades without being cut, and who gave similar explanations for her abilities.

Other examples are found in studies by Michael Murphy and Rhea White, who reviewed the peak experiences and psi experiences reported by athletes. They describe highly unusual feats of strength and agility that far transcend ordinary human abilities.

CASE: Patsy Neal, Professor of Physical Education, describes a remarkable experience while competing in the Free-Throw Championship at the National AAU Basketball Tournament during her freshman year at college. She had practiced diligently for this event and came into the tournament confident she could score well. However, she found herself too nervous to score in the early competition rounds. The night prior to the last round she prayed for assistance and did her best to image herself being calm even though she was performing in front of the crowd – but could not dissipate images of failure. Falling asleep, she had a dream:

> I was shooting the free-throws, and each time the ball fell through the goal, the net would change to the image of Christ. It was as though *I* was flowing into the basket instead of the ball. I felt endless, unhampered... and in some way I was connected to the image of Christ that kept flowing from the basket. The sensation was that of transcending *everything*. I was more than I was. I was a particle flowing into *all* of life. It seems almost profane to try to describe the feeling because the words are so very inadequate.

Next day, the feeling persisted after she woke. She felt as though she was floating through her day, rather than just living it. When she shot her free-throws that evening in the finals, she felt she was probably the calmest she had ever been in her life.

> I didn't... see or hear the crowd. It was only me, the ball, and the basket. The number of baskets I made really had no sense of importance to me at the time. The only thing that really mattered was what I *felt*. But even so, I would have found it hard to miss even if I had wanted to.
>   ... I know now what people mean when they speak of a "state of grace." I was in a state of grace, and if it were my power to maintain what I was experiencing at that point in time, I would have given up everything in my possession in preference to that sensation. (P. Neal, p. 167)

She scored 48 out of 50 baskets, winning the championship.

Many similar accomplishments are reported by Oriental athletes, who relate to sports as meditative practices. Their athletic performances are routinely conducted while they are in alternative states of consciousness (ASCs). Until recently, Western athletes also reported ASCs which sometimes accompanied exceptional physical performances, but only as rare, unsought occurrences. Today, athletes often speak of getting into a *flow* state, where they are exclusively aware of the physical activity in which they are engaged. Tiger Woods' fierce concentration on his golf strokes is a legendary example of this sort of focus. They also commonly speak of peak experiences. These are directly analogous to meditative states.

> *They can because they think they can.*
> – Virgil

How do they do that?
Such extraordinary feats are difficult to comprehend, or sometimes even to believe. Stelter hypothesizes that firewalking may involve the production by the body of a substance that psychically coats the feet to protect them from the hot coals. He takes as his paradigm the materializations of *ectoplasm* by mediums,

which have been observed under sufficient scientific scrutiny to leave little doubt, in his opinion, that they are in fact real.[38] However, no direct evidence for such materializations in firewalking has yet been reported.

Others have suggested that a layer of sweat on the foot may protect the skin, much as a drop of water will scoot across a hot griddle when a layer of steam is formed under it. I feel that this explanation is untenable, because most firewalkers have dry skin on their feet, and because in any case, steam scalds the skin, and evaporates quickly at high temperatures. Another hypothesis is that ash forms an insulating layer over the hot coals. This does not appear likely, as coals with ash on them can still burn people, including some of the firewalkers. In the latter instances, several of the burned firewalkers indicate that they were unable to hold the safe, firewalking state of consciousness in their minds while crossing the bed of coals. If they relinquished this special alternative state of consciousness even for a moment, their feet were burned.

Of the thousands of firewalkers in America, only a handful have been burned, according to Larissa Vilenskaya, a psi researcher and firewalk instructor. In my own experience, I could not hold my hand closer than six inches from the coal bed without feeling serious pain from the heat. Yet my feet and ankles felt no heat when I walked across the coals. The fact that some have been burned during firewalks appears to confirm that those who *are* successful demonstrate an unusual ability. Schwarz's reports on the clothing and oil that did not ignite while in contact with the bodies of the fire handlers may support Stelter's hypothesis regarding an emanation of ectoplasm that prevents the fire from harming the body. Perhaps a substance or an energy field is produced that protects against heat.

Most of the above reports have several factors in common. The subjects all claim that they engage in mental exercises in order to be able to achieve the physical feats of being uninjured by sharp objects or by hot materials. They visualize themselves as being at one with the heat or blade, tenaciously hold onto a belief that they cannot be harmed, or enter alternative states of consciousness (ASC). In their *conscious* awareness, they hold firmly to their belief that they are capable of these unusual physical feats.

Further evidence for the ability to change one's body through beliefs and visualizations can be found in reports of exceptional athletic accomplishments. When unusual athletic prowess is exhibited it is often associated with an ASC. The ASCs described by Murphy and White appear similar to, if not identical with, the mystical states described by meditators.[39] Common characteristics include a sense of being one with a higher sentience, or knowing in a profound way one's relationship with the world. This all seems to point to the existence of an alternate reality, which may overlap with the trans-dimensional realities that Lawrence LeShan associates with spiritual healing.[40] The ASC seems to enable people to alter their body's capabilities. Strength, speed, coordination and dexterity all seem to be enhanced. It is not clear whether the ASC is required before the physical feats can be accomplished or whether it is a result of the extraordinary performance. The former seems more likely, judging from the available reports.

When we change the ways in which we perceive and relate to the world, we apparently can alter our relationship with the world – including alterations in our body and its ways of functioning. Enhancing the body's physiological mechanisms during ASCs can improve abilities to recuperate from a variety of body dysfunctions, and by implication from various diseases as well. The athletics-ASC appears to include an anesthetic component, as it is well known that athletes may not feel pain *until after their performance* if they are injured during sports events. Reports of people who painlessly pierce their flesh with swords and needles indicate that the body can be prevented from responding to injury with pain and from becoming infected, and can mend itself very rapidly and completely. The parallels with spiritual healing are clear – our state of mind can profoundly influence our body functions.

I can add to these reports my own experiences in playing racquetball. I decided to apply relaxation exercises whenever I sustained an injury. Since racquetball is played at high speeds in a closed court, I often found myself bruised by balls that struck me with considerable force. So I decided that the next time a ball hit me, I would immediately pause, breathe deeply and tell myself to relax. I found that the pain went away almost instantly. There was redness at the place of impact, but there was very little subsequent discoloration, and what there was cleared up in two days – in contrast with the week or more that it had taken previously for such bruises to resolve.

I feel that the greatest part of my success (which was often repeated, with ever-increasing competence) derived from my conscious relaxation at the time of injury. I have asked myself whether perhaps the blows I sustained during this period were less severe than earlier ones, and in at least one case I can definitely state that this was not so. My partner unexpectedly turned and hit the ball toward the back wall instead of the front, a shot that requires extra force to rebound the ball to the front wall. The ball struck me a resounding blow on the cheek that stunned me and alarmed my partner. But after applying my (by then well-practiced) routine, I was able to relax and even joke about the unexpectedness of his move. The pain rapidly abated and I experienced no subsequent black-and-blue discoloration whatsoever.

The feats of the Sufis described in the Parmann Project may be an exception to the ASC hypothesis. It is possible that they represent rapidly induced ASCs, similar to rapidly induced hypnotic inductions. The statement by the South Seas fire-handler that he needed to be sure he was not hurting others before he could "be one with the fire" parallels the observations of Eastern mystics that the state aimed for in meditation is one of detachment from worldly concerns. Seemingly, in order to achieve such exceptional feats, some adepts must be totally absorbed in the task at hand, and unencumbered by even an unconscious hint of the nagging, unfinished business of the everyday, sensory-reality world.

Athletes echo this observation in another context, reporting that during peak athletic experiences they are completely absorbed in their actions. They are not thinking *about* what they are doing. They are *simply doing it*. Similarly, total absorption in a mental focus is probably a major contribution of meditation to the achievement of healing states. This absorption appears to facilitate and enhance the body's functions, be they physical action or self-healing.

A transpersonal component is also reported with peak experiences. There is a feeling of being one with the flow of whatever you are doing; being an integral part of a greater whole; or being aware of the scene as though you are viewing it in its entirety, rather than just from your own personal vantage point. This might be described as a sort of dance, in which the dancers are so much a part of the action that they seem to function as a unified organism.

> *O body swayed to music, O brightening glance,*
> *How can we know the dancer from the dance?*
> – W. B. Yeats

Athletes may even feel that they are somehow united with their sports equipment (such as a bow and arrow), or animal trainers with their horses or show dogs during competitive events, and that these interactions which reach beyond their physical boundaries are somehow extensions of themselves. Again we see parallels with spiritual healing experiences. One of the ways in which healers describe the healing state of awareness, as detailed by Lawrence LeShan, is that they become one with the healee and, at the same time, one with the All.

Many questions remain to be clarified, such as: What states of consciousness are most conducive to healing? Does the effectiveness of an ASC relate to the personality types (e.g. in regard to Jungian polarities and extraversion/ introversion)? Are mental images subject to enhancement through group inputs, as in group meditation or to increases in potency over time through Rupert Sheldrake's morphogenetic fields? Are there self-healing capabilities that can be conferred rapidly by particular adepts without the benefit of ASCs?[41] These questions invite us to explore further in the realms of self-healing and healer healing.

SPECIAL BRAIN AND BODY FUNCTIONS

> *In our efforts to explore human illness we have looked where the light is*
> *good. In some cases we have been fortunate enough to find valuable lost*
> *keys... But the problem in most diseases is that the key seems to be lost in*
> *many places at once, and the search leads us deeper into the dark where*
> *the chains of causation weaken and break.*
> – Larry Dossey 1982

Several special functions of the brain and body are helpful in understanding further aspects of healing. This section will briefly examine the perception of pain, special functions of the skin, and brain hemispheric functions.

Pain

> *Illness is the doctor to whom we pay most heed;*
> *to kindness, to knowledge we make promises only;*
> *to pain we obey.*
> – Marcel Proust

C. Norman Shealy, reviewing the *Nuprin Pain Report* – a survey of pain in the

US in persons aged 18 and older – notes that in the course of a year 73% of the general population had one or more headaches; 56% had backaches; 51% had joint pain; 46% had stomach pain; 40% had menstrual pain; and 27% had dental pain. An estimated four billion workdays were lost annually, for an average of 23 days per person per year.[42] While pain is generally treated as a physical problem, we shall see that is an enormously complex phenomenon.

Perception of physical pain is not a simple process, since many factors are involved. These fall into three broad categories defined according to the physical origins of the pain the degree of sensitivity to pain and spiritual factors related to pain.

1. Pain perception is initiated by stimulation of nerve endings in the various organs of the body. Sources of stimulation can include:

a) mechanical factors – trauma ranging from chronic external pressure to acute blows or cuts; internal trauma from heavy use of the musculoskeletal system beyond its natural capacities; and swelling or other deformity of organs and tissues from factors such as edema (excessive body fluid), infection, and direct trauma to nerves;

b) chemical or metabolic factors – caustic external substances or toxins that damage tissues or cause muscle spasms; and accumulations of physiological toxins within the body;

c) thermal or electromagnetic stimulation – reactions range from unpleasant sensations, through muscle spasms, to coagulation of tissues;

d) *infections* – direct inflammation of nerves or indirect pain via swelling of tissues and organs;

e) neoplastic – tumors with invasions of tissues and nerves, or indirect pain via swelling of, or encroachment upon, tissues and organs, especially nerves and bones;

f) degenerative factors – wearing out of tissues and articulating surfaces, with pain felt as the body "complains" about overuse;

g) immune system responses – swelling or inflammation of tissues because of allergic reactions that produce inflammation (rheumatoid arthritis is included here because it is thought to be caused by the body's allergic reaction to parts of itself, as though they were foreign intruders);

h) neurophysiological factors – malfunctions of the nervous system, leading to tension in muscles, which eventually tire or spasm, producing pain, which in turn creates the vicious circle considered previously; and

i) psychological factors – muscle spasms resulting from tension or conditioned responses; metaphors for emotional problems; and *phantom limb* phenomena following amputations. This category is given a finer analysis in the following section.

2. Pain perception is more than a simple chain of cause and effect relationships. One person may have little reaction to a given pain stimulus, while another may writhe in agony under the (apparently) same stimulus or condition. Psychological factors influencing pain perception may involve:

a) innate differences in pain thresholds – one person may have less or more sensitivity to certain stimuli than another;

b) general state of the nervous system (whether affected by tiredness, stress, anxieties, or other psychological factors) – this may relate to altered sensitivity thresholds, or to the amounts of emotional and biological energies a person has for coping with the added stress of pain;

c) specific psychological factors – for example, people may tolerate post-surgical pain well if they know that the operation has resulted in a cure of their illness, or they may tolerate the same pain poorly if they hear that the surgery brought only a diagnosis of incurable disease;

d) cultural conditionings – which teach a person to be stoic or vociferous in dealing with pain;

e) attention factors – in the height of an emergency or exciting situation (accident, sports event), while engrossed in achieving an immediate objective, a person might not feel a pain despite a severe injury. Only later, when attention is focused on the wound, is pain perceived. People who have a goal to work toward may focus all their attention on this and even deliberately ignore their pain, subsequently finding that they also feel the pain less;

f) mood factors – may influence responsivity to pain (anxiety and depression may increase pain, tranquility and joy decrease it);

g) rewards associated with the expression of pain – may influence the frequency of its occurrence and the severity of its expression.

A person who unconsciously enjoys some benefit (secondary gain) from a pain, such as avoidance of unpleasant tasks or extra attention from family members, is likely to experience more pain. People who anticipate compensation following accidents are likely to relinquish their pains slowly, if at all.

> *I enjoy convalescence. It is the part that makes illness worth while.*
> – George Bernard Shaw (1921)

h. phantom limb phenomena – persistence of perceptions in a part of the body (e.g. limb, breast) that has been amputated, often with pains that are experienced as though the limb were still present. Paraplegics may have phantom limb pain, even when their spinal cords have been severed so that no ordinary sensations are felt from beyond the level of the nerves that were cut. Similarly, phantom limb sensations are reported in people with congenital absence of limbs; and

i. fantasy pains – sensations seemingly created by the mind, where no objective causes can be identified. These are essentially body metaphors for anxieties, emotions and traumatic experiences.

3. Transpersonal or spiritual awarenesses may contribute to how we experience and comprehend our pains.

a. Pain may be a stimulus for us to pray, or to question why we are suffering, and to ask God for help in understanding and dealing with our injury or illness. At the very least, pain may be the unconscious mind's way of forcing us to take a break from stresses or lifestyles that are in some way harmful.

Many people who have serious health issues come to feel that their illness led them to re-examine their lives, and to make enormously enriching decisions for better relationships and more emotionally satisfying and rewarding careers, not to mention healthier lifestyles. This life-transforming process may come as a response to the physical challenges that force us to face our mortality and ask questions about the meaning of life.

b. We may come to feel a spiritual causality that underlies and guides major life challenges, sensing that we might have been deliberately invited or pushed into such experiences by our higher self, by spirit or angelic guides, or by the Infinite Source – as a way of deepening our spiritual quest in life. Pain may be related to lessons chosen by our higher self or soul for our spiritual growth. When we are free of pain we tend to be complacent, and coast along, enjoying life but not learning very much. When we are in pain we are challenged to find new solutions to our problems, to plumb the depths of our being, and to push beyond the limits of our ordinary capabilities and awarenesses.

> *We are not human beings having a spiritual experience, but spiritual beings having a human experience.*
>
> – Pierre Teilhard de Chardin

c. Pain may be a residual from a previous incarnation, which invites us to explore this dimension of our existence and to resolve ancient emotional scars.[43]

Assessments of pain

Clinicians do not agree on methods for the assessment of pain. Pain is a completely subjective experience, and there is no direct, objective way to measure it. Subjective evaluations rely on people's self-assessments, which may be as varied as human experience itself. Stoics and people with apparently high thresholds for experiencing pain may report minimal discomfort from injuries and stresses that others may find very painful, either because they have low pain thresholds or because of characterological or habitual emotional intensity – as listed at the start of this discussion on pain.

Cultural factors may play a role here. During my medical training I was challenged by the differences in apparent pain tolerance of Caucasian, Black and Hispanic women who were in labor. The Hispanic women would moan and scream with pain much more than the Caucasian or Black women. My initial impulse was to prescribe more pain medicine. The nurses, who had worked in the delivery room for a good while longer than myself, cautioned me against this. Pain medicine can often be sedating and can prolong labor if given injudiciously. Assessment of pain by anyone other than the people who are themselves experiencing it is therefore fraught with potential inaccuracies due to cross-cultural differences.

Serial assessments of pain with standardized testing instruments, in which people serve as their own controls for several treatment interventions, would appear to offer the best approach for testing treatments for pain. In this way one can have some degree of assurance that a change in the test response represents a real difference in pain levels related to a treatment given, rather than to differences between various people's responses to pain.

Two types of pain assessment are in common use. The first relies on standardized self-assessment questionnaires that have been given to many people in order to derive standardized norms for responses. With this method, researchers get a rough idea of the intensity of pain levels reported by subjects in a given study. This assumes that there are no cultural or other differences between the standardization groups and the experimental study subjects that might make the standardization irrelevant to the study group.

Another test of this type is the Visual Analogue Scale (VAS). The VAS requires that people put a mark on a line of standard length (commonly 10 cm), where one end of the line represents no pain and the other end "the worst possible pain." It has been shown that this test is generally as reliable as any other pain assessment. The advantage of the VAS is that is very quickly administered and scored, compared to other types of tests.

The second approach is to measure objective body variables that tend to parallel the subjective experience of pain, such as muscle tension and skin resistance. Although these provide objective measurements, they are not all strictly related to pain, and may be influenced by other factors – such as anxiety, muscle strain, tiredness, and the like.

There is thus no measure of physical pain that is both direct, entirely reliable and free of confounding influences. My personal impression is that the VAS is as good as any of the available methods, and by far the easiest to use.

Even more difficult to assess is emotional pain. A Visual Analogue Scale can readily be used for tracking pain in individuals, but comparing emotional pain between different people is fraught with problems.

> *Why is it that I'm most aware of my body only when it's not working properly?*
>
>   – Ashleigh Brilliant

The conventional medical view is that pain is usually a symptom of physical dysfunction. The physiological cause(s) of the pain, per the list above, must therefore be identified and treated in order to relieve or eliminate the pain. When specific physical causes for the pain cannot be identified, or when the pain does not respond to pain medications, many doctors raise their hands in surrender and refer the patient to a psychotherapist.

With luck, the patient may find a therapist who knows to ask, "What is your pain saying?" Often the answers lie in emotional conflicts that produce chronic tensions in the body, which end up being expressed as pain. In such situations, the pain is acting as a call from the unconscious mind, to bring attention to those factors that are producing chronic tensions. Often, the mind-body connection for the pain is metaphoric, as described above. Michael Greenwood points out that pain may be a doorway into places where the ego doesn't normally want to go. It can be a way for the unconscious mind to speak to us through our bodies, to insist that we attend to dis-ease in our emotional, relational or spiritual life before chronic tensions result in disease that could gallop out of control in our physical body.

When a wholistic therapist can help us find the inner meanings of our symptoms, we can also find the reins which enable us to regain control and redirect our lives. The responsibility of the therapist is to guide people to identify the causes of their own pains.

... Physicians are released from the need to pretend they know what to do, or to diagnose and treat what they cannot entirely understand – and patients can reclaim their own authority and learn to honour their own intuitions and hunches. Both are freed to follow whatever direction seems appropriate to the needs of the moment; and at that point, true healing can begin.

– Michael Greenwood 1998 (p. 55)

Pain and CAM therapies

Sickness and disease are in weak minds the sources of melancholy; but that which is painful to the body, may be profitable to the soul. Sickness puts us in mind of our mortality, and, while we drive on heedlessly in the full career of worldly pomp and jollity, kindly pulls us by the ear, and brings us to a proper sense of our duty.

– Richard E. Burton

Acupuncture is well known and well researched as a treatment for pain relief.

While no research has been published as yet on self-healing for pain through acupressure techniques, there is a wealth of clinical literature supporting this modality. My personal experience in helping people to deal with pain using one of these approaches, WHEE,[44] has convinced me of its effectiveness.

CASE 1: A psychiatric resident came to work one day with that look on her face which said, "No loud noises, please, and no bright lights! I'm having a serious migraine attack." After a weekend in bed, with all of her migraine and pain medications, she estimated the severity of pain was still at a level of "8" out of a possible worst level of pain at "10." Within three minutes of tapping on acupressure points, while reciting a simple affirmation, her pain was down to a much more tolerable "3."

CASE 2: A secretary in the clinic where I worked was hobbling around with pain in both knees due to osteoarthritis. She had suffered these knee pains for 17 years, and when I offered to help her, the pain was at a level of "7." Within 10 minutes of using WHEE, the pain was down to a "2."

Spiritual healing is especially effective in relieving the physical pain that is experienced with acute and chronic conditions.

Healers report anecdotally that pains of every sort respond well to healing. Controlled studies have shown that spiritual healing is effective for tension headache and backache. Healing can prolong the time between doses of pain medication required after surgery; but it does not seem to be as good as standard pain medications for postoperative pain.

My impression is that the easing of pain by healers is attributable both to spiritual healing and to suggestion, but that healing is actually the more potent factor. Many anecdotal reports are available of patients who respond to spiritual healing after suffering from chronic, severe pains due to objectively verifiable illnesses, when previously obtained no relief from many medicinal, physical and psycho-therapeutic treatments over long periods of time. These patients should have experienced some reductions in pain from the conventional measures if they were amenable to relief of pain via suggestion. However, their subsequent response to a healer could still be due to special rapport, particular expectations, or other factors of suggestion that might have been present in the spiritual healing situations.

Chronic pain is a problem in and of itself, but it also has secondary effects. It is physically and emotionally draining, and often produces depression. When pain is a manifestation of serious illness, such as cancer, it can also raise anxieties and fears about death. Spiritual healing can help with these secondary problems.

It is not death or pain that is to be feared, but the fear of pain or death.
– Epictectus

Eric Leskowitz found that phantom limb pain responds to healing, where no other conventional techniques have helped.

From the above it is obvious that one cannot easily evaluate healees' responses to a healer in terms of what happens to their physical pain. Diverse factors may cause either increases or decreases in pain. Only through studying numerous similar cases of painful conditions treated by healers, including experimental and control groups, can one hope to arrive at some assessment regarding the effectiveness and efficacy of healing in treating pain. For instance, it would be helpful to have a study of hypnosis compared with spiritual healing, for surgical pain.

Anecdotal reports abound on the benefits of spiritual healing in the treatment of emotional pain. Formal studies show that Therapeutic Touch was helpful in alleviating post-traumatic stress following Hurricane Hugo in the US and that SHEN therapy was helpful for families of victims of a school massacre in Ireland. My personal experience as a psychotherapist and healer is that healing eases emotional pains dramatically.

Perspectives of healers regarding both physical and emotional pain may differ considerably from those of allopathic medical practitioners and conventional psychotherapists. Within the belief system of many healers, pain may be viewed as one of life's most valued lessons.[45]

Suffering presents us with a challenge: to find goals and purpose in our lives that make even the situation worth living through.
– Victor Frankl

Pain calls us to examine what is out of harmony and therefore producing tension in our lives. In my practice of psychotherapy combined with spiritual healing, I find that the healing encounter may facilitate identification of sources of distress underlying pain. Psychotherapy then helps to sort out solutions to the emotional conflicts.

Pain (and illness in general) may also cause us to pause and ask what we are doing with our life, or to consider what life is all about. In doing so, we may be able to connect with our personal spiritual awareness. Ram Dass observes that all acts of healing are ultimately our selves healing our higher Self.[46]

Sometimes physical pain has known causes, but may be unresponsive to physical, psychological, and healing interventions. Certain injuries, as well as neurological, degenerative and cancerous causes for pain, have no cure. Here, spiritual healing can be a great help in palliating and learning to live with the pain.

To some readers, much of the above may seem far-fetched. It may challenge your belief systems to consider that your body may speak to you through pain and other symptoms.

Others may feel blamed if someone asks them what their unconscious mind is saying through their pain (or other symptoms) – interpreting the questions as accusations that they are *imagining* the pain. Doctors may unwittingly precipitate such feelings when no physical cause can be found for pain, and they therefore suggest psychological counseling.

> *There was a faith healer of Deal,*
> *Who said, "Although pain isn't real,*
> *If I sit on a pin*
> *And it punctures my skin*
> *I dislike what I fancy I feel!"*
> – Anonymous

Pain, whatever the cause, is always real but even when the primary cause is clearly physical, psychological components may contribute to perpetuating or worsening the pain, or can influence the way we respond to it. Counseling can uncover such factors and can relieve the pain or help us manage it.

In my personal experience and in the lives of many I have met – both as friends and as clients – I have found that pain can deepen our appreciation for life. It certainly heightens our empathy for others who are in pain and distress.

> *Your heart is not living until it has experienced pain...*
> – Hazrat Inayat Khan

Special skin functions

The skin may serve as far more than just a barrier between people and their environments, or a simple sensory organ. It is also an important interface for communicating with others.

Touch is an extremely potent mode of communication, though relatively little research has been done in this area. Caressing and soft touch are important to the normal development of infants, although studies on humans have not been conducted to differentiate this single factor from social attention in general. Studies with apes indicate that touch is vital to normal development. Apes raised without a soft surface to cuddle up to will become psychologically disturbed.[47]

> *The greatest sense in our body is our touch sense. It is probably the chief sense in the process of sleeping and waking; it gives us our knowledge of depth or thickness and form; we feel, we love and hate, are touchy and are touched, through the touch corpuscles of our skin.*
> – J. Lionel Taylor

Many psychotherapists comment on how good people feel when they are touched. Massage and aromatherapy are among the most popular of complementary therapies. The nonverbal message of interpersonal openness, acceptance and caring conveyed by touch has a potent effect on clients. Their perception of the therapist is altered from that of a distant, analytical, uninvolved professional to one of a caring, compassionate and accessible person.

This observation has also been successfully applied by salespersons and others for whom making contact is important. It is well known that even a casual contact by touch between a salesperson and customers will significantly increase the number of sales.

It is very sad that the fear of being sued for sexually inappropriate behavior has led legislators in many states to rule that touching must be prohibited in the psychotherapeutic encounter.

Touch, skin sensitivity and spiritual healing

One possible mechanism whereby laying-on of hands healing may be effective is simply through the power of touch, unrelated to spiritual healing. Conversely, part of the potency of touch may reside in spiritual healing effects, which may occur even without the conscious knowledge or intention of the practitioner.

Studying the skin may contribute further to our understanding of healing. Sensations experienced by healers and healees during touch and distant healings have not been explained. These include sensations of heat, cold, tingling, "electricity-feeling," vibrations and others. The skin may actually have special sensory receptors for healing energies. Moreover, the skin could conceivably emit such energies.

Cases of paranormal perception of color via the skin, commonly termed *dermal-vision*, have been reported over the past two decades. Subjects typically describe the color of an object without receiving any visual cues, when the object is either touching or merely close to their skin. With practice they can even identify various sensations that they associate with different colors. Red may be "stickier" than blue, or yellow may be "rougher" than another color. Lab tests of abilities to identify colors by this method have shown significant results. Some people have even achieved sufficient sensitivity to be able to read large letters using their skin as the sole sensor.

Yvonne Duplessis took this research a step further. She found that subjects could identify colors from several feet above the colored target. Different colors appeared to radiate to different heights, and the relative heights differed consistently according to whether the testing was done in daylight or artificial light. Even more interesting, *wood and metal sheets interposed above the targets did not block or alter the sensations or the heights at which they could be perceived.*

These dermal perceptions are considered *synesthesias,* or cross-sensory perceptions. Colored light impinging on the skin probably stimulates nerve endings that are normally used for sensing touch. When the light rays are perceived by the skin sensors, they are translated by the brain into perceptions that are familiar from previous sensations under other types of stimuli. Subjects who feel the light on their skin use the "vocabulary" of touch to describe the light, because that is the range of sensations they are used to receiving and interpreting through their skin.

Another explanation for dermal vision is that in the embryo stage of development, the ectoderm (outer cell layer) is the origin for neural and sensory organs as well as for skin. The skin may therefore possess latent sensory abilities usually thought to reside only in the specialized sense organs (e.g. eyes, ears) which originated during their development in the embryonic skin.

This may explain feelings of heat, cold, tingling and "color" reported by healers and healees during healing. The skin may be stimulated by healing energies, but the brain may be interpreting the stimulation in its more familiar vocabulary of touch sensations, as with dermal optics.

A spiritual dimension to dermal optics was reported by Si-Chen Lee and colleagues in Taiwan. They found that children between 6 and 13 years old can be trained in finger-reading. These children could identify complex Chinese ideograms and reproduce them with great accuracy.

Using sophisticated measuring devices, they found that blood flow to certain parts of the brain as well as electroencephalogram patterns shifted at the time their best subject reported she was perceiving the images through her fingers.

They were surprised to find that "when certain special words related to religion - such as Buddha, Bodhisattva, or Jesus (in Chinese), 'I am that I am' (in Hebrew, meaning God) - were presented for finger-reading, these youngsters saw extraordinary phenomena, including bright light, a bright and smiling person, a temple, the Christian cross, or heard the sound of laughter. These responses are completely different from responses to other, ordinary, non-religious words." If the spiritual words were in separate pieces (e.g. "Bud" and "dha"), the children read the characters alone and did not identify these as spiritual names.

Viktor Adamenko, a former Russian researcher now living in Greece, goes much further in speculating on possible properties of the skin. He suggests that the skin may act as an antenna. This hypothesis might explain the following reports:

> 1. People have claimed that they heard peculiar sounds or smelled a sulphurous odor prior to the arrival of meteorites.
> 2. High-frequency transmitters can produce auditory sensations of humming, whistling, or crackling, at frequencies that are clearly outside the range of normal hearing. The frequencies of 425, 1310 and 2982 megacycles seem particularly likely to produce such effects.

Adamenko feels that smell may be dependent on the resonation of molecules. Minute vibratory "sounds" may be what we sense, rather than particular configurations of molecules acting via chemical stimulation of sensory nerve endings in the skin of the nasal mucosa. If one part of the skin is sensitive to such electromagnetic resonation, the rest of the skin may be similarly sensitive.

He further suggests that the perception of sounds associated with meteorites may be due to low-frequency oscillations produced by the meteorites. This hypothesis is supported by the following unusual experiment, reported by Adamenko:

> If two subjects tightly grasp wires connected to a radio receiver which has no loudspeakers, and lean ear to ear, they can hear music and words picked up by the receiver. Each subject's eardrums apparently function as a loud-

speaker for the other because of the low-frequency current picked up via the wires. If the two subjects hold hands, the sound disappears. The human body appears to function to some degree as a radio receiver.

Sound and spiritual healing

Certain kinds of sound can produce healing effects. Lu Yan Fang Ph.D., of the National Electro-Acoustics Laboratory in China, recorded infrasonic sound emitted from the hands of qigong masters[48] during external qi healings. She was able to produce healing effects with synthetic infrasonic sound at similar frequencies, and reported benefits for pain, circulatory disturbances and depression. On the basis of these explorations, the infrasonic emitting machine is now being studied in America.

The frequency emitted by this machine is similar to that of alpha brain waves. This suggests that infrasonic sound emitted by the healer may be an active force in bringing about changes in nervous system activity. It would be of great interest to determine how the healer emits the infrasonic sound.

It is still too early to know whether infrasonic sound conveys the full effect of spiritual healing. Anecdotal reports that I have heard indicate that only partial healing can be achieved with devices that produce infrasonic sound. My expectation is that the human instrument is far more subtle and potent than any mechanical substitute.

I would also question whether the infrasonic devices act purely in and of themselves, or whether they might be variations on radionics devices (instruments which project healing without emitting any known form of radiation), and are known to produce effects that are linked to the operators of the devices. That is, the radionics devices seem to amplify the healing powers of the operators, projecting them to any location around the globe. Clearly, infrasonic waves could not project healing effects at a distance of more than a few yards, so they cannot provide the sole vehicle for the entire range of known and scientifically demonstrated healing effects.

Various reports hint that parts of the skin may be involved in complex interactions with sound. An article in the journal *Brain/Mind* (1983, V.8) discusses a discovery in the field of audio recording called *holophonic sound*. Developed by the Italian scientist H. Zuccarelli, this method includes a reference tone along with the recorded sounds, so that an interference pattern is created in sound waves. This seems to add extra dimensions to recorded sound, making it appear more realistic. Listeners report that they can sense a directionality in such recordings that far exceeds the quality of stereophonic recordings. Subsequent investigations have demonstrated that *the ear emits a tone that seems to function as a reference tone for itself.*

A report by Walter and Mary Jo Uphoff indicates that during *thoughtography* (the production of pictures on film via psychokinesis),[49] sound waves are sometimes detectable emanating from the head of the subjects. This was a serendipitous observation made by scientists who were investigating a Japanese youth, *Masuaki Kiyota*. The scientists were looking for radioactive emission from his body, to explain his ability to produce pictures on film that was shielded by metal. They did not find any evidence of such radiation, but their microphones picked up an unexplained noise during taping of the experimental sessions. Subsequent investigations showed that the sounds were in the vicinity of 30-34.5 megahertz, that they occurred only during periods when Kiyota was concentrating in order to produce PK phenomena, and that they appeared to originate in the left frontal lobe of his brain.

Theories to account for the production of sounds from ear and brain have not yet been proposed. Nevertheless, the discovery of this phenomenon opens up further possibilities for investigating the means by which a healer may influence a subject, particularly in view of the evidence for energy fields or energy bodies surrounding the physical body. Healers may influence healees' biological energy fields via such emissions. The healees' adjusted energy fields could in turn influence their physical conditions, resulting in healing effects.[50]

BRAIN HEMISPHERIC FUNCTIONS

Widespread investigations are currently being conducted to clarify the distinctly different functions of the right and left hemispheres of the brain. (In this discussion, the subjects studied are assumed to be right-handed. For left-handed people, the brain hemispheres involved in various functions may be reversed to varying degrees.) Experiments have shown that the functions of analytical, logical, intellectual thinking and expression of language are carried out in the brain's left hemisphere. The right hemisphere of the brain performs intuitive, artistic, symbolic and analogical thinking functions. (See Table II-4.)

Every 90-120 minutes the dominant activity in the brain hemispheres alternates from one side to the other. Although Eastern meditation experts have known of these shifts for millennia, Western science has only recently become aware of them. When hemispheric functions are predominating on a particular side, the nasal passage on the opposite side is markedly more open. That is, when your left nostril is open, your right hemisphere is "in gear," and conversely for the opposite nostril and hemisphere. This is called the *ultradian rhythm* of the brain.

Our brains tend to focus primarily on one hemispheric mode or the other when we are engaged in a specific task, and we tend to have characterological preferences for one or the other mode of functioning. We are all familiar with extremes of such types – for instance, the typical left-brain character is unemotional, logical, and always analyzing what is going on. These are people who have difficulty answering when asked what they are feeling about a given situation, and they are commonly accountants or scientists by profession. Their right-brain preference counterparts, the emotional, intuitive, impressionistic folk, are commonly poets or artists who may have problems dealing with facts and figures.

Thank God for making reality, and for giving us means of escaping from it.
– Ashleigh Brilliant

Fredric Schiffer, a psychiatrist at Harvard University, has explored simple ways in which to identify for yourself whether you have strongly divided functions

Table II-4. Brain Hemispheric Functions

Left	Right
Rational/ Logic/ Cognition	Intuitive/ Emotion/ Feeling
Differential	Existential
Detail-oriented/ absorbed	Gestalt-oriented, bored
Time sense (past, present, future)	Present-oriented
Paced by rules (acts with time awareness)	Impulsive (acts on present awareness)
Directed/ controlled by rules	Spontaneous
Bound	Expansive
Aims/ Goals oriented/ Planned progress	Instant gratification/ Impatient
Cautious/ Inhibited	Over-reacting
Product	Process
Temporal/ Partializing	Spatial/ Wholistic
Sequential aspects of math (e.g. algebra)	Spatial aspects of math (e.g. geometry)
Sequential (slow)	Parallel (fast)
Discrete	Continuous
Successive (either/ or)	Simultaneous (both/ and)
Focal	Diffuse
Explicit	Tacit
Objective	Subjective
Convergent approach	Divergent approach
Conscious	Unconscious
Language comprehension abstract	Language comprehension concrete
Speech content	Voice intonation
Rhythm	Melody, pitch
Linguistic	Pantomime, kinesthetic, musical
Grammatical	Visuo-spatial
Abstract models	Perceptual-synthetic
Synthesis	Creativity
Relatively narrow arousal level range over which hemisphere can function	Relatively wide arousal level range over which hemisphere can function
Evolutionarily newer	Evolutionarily older

Adapted from: Thomas H. Budzynski 1986.

between your left and right brain hemispheres. Think about a problem or memory that disturbs you (with feelings of hurt, anger, or remorse, etc.). Now, use your right palm to completely cover your right eye, and your left palm to cover all but a little of the ear-side of your left eye. This will allow a little light in from the left side of your left eye, which will stimulate and activate your right hemisphere. Spend a few moments exploring your feelings regarding the issue you have chosen to focus on. Then reverse the process and cover your left eye entirely, leaving only a little of the ear-side of your right eye uncovered, and spend a few minutes exploring how you feel about the same issue.

About 60 percent of people will notice a distinct difference, sometimes quite a strong one, between the responses of their right and left hemispheres to this type of stimulation while focusing on an emotionally distressing issue. For most, the left, thinking hemisphere is more rational and can sort out how to deal with the issue, while the right brain tends to be emotional, and when it is activated, they may feel quite upset about the issue. [51]

Schiffer finds that some people he sees in psychotherapy have distinct personalities that are evoked when the left and right brain hemispheres are stimulated. In some of his clients there is a very wounded, angry, immature, self-destructive personality that is more often evoked by stimulating the right brain, and a more mature, composed, rational, constructive personality, evoked in the left brain. This knowledge can allow the therapist to selectively access the wounded personality and thus facilitate releases of psychological traumas. The constructive personality is encouraged to provide support and control over the life of a person who may otherwise be dominated by the emotions of her wounded side, and may therefore be self-destructive.

CASE: Schiffer gives the example of "Harold," a brilliant newspaper reporter in his fifties, who was extremely ambivalent about his relationship with his girlfriend. Harold's mother had had unrealistic expectations of him in his childhood, and rejected him when he could not satisfy her need for him to bring her vicarious glory through successes that were beyond his abilities. In his right brain hemisphere, Harold carried severe hurts from this experience. In therapy he was able to identify what he called his immature self, which constantly anticipated rejections like he had experienced from his mother. These feelings were particularly strong whenever he was close with his girlfriend. Schiffer was able to help Harold strengthen his mature self and release the hurts of the immature self, so that Harold was no longer living in the past. Harold went on to overcome his doubts and fears that his girlfriend might hurt him in the same way as his mother had.

Schiffer patented special eyeglasses with shaded tinting from right to left, which can stimulate the appropriate brain hemisphere to activate the more constructive personality, and promote its healing contribution to the patient's life. You can make a simpler version of these glasses with two pairs of safety goggles and some duct tape. (See exercise in Chapter 5.)

Daniel Goleman's bestseller, *Emotional Intelligence*, points out how Western society has emphasized left-brain functions to such a degree that right-brain functions are now given far less importance. He argues persuasively that right-brained, intuitive and feeling awarenesses are vital to the development of our self-image, and may often be more accurate in assessing social and relational situations. This book is very highly recommended reading for anyone who is interested in this subject.

Not all researchers agree about the importance of right/left brain function distinctions. For instance, some point out that while artistic functions might be initiated in the right hemisphere, verbal expressions of creativity involve the left hemisphere as well. These criticisms do not invalidate the observations of discrete right and left brain functions, which are distinguishable, but may sometimes act in synchrony or harmony with each other, and at other times may conflict.

> *We should be passionate about our profession, and professional about our passion.*
> – M. Leon Seard II

Eye Movement Desensitization and Reprocessing (EMDR), developed by Francine Shapiro, a Californian psychologist, is a new psychotherapeutic approach that appears to be related to the integration of right and left hemispheric activities. EMDR is an extremely potent method for treating stress disorders. In classical EMDR therapy people are instructed to focus upon their negative experiences, negative feelings and self-critical beliefs about themselves, while moving their eyes rhythmically from left to right and back a number of times. For reasons that have not as yet been explained, the negative feelings attached to the traumatic memories diminish within minutes. When the negative feelings have been dissipated, positive feelings and affirmations are implanted and enhanced using the same technique.

It is hypothesized that in EMDR, the back and forth eye movements help to integrate the thinking and feeling aspects of our experiences. This may be similar to what happens during dreams when we have rapid eye movements (REM). It has been postulated that REM periods during sleep reflect the integration of recent and long-term memory. Perhaps EMDR will further clarify the function of REM.

People with the most severe emotional post-traumatic stress disorders (PTSD) deriving from horrendous war experiences or rape, as well as people with lesser stress reactions, have been helped by EMDR.

Following the initial development of EMDR, it was found that alternating stimulation of the right and left sides of the body by touch and sound could produce the same effects. A common way to do this is to pat your hands on right and left thigh as you sit in a chair, or to fold your arms and alternate patting each bicep. (The latter has been called the *butterfly hug*.) This is particularly helpful for people who experience nausea, similar to seasickness, from moving their eyes back and forth. It is also helpful in treating children, for whom the touch aspect of the butterfly hug is self-comforting and a helpful form of self-healing.

I have explored this method with my psychotherapy/ healing clients and with my own personal stresses and painful past experiences. The rapidity and thoroughness of the clearing of negativity and acceptance of positivity is astounding. I have helped many clients achieve major transformations in their fears and emotional defenses within minutes.

The curious paradox is that when I accept myself just as I am, then I can change.

– Carl Rogers

When EMDR is used alone, there can be intense releases of emotions which may have been buried for many years. For this reason, it is strongly advised that you use EMDR only in a therapist's office and not on your own.

I have developed a hybrid of EMDR and another self-healing approach, *Emotional Freedom Technique (EFT)* – described in Chapter II-2. This method does not produce intense emotional releases and is safe to use on your own. (See WHEE experiential exercises based in Chapter 5.)

Laural Parnell finds that during the course of EMDR treatment clients may have transpersonal and psychic experiences, opening their minds into creativity and deeper awarenesses of love, forgiveness, and enlightenment.

I have also encountered similar transpersonal awakenings in my practice with EMDR, and now with WHEE. I was pleasantly surprised to find that in addition to helping people release chronic anxieties, phobias, poor self images and the like, WHEE brings about an incredible feeling of calmness. In some people this sensation is so profound that it is unsettling, because they have not known such peace for as long as they can recall. In addition, as people reach a deep state of acceptance of themselves and of others, they may feel a spiritual opening – a profound sense of knowing that they are okay, lovable, free of sin/ guilt, and in touch with the Infinite in a personal way.

Brain and body laterality and spiritual healing
The tendency for one side of the brain, connected with the opposite side of the body, to process and express different sets of functions is referred to as brain and body laterality. There are several different ways in which this may relate to spiritual healing.

For one thing, there appear to be projections of the qualities of brain laterality to the body. Intuitives report that the right side of the body expresses masculine energy, and the left side of the body feminine energy. The right side of the body is linked to the left brain, whose functions are specialized in linear thinking. Linear thinking is more characteristic of men than of women. Conversely, intuitive and feeling expressions, more common in women, are functions of the right brain. The right brain links to the left side of the body, hence the association of the left side with feminine characteristics.

Mona Lisa Schulz, a neurologist with very strong intuitive gifts, reviews fascinating research to support such divisions of the two sides of the body into masculine and feminine functions. For instance, in hermaphrodites, (people who have dual sexual characteristics), the male sexual organs are usually found on the right, while the female organs are on the left. The right testis generally develops first, whereas it is the left ovary that is the first to develop. Bowel cancers develop in men more often on the left side and in women more often on the right. Premenopausal women who are right-handed get breast cancers more often on the left, while postmenopausal women are more prone to cancers on the right. Women who are left-handed have the opposite frequencies. Schulz notes that pre-

menopausal women are more involved with nurturing activities of raising families, and nurturing is more associated with the emotional, right side of the brain

You can do a simple exercise that may help you to perceive your own right and
left brain modalities. See the procedure suggested by Schiffer, above, for stimulation of right and left sides of the brain while thinking of a problem that upsets
you. (The exercise is detailed in Chapter 5.)

Psi abilities may also be linked with right brain functions, because they are more
likely to occur in nonlinear states of consciousness.[52] They are often experienced
as intuitive perceptions. Researchers are still debating the interpretations of their
studies of psi and laterality.

Western society has overemphasized left brain thinking as the "correct" or
"proper" way to analyze situations and to function in the world, and as the only
road to success – particularly through linear achievements on tests and in employment. At the same time we discount intuitive functions, relegating them to
"less serious" activities such as leisure-time artistic pursuits. These functions are
seen as "unscientific" or un*reason*able. (Clear left brain language biases.)[53]

We ought to learn to become human beings rather than human doings.
                                                      – Anonymous

Notwithstanding the historical reasons behind this tradition,[54] the fact remains
that most of us who are raised in Western cultures have deeply ingrained habits
and prejudices toward left brain functions and against right brain ones. This may
help to explain why psi powers seem so alien to us. It may also be why spontaneous expressions of psi abilities are less commonly reported in a Western context
than in non-Western cultures. Eastern teachings emphasize intuitive, holistic
modes of perceiving the world. In some cultures this awareness has been carried
to the opposite extreme. Meditative contemplation and passive receptivity have
been stressed to the neglect of logical, linear thinking and planning.

This Eastern approach has produced a wealth of information about inner states
and spiritual development, but it has been at the cultural expense of inertia and
apparent ineptness – by Western standards – in dealing with material problems.
However, one aspect that is overlooked in these analyses through Western eyes is
that many of the non-industrialized, intuitive-sensitive cultures live in harmony
with their environments. Though they are subject to the vagaries of weather and
availability of food supplies, prior to being "modernized" they do not despoil
their worlds through excesses of exploitation and control.

What seems both logically and intuitively reasonable is that human beings
should develop a balance between their hemispheric functions, both in terms of
their inner world and in terms of their interaction with the environment.

*In a strange way, analog associations are never wrong: they are just
nearer or farther from the central truth, as though accuracy moves in resonant rings of propinquity that can get warped when too far from the center.
To notice analogs and heed them accurately, one must true up the inner
gyroscope and walk into the echoing halls of intuition toward a central
truth along the resonant labyrinth of the right brain hologram. Seeking*

truth in here is scary for those who shun dreams, neglect their dark side, disown shadow. But the analog domain can become rich and beautiful, a place of inspiration and creation. Its analog richness, however, should always be examined and paralleled against the left brain's logic, to see whether the whole is split and divided against itself... or if its view of reality is congruent and harmonious.

– Katya Walter (p. 174)

Recent research suggests that healing is correlated with an integration of both hemispheric functions. The work of Maxwell Cade and Geoffrey Blundell on the *mind mirror* has demonstrated that effective healers show symmetrical patterns of EEG (brain wave) activity during healings. Some even are able to maintain this balance while engaged in casual conversation and other activities unrelated to healing. This lends support to speculations that brain hemispheric synchronization is relevant to healing ability. It was also found that EEG frequency patterns of the healer and the healee would occasionally synchronize during healings, but it is unclear whether this is related to hemispheric synchronization within the same person.

Mind mirror studies of yoga and meditation adepts, along with studies of people who are successful in their chosen careers, also show a balanced hemispheric pattern. Meditation may be one method for bringing the brain hemispheres into synchronous activity. This state may reflect a more comprehensive mode of brain function, and this may explain why people who are able to activate both hemispheres simultaneously are able to do things that others, who are limited to a single primary hemispheric mode, cannot do.

Further research is needed to clarify these early observations and speculations.

SELF-HEALING PROGRAMS

Every day, in every way, I am getting better and better.
– Emile Coué

There is a plethora of self-help approaches available for treating and curing one's own disease and dis-ease. Some of these primarily involve attitudinal changes. If you attend more to positive developments than to negative ones, in your life, or even if you simply make a point of smiling more, you will feel better.

Many books, such as Norman Cousins' *Anatomy of an Illness,* describe active self-help methods. Cousins' method of laughing himself to health is highly original. When diagnosed with scleroderma, a medically incurable illness, he refused to accept his medical death sentence. He watched numerous humorous films starring Laurel and Hardy and other comedians and managed to release whatever negative energies were causing and maintaining his disease – making an otherwise unexplainable recovery.

Self healing is not an uncommon experience. Other practitioners have systematically applied knowledge obtained from behavior modification, biofeedback, autosuggestion, visualization and numerous relaxation techniques with similar results. Most of the books in this category relate principally to relaxation of emotional and physical tensions.

Meditation can promote relaxation and have other, far-reaching effects. It can often bring about subtle, qualitative alterations leading to the development of more positive attitudes towards oneself and others. These effects are difficult to describe, and even more difficult to quantify and measure.

Self-healing can accelerate recuperation from most illnesses. I will discuss heart disease and cancer as the most challenging of these. (AIDS is similarly problematic, but it has not yet been as well researched.)

Self-healing with cancer

Conventional treatments for cancer include surgery, chemotherapy, and radiotherapy as therapeutic and palliative interventions, with pain killers prescribed to treat the most common and most feared problem. All of these treatments carry severe side effects. Chemotherapy and pain medications in particular may impair quality of life, which is a sad prospect when one's remaining time is limited.

It is astounding to note that many of the chemotherapy agents administered routinely have not been studied in controlled experiments to demonstrate whether they are beneficial in prolonging life. If these agents are shown to *shrink* tumors it is assumed that they are beneficial. In fact it has never been clarified in controlled trials whether people with cancer would survive as long if they did not receive chemotherapy. It is considered unethical to conduct studies in which some people with cancer would not be given what *may be* effective treatments.

Screening for cancer is touted as offering the prospect of early identification of the disease, which can allow for earlier, presumably more effective intervention. However, this is not always the case. For instance, with cancer of the cervix this is only a partial truth. Surgery is frequently recommended for mild to moderate abnormalities on cervical smear tests. It is far from certain that this is necessary, and the surgery carries a small but significant risk of complications.[55]

The costs of cancer screening are considerable. In women under 55, for instance, it has not been shown that regular mammograms increase the success rate of diagnosing cancers. There is also the added factor of the increasing risk of cancers with repeated exposure to x-rays.

Daniel Greenberg summarizes twenty years of experience in the American "War on Cancer," which was declared by President Richard Nixon and Senator Edward Kennedy, and affirmed by the National Cancer Act of 1971. The results of pouring about $520 billion into research, mostly on the physical treatment of cancer, are unimpressive. Fears and desperation in people with cancer, rigid approaches on the part of conventional medicine, and profit motives of the drug industry are the active forces in the politics of cancer, just as they were at the start of this "war." Greenberg points out that Congress was inspired and misguided by the success of the American moon-landing in 1969and sought to conquer cancer as it had conquered the problems of lofting space vehicles into orbit. "... A few sensible voices cautioned that the Manhattan Project and the Apollo program were engineering feats based on existing scientific understanding. Cancer, they pointed out, was not understood... " Though there has been a slight reduction in cancer mortality for patients below age 65, the overall incidence of deaths from cancer in the US has risen from 335,000 in 1971 to 553,000 in 2000. Minority groups were also noted to be suffering greater incidence and mortality rates for cancer. Greenberg points out that Congress has continued to pour funds uncritically into this "war," despite the lack of any evidence that it is being won.

However there is increasing evidence that through self-healing approaches, it is possible to ameliorate symptoms of cancer, reduce the morbidity involved in toxic cancer radiotherapy and chemotherapies, and in some cases, to increase survival time or even effect total remissions of the disease.

Until recently the diagnosis of cancer has held a very negative prognosis. Patients could expect to suffer from the pain associated with the disease, from toxic therapies, and from fear of recurrence or impending death. Self-healing methods offer a variety of approaches to deal with these stresses and fears.

It is generally assumed that cancer is a scourge to be fought in every possible way – to be extirpated, poisoned, irradiated and eliminated at any cost. However, when people with cancer are invited to discuss their illness they often show another side to this picture.

> *... Most people experiencing cancer or other life-threatening illness will tell you they came alive under the crisis of the diagnosis. Priorities were suddenly revalued. The petty and infantile were discarded for the meaningful and fulfilling. Relationships that had been taken for granted were heightened. Other relationships, long dead, were discarded.*
> – W. Brugh Joy (1990, p. 149)

Psychological explorations are now uncovering ways in which people allow their illnesses to develop, as well as ways to help people deal with them.

Bernie Siegel, a surgeon in New Haven, Connecticut who treats many people with cancer, is a naturally gifted counselor and a very loving human being. He advocates wholistic approaches to involve cancer patients more fully in their own treatment. He even coined the term *respant* (for *responsible participant*) to replace *patient*. He asks his respants the following questions:

1. Do you want to live to be 100?
2. What has happened to you in your life in the year or two prior to the illness?
3. What does the diagnosis mean to you?
4. Why did you need this illness?

In discussing the answers to these questions with his respants, Siegel helps them to discover why they may have allowed cancer to develop, how they can change their unhealthy attitudes and how they can find new reasons to live. Typically, they found themselves in a job or in a personal relationship that was unbearable, but they couldn't see any acceptable way of leaving. In group therapy some come to realize that they have allowed the cancer to develop as a socially acceptable form of suicide.

One of Siegel's most potent techniques is to ask respants to draw pictures of themselves, of the cancer, and of their cancer therapies. From the drawings he can assess whether the respant is a good risk for surgery, whether chemotherapy and/or X-ray therapy are likely to be successful, what conflicts might underlie the illness and what hopes there are for recovery. Siegel found that only a few exceptional people will elect to work with his approach to overcome their disease through active efforts on their own part.

Another pioneer in psychological treatments for cancer is Lawrence LeShan (1989), who has been exploring for forty years how intensive psychotherapy can help people suffering from a variety of terminal cancers. LeShan describes life patterns and a personality type that seem particularly susceptible to cancer. Common catalysts for developing illness can include a loss of *raison d'être* (reason for *being*) and an "inability to express anger or resentment... in their own defense." LeShan feels that a sense of joy and purpose in life is essential for improvement.

LeShan reviews cancer mortality rates around the world, finding that many studies support the predictions drawn from his observations. He reports in detail on a number of individuals who experienced a remission of their cancer linked with shifts in their attitudinal patterns during psychotherapy. These clinical observations strongly suggest that people may contribute to the development and/or remission of their own cancer.

Siegel and LeShan are only two of many explorers in this field of self-healing. Several common denominators in their approaches are emerging. Self-healing therapies require that people regularly practice relaxation, meditation, imagery or other techniques, and that they attend to the basic lifestyle factors of diet, exercise, and avoiding toxins (alcohol, tobacco, and various environmental toxins). Deeper self-healing may be achieved if they can identify and deal with the stresses and conflicts that may have led them to permit the cancer to develop.

How can these methods succeed? How is it possible that psychological interventions will halt or reverse the development of cancers of all sorts?

The *surveillance theory* hypothesizes that cancerous cells are constantly appearing in every individual, but that in most people they are quickly destroyed by the immune system. Combinations of physical factors such as radiation exposure, genetics, diet and contact with carcinogenic substances can predispose certain individuals to develop clinical cancer. O. C. Simonton and colleagues describe a number of helpful psychotherapeutic techniques including relaxation, focusing on positive mental images and goals, exercising, and working with family support systems. Visualization techniques invite people to develop mental images of their immune system fighting the cancer (e.g. they may see white blood cells as white knights, sharks or soldiers. attacking the cancer cells and destroying them).

O. Carl Simonton et al. reported from their pioneering explorations:

> In the past four years, we have treated 159 patients with a diagnosis of medically incurable malignancy. Sixty-three of the patients are alive, with an average survival time of 24.4 months since the diagnosis. Life expectancy for this group, based on national norms, is 12 months. A matched control population is being developed and preliminary results indicate survival comparable with national norms and less than half the survival time of our patients. With the patients in our study who have died, their average

survival time was 20.3 months. In other words, the patients in our study who are alive have lived, on the average, two times longer than patients who received medical treatment alone. Even those patients in the study who have died still lived one and one-half times longer than the control group.

Three years later, the status of the disease in the patients still living was as shown in Table II-5.

Table II-5. Status of four-year cancer survivors

	No. of patients	% of total
No evidence of disease	14	22.2
Tumor regression	12	19.9
Disease stable	17	27.0
New tumor growth	20	31.7
Totals	63	100.0

All of these patients were at one time considered medically incurable.

Although these results are not from a rigorous study, they strongly suggest that self-healing for cancer is possible. Most impressive are reports of self-controlled cases in which discontinuation of Simonton techniques led to more rapid tumor growth and, conversely, resumption of therapy led to slowed growth and/or regression of tumors.

Jean Bolen (1973) summarizes the results of Simonton's treatment of 152 patients in Table II-6.

Simonton and Matthews-Simonton replicated the above-mentioned study with patients who had advanced breast, lung, and bowel cancers. They reported that group therapy and counseling increased the mean survival time to twice what is expected for patients with these cancers in the US. However, no statistical analyses supported their findings, and again, selection factors may have biased the results.

Stephen Levine and other therapists have found that for many respants visualizing aggressive imagery of fighting the disease does not work as well as meditation for harmonizing oneself with both one's inner self and one's environment.

CASE: A Quaker attended a workshop on developing imagery for fighting cancer. He felt he was a complete failure when he simply could not muster up aggressive imagery of his body fighting against the cancer – because this completely contradicted his pacifist principles, and he thought he would reluctantly have to give up on these methods. But after sleeping on the problem, he was pleased to awaken the next day with the mental imagery of small but strong gnomes who came along and firmly grabbed the cancer cells and carried them to the kidneys for elimination.

Table II-6. Two-year study of patients treated by O. Carl Simonton, MD

	Uncoop-erative, does not follow instruc-tions	Uncoop-erative, rarely follows instruc-tions	Usually follows instruc-tions	Follows instructions and shows some initia-tive	Full coop-eration, follows instructions implicitly, is enthusiastic about get-ting better	Totals
Patient response	- -	-	+ -	+	+ +	
Excellent: Marked relief of symptoms and dra-matic improve-ment of conditions	0	0	0	11	9	20
Good : Relief of symptoms and gen-eral condition improved	0	2	34	31	0	67
Fair: Mild relief of symp-toms	0	14	29	0	0	43
Poor: No relief of symptoms	2	17	3	0	0	22
Totals	*2*	*33*	*66*	*42*	*9*	*152*

Larry Dossey (1991, p. 197) presents similar observations:

> The message being delivered today to many sick persons is... that only if they demonstrate an antagonistic, robust "fighting spirit" will they have a chance to "beat cancer" or recover from heart disease or some other mal-ady. But there are other ways to "fight"... These ways require giving up the hubristic, arrogant, and narcissistic belief that the universe revolves around our own condition and should invariably dance to our tune. They require that we cease dictating our own terms to the universe, that we hush our petulant little "I want it thus," that we stop our incessant efforts to beat the world into line. This cessation can ideally create a vacuum or an empti-ness into which healing *can* flow.

What is advocated in these psychological approaches to treating cancer is an atti-tude of asking for and expecting help via inner resources of self-healing, and via one's higher self/ cosmic energies/ Divine intervention. This sort of surrender to a higher power is quite the opposite of giving up hope, which is a more common response to a diagnosis of cancer.[56]

Positive imagery works not only with combating the illness but also with managing the toxic side effects of some therapies. Nausea caused by chemotherapy and radiotherapy may be markedly reduced through mental imagery which supports the expectation that the body is working in concert with the external agents to fight the cancer. People who draw pictures of their radiotherapy as magic bullets that are guided to strike all the cancer cells find that they weather their radiotherapy in better shape than expected.

How can mental exercises change the course of cancers? It is possible that visualizations increase the activity of the body's immune system. Steven Locke and Mady Hornig-Rohan review 1,453 professional articles on this subject in an outstanding annotated bibliography, and Jeanne Achterberg (1985) presents a most readable and thorough discussion on the subject. Achterberg finds that this approach has been honed to such a degree that the course of illness in people with cancer can now be predicted through analysis of their visual imagery regarding the state of their cancers and the state of functioning of their immune systems. Sadly, very few medical cancer therapists have used these tools to help their patients.

Developing on the work of Simonton and colleagues, other researchers have explored the effects of psychosocial factors in influencing cancer and heart disease. Just a few of the many available reports are reviewed here.

Amanda Ramirez et al. investigated the possibility that stresses might worsen the prognoses of women who have had surgery for breast cancer, finding evidence to support this likelihood. Adverse life events and difficulties occurring during the postoperative disease-free interval were recorded in 50 women who had developed their first recurrence of operable breast cancer and during equivalent follow-up times in 50 women with operable breast cancer who were in remission. Severely threatening life events and difficulties were significantly associated with the first recurrences of breast cancers. Highly significant correlations were found between adverse life events and the subsequent development of the cancers.

Another fascinating and encouraging report on self-healing for cancer comes from David Spiegel, a psychiatrist at Stanford University. Together with several colleagues he set up a weekly support group for 86 women who had metastatic breast cancer, to provide instruction in self-hypnosis for pain relief. At the end of a year the women who participated in the group intervention were coping better with their pain than 36 women who did not have a similar support group. Much later, the investigators heard reports of people who seemed able to prolong their lives through relaxation and imagery, so ten years after the study they checked up on how these 86 women had fared. They were amazed to find that the entire control group had died within four years, but a third of the treated group were still alive at four years and three had survived ten years. The effects of treatment had become apparent 20 months into the study, which was 8 months after the end of the therapy group.

Fawzy et al. (1993) replicated Spiegel's study, with 35 patients who had malignant melanomas (skin cancers) in early stages of development. There were lower rates of recurrence and death for the treatment group, compared to a randomly chosen group of patients with melanomas who did not receive this treatment.

Both Spiegel's and Fawzy's studies have been criticized for the small numbers of patients studied and other research procedures.

J. L. Richardson et al. found that cancer patients who had been given education and support, designed to enhance medical compliance, survived longer than controls who had not had these interventions. However, the longer survival times were not correlated with the degree of medical treatment compliance. The researchers' impressions were that the critical factors increasing survival were the greater social support and sense of being in control of their situation, along with improved self-care habits.

Linn, et al. studied the effects of individual counseling on people with advanced cancers. This randomized study found enhanced *quality* of life, although no significant *prolongation* of life. These researchers concluded that psychosocial interventions late in the course of cancer could not be expected to affect the survival time. However, this study did not include the full range of psychosocial support and education that were provided in the studies of Spiegel et al. and Fawzy et al.

Dean Shrock et al. studied the effects of a series of six Health Psychology classes on breast cancer and prostate cancer patients. Each class was two hours long, offered weekly over the course of a year. Participants were encouraged to attend as often as they wanted, together with family and others in their support network. From 5 to 50 participants attended any one class, with a mean participation of 16. In addition to giving lectures, group leaders also encouraged discussion and socialization. A guided imagery audiotape was provided, including exercises in relaxation and imagery to enhance immune functions. Participants were also encouraged to engage in joyful and meaningful activities, and not to be critical of themselves if they failed to adhere to the program schedule or heed the advice provided. The death rate at five years was significantly higher in the control group

Schrock and colleagues propose that several mechanisms, which are not mutually exclusive, may explain the positive effects of psychosocial interventions in prolonging survival of people with cancer:

1. People are encouraged to comply with effective conventional medical advice and treatments.
2. Suggestions for improvement may increase self-healing. These interventions may act as potent placebos.
3. Increased social support, with the opportunity to share and vent emotions in a safe setting, can reduce stress while increasing hope and enhancing feelings of being more in control of one's life. All of these factors can enhance immune responses.
4. Strengthening hope can enhance immune functions, possibly through neuorimmune or neurohormonal pathways.
5. The factor most often cited by participants in these cancer psycho-educational programs is that they encounter others – both peers and health caregivers – who listen to them, support them, and care about them.

David Spiegel (2001) summarizes this research, noting that five out of ten of the trials found that various forms of psychotherapy enhance survival of patients with cancer The benefits were greatest among those who showed the most initial anxiety and depression. Linn et al. also showed positive psychological effects, but no somatic ones. Three of these studies reported only transient psychological benefit or none of any kind Spiegel notes:

> The difference between the findings of the two studies may be explained by changes in treatment during the past several decades. First, the medical treatment of breast cancer has improved substantially, and the notable reduction in breast-cancer mortality that began in the late 1990s undoubtedly reflects the earlier detection of cancer, the use of selective estrogen-receptor modulators, and the development and use of more effective chemotherapy.
>
> Second, psychosocial support for patients with cancer has also improved substantially. Emotional support for patients with cancer is far more readily available than it was decades ago. Because medical and surgical treatments are better now and emotional support has improved, the effect of formal psychosocial intervention on survival time that was found in earlier studies is difficult to replicate.

Another factor influencing the severity of patients' response to cancer is a history of previous traumatic stress. Lisa Butler and colleagues found that where people had experienced severe stress earlier in life, there was greater likelihood of responding to the cancer with avoidance, and anxieties about the cancer were likely to be more intrusive.

Future research might therefore focus on those people with cancer who are more anxious, and who have previously experienced serious life stresses.

Believe that life is worth living, and your belief will help create the fact.
– William James

Self-healing for cardiovascular disease

Dean Ornish, an Internist at the University of California, San Francisco, developed a group therapy approach for people who have severe heart disease. Ornish has shown that with regular practice of relaxation, meditation, low fat diet, exercise and group therapy, people not only can arrest the progress of their heart disease, but can prevent damage in their cardiac arteries. This even helps to avoid cardiac bypass surgery.[57] After one year of participation in his group, many people had reversed the atherosclerotic arterial hardening that was causing their cardiac symptoms of pain and severe limitations in their abilities to tolerate exercise. Prior to the development of the Ornish approach, it had been considered impossible to bring about such changes without medication or surgery. Further studies have shown that the improvements are progressive if people continue with the self-healing regimen.

H. J. Eysenck (1992) summarizes a series of studies supporting the following hypotheses:

1. Psychosocial factors (personality, stress) play an important role in the development of cancer and coronary heart disease.
2. These factors are different for cancer and heart disease, and can be measured in healthy people as well, leading to the postulation of personalities that are particularly prone to cancer or coronary heart disease.
3. The cancer-prone personality is characterized by suppression of emotion and inability to cope with interpersonal stress, leading to feelings of hopelessness, helplessness and eventually depression.
4. The coronary-heart-disease-prone personality is characterized by strong reactions of anger, hostility, and aggression.
5. Appropriate behavior therapy (stress management) can be an excellent preventive intervention to make people who are prone to cancer or coronary heart disease less likely to develop other diseases.
6. Similar types of treatment can prolong the lives of patients with inoperable cancer.
7. Risk factors (psychosocial, genetic, behavioral etc.) are synergistic, not additional.
8. Cancer and coronary heart disease are each influenced differently by consumption of coffee, cola, and alcohol, in line with theoretical expectation.

Eysenck (1992) argues convincingly against criticisms of these studies by other researchers:

> ... The results of a prospective, multidisciplinary study of women with early breast cancer... indicated that psychological responses to cancer diagnosis, assessed three months postoperatively, were related to outcome five years later (Greer, et al.). Recurrence-free survival was significantly commoner among patients who reacted to cancer by denial or "fighting spirit" than among patients who responded with stoic acceptance or feelings of helplessness or hopelessness. Ten years since our cohort of patients was recruited, we have re-examined the association between psychological response and outcome. Although there was a higher mortality rate in the second than in the first five years, a favorable outcome is still commoner among those whose responses were categorized as fighting spirit and denial (11/20, 55%) than among those who showed stoic acceptance or helpless/hopeless response (8/37, ... 22%) ...

Worthy of brief mention here are early reports indicating that imagery, relaxation, and meditation can be effective in treating AIDS as well as cancer.

Psychoneuroimmunology (PNI)

A whole new medical specialty called *psychoneuroimmunology (PNI)* is developing around these findings.[58] PNI techniques include relaxation, meditation and imagery, combined with a support group. PNI is helping to clarify the broad extent of the mind's influence over the production of hormones, antibodies, white cells and other factors that are essential to health and to coping with illnesses such as cancer and AIDS (P. Solomon). As explained earlier, white cells contain some of the same neuropeptides that are present in the nervous system, and we are finding that the immune system interacts far more intimately with the nervous system than was previously appreciated. As discussed earlier, some suggest that the immune system is actually an extension of the nervous system. This might help to explain the body's "memory" for immunizations and infections over many years.

Although much is known about the processes involved in the immune system's protection of our bodies from disease, it is not clear what factors are responsible for regressions of cancers. Possible mechanisms could include:

1. *Starvation* of the cancers' blood supply through selective constriction of blood vessels that nourish the tumor;
2. *Activation of immune mechanisms,* including antibodies and white blood cells, which can attack the cancer with enhanced vigor;
3. *Alteration of hormonal and/or other physiological conditions conducive to tumor growth* - such factors may also be associated with emotional states of fear, anxiety, depression and despair;
4. *Restructuring* of the body via *visualization* of new self images; and
5. *Other psi and bioenergy self-healing mechanisms.*

Mechanisms (4) and (5) could support the hypothesis that there is an energy template for the body that can be altered through mental imagery.[59]

The medical community is unfortunately unreceptive, for the most part, to approaches that rely on psychological techniques, and which place a substantial measure of responsibility for recovery on the respant. Doctors are used to prescribing physical and chemical measures for cancer therapy. Psychotherapy and self-help approaches for cancer sound incredible to them, and are thought to be placebos (used here as a pejorative term to mean a non-effective treatment rather than a self-healing approach) within the conventional allopathic system.

Doctors often fear that their patients will delay conventional therapies past the point at which they could be effective, or reject them entirely because of their distaste for undergoing mutilating, painful and toxic treatments. Many physicians believe that patients who resort to spiritual healing are grasping at less threatening, but ineffective straws.

Critics of conventional cancer therapies have observed that treatment of cancer has become an industry. Like any established institution, this industry tends to perpetuate itself and to resist approaches that might encroach on its territory.

Another factor plays into this conflict between conventional therapies and self-healing approaches. The fear of death in patients and in medical staff is poorly managed.[60] Doctors are trained to diagnose and cure disease, and they often feel that they have failed when they find themselves confronted by a medically incurable illness. They are likely to ignore the obvious, as is pointed out by Bernie Siegel: "Life is invariably fatal. A doctor ought to be aiming to improve quality of life, not simply to prolong it."

Self-healing CAM therapies face a major challenge in proving their worth through objective research. The selection of patients with cancer who are willing to participate in complementary cancer therapies is problematic. I was surprised to hear that in various studies the percentage of cancer patients willing to explore such self-healing therapies ranged from a high of 10-20% to a low of less than 1%. Much of the research to date has therefore been based on a highly self-selected group of patients who agree to practice these new methods. The prognosis for those who consent to participate may already be better than expected because these patients tend to be *fighters*, have a greater will to live, and perhaps are less depressed. This feeds the doubts of skeptics, who do not want to encourage false hopes in cancer patients who might not be predisposed for success in self-healing.

Sadly, all of these factors have combined to severely limit the availability of PNI practices for patients with cancer, cardiovascular disease, AIDS and other illnesses.

Much of Western medicine is focused on putting more days into our lives, at any cost. But a major shift toward putting more life into our days can be brought about through better attitudes toward serious and fatal illnesses. Cancer and other life-threatening illnesses can be challenges that lead to positive emotional changes. Hervé Guibert observes that cancer is "An illness in stages, a very long flight of steps that led assuredly to death, but whose every step represented a unique apprenticeship. It was a disease that gave death time to live and its victims time to die, time to discover time, and in the end, to discover life."

People with fatal illnesses may come to a state of mind in which they feel grateful for the positive changes the illness has brought into their lives. I myself found it difficult at first to believe reports of this kind of positive acceptance. It is only in working closely with people who are struggling with cancer and AIDS that I've come to understand this. When we realize that there is very limited time left to live, we are forced to choose carefully how we budget our precious remaining minutes on this earth. Many problems that may have seemed important before, now shrink to insignificance – when we ask ourselves if we truly want to spend our limited remaining time attending to them. Sorting out relationships becomes much more important – with our own past and with significant others in our lives. It becomes easier to let go of old emotional dross and urgent to put our personal relationships into the best possible order. Sorting out unresolved issues and saying goodbyes can be a great blessing to friends and family as well.

When we process all of these issues, our *quality of life* is dramatically improved. We feel much more alive when every minute is being lived to the maximum, when we are no longer wasting time on outdated *shoulds* and *shouldn'ts* – old habits that may have been programmed into our personal life computer many years earlier by our child selves or by parents, teachers, religious institutions and others who couldn't know then where we would be today.

Spiritual questions arise as we ask ourselves what may await us when we close our eyes for the last time and release our final breath. We may find comfort in the religious teachings and practices of our upbringing or of our choice. Recent studies suggest we may be blessed with pre-death visions of spiritual vistas that seem as real – if not more real – than anything we have experienced in the flesh. We may look forward to being welcomed by the spirits of those who have preceded us across that mysterious divide between life in the flesh and pure spirit existence.

And almost every one when age, disease, or sorrows strike him,
Inclines to think there is a God, or something very like Him.
                                          – Arthur Hugh Clough

Death is only frightening to those who run away from it. Reports by people who have had near-death experiences, spirit communications and reincarnation memories uniformly confirm that the transition is painless, and that the spiritual dimensions are far more pleasant than life in the flesh.[61]

Despite all of the above, few of us rush to abandon our physical existence. We hang onto life because that is what we know. Healing is largely a matter of making the best of the life we have been given.

SPONTANEOUS REMISSIONS OF ILLNESSES

Give it a name, any name, and we feel we understand what we're talking about.
                                          – Anonymous

Tilden Everson and Warren Cole reviewed the medical literature on cancer from 1800, and identified 176 cases *of spontaneous remission.* They suggest that modern isolated "cures" of cancer via unorthodox therapeutic measures might actually be spontaneous regressions of cancer. That is, the natural progression of the disease in some instances might include remissions that could be unrelated to therapeutic interventions. They propose that the following factors might contribute to such remissions: endocrine influences; fever and infection; allergic or immune reactions; disruption of the nutrition of the cancer; removal of the carcinogenic agent; unusual sensitivity to therapy that is normally inadequate; complete surgical removal of the cancer (where it had been presumed that the removal was incomplete); and incorrect histologic (microscopic pathology) diagnosis of malignancy.

Although estimates of the frequency of spontaneous regression of serious illnesses are greatly speculative, all sources agree that it is extremely rare, possibly in the range of one case per 80,000 to 100,000.

Everson and Cole had to rely on retrospective reports from a variety of sources, spread over many decades. Duration of the spontaneous remission was of necessity determined by the publication date of the report, except in the cases where death was recorded.

Brendan O'Regan and Caryl Hirshberg, with the advantage of computer-assisted library searches, undertook the Herculean task of reviewing 3,500 case reports of *spontaneous remission,* many from more recent years. About three-quarters of these remissions were from various types of cancers. They point out that spontaneous remissions may occur without allopathic treatment; may be associated with treatments by allopathic or complementary therapies; or may be associated with spiritual cures –sometimes labeled as *miracle cures.* They most often occur gradually, over days or months, but may also occur rapidly, within minutes or hours.

> *You see things; and you say "Why?" But I dream things that never were;*
> *and I say "Why not?"*
>
> – George Bernard Shaw (1921)

According to O'Regan and Hirshberg, spontaneous remission has been largely overlooked by medical science for several reasons:

1. remissions are usually identified after the fact, which makes the processes involved in these unusual cures difficult to study;
2. quality of reports varies in so many respects that it is difficult to assess their frequency or accuracy;
3. doctors suspect that there must have been errors in the initial diagnosis;
4. clinicians are reluctant to report such remissions – wary of skepticism, and afraid of being criticized for poor initial diagnosis or other similar errors;
5. clinicians treating physical conditions often omit details of patients' personal histories, and clinicians addressing psychological aspects of illness rarely include documentation about the physical conditions; and
6. skeptics suspect that all such remissions will be temporary.

O'Regan and Hirshberg's survey is a monumental work. However, it focuses heavily on remissions of physical illnesses, with minimal consideration of psychological aspects of remission. The next reference amply redresses this deficit.

  Caryl Hirshberg and Marc Ian Barasch reviewed *remarkable recoveries* from a broad spectrum of illnesses. Great attention was given to people's descriptions of their beliefs about illness, how they received their treatments – both conventional and complementary – and how they understood their transformations. I have selected a few examples from among their many helpful observations. The study contains numerous other discussions and fascinating individual accounts of personal health challenges that were met with courage, and were dealt with through a spectrum of wholistic healing approaches.

  Hirshberg and Barasch noted that certain characteristics appeared frequently among the large number of people they interviewed:

1. They had a strong sense of their *selfhood*.
2. They demonstrated qualities of *congruence*, being true to themselves in the emotional, cognitive, and behavioral aspects of their lives.
3. They did not cluster in particular personality styles. "[I]t may be more a matter of finding an individual 'right path' than having the 'right stuff.'" (p.152)
4. They were *determined to improve*, and *assertive* in exploring therapeutic alternatives and implementing them.
5. They refused to accept dire prognoses from doctors, sometimes even deciding to fight their illnesses to spite their doctors' predictions. Such *constructive denial* might even include refusal to equate a serious diagnosis, like cancer, with death.
6. They developed reasons to live and to enjoy life.
7. They had spiritual experiences, often associated with profound personality changes, as a result of their illnesses.

In the foreword to this outstanding book, Larry Dossey observes:

> Because remarkable recoveries often occur unbidden and out-of-the-blue, they appear to be a blessing, a grace. We do not know the buttons to push to make them happen; we cannot compel them to our bidding. This means we cannot control them. Control has become immensely important to generations of scientifically trained physicians. Could it be that we modern doctors, so desperate to control nature, have shunned these marvelous events because they are so uncontrollable? (p. xii)

This book contains a wealth of information for anyone who is interested in spontaneous remissions and remarkable recoveries from illnesses. It strongly suggests that self-healing mechanisms are at work when people experience unusual recoveries from illness. Clearly, some of the processes and many of the mechanisms in these self-healing experiences do not take place within the conscious awareness of the people experiencing them, nor are they evident to those studying them, and in that sense these remarkable recoveries appear to be "spontaneous." However, in broad terms it can be hypothesized that some of the factors related to the occurrence of such remissions include: changing one's attitudes and beliefs about one's illness; releasing blocked emotions; finding joy, and changing one's relationships, life course and styles of handling emotions in order to facilitate release of tensions, conflicts and resentments.

A final strong recommendation for further reading is the personal account of Marc Ian Barasch (1993) in his search for ways to deal with a thyroid tumor. Barasch includes brief vignettes of many others who faced the challenges of serious illnesses and transcended them. This is a masterful presentation, full of helpful information about dealing with these issues, and a good read besides.

> Almost all the journeyers I interviewed discovered that new life can grow from the same painful roots that may have contributed to their disease. For if some disease springs in part from an early-thwarted need for love and relatedness, a soul-growth denied, then the roots of illness are, paradoxically, the very roots of life.
>
> – Marc Ian Barasch (p. 99)

So-called spontaneous remissions may represent self-healing, perhaps through some of the mechanisms suggested by the above-mentioned authors, or through spiritual healing, which Everson and Cole did not examine and O'Regan and Hirshberg considered only in an extremely limited scope. They made no attempts to investigate psychological correlates of cancer regressions. This would be impossible in any case in such retrospective studies, since psychological (not to mention PNI and psi) factors of disease have not been in the forefront of medical awareness, and thus have been under-reported.

Once we become aware of spontaneous remission, we must ask whether remissions reported by various therapists are anything more than this. The reported rates of improvement with Simonton-type techniques and other PNI approaches appear to exceed the rate for spontaneous remission, but because subjects self-select for these treatments, it is difficult to be certain of this.

Conventional cancer treatments usually include chemotherapy. Modern medicine has readily embraced this mode of treatment despite its terrible morbidity, including nausea, vomiting, diarrhea, hair-loss and more.

It is rather shocking to realize that this drastic method of treatment has been widely used even though controlled studies of chemotherapy have in most cases been methodologically flawed in ways similar to the Simonton studies. Robert Oye and Martin Shapiro found that:

> ... Of 80 studies, 95% reported response to chemotherapy as an end point. Of 38 studies demonstrating 15% or greater objective response, 76% reported significantly greater survival of responders than of nonresponders. Of 21 studies containing statements supporting treatment effectiveness, 95% based this claim at least in part on the superior survival of responders compared with nonresponders. Because responders may have lived longer without treatment, such comparisons are not valid and may lead to overly optimistic views of chemotherapy effectiveness.
>
> ... No study confirmed survival of responders as superior to that of a favorable subset of untreated patients.
>
> ... None of the studies systematically examined quality of life in the patients treated with chemotherapy.

For all the researchers know, the responders in these studies might have done equally well without treatment (perhaps even better!). Non-responders might be selectively poisoned by chemotherapy, and might therefore do worse than responders, rather than vice versa. To prove chemotherapy effective, a group of treated patients with positive prognoses should be compared with a similar untreated group. The medical profession, having assumed that chemotherapy is effective, considers such a study unethical. They are also afraid of being sued by patients who could complain that they were not given the best available treatment.

This is condemning evidence against the common-practice standard of acceptability in Western medicine. It is distressing that cancer patients are being subjected to the torment of treatments that have not been properly demonstrated to be effective.

One may only hope that spiritual healing, clearly a non-invasive, non-toxic therapy, will be increasingly used in the treatment of cancer, along with more accepted modalities. This is not to say that healing must replace chemotherapy and radiotherapy. It may be that healing could be effective in combination with them, certainly in reducing toxic side effects and possibly in potentiating the actions of more accepted treatments – assuming that they are in fact effective.

A FEW WORDS IN SUMMARY ABOUT PSYCHOTHERAPIES

The variations on the themes of psychotherapy are as infinite as the creativity of therapists and the countless manifestations and resolutions of the suffering of mankind. It is impossible to say in all cases which treatment method may be the best for any given problem, because health problems are manifested through the complex interplay of genetic endowments, personalities, relationships and cultural settings within which they occur.[62]

In many ways, the person who is the instrument of the therapy is as important as the methods that she applies. The more work therapists have done on themselves in their own paths through life, the better instruments they will be in helping clients to change. Ram Dass (1996, p. 75) observes, "The mistake of therapists is in thinking they do something *to* other people. I don't have that sense of doing anything *to* anyone else. I have a sense that I am an environment, and people do it to themselves."

The indefinable *chemistry* of relationships between therapists and clients also influences the clients' openness to growth and change. In the most profound therapeutic relationships, therapists open their own hearts, and learn and grow as much as their clients do.

These observations apply all the more in spiritual healing, where the subtle energy interactions and spiritual dimensions of the encounter can add to the complexity of the therapeutic relationship. Swami Satchidananda (1996, p. 227) advises, "If we don't experience that God in us, we will never see God in anyone else because we have no eye to see." Everyone must work on the shadow aspects in every level of their being, in order to provide as clear a channel as possible for healing.

THE MIND AND THE BRAIN

The brain is the organ through which we think that we think.
– Ambrose Bierce

Where the mind actually resides is far from obvious. The structure and processes of the brain are by necessity much easier to define. It is clear that if the brain is awry physically, biochemically or electrobiologically, the expression of mind is distorted or impaired. Doctors have discovered much about how the brain functions through examining people whose brains have been injured by trauma, vascular disease, tumors, infections or surgery. The resultant psychological and physical deficits reveal the functions of the damaged or missing portions of the brain. Further information can also be obtained during neurosurgery – which is usually performed under local anesthetics because the brain does not hurt when it is probed. Neurosurgeons can carefully stimulate selected portions of the brain electrically and obtain information about their function by observing patients' responses.

Biochemical studies of the brain have shown that it performs numerous chemical and hormonal processes that are maintained in a delicate, homeostatic balance. Even minor chemical changes can produce serious brain dysfunctions. Medicines and drugs can likewise alter brain functions, for better or worse.

EEGs and new computerized electromagnetic and radioactive imaging devices[63] allow researchers to study the living brain in incredible detail. With special techniques they are also able to assess changes in brain functions during various mental activities and processes. Studies of humans have been supplemented with numerous experiments on animals, whose brains are sufficiently similar to human brains to permit deductions and inferences as to how the human brain works.

Using these methods, very detailed physical, biochemical, and electrobiological maps have been drawn of many brain processes. Based on these studies there are those who hold that "mind" is primarily or even purely a function of the brain. They point out that particular reactions are elicited, including motor responses, sensory perceptions and emotional tones, when particular portions of the brain are stimulated electrically with a surgeon's probe, or if particular drugs or hormones are present in the brain. They therefore conclude that consciousness is a product of brain bioelectrical activities.

Yet there is also strong evidence suggesting that mind is not necessarily the product of brain. Among the more interesting of these, consider the following:

1. During anesthesia, when people's conscious awareness is asleep, they may still hear and respond to what is taking place in the operating room. Cases are reported in which a surgeon made negative comments such as, "Too bad! There's nothing more we can do. The cancer has spread too far," and within moments the patient's heart stopped beating. Conversely, suggestions may be given while patients are under anesthesia that they will have less post-surgical pain and other complications. Sometimes they respond so well to these suggestions that they may be discharged from the hospital sooner than expected.
2. Many cases of out-of-body (OBE) viewing of the operating room during surgery while patients are under anesthesia have been reported.[64] In such OBE experiences, patients feel themselves floating as a point of consciousness or a ghost-like being near the ceiling of the operating room, looking down at their physical body, on which the surgical team is still operating. They will often be able to recall in minute and accurate detail various actions that occurred and words that were said during their operations (sometimes to the embarrassment of their surgeons!).
3. Research on reports of near-death and reincarnation experiences suggest that there is more to the mind than the brain that exists in one's current life can account for. For example, children and adults who live in countries where they have no access to newspapers or media have reported details of previous lives that have been verified – when there was no known way in which they could have obtained the information in question. In occasional instances these reports include the use of languages that the speakers have never learned.
4. There are people who have grown up with unidentified hydrocephalus, which has left them with such large ventricles (fluid filled-spaces within the brain) and such a thinned cerebral cortex that they should be imbeciles (as it is assumed that an intact cerebral cortex is required for thinking), yet they have become successful university students.

The alternative view, supported by these sorts of observations is that the mind exists outside of the brain, or overlaps several dimensions to include the brain, which acts like a radio receiver for mind.

In this view, mind resides on some non-physical plane(s) but expresses itself via transformations of energy or information through the brain. The brain contains an estimated 10 to 14 billion nerve cells, and there is a constant interplay of electro-chemical messages between its countless cellular interconnections. It is possible that the brain may readily be influenced by outside energies that can modulate some of this ongoing intercellular activity. A minimum of energy input might be required to influence any of the multitudes of brain cells that are frequently standing on the threshold of emitting impulses. Thus the brain could readily act like radio or TV receiver.

All the body is in the mind, but not all the mind is in the body.
– Swami Rama

Philosophical speculations have gone even further. Consider the following observation from the psychologist Keith Floyd: "Contrary to what everyone knows is so, it may not be the brain that produces consciousness but rather, consciousness that creates the appearance of the brain matter, space, time and everything else we are pleased to interpret as the physical universe."

While such statements – based on evidence from neurobiology and psi research – might appear speculative, well-substantiated research from quantum physics suggests similar conclusions. Quantum physics has shown that the consciousness of the observer determines that which is observed. Consciousness therefore appears to shape matter. While this doesn't prove that the consciousness is primary and brain secondary, it lends support to this possibility.[65]

The physicist does not discover, he creates his universe.
– Henry Margenau

These questions are highly complex. The evidence for theories of mind influencing brain, and possibly even creating reality both internally and externally, deserve far more consideration than is practical in the context of this volume. It may eventually prove impossible to arrive at definitive answers to some of these questions, but in my opinion, the theory of mind being the primary agency is consistent with the greater weight of evidence.

TRANSPERSONAL PSYCHOTHERAPY

Much of what we think is extraordinary in another plane is just the ordinary - not understood or experienced.
– Ted Kaptchuk

Most conventional psychotherapists are trained to help people suffering from distress in their inner psychological worlds. Some therapists extend treatment to involve relationships with other people, as in couples, groups and family therapy. Spiritual awareness is usually relegated to ministrations of the clergy, and is dismissed by many psychotherapists as fantasy, wishful thinking, the beliefs and habits resulting from religious upbringing, or a manifestation of the denial of death. The most damning criticism of religion by psychology and philosophy (Ferrer) is that there is no way to prove it is intrinsically valid rather than a mental construct.

We tend to overlook the fact that psychology[66] is based on unprovable basic assumptions, just as religions are. In fact, there are probably more theories in psychology than there are religions. Frances Vaughan observes, "Psychology, like exoteric religion, is an expedient rather than a final teaching."

Ordinary people (who are not trained in specific academic disciplines that specialize in *parts* of human experience) often view spirituality as an important lining to the fabric of their lives, inseparable from their other experiences.

> *... The older I became, the more the intimation grew that the deepest longing in the universe of the unconscious, in fact the greatest of all the urges in the collective unconscious, was the strange, irresistible longing to become more conscious: that and not the unconscious, was the real life-giving mystery...*
>
> – Laurens van der Post (1994, p. 21)

A new *transpersonal* branch of psychology has emerged that includes in its practice meditative techniques, explorations of alternative states of consciousness, and integration of spiritual, mystical and religious teachings and rituals. These practices all seek to heighten people's awareness of aspects of their beings that partake of the Infinite Source. Transpersonal awareness suggests that each of us is a part of a vast whole – an intricate network of which we are usually but dimly aware. If we see our lives in relation to the All just as the life of a cell is in relation to our whole body, then our lives may take on a deeper meaning. Such awarenesses are better experienced than articulated in words. They partake of the essence alluded to by F. David Peat in discussions about the elements of the unconscious, in which he suggests that there is a higher self:

> [T]he archetypes leave their footprints in the mind and project their shadows across thought. While it is not possible to observe the archetypes directly, their movements can be sensed through the numinous images, myths, and happiness that enter consciousness...

At the very least, transpersonal approaches can provide an expanded perspective from which to view our own problems. Anxiety or depression may not appear so onerous when they are placed in these temporal, spiritual or priority frameworks. These dimensions of therapy can also provide discipline, inspiration, courage, hope, and community with other people or higher powers.

> Break*down* may be a break*through.*
> – Anonymous

For some, transpersonal approaches can be transformative, especially when we have "hit bottom." We may emerge from "the dark night of the soul" through transpersonal therapy into completely new modes of interacting with the world.

To illustrate how transpersonal awareness can be accessed for healing let us consider a few salient examples of such approaches. The most common of these is meditation.

Meditation leads us inward to Alternative States of Consciousness (ASCs) in which we can find relaxation, peace, release from worldly cares, emotional release of buried hurts, serenity, inspiration, and connection with our higher selves and with the Divine. Because these ASCs and inner worlds are beyond the descriptive powers of linear words and concepts, it is difficult to articulate them. Of the many writers on meditation I particularly recommend Daniel Goleman and Ken Wilber.

Daniel Goleman follows classical Eastern meditative practices in describing two paths for meditation.

The *path of concentration* involves focusing undivided attention upon an object, either in the world outside or within the mind (Goleman 1977). With practice, one reaches successively deeper meditative stages.[67] The first is a merging with the object. "Rapture at the level of the first stage is likened to the initial pleasure of excitement at getting a long-sought object; bliss is the enjoyment of that object." (p. 14) At the second stage the meditator stops focusing on the object and identifies with the rapture, freeing the mind of all concrete thoughts. At the third level the meditator attains equanimity, or an even-mindedness that exists beyond the rapture and produces an encompassing bliss. Going deeper, the fourth stage brings cessation of all thought and sensation, and even of breathing. "The meditator's mind at this extremely subtle level rests with one-pointedness in equanimity." (p. 17)

Further stages on the path of concentration are formless. The meditator's concentration cannot be disturbed. He comes out of the meditative state according to his intention, which he determines prior to entering the meditation. At the fifth stage the meditator becomes aware of the space that the object of focus occupies, with only the dimmest remnant of perception of the object itself remaining at the periphery of his concentration. The sixth stage extends awareness into the infiniteness of space. Then, abandoning the focus on space, the meditator reaches infinite awareness. The seventh stage is the void. The eighth and final stage is awareness of the peacefulness of the void, without even the desire to attain this peacefulness. Only the faintest residual mental processes remain.

On the *path of insight* the meditator focuses awareness on perceptions of body, feelings, mind or mind objects, but does not analyze them in any way. Should a thought about a perception occur, then the thought itself becomes the subject of concentration. Without judgment, the meditator releases each perception after contemplating it. A degree of facility in concentration is required for insight practices, so that these will follow naturally upon the practices of the *path of concentration.*

Any of these techniques of *mindfulness* will break through the illusions of continuity and rationality that ordinarily sustain our mental life. In *mindfulness*, the meditator begins to discern the random units of mental perception from which her reality is built. From these observations emerge a series of realizations about the nature of the mind. Through this process, *mindfulness* matures into *insight*. The practice of insight begins at the point where mindfulness continues without interruption or time lag. In *insight meditation* awareness fixes on its object so that the contemplating mind and its object of contemplation arise together in unbroken succession. This point marks the beginning of a chain of insights – mind knowing itself – which eventually can lead to the *nirvanic* state.

The first step in mindfulness is to realize that the mind is distinct from the phenomena it contemplates. Next, the meditator notices that she is not willing these processes, but that they proceed on their own. She realizes that the "I" does not really exist. Reality shifts with endless perceptions from moment to moment, and she experiences only the state of impermanence. The constantly changing nature of reality leaves nothing to which one needs to remain attached. Eventually a state of detachment is reached in which the mind is perceived as a source of suffering.

> *We are all serving a life-sentence in the dungeon of self.*
> – Cyril Connolly

As the meditator continues through this development of awareness, various visions and rapturous feelings begin to arise. Goleman labels this *pseudonirvana,* because it is really only a stage on a longer path. Though the meditator may be tempted to enjoy these distractions, he must simply focus on his attachment to them, rather than on the feelings themselves.

More difficult stages follow, in which the disappearance of awareness becomes more distinct than one's perceptions of both the object and one's contemplation of it. At this point, all awareness loses its attraction, and stopping mental processes appears to be the most attractive goal. Painful feelings may assail the body and suffering may become intense. As the meditator continues simply to note these feelings, they eventually cease. Contemplation then becomes automatic and focus clears. Each transient moment is simply noted and released, and no deliberate effort is needed to maintain a detached meditative state.

> [A] consciousness arises that takes as its object the signless, no-occurrence, no-formation: *nirvana*... . Awareness of all physical and mental phenomena ceases entirely.
> [N]irvana is a "supramundane reality," describable only in terms of what it is not. Nirvana has no phenomenology, no experiential characteristics. It is the unconditioned state. (Goleman 1988, p. 31)

With *nirvana* a natural moral purity emerges which eliminates all emotional attachments. The earlier stages suppress rather than eliminate these factors. "... Entering the nirvanic state is... 'awakening'; ... subsequent stages are... 'deliverance'." (p. 33) With deliverance, the meditator relinquishes ego attachments to achievements, pleasures, emotions and possessions. Moral misbehavior is no longer within the spectrum of his conduct. Deliverance is experienced in an initial, partial state, and then it becomes permanent. Fully developed, the meditator becomes an *arahant* – an awakened being or saint.

The paths of contemplation and insight may be different for Eastern and Western meditators, and I will discuss this further below.

A second analysis of meditation may help to clarify some of the intricacies of this finest of human endeavors and greatest of human challenges.

> *Who is brave? The person who conquers his own spirit.*
> – Jewish saying

Ken Wilber is a world expert on meditation. He views consciousness as extending beyond ordinary awareness – largely through the unconscious mind – into transpersonal and cosmic awarenesses.[68] This is in contrast to conventional psychology, which views the unconscious as a sort of computer – a storehouse of material that may be perceived consciously or subliminally and is then screened and repressed. Within this framework, the unconscious is considered an *automatic pilot* for repetitive responses and behaviors of mind and body. Meditation is acknowledged by psychologists as a tool that can be used to penetrate repressions, stop filtering and de-automate responses. Wilber's approach is much less mechanistic; he emphasizes that meditation is, most importantly, a path towards transcendence.

Wilber details a very complex analysis of how children grow through various maturational levels during their psychological development. At a given level the child *translates* emotional drives and cognitive needs into various behavioral expressions. At a given level of development the child is capable of analyzing and understanding inner and outer experiences that are within the range of her comprehension, at that particular level of development. As the *translations* that characterize a given level of development become outmoded in the process of conceptual and emotional maturation, her consciousness is *transformed* into a higher level of organization and functioning. "There is differentiation, dis-identification [with outmoded coping mechanisms], transcendence and integration" (p. 93).

These maturational processes of *translation* and *transformation* are like the risers and steps in a staircase. The periods of translation are plateaus where a person explores and consolidates each of their successive levels of awareness. Then comes a rise through transformation to a new level, which is qualitatively different from the previous level. This is followed by successive alternating steps of translation and transformation as a person's awareness matures and deepens. Adults may continue to develop and deepen their awareness or may stop at a given step.

Throughout the ages, many religious and mystical traditions have invited people to explore various ways to facilitate the transformation process which reaches into higher steps of spiritual awareness.

Meditation is the path to transformation that has been explored in the most systematic way. Meditation can take a person into deeper levels of awareness, through a variety of approaches. Meditation masters can frustrate and block the customary *translations* and undermine emotional resistances, while introducing symbols that embody aspects of the higher levels of consciousness, which are then used as the focus of meditation. Practicing the higher meditative translations helps to induce spiritual transformation. Such translations may include awareness of timelessness, avoidance of attachments, uniting with objects outside oneself, accepting unconditionally everything that enters consciousness, and holding awareness of love in one's consciousness.

Concentrative meditation stops the ordinary, distracting activity of translation. By concentrating on a particular image, word, chant or other focus, the mind is occupied and stops its wandering.

Receptive, *observing meditation* defocalizes attention, with the mind observing its own mental processes but not engaging in any of them – simply letting them drift by. Both these forms of meditation place meditators at a higher level of awareness than their customary conscious translations, while breaking down the lower order of translations.

Wilber identifies three classes of meditation:

1. Meditation may focus on the body, as in various forms of yoga, with the goal of transmuting body energies into lower subtle regions of awareness.
2. Meditation may focus on higher subtle regions beyond the crown chakra.
3. The meditator may focus on "inquiry into the causal field of consciousness itself, inquiry into the I-ness or the separate-self sense, even in and through the Transcendent Witness of the causal region, until all forms of subject-object dualism are uprooted." (p. 96)

Any of these paths can lead to the highest states of meditative consciousness. Ultimately, individual consciousness unites with the cosmic consciousness.

> And so proceeds meditation, which is simply higher development, which is simply higher evolution – a transformation from unity to unity until there is simply Unity, whereupon Brahman, in an unnoticed shock of recognition and final remembrance, grins silently to itself, closes its eyes, breathes deeply, and throws itself outward for the millionth time, losing itself in its manifestations for the sport and play of it all. Evolution then proceeds again, transformation by transformation, remembering more and more, until each and every soul remembers Buddha, as Buddha, in Buddha – whereupon there is then no Buddha, and no soul. And that is the final transformation... (p. 99)

Wilber believes that the ultimate healing is Unity with the All[69]. He views psychological growth in terms of its progress towards this goal. However, unconscious resistances to meditative progress are many and strong. This makes the practice of meditation a challenge that may require years of practice to master. Most commonly,

> Because man wants real transcendence above all else, but because he cannot or will not accept the necessary death of his separate-self sense, he goes about seeking transcendence in ways, or through structures, that *actually prevent it and force symbolic substitutes*. And these substitutes come in all varieties: sex, food, money, fame, knowledge, power – all are ultimately substitute gratifications, simple substitutions for true release in Wholeness... (p. 102-3)

Wilber is describing what has been called in psychological terms *Eros*, the drive to wish, desire, seek, grasp, possess and so forth. Eros is dealt with through concentrative and receptive meditations.

A major anxiety encountered during meditation is *Thanatos,* the fear of dying, and thus of losing one's awareness of self. This occurs to some extent with each advancement and growth from one meditation level to another. It is a natural fear, quite distinct from psychopathological anxieties and fears. This fear is inherent in developing a growing sense of being a separate self, and it finds expression at each level of development according to the translations appropriate at that level. The challenge is to transcend this fear in order to ultimately relinquish all sense of self and unite with the All.[70]

> ... Only at the end of psychological growth is there final enlightenment and liberation in and as God, but that is the *only* thing that is desired from the beginning...
>
>   The point is that each stage or level of growth seeks absolute Unity, but in ways or under constraints that necessarily prevent it and allow only compromises: substitute unities and substitute gratifications... (p. 101)

The climb up the stairway to spiritual awareness can be accompanied by resurgences of repressed memories and emotional releases. Wilber cites M. Washburn, who suggests that only the receptive type of meditation opens directly into the unconscious. This receptive, absorptive meditation focuses so completely on the object of concentration that everything else, including unconscious material, remains outside of the meditator's awareness during the meditative practice. In absorptive meditation, unconscious materials are confronted only after the meditative object is relinquished or the meditative practices are concluded. Wilber feels that this advantage of receptive meditation definitely applies in accessing the shadow aspects of the unconscious but not in exploring the emergent, higher aspects of the unconscious that develop as a result of meditation. (In view of the greater emphasis placed upon "clearing the psychological shadow" in the West, it would seem to me that this is a very important consideration in choosing a path of meditation.)

Deeper meditative practices can take us into realms of consciousness that are hard to define or describe. Eastern meditative masters have been teaching meditation for many hundreds of years, and they find that students of meditation regularly go through specific phases of awareness as they deepen their meditative practices. Eastern terms for these stages can be difficult for westerners to understand, as you may have found with Goleman's explanations. Wilber (1980) proposes a map of this inner territory in terms that represent extensions of the stages of growth as defined in Western developmental psychology.

Wilber suggests that human consciousness develops in a stepwise fashion through what he calls the *outward arc*, and that meditation can extend consciousness into dimensions beyond our ordinary awareness through the *inward arc*. (See figure II-5, from Wilber 1980, p. 5)

Conventional psychology has identified stages of cognitive development; psychosexual development; emotional/ affective development; formation of family relations; moral maturation, and more. Wilber considers all of these to be on the *outward arc* of human consciousness, even though they are processes that may extend to the end of a person's physical existence.

Wilber created his own terminology for the developmental stages that he considers significant.[71] These stages and their progressive evolutions from one to another are well worth considering – if you want an in-depth understanding of the meditative process. However, Wilber's terminology and explanations are quite challenging to follow, so if you find this more detailed than you want or need to know, you might just skim this section or even skip ahead to the big asterisk on page 148.

Figure II-5. The complete life cycle

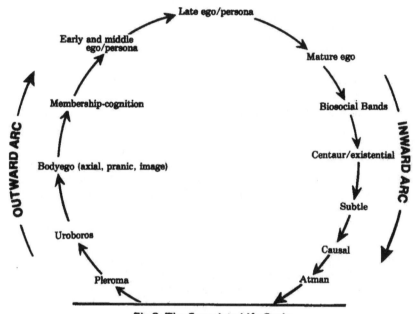

Fig 2. The Complete Life Cycle

Wilber starts with the *Pleromatic Self* of the fetus and newborn infant, who does not differentiate between the self and the material world. Consciousness is autistic, relating to the world without any appreciation of space or time, and assuming itself to be the center of the universe.

The first task of the infant is to differentiate between self and others, usually through the relationship with its mother. This leads into the next stage of the *Uroboric Self* (named for the mythic serpent that is pictured eating its own tail). The infant develops a dim and poorly differentiated awareness of self as differentiated from the mother's breast. There is still no sense of time, nor any real appreciation of the nature of others as existing for any reason other than to satisfy the infant's needs.

In the stage of the *Typhonic Self* the infant develops awareness of its physical body as separate from its physical environment. In this stage only objects that are present remain within the infant's awareness – out of sight is truly out of mind. In the early *typhonic* stage the self simply *is* in whatever state it finds itself.

Next, the child's awareness of a *Pranic Self* develops through the experience of basic emotions. In the earliest stages there is only a primitive awareness of hunger, tension, anxiety, anger, while satiation/ pleasure, and causality is still beyond conceptual awareness.

The infant develops its ability to conceptualize imagery when it is around seven months old, and it begins to separate out objects in its environment, though it still does not connect them causally. They simply are or are not there. Classes of objects may be identified according to individual parts, with only partial understanding of categorization. This is called *prelogical*, *part-identity* or *parataxic* logic. In this *primary process* thinking, self and objects in the outside world may be confused.

The infant then develops an *image-body* awareness. The baby is highly sensitive to the quality of caring received, and is vulnerable to adopting a positive or negative self-concept, depending upon the treatment it receives from its mother. As imagery can be invoked internally, this imagery can also evoke emotions, and imagined anxieties become possible. Wishes and desires may also be fulfilled by imagined pleasures.

As the infant learns to distinguish itself as being separate from objects, the self *transcends* those objects and can then operate upon them through the mental structures that have differentiated at that level of development.

The *Membership Self* evolves as language learning introduces new capabilities, including an expanded appreciation of time, a deeper and more complex emotional life and basic elements of self-control – all in all, a higher order of self-awareness. The details of development at this level are very much shaped and limited by the participation of the individual in a particular family and culture. This has been identified as *secondary process*; and *realistic thinking*.

This stage takes a relatively long time to develop. In the intermediate period there is a mixture of logic and magical thinking, termed *precausal*; *prelogical*; or *autistic language*. Thinking at this level is mostly auditory and verbal.

As logical awareness matures, children achieve a greater degree of consensual reality testing within their culture. While this is clearly advantageous and necessary, each step forward may require considerable readjustments. For instance, an awareness of oneself as being separate from others enables one to engage in more realistic interactions with them, but this individuation may be frightening at first.

The *Mental-Egoic Stages* introduce further elaborations of self-awareness. A thinking-self develops as a self-concept or *ego*. Wilber identifies an *early ego* (age 4-7), *middle ego* (7-12), and *late ego* (from 12 years to the start of the inward arc, if and when the person commences on this path, usually after age 21).

Using the language of Transactional Analysis (I. Stewart/ Joines), Wilber describes how subdivisions of functions evolve within the ego. One of these is an emotional *child* part that is highly interactive with other ego subsections. This is the aspect of the self that seeks immediate pleasure and avoids pain, that wants to be accepted by parents and parent-figures, and fights and rebels against authority for its independence while at the same time seeking the security of external limits.

An *adult* part assumes the tasks of logical analysis and prioritizing inner and outer needs and wants, relative to costs. A *parent*, or *super-ego* part internalizes attitudes and behaviors that are approved or forbidden by parents and society.

Every individual has to modify his behaviors in response to his environment. Aspects of the self that are uncomfortable to the conscious self may be repressed in unconscious parts of the mind. The repressed parts of the self constitute the *shadow*, and the remaining, "fraudulent" self or "social mask" is termed the *persona* (Jung's term).

Wilber examines the transitions from one stage of development to another, and finds that the self must dis-identify with its current structure in order to identify with the next higher level.

> [B]ecause the self is differentiated from the lower structure, it *transcends* that structure (without obliterating it in any way), and can thus *operate* on that lower structure using the tools of the newly emergent structure (p. 80). [A]t each point in evolution or remembrance, a *mode* of self becomes merely a *component* of a higher-order self (p. 81).

Each level has a *deep structure*, which defines the inner nature, functions and limitations of that level, and a *surface structure*, which is the outward expression of the deep structure. Wilber uses the analogy of a building, in which each floor represents the structure of a given level. The rooms, their contents, and the activities that go on within them represent the surface structures of the self. He calls movement within surface structures *translation*, and movement from one deep structure to another *transformation*. Translation involves various expressions within the same level. In lower levels, the oceanic awareness of the *uroboric* self is transformed, as the axial self-image develops into an awareness of bodily pleasure. At a higher level, a little girl may experience anxiety on the level of the *typhonic* self if she receives insufficient attention from her mother. This could be experienced as physical tension, emotional irritability or crying – all of which are translations of the original discomfort. Endless translations occur within the range of capabilities at any given level.

If the stress continues in the little girl's experience, a transformation may be precipitated. In a regressive transformation the girl would withdraw into herself and stop communicating with the outside world, turning inwards, shutting off her emotions from her own awareness, and seeking satisfaction through doll play and fantasy. A progressive transformation could be to develop mental explanations to rationalize the distress and soften the anxieties, tensions and emotional pain that it invokes. The latter process involves transformation into the mental levels. The child could say to herself, "I must be a bad girl if Mommy doesn't want to pay attention to me. I'll have to work very hard to be good and do everything Mommy wants." Or she could displace her frustration and anger onto objects in her environment, or engage in any of the myriad of possible translations within the mental level of development, which represent the immense diversity of human expression. All of this would occur within her unconscious mind.

When direct expressions of needs are diverted through defensive translations, developmental progress is distorted and may even be arrested. Normally, when feelings arise and seek expression, a *sign* comes into conscious awareness regarding the discomfort at that level, and appropriate action is taken to relieve the discomfort. When a category of need has been blocked at a previous level, its expression cannot be sought directly at a later level because it is kept out of conscious awareness. The unconscious mind continues to work hard to repress the memories of the distressing material from awareness and thereby to diminish pain. At the same time, the unconscious mind will send *symbols* regarding the buried conflict into awareness, hoping that the conscious mind at its new level of awareness will find more productive ways to sort out the discomfort – which will not leave pains buried from awareness but forever present in the unconscious mind. These symbols can take the form of irrational thoughts, inappropriate behaviors, physical symptoms and the like. People forget how they translated their original stresses into defensive patterns of reactions, and even *that* they did so. Psychotherapy can help people to translate symbols back into their original signs, complete with the feelings that were involved. This then enables a completion of the translational development that was blocked by the inner conflict.

When the body, ego, persona and shadow are harmonized into a unified whole, a *Centauric Self* emerges. This is an existential level at which the lower levels are not ignored but are viewed dispassionately as past experiences. The person is no longer distracted, dominated or driven by memories or symbols from the lower levels. This is the level of existential psychology in which the whole person is integrated and the total is more than the sum of the parts – having progressed beyond the ego and persona levels of development/ awareness. It is here that the *spontaneous will* of the whole self originates. Beyond the *membership* level of self, but still linked with body awareness, are the "realms of being that transcend conventional, egoic, institutional, and social forms" (Wilber 1990, p. 56). Existing in the *now*, fully aware that all time is *present*, is another characteristic of the *centaur* level.

> *[T]he nowness of everything is absolutely wondrous.*
> – Dennis Potter

Transpersonal aspects of the centauric level have parallels with the pre-personal levels of development as defined by Freud, but these two states are clearly distinct. Wilber emphasizes that psychoanalysis has mistakenly presumed that transpersonal awareness represents a regression to infantile, wish-fulfilling fantasies – of an all-knowing, all-caring parental figure that is mistakenly projected as a God-figure. Wilber marshals reasons and evidence to refute this assertion.

Wilber points out that imagery and fantasy provide modes for transition through the existential and into the transpersonal levels. Lower fantasy is focused on the body-self, while higher, mature fantasy looks toward higher modes of awareness and being, which transcend physical existence. Symbolic imagery is the language used by our brain to translate transpersonal perceptions into conscious awarenesses that we can begin to appreciate, though we may not comprehend them in their entirety.

Mircea Eliade (1970) comments:

> ... The symbol reveals certain aspects of reality – the deepest aspects – that defy any other means of knowledge. Images, symbols, and myths are not irresponsible creations of the psyche; they respond to a need and fulfill a function, that of bringing to light the most hidden modalities of being.

As the individual opens to the centauric levels, intuition and higher energies become more easily available to conscious awareness. Intuition may exist on lower, psi levels and may also extend to the higher awareness of a Divine presence.

All of the stages described above belong to the *gross realm* of being that Buddhism considers "the realm of ordinary waking consciousness." As we stretch to experience the transcendent from the gross realms, we move into regions that are even more difficult to describe.

Wilber identifies *subtle realms* that are beyond words. The *lower subtle* is associated with the brow chakra, or *third eye*, and connects to psi and astral awareness. The astral realm includes out-of-body experiences and aura perception, which Wilber acknowledges are often considered to be elements of psi awareness.

The *high subtle* realms start at the crown chakra and extend into seven transcendent levels. In the first four we may encounter intuitional inspiration, spirit guides, angels, devas and the like, extending to archetypes of God. Wilber views all of these phenomena as parts of one's own higher self. The highest three realms are entirely beyond the descriptive power of language. In these realms, consciousness differentiates itself completely from the lower mind and self.

> [I]t is God as an Archetypal summit of one's own Consciousness... At its peak, the soul becomes one, literally one, with the deity form... with God. One dissolves into Deity, *as* Deity – that Deity which, from the beginning, has been one's own Self or highest Archetype... (p. 69)

The *Causal Region* lies beyond the high subtle realm. The *low causal* is "the Pinnacle of God-consciousness, the final and highest abode of Ishvara, the Creatrix of all realms." At this level:

> [the] deity-Archetype itself condenses and dissolves into final-God, which is here seen as an extraordinarily subtle audible-light... from which the individual... Archetype emerged in the first place. Final-God is simply the ground or essence of all the archetypal and lesser-god manifestations which were evoked – and then identified with – in the subtle realms. In the low-causal, all of these archetypal Forms simply reduce to their Source in final-God, and thus, by the very same token and in the very same step, one's own Self is here shown to *be* that final-God, and consciousness itself thus transforms upwards into a higher-order identity with that Radiance. Such, in brief, is the low-causal, the ultimate revelation of final-God in Perfect Radiance and Release. (Wilber 1990, p. 71)

In the *high causal* region:

> ... all manifest forms are so radically transcended that they no longer need
> even appear or arise in Consciousness. This is total and utter transcendence
> and release into Formless Consciousness, Boundless Radiance. There is
> here no self, no God, no final-God, no subjects, and no thingness, apart
> from or other than Consciousness as such. (p.72)

Beyond this level:

> ... Consciousness totally awakens as its Original Condition and Suchness...
> which is, at the same time, the condition and suchness of all that is, gross,
> subtle, or causal. That which witnesses, and that which is witnessed, are
> only one and the same. The entire World Process then arises, moment to
> moment, as one's own Being, outside of which, and prior to which, nothing
> exists. That Being is totally beyond and prior to anything that arises, and
> yet no part of that being is other than what arises.
>
> And so: as the center of the self was shown to be Archetype; and as the
> center of Archetype was shown to be final-God; and as the center of final-
> God was shown to be Formlessness – so the center of Formlessness is
> shown to be not other than the entire world of Form. "Form is not other
> than Void. Void is not other than Form," says the most famous Buddhist
> Sutra... At that point the extraordinary and the ordinary, the supernatural
> and mundane, are precisely one and the same...
>
> This is also... the Ultimate Unity, wherein all things and events, while
> remaining perfectly separate and discrete, are only One. Therefore, this is
> not itself a state apart from other states; it is not an altered state; it is not a
> special state – it is rather the suchness of all states, the water that forms
> itself in each and every wave of experience, as all experience. It cannot be
> seen, because it is everything which is seen; it cannot be heard, because it
> is hearing itself; it cannot be remembered because it only *is*. By the same
> token, this is the radically perfect integration of all prior levels – gross,
> subtle, and causal, which, now of themselves so, continue to arise moment
> to moment in an iridescent play of mutual interpenetrating. This is the final
> differentiation of Consciousness from all forms in Consciousness,
> whereupon Consciousness as Such is released in Perfect Transcendence,
> which is not a transcendence from the world but a final transcendence as
> the world. Consciousness henceforth *operates*, not on the world, but only
> as the entire World Process, integrating and interpenetrating all levels,
> realms, and planes, high or low, sacred or profane. (p. 73-4)

*

Others have made observations similar to Wilber's. All agree that transition from
one level to another requires a release of previous patterns of belief. This *letting
go* is often experienced as a little death. Our little deaths prepare us for our
physical death, particularly if we are working on our inner awareness and
developing transpersonal awareness.

Death is only what shoves life along its way. It is a doorway to something new. Nothing is annihilated or lost or forgotten. All is carried on to the next place and all experience is shared and remembered. It is a great trick to learn to use this doorway. You must face, confront your death, prepare to die. This changes your place among the webs, gives you courage, shows you how living is a matter of attention.

– Kay Cordell Whitaker

Marie-Louise von Franz (1987), a gifted Jungian teacher and writer, presents further parallels to Wilber:

All of the symbols which appear in death dreams are images that are also manifested during the individuation process. (p. xiii)

Wilber (1980) explains that in Buddhist tradition, immediately after physical death each person opens to ultimate Consciousness. The average person is not prepared for this level of awareness and holds on to perceptions of personality, earthly thoughts, and so on. These draw them away from the infinite light.

Contracting in the face of infinity, he turns instead to forms of seeking, desire, karma, and grasping, trying to "search out" a state of equilibrium… [T]hese karmic propensities couple and conspire to drive the soul away from pure consciousness and downwards into multiplicity, into less intense and less real states of being (p. 164).

Fear of dissolution into the infinite All continues to drive people back from enlightenment, to the point of involution – when they are reborn, repressing (but not entirely forgetting) memories of this process.

A person can step off this wheel of life, death and rebirth through dedicated meditation. The potential is there at every moment, as consciousness is constantly shifting, at every instant, from ordinary awareness to infinite awareness. "This moment-to-moment phenomenon we call 'microgeny' – the micro-genetic involution of the spectrum of consciousness" (Wilber, p. 175).

As intricate and detailed as Wilber's analyses of meditative stages is, sometimes we can sense deeper truths more directly - in and between lines from experienced meditators:

… This noting of mental states encourages a deeper recognition of what is happening while it is happening. It allows us to be more fully alive to the present rather than living our life as an afterthought. It enables us to watch with mercy, if not humor, the uninvited swirl of "mixed emotions" not as something in need of judgment but as a work in progress.

– Stephen Levine 1997 (p. 35)

[M]editation is the practice of the art of dying, of letting go into the vast unknown.

– Stephen Levine (1997, p. 62)

... Healing awareness is a noninterfering attention that allows natural self-healing responses to take place...

... When consciousness itself becomes the object of attention, the necessary conditions for healing may become apparent...

– Frances Vaughan (1995, p. 59)

Those who justify themselves do not convince. To know truth one must get rid of knowledge. Nothing is more powerful and creative than emptiness.

– Lao Tsu

[E]ach technique needs to be done with balance and heart for the practice to take one beyond the method itself. For one not to be only a meditator but to become the meditation itself...

– Stephen Levine (1991, p. 14)

[T]he self as a subject cannot be known without turning itself into an object, thereby separating itself conceptually form the whole, apart from which it does not exist. One may nevertheless persist in treating oneself as if one were a distinct separate entity looking for its true nature. Just as the eye cannot see itself, the Self cannot find itself. As soon as I see myself as an object, I have made myself into an entity which exists only as a concept in my mind. The ego, insofar as it is known or perceived as an object, becomes the object of an unknown and superordinate subject, namely the Self. This self can be experienced, but cannot be known as an object.

– Frances Vaughan (1995, p. 53)

The earth is rapidly entering a new field of consciousness that is bringing it back into resonance with primal rhythms of creation. This new consciousness is rooted not in the historical human understanding of God but in an intelligence that resides within the very animating current of the universe. It is rooted in the informational reality of a universal Presence whose awareness and memory is awakening inside human time, awakening and gazing forth from within each vested interest, each player in this planetary field, helping people to understand the greater context in which they move the board, the other players, the rules of the Primate into Universal Species game.

– Ken Carey (p. 101-102)

Another avenue to transpersonal awareness is through bioenergy therapy. John Pierrakos (1974) discusses his views of the mind-body connection:[72]

With Reich, I recognize that the human character has three layers of development: the innermost, where spontaneously decent impulses originate; a middle layer, which Reich identified with the Freudian repressed unconscious, and where negative and destructive impulses germinate; and the outermost layer, the external behavior that the person interposes between the inner impulses and the outside world. Willfulness appears most strongly in this outer shell, maintaining the facade of manners and mores required by society. But volition penetrates through the interior layers too, because of the person's psychosomatic identity; and as it can work to perpetuate blocks, so can it work to remove them.

Bioenergetic therapy begins with the practitioner exploring the characterological symptoms that are perceptible both on the surface and below it. Vocal tones, body postures and gestures, skin texture and resilience, hair quality, eye luster, and other evidence reveal the location of blocks, their intensity, their interrelationships, something of their etiology, and their overall configuration – the type of character structure.

Pierrakos uses physical exercises (similar to those of Reich and Lowen) to help clients to understand their body *armoring* and defensive tensions, and to loosen up so that core energies can be mobilized. He emphasizes the element of willfulness in holding on to illness, when people elect to maintain their symptoms (despite their discomfort) rather than face the core emotions that may lie behind them.

He proceeds with discussion of integration of elements that extend beyond the individual person, into the *trans*personal.

> I found that almost all patients increasingly sensed a lack of deep fulfillment as they progressed toward the freeing of their functioning and improved their life situations. They showed this invariably as a yearning for greater unification with external reality.
>
> [T]he human energy system is by nature a creative design of forces working bidirectionally to integrate the self within and fuse the self with the environment.

In other words, our bioenergies coordinate our inner worlds of the body and mind, while at the same time linking us energetically with the environment – with which we are in constant bioenergetic interaction.

> [T]he mass of the living energy is the quantity of the person, and the consciousness of the living energy is the quality of the person. We do not therefore have a body and a spirit; we have a vital substance that in structure is the body and in function and perception is the spirit. The substance, under its two aspects, composes the core of the human being. The physiological body is energy slowed down into a denser, stable form rather as ice is water solidified. It swims in the energy body and is distinct from it only in degree of energetic vibration, not in substance.
>
> This definition accords with the findings of the physical sciences. We know that man is made of billions of cells that cohere structurally and functionally in an ascending order of complexity, from cells to tissues, from tissues to organs, from organs to systems, from systems to the entity who is the self. Under a microscope with the power to multiply, say, 500,000 times, the body would look rather like a galaxy, the cells spread out with spaces between them but uninterruptedly exchanging energies.

Pierrakos is speaking here of the same hierarchy that Gary Schwartz described earlier in linear terms, functioning as a system that is linked by imagery.

> ... Every minute cell knows exactly what it is doing – it is aware, and it acts as an individual. The same is true of all the structural components, up to the complex that is considered the seat of feeling, thought, and decision, the brain. But consciousness is not only the operation of the faculties of the mind. It is the unified whole of the power of knowing, from the cell's to the mind's and more: it includes the innate movement of the core outward from the self, the movement of the soul.
> The core of the person reaches toward infinity...

While it may seem that Pierrakos is using a metaphor of energies to link the elements in the hierarchy, he is actually speaking from his personal perceptions of these energies. Pierrakos is able to see auras, the halos of color, which are the energy fields that surround all objects (especially living ones). He describes several ways in which he correlates auras with his therapy:

> Any significant blocks disturb the entire energy system, not just the regions where they are located. This shows in the centrifugal outflow that makes up the aura.
> The organism as a whole, then, exhibits the three-beat pulsatory rhythm, just as does each miniscule cell – the assertive phase that carries energy outward from the body, the receptive phase that pulls energy into the body, and the rest phase that completes the cycle.
> The flow rate ranges from a low of about 15 pulsations per minute to 40 and above when the person is highly charged, as in sexual communion.[73]
> In an armored person, conversely, the energy flow in both directions is visibly sluggish at the sites of blocks, and the overall rate of pulsation in a neutral state is unnaturally high or low.

The phenomenon of the aura, which is an apparent visual perception of the energy component of matter, suggests the existence of energetic aspects to physical bodies. In Chapter 3 there is a wealth of evidence confirming the presence of such fields, suggesting that they may represent an energetic embodiment of our transpersonal selves. Pierrakos's core therapy integrates many levels of perception and awareness in both the therapist and the healee.

If each of us has a bioenergy self as well as a physical self, this could explain a variety of transpersonal theories and experiences, including out-of-body experiences, near-death experiences, survival of a spirit self beyond physical death, ghosts, channeling, and reincarnation. This is reflected in several ways in transpersonal psychology.

Many transpersonal therapists are now addressing clients' awareness of past life experiences in their practice. Though this may seem far-fetched, there is ample evidence to support the therapeutic benefits of such work.

The most remarkable evidence for psycho-spiritual residues that reach across linked lifetimes has been gathered by Ian Stevenson, a psychiatrist at the University of Virginia.[74] What I find most fascinating and convincing are his investigations of a series of birthmarks that correlate with physical traumas recalled from past lives by the people who bear these marks. For instance, a man had a small birthmark on the right side of his neck and a larger one on the left side of the back of his head. This corresponded with his memories of having committed suicide by shooting himself with a rifle that he had held under his chin, pressing the trigger with his toe. Stevenson was able to verify that a person fitting the past life memories of this man had in fact killed himself in just the manner described.

Within this framework of understanding, problems in our current lives may reflect physical and emotional traumas that have left scars in the surviving consciousness or in the energy body from past lives.

> *Every problem is an assignment from your soul. Therefore, acknowledge that a purpose is being served by your problem, your wound, your illness, your disability, your terminal condition, and try to align with it; that is, seek what it is trying to teach you. Remember that from the soul's perspective, a change in consciousness is of far greater value than a "cure." Therefore, follow King Solomon's wise injunction: "With all your getting, get understanding." Make that understanding the object of your quest and be optimistic that you will be rewarded.*
>
> – Robin Norwood

Psi and spiritual healing in psychotherapy

Several pioneering therapists are now incorporating aspects of psi into their work. This is an enlightened step, bridging a gap that heretofore has been filled primarily by many types of psychic *readers*. Through telepathy, clairvoyance, precognition and retrocognition, as well as through awarenesses of transcendent realms, psychic counselors can markedly deepen and quicken the psychotherapy – tuning in to issues that underlie people's problems. While no research has been done as yet to confirm this, it is my clinical impression that without such intuitive insights, it may take many more weeks and months to achieve the same progress. Furthermore, without the inputs through the intuitive impressions from transcendent realms there may be many subtle causal factors which could be completely missed.[75]

A caution is in order here. Many intuitive readers do creditable jobs, but some offer "shoot-from-the hip" insights without the benefit of proper psychotherapeutic processing of the materials. This can be unsettling and upsetting to those clients who are unprepared for intense emotional releases, and who are left without the benefits of counseling to sort out their emotions.

As a psychiatrist/ healer I am very interested in exploring cross-fertilizations between the practices of healers and psychotherapists. Let me share some of my early impressions.

One of the areas where healing can be helpful in psychotherapy is the alleviation of anxiety. This facilitates the process of therapy, making it easier for careseekers to deal with distressing emotional material. One of the nicest aspects of spiritual healing in this regard is that it is not habit-forming and has no dangerous side effects – in contrast with many of the medications that are used to treat anxiety.

There is a secondary level of anxiety that responds particularly well to healing. This type of anxiety may arise *from* people's basic conflicts and concerns. When people become upset or ill they tend to become anxious about being dis-eased. I call this level of worry *meta-anxiety* because it functions at a level of abstraction once removed from the original problem. Meta-anxiety frequently becomes part of a vicious circle of tension → worry about the tension → more tension → more worry → worry about the worry, and so on. At times this cycle can lead to panic. This is the level where people say in distress, "I can't stand this tension any more! I'm going to explode if this continues!" or "I'm going crazy!" or even, "If this depression continues, I'm going to kill myself." If therapists are uncomfortable with their clients' emotionality or with their meta-anxiety, they may consciously or unconsciously convey their uneasiness to their clients, whose meta-anxiety may then escalate to unmanageable proportions. Conversely, if therapists are not upset by strong emotional releases or panicked by the meta-anxiety, they can help their clients endure the anxiety-laden process of facing their fears and emotional hurts and assist them in restructuring their unconscious mind's defenses – enabling them to process and deal with the issues at hand. Their clients will thus be reassured that they need not panic, since they will not be struggling alone.

> *It isn't what happens that bugs you, it's the things that you say in your head about what happens that makes all the machinery get messed up, and leads to varieties of disease.*
> – Wallace C. Ellerbroek

Suggestion in all its forms can alleviate meta-anxiety, whether it be through a visit to a physician or healer; a diagnosis that transforms one's nameless fears into medically recognized syndromes (even if the obscure medical terminology is incomprehensible!); or simply the belief that the healer is healing us. Healing may thus be effective in part because of its relief of meta-anxiety through suggestion.

My clinical impression from speaking with many other healers, as well as from the experience gained in my own practice of psychotherapy combined with healing, is that *healing is specifically effective in relieving meta-anxiety, above and beyond the suggestion component.*

I have witnessed powerful emotional releases during healings, especially with *Reiki* and *Mariel* techniques, and I have heard similarly positive reports about SHEN healing methods. When people experienced these releases during healing, they did not come close to the meta-anxiety levels that I would have anticipated from similar emotional releases in a conventional therapy environment. Even patients who had previously denied having emotional difficulties, and had refused psychotherapy were helped though these techniques.

In these cases, the repressed emotions simply well up and pour out during healings. Sometimes they are digested without discussion or apparent conscious processing of the traumas. At other times there are spontaneous developments of insight and understanding by the healees, on their own or with the aid of counseling from the healers.

I propose that several mechanisms may contribute to these effects. First, healers and healees trust that whatever happens during healing is directed by a higher power, and is therefore sure to be beneficial. Second, healers and healees communicate on very deep levels during healing (probably including telepathy and/ or clairsentience) so the healees do not feel alone with their anxieties, and can draw directly and deeply on the healers' confidence in their ability to deal with these powerful emotions. Third, and most important, the healing process itself appears to help healees deal more effectively with their primary-level emotions, thus eliminating the meta-anxiety and panic.

Many healers report that one of the most noticeable effects of healing is a feeling of relaxation, with deep breathing and a sense of warmth or tingling. Controlled studies of healing for anxiety produced highly significant results,[76] confirming similar anecdotal reports. Clearly, this effect can help healees to break vicious circles of anxiety → tension → pain → etc. This seems to be an effect of spiritual healing per se, above and beyond those provided by conventional interventions already mentioned.

The usual assumption in psychotherapy is that people are cured once the problems that are bothering them are eliminated. But another possibility exists – as this apocryphal story illustrates:

CASE: John met his friend Henry at their ten-year high-school reunion. Discovering that Henry was unmarried, John asked him why. With some embarrassment, Henry revealed that he avoided serious relationships because he feared they would result in the woman discovering that he was a bed-wetter. He felt he could not endure such mortification. John then told Henry about his successful psychoanalysis for much more difficult problems, and recommended several good therapists.

When Henry arrived with his wife at the twentieth high-school reunion, John pulled him aside, saying, "I guess the psychoanalysis got rid of the bed-wetting?" "No," replied Henry. "Now I'm proud of it!"

People completing therapy may simply have learned to accept and live with their difficulties. Healers, who have broader worldviews than most psychotherapists and conventional doctors, may introduce new perspectives that permit clients to accept rather than fight against their symptoms. Spirituality may teach patience, tolerance, forgiveness, willingness to transcend one's travails and to help others, and more – while encouraging clients towards greater self-acceptance.[77]

A psychological problem can also be transformed into an asset. Psychology refers to this process as sublimation. For example, mentally ill people can transform their fantasies into artistic creativity (technically termed *regression in the service of the ego*), and hyperactive people can channel their energies into productive work. Katya Walter makes a strong case for combining our logical and linear potentials as *analinear* awareness:

> ... Logic has often labeled those who gather in the liminal twilight bordering the dark unconscious as deviates on the fringes of society, as romantics and degenerates and witches and spellbinders and dangerous lunatics escaped from the linear highways of traditionally sanctioned thought. Yet these people can enrich us even as they are despised for going beyond the

pale and over the linear edge. They stride into the boundless nightways of creation where darkness bestows creative riches and hidden truth.

Seers and artists and shamans could be an integral part of our society. Dark resonance could be acknowledged and discussed and harmonized within the culture, and in oneself. Dreams could be understood and heeded. Drugs could be dropped for the true high of a meaningful life that is not just touched by god, but nestled in god. (p. 145)

Healers are good at suggesting ways to sublimate problems, by opening healees to an awareness of the lessons that an illness may bring to the sufferer. They refocus healees' outlook from *fighting* their illness to *listening to what messages it is conveying and what lessons it is inviting the healee to learn.* They also may introduce alternative cosmologies such as reincarnation and astrology. These may at least provide people with explanations for their problems, and give them hope that things can change with understanding, patience, altered behavior, and the shifting of planets in the heavenly spheres. On deeper levels, these cosmologies remind us of our interrelationship with the All.

Sometimes physical symptoms may not respond to healing because they are rooted in such deep and pervasive disorders that to relinquish them would require intolerable changes in their underlying emotional condition. This may be one factor in some failures of spiritual healing – some healees may simply not be ready to relinquish their symptoms. In such cases healers can at least help people to bear their cross of suffering. Some of the more potent healers and some of those who are more gifted in counseling have effected dramatic changes even in such difficult cases, though not, by any means, in all of them.

On the other hand, many healers I have spoken with shy away from working with clients who have emotional problems. The healers have little understanding of the psychological processes involved. More enlightened healers refer these healees for counseling or therapy, while unenlightened healers simply ignore emotional problems. Sadly, many unenlightened doctors and nurses do the same.

The healing of psychological disturbances alone – that is, emotional distresses that are unconnected with physical problems – is scantily reported in the anecdotal literature on healing. There are relatively few articles written on healing for anxiety, depression and other emotional issues. An interesting exception is described by Alberto Villoldo and Stanley Krippner (1987). They describe a Brazilian surgeon who is now a healer working primarily with schizophrenics and epileptics. Kyriakos Markides describes a very remarkable Cypriot healer, the late Daskalos, who addressed serious emotional problems, sometimes identifying karmic components.[78] I am personally familiar with a growing number of other, less well-known psychotherapists who are also healers, who are very capable, sometimes actually gifted, in treating emotional problems. Through the addition of healing to their therapy, they appear able to facilitate much more rapid and deep developments of insights and emotional changes in their clients.[79]

No scientific studies of these types of healing have yet been reported. Therefore we cannot say with certainty whether the application of healing for anything more than reduction anxiety or depression is truly effective, though this seems highly likely.

The combination of healing with psychotherapy raises many controversial issues. Let me share some questions that I am struggling with as I expand my practice of psychotherapy combined with spiritual healing. My training led me to believe that people must understand the roots of their problems in order to receive the full lessons of their illness. Yet there are potent healers (such as the late Harry Edwards)[80] who primarily address the physical component of illness, and bring about rapid, dramatic, physical improvements without the benefit of psychological understanding. Some have suggested that insight, along with spiritual growth, will naturally follow of its own accord and in its own time. I feel that this is an important question to study, with far-reaching implications. I also would like to study healers and healees who do and do not address psychological components of illness, to learn whether there are quantitative and/ or qualitative differences in their healings.

Healers also offer dimensions of spiritual healing and counseling for the dying. A good death in itself is seen as the final healing.[81]

All of the factors mentioned above are at play in any therapeutic interaction. Suggestion is one of the most important of these, and one that makes many contributions to healing, so it has been discussed in greater detail above. Spiritual healing, likewise, is an inevitable aspect of therapeutic interactions.

COLLECTIVE CONSCIOUSNESS AND SPIRITUAL AWARENESS

Diverse evidence suggests that our minds can reach beyond the realm of our own individual consciousness.

Carl Jung described what he called the *collective unconscious*, exploring this shared pool of awareness as mirrored in the dreams and mental imagery of his psychoanalytic patients. This collective awareness manifested in universal *archetypal images* that often were not meaningful to his patients until Jung identified their mythic significance, at which point the messages from their unconscious minds were clarified, and their emotional problems were resolved.

> I vividly recall the case of a professor who had had a sudden vision and thought he was insane. He came to see me in a state of complete panic. I simply took a 400-year-old book from the shelf and showed him an old woodcut depicting his very vision. "There's no reason for you to believe that you're insane," I said to him. "They knew about your vision 400 years ago." Whereupon he sad down entirely deflated, but once more normal.
> – Carl Jung (1964)

It appears that mythic, archetypal imagery resides in a collective conscious of mankind, available as a vehicle for expressing and processing emotions and conflicts. There may be layers and layers of interconnectedness. Marie Louise von Franz (1980) suggests there is a core layer of the mind in which universal consciousness resides, a layer in which all of mankind participates, and that extending out from this core are increasingly developed and localized layers, each limited in their scope of awareness to particular transpersonal levels. People connect with whatever layers they are sensitive to, according to their degree of psychological and spiritual development.

> Our personal psychology is just a thin skin, a ripple on the ocean of collective psychology. The powerful factor, the factor which changes our whole life, which changes the surface of our known world, which makes history, is collective psychology, and collective psychology moves according to laws entirely different from those of our consciousness...
> – Carl Jung (2000, Vol. 18; 371)

This all sounds very grand, but how can we explain the collective unconscious?

The most basic elements contributing to the collective unconscious are the psi powers of telepathy, clairsentience (perceiving objects in the world without outer sensory access to them), precognition (knowing the future) and retrocognition (knowing the past).[82] If we can communicate with others telepathically, and they with us, then our minds have the potential to link with others in a network that forms a collective consciousness.

Spontaneous psi interactions between people often occur during dreams, and psi perceptions often come to us as metaphoric imagery. The similarity between dream imagery and psi imagery suggests that both may occur in the same parts of the brain and/or mind, in the deeper layers of our awareness, below conscious perception and cognition. Our unconscious minds are in more immediate and intimate contact with the world beyond ourselves than our conscious minds are aware of. Our psi awareness is frequently (perhaps even constantly) functioning below our conscious awareness. We are thus intimately linked to the minds of everyone else in the world through telepathy, as well as to the inanimate world via clairsentience, in a vast interconnected network. Precognition and retrocognition extend our awareness backwards and forwards in time, so our consciousness can extend anywhere and *anywhen*. In essence, there is a cosmic data bank to which we all have access through our personal participation in its creation and maintenance – though each of us sees only portions of it, and these are generally perceived indistinctly.

You might think that such speculations are far-fetched, but various experiments have confirmed that it is possible to bring these psi perceptions into conscious awareness. For instance, remote viewing studies by Robert Jahn and colleagues at Princeton University School of Engineering have shown that subjects sitting in a laboratory can accurately describe what is transpiring at distant locations, *before* the verifying observers choose the locations and then go there to validate the predicted psi perceptions.[83]

Rupert Sheldrake hypothesizes that specific files in the cosmic data bank are reserved for the use of each living species. Individuals within a species contribute information to their species' file and can also read information that has been accumulated within the file. This would explain such phenomena as the migration of birds, which can fly accurately to their species' nesting grounds without instructions from others of their species.

Laboratory experiments provide further support for Sheldrake's theories. The most striking demonstrated an ability of highly inbred strains of laboratory mice to learn mazes. In the US, mice from one of these strains were taught to run particular mazes, and successive generations learned them faster than their forbears. This was at first explained away as social learning that was transmitted from parents to offspring. However, years later, scientists in England tested mice of the same strain, who were very distant cousins of the original US mice that had learned the mazes. Though they had common ancestors, the English mice were not direct descendants of the US mice and could therefore not have acquired their maze knowledge through genetic inheritance or social learning. Nevertheless, some of the English mice ran the same mazes correctly on their first trial. Sheldrake's theory of a species-specific intuitive data bank could explain these findings.

Sheldrake also suggests that data on the body shape, size and functions of each species are stored in some of these files, which he calls *morphogenetic fields*. These could serve as cosmic information centers that track the development of species over time.

Spiritual awareness seems to reside in a similar transpersonal cosmic library. We can tap into this resource if we first clear our inner computer screen, as in meditation, or if we pray to be linked into the grid of collective consciousness. Prayers and rituals that are repeated many times may become morphogenetic paths towards spiritual awareness. These subjects are discussed further in Volume III.

PREVIEW OF AN ENERGY HEALING MODEL

Let us briefly review the discussion so far of mind-body links.

Interactions between the mind and the body are pervasive and complex. At the simplest level, we see that emotions are expressed by the body in nonverbal communication.[84]

At a more organic level, memories may be stored in association with, if not actually within, various tissues and organs of the body – particularly in muscles and tendons, as witnessed in the emotional releases that are common during massage and other *bodymind* therapies. Several psychophysiological mechanisms for this storage are possible. There is strong evidence that psychological conditioning can imprint information in the body. This occurs through nerves, muscles and hormones. Emotional stress may produce localized or generalized physical tensions, accompanied by pains or other malfunctions in many parts of the body, such as muscle and joint aches, hypertension, asthma or ulcers. The immune system may also participate in these bodymind interactions.

Conversely, problems in the body may also influence our awareness and emotions. Illnesses caused by known physical agents and processes may be accompanied by emotional and physical tensions. If these are chronic, they can produce pains that lead to vicious circles of pain → anxiety → tension → more pain → more anxiety → etc. Such tensions may present as simple muscle tightness (e.g. headaches, backaches, stomach aches, etc.), or they may exacerbate other illnesses, as in the case of emotional disturbances that worsen existing diabetic metabolic disorders, or set off thyroid dysfunctions.

Many aspects of these discomforts may be relieved through a variety of conventional psychotherapy techniques, including talking psychotherapy, suggestion (generated by oneself or by others), placebos, hypnosis, relaxation techniques, meditation, biofeedback, and medications (e.g. tranquilizers, pain medicines and muscle relaxers). These interventions block the recurrent loops of the vicious circles.

In addition to the bodymind mechanisms that have been discussed in this chapter, numerous complementary therapies (discussed in Chapter II-2) demonstrate that the mind may influence the body through *subtle energy* aspects of the body. That is, there are subtle biological energy fields around and within the body that may be influenced by the mind, and that may reciprocally influence the mind. These fields appear to control various functions of all levels of our being.

Many conventional medical practitioners find it difficult to understand subtle energy medicine. This is partly because they tend to focus on one particular mode of complementary therapies, or even on a partial aspect of a method, and forget that other factors may simultaneously be playing an equally important role. Biological energy interventions have been ignored by conventional medicine, and it has been assumed that spiritual healing is no more than massage, soothing touch or suggestion. The subtle energy aspect of healing has been largely overlooked.

> *If all you have is a hammer, then everything looks like a nail!*
> – Abraham Maslow

It may be that aspects of mind function as an energy field, with the brain serving as a transducer for this field. Healers go even further and suggest that the energy field is where a person's *being* resides, and that this is a template for the physical body. Looking at it from the other side, the body can be seen as the expression of a person's spirit. It is like a sort of metaphysical garment that is worn while receiving a lifetime of lessons (which may include illnesses) and then discarded, to be replaced in future lifetimes by other garments that are appropriate to further lessons. These spiritual and philosophical aspects of subtle energies and healing are discussed in Volumes III and IV of *Healing Research.*

Self-healing may be brought about by a change of mind that alters subtle energy fields, which subsequently causes changes in the body.

If we accept that spiritual healing may be projected by healers in the form of energy fields,[85] we can postulate that it might act on the body in further ways. It could release old, maladaptive mental and emotional patterns; permit natural, healthy patterns to reassert themselves; and/ or insert new, healer-inspired, healer-generated or healer-transmitted patterns in the bodymind of the healee.

Moving from purely psychological problems to psychosomatic ones, we find additional levels of complexity. Spiritual healing may be directly effective in alleviating body tensions and releasing memories stored within the body, bypassing the conscious mind.

> *It appears possible that consciousness may extend beyond the brain to include the whole body.*
> – DB

There will be further discussion of biological energy fields in Chapter II-3, following a review of many of the established techniques of wholistic energy medicine in Chapter II-2.

> *Our genetic heritage endows each of us with a series of emotional setpoints that determines our temperament. But the brain circuitry involved is extraordinarily malleable; temperament is not destiny.*
> – Daniel Goleman

CHAPTER 2

Wholistic Energy Medicine

The part can only be known
when the whole is apparent.
— Ted Kaptchuk (p. 142)

As you read this chapter, I hope you will attend in particular to the manners in which various therapies conceptualize and address problems. None has the exclusively correct approach for dealing with every health issue. Each offers a window of understanding and a doorway for therapeutic interventions in the house of healing.

Healing may be defined as the movement toward wholeness – through enhanced and harmonized awareness and function of body, emotions, mind, relationships and spirit. The ancient Germanic and English roots of the word "healing" derive from *haelen*, meaning "to make whole." To emphasize this point, I use the term *wholistic healing* to mean whole-person care.

At its best, wholistic medicine[86] is whole-person healing. This appeals to people who are discouraged by conventional, allopathic medicine's heavy focus on the body – on the *physical* aspects of illness. Ruth Benor Sewell, worked a lot with women who had breast cancer. Their nearly universal complaint was that their breasts were being well cared for, but the doctors seemed to forget that there was a woman attached to the breasts that they were probing and x-raying and needling and cutting and reconstructing, while prescribing toxic chemicals in hopes of curing the body of its disease.

Whole-person care has often been addressed under the popular term *holistic* (without the "*w*") care. These days, this term has come to have different meanings in various contexts. Often, it refers only to the use of isolated elements of a few complementary/ alternative medicine (CAM) therapies (such as acupuncture, osteopathy, herbalism and others) – which are often offered in very abbreviated and versions of the original practices, without including their rich roots in diverse ancient and modern treatment philosophies. Too many allopathic therapists go on weekend courses to learn about these modalities and immediately start applying fragments of the methodologies from these traditions. The *methodologies* are viewed as the whole therapy. The fuller essences of the therapeutic practices are ignored or discarded and much of their benefits are lost.

> *We have spent too much time criticizing healers because they are not doctors and not enough time criticizing doctors who are not healers.*
> – Jesuit Father Louis Beirnaent

Complementary therapies offer extensive systems for conceptualizing *dis-ease* and disease. These systems differ substantially from the traditions of Western, allopathic medicine in their approaches to problems of physical, psychological and spiritual health and illness.

Some of the explanations offered by CAM therapies may appear strange – within Western systems of analyzing the world. I urge you not to reject them on this basis. At the very least, there may be elements within these CAM approaches which could be understood within conventional medical science. Herbal remedies may contain medicinal substances. Massage therapies may work through relaxation of the body, which in turn improves circulation, decreases levels of stress hormones, and enhances the "feel-good" levels.

If you hold an open mind, you may also find that CAM therapies suggest ways for expanding our understandings of health and illness. Western medicine focuses almost exclusively on the body – as a *physical* organism. Its interventions are primarily physical – through medications, hormones, surgery, and recently expanding into genetic manipulations. CAM therapies address the subtle energies that hold body, mind, relationships and spirit together.

If these systems feel to you more like myths than reality, consider the possibility that Western explanations of the world may also contain many elements of myth. It is widely acknowledged that half of all medical beliefs and practices are wrong... and that we have no way to identify at any point in time which ones are correct and which are not! Assessments of medical practices at intervals as short as ten years will reveal many of the false beliefs – clarified in the light of new discoveries and new theoretical explanations.

And myths should not be dismissed as useless folktales. Myths guide and shape our lives in obvious and subtle ways. The myth that Western science will one day understand everything about the universe through analysis of the material world has led to many discoveries that make our world more habitable, predictable and safe. However, this myth is so pervasively prevalent that to question it almost seems to be a heresy. This very same myth leads us to seek to gain control nature, just as we seek to gain control over our physical bodies – rather than seeking ways to live in harmony with nature. In addressing illnesses, many CAM therapies (notably Native American and Traditional Chinese Medicine) advocate strongly for explorations of our place in the broader world around us, seeking to understand what is out of harmony in our relationships with each other and with nature when we suffer from diseases. Within these systems, disease is a manifestation of dissonance between the individual and the world around her. Treatments may be directed to the community as well as to the individual, restoring harmony on more than one level. Western science is beginning to acknowledge that such factors may contribute to health and illness – when conceptualized and analyzed from perspectives of systems theory, chaos/ complexity theory, and studies of subtle biological energies

CAM therapies not only offer contrasts to conventional medicine, they also suggest ways in which conventional medicine might broaden and expand its own interventions.

In our focus on the goal of *curing* illness, we too often overlook the healing effects of *caring* that make the journey towards wholeness a healing one. Rudolph Ballentine (1999; 2001) has excellent discussions on conventional medicine's heavy emphasis on *effects* of underlying problems that manifest as symptoms and illnesses, and *effects* of discrete medical and surgical interventions that are meant to address these surface manifestations of deeper issues.

Conventional Western medicine has concentrated on treatments of the body, viewing psychological issues as peripheral to medical practice. This attitude permeates medical training, where students are drilled in finding the correct physical diagnosis and prescribing the best physical interventions.

I was distressed in medical school when I attended a well-baby clinic. The pediatrician was an absolute joy to observe. He obviously loved helping the babies and mothers who came to him for guidance, reassurance and clarifications of their maturation and health issues. Equally, the mothers, babies and children loved coming to visit him. This was such a breath of fresh air to me – in the otherwise dehumanizing process of medical education that focused on diagnosing and curing illnesses rather than treating people with dis-ease. My distress was over the attitudes of my fellow-students. They felt it was a waste of time sitting around with babies who were mostly healthy and mothers who were often anxious over problems which were not life-threatening.

Wholistic medicine views people as complex organisms whose minds, emotions, relationships and spiritual selves are as much a part of whatever they are experiencing as their physical bodies are.

This volume of *Healing Research* explores how consciousness can influence states of health and illness, acting directly through neurological, hormonal and immune mechanisms, as well as through biological energies. Psychological *dis-ease* manifests as *disease*. Physical problems are often a wake-up call from the unconscious mind, for the conscious mind to become aware of inner disharmonies and conflicts.

It is not surprising that about half the prescriptions written by family practitioners go unfilled or unused. People realize (consciously or unconsciously) that the symptoms the physician is addressing are not the real issue. What they really need is something that the doctor is not providing.

Wholistic healing helps people to become aware of their whole selves on all levels, and then to discover the disharmonies that are manifesting as problems in their lives, so that they can sort out how to address them. In many cases it is not just a matter of treating the symptoms of physical pain, fatigue, or trauma. These symptoms invite us to explore the underlying tensions that have created them, as discussed in Chapter II-1.[87]

Facilitating self-healing and whole-person care is a creative challenge to wholistic health caregivers. They must be educators as well as prescribers and providers of direct interventions. This is in sharp contrast with the physician's traditional roles of *prescribing and administering treatments* within the prevalent model of Western allopathic medicine. These issues will be discussed in greater depth in the concluding sections of this chapter.

Strengths of conventional, allopathic medicine
Wholistic health care need not conflict with good allopathic medical care.

The strengths of conventional allopathic practice are in making precise diagnoses and prescribing specific therapies. To arrive at a diagnosis, doctors rely on the history of symptoms, on physical examination and on the results of laboratory tests that may be quite sophisticated. Preventive interventions have also been a major contribution of modern medicine, particularly in improving hygiene and sanitation.

For many years allopathic medicine rejected complementary therapies because there had been little or no rigorous, Western-style research to validate the efficacy of their approaches. Western doctors (including myself) thought that these were spurious interventions – no better than placebos that could lead to improvement through the potent powers of suggestion.

> *Formerly, when religion was strong and science weak, men mistook magic for medicine; now, when science is strong and religion weak, men mistake medicine for magic.*
> — Thomas Szasz

Allopathic medicine recommends *evidence-based* practice. Ideally, new therapies should be carefully researched before they are accepted into the medical armamentarium to help fight against disease. Doctors and nurses are cautious against making the *Type I research error* of accepting as valid a therapy that is not truly effective.[88] We know that therapies may be effective simply because patients and doctors *expect they will work*, whether or not they are intrinsically beneficial. This is called the *placebo effect*. Roughly 30% of patients suffering from almost any illness will show some symptomatic improvement with any treatment whatsoever. This appears to be due to the effect of psychological expectations, working in combination with the patients' own self-healing capacities.

Conventional medical practitioners have regarded these *placebo* responses as something of a nuisance, feeling that they interfere with efforts to determine the effects of what Western medicine considers *real* therapeutic interventions, particularly when medications are involved.

Various research strategies have been devised to test the effectiveness of treatments, taking into consideration the placebo response.

Research approaches
Randomized controlled studies: To guard against Type I errors, researchers have devised the *randomized controlled trial* (*RCT*). A treatment modality (medication, surgical procedure, psychotherapeutic method, or complementary therapy) must

pass a battery of stringent RCTs before it can be accepted as a legitimate therapy. In an RCT, a group composed of patients who have the same diagnosis and severity of illness is randomly divided into sub-groups. One of the subgroups is given the therapy under study and another group is given a known placebo. A third group may be given a therapy of proven intrinsic value (a medication, massage, etc.). The groups receiving comparison treatments are called *control* groups. Therapists, researchers and subjects in the study are kept *blind* to which of the treatments (experimental therapy, placebo, or intervention of known value) is being given to any one subject. This minimizes the effects of suggestion, which might influence subjects to feel better or worse in response to the expectations of the therapists or researchers, or according to their own expectations of improvement with a given therapy. Assessments of symptomatic change, whether negative or positive, are likewise made by diagnosticians who are blind to the particular therapy being given, for similar reasons. Where therapists and subjects are blind to the treatment given, it is called a *double blind* study.

Therapies are administered within a standard protocol that is determined prior to the start of the study, so subjects within treatment groups will receive similar doses and durations of interventions. This assures that the treatments under study are of known quality and quantity and it allows other researchers to replicate the experiment under a similar protocol.

When the study is completed, statistical analyses are prepared, based on the results. These provide estimates of the possibility that the results of the RCT might have occurred by chance. The most common statistical standard for a treatment to be accepted as a valid finding rather than a chance occurrence is that it must be effective beyond the statistical probability of five times in a hundred. That is, there is less than a chance of 5 times in 100 that the results could have occurred randomly. (This is expressed as *p less than .05*, or *p < .05*). Naturally, if the same results would only occur by pure chance less than one time in a hundred ($p < .01$) or one time in a thousand ($p < .001$) and so on, they are that much more impressive.

> *The aim of science is not to open the door to infinite wisdom,*
> *but to set a limit to infinite error.*
> – Bertolt Brecht

At the end of the study, subjects in the various groups are checked to see that there were no differences between the groups in respect to any clinically important variables. For instance, there might have been one group in which the subjects had more severe symptoms than another group – which would have biased the comparison between groups in their responses to the different therapies that each group received.

The initial randomization of subjects into the various groups is meant to guard against this possibility. Assigning subjects randomly to each group makes it statistically more likely that equal numbers of subjects with any given symptom or characteristic will be assigned to each group and therefore that the groups will be closely equivalent at the start of the study.

In some studies the same subjects are consecutively given active treatments and placebos, also under double-blind conditions. Subjects thereby serve as their own control group, thus eliminating the risk of variations in the composition of different groups. The difficulty with this approach is that there may be effects of a treatment that could carry over from one period of intervention to the next, thereby confounding the final results. In addition, subtle factors might bias each treatment period differently. For instance, there could be a change in personnel or other factors that differ for various subjects over a period of time. There might thus be more (or less) sympathetic clinical or research personnel present in either the treatment or control periods, which could bias the results through suggestion effects that would differ in the different treatment and control periods.

Despite the best efforts of scientists to establish a research protocol that will protect against Type I research errors, it is still possible that errors may occur. For example, there could be confounding differences between groups which are not identified and which bias the responses of some or all of the subjects for better or worse. This could mislead researchers into believing that the therapy caused (or failed to cause) various effects, when in reality the observed effects were due to unequal distribution of symptom severity between groups (or some other biasing influence – perhaps age or sex), which led to the different responses between the groups. If such an error leads to the rejection of a therapy as being ineffective when it *is* actually a potent intervention, it is classed as a *Type II research error*, which is an error of *rejecting as false something that is actually true*.

Notwithstanding its stated good intentions and best efforts, the actual practice of evidence-based medicine remains elusive. Conventional medicine generally overlooks the fact that the majority of accepted medical treatments have not been subjected to this careful scrutiny. Furthermore, medical research is challenged by the enormous complexity of the human organism, which eludes the best efforts of studies that are intended to clarify its nature. It is impossible to account for every relevant variable that might influence a given symptom or illness. Many studies, even when performed to the highest scientific standards, remain open to questions and criticisms regarding confounding variables that might have accounted for or at least influenced the observed results.

There is also a growing trend in America for medical advertising and promotional companies to commission medication studies. This introduces serious issues of researcher bias in performing and reporting the research.

Even without all of the above methodological problems, the results of studies are frequently open to more than one interpretation. The practice of medicine therefore remains as much an art as a science.

The tendency in conventional medicine is to err in favor of caution and not to accept new therapies until there is a convincing body of evidence with minimum risk of Type I research errors. Even leaving aside consideration of complementary therapies, many are questioning the validity of relying so heavily and exclusively on controlled studies, pointing out that the focus of RCTs is too narrow.

The U.S. Food and Drug Administration (FDA) licenses the prescription and sale of new medications and therapies on the basis of such research. The costs of building a body of evidence for FDA approval amount to hundreds of millions of dollars for each treatment. Needless to say, only pharmaceutical companies and other organizations with enormous financial resources can afford such expenses.

It is not suggested that RCTs should be abandoned. There are, however, other research approaches that can round out the picture, particularly with CAM therapies.

Observational studies: Anecdotal evidence from reports of individual therapists is also useful in sorting out which therapies are of benefit. However, there are countless difficulties involved in accepting any individual person's positive response to a treatment as evidence for the efficacy of that treatment. Possible confounding variables that may contribute to an individual's improvement include: spontaneous waxing and waning of symptoms over the normal course of the illness; constitutional or psychological strengths of that particular person which may exceed the average; unknown variables of diet, activity, or other therapeutic interventions; changes in psychological stresses or in social support; and so on.

Anecdotal reports are strengthened when a series of subjects' responses to treatments is presented. If several people had similar results, it is more likely that the observations are valid.

A further caution, however, with anecdotal evidence is that the professional training, views and personal experiences of the reporting observer may bias the report.

Nevertheless, anecdotal evidence provides the necessary initial observations of a new therapy and if these reports suggest that the therapy may be helpful, they encourage further study.

In addition, anecdotal reports are usually rich in details of a personal nature – details that tend to be lost when the responses of large numbers of people are statistically analyzed.

Qualitative studies analyze individual responses to treatments, while still guarding against Type I errors. Small numbers of people with a common problem are given a particular therapy and their reports are studied in great individual detail. Analyses of these details provide a basis on which to build theories about *how a therapy may work to make a person better.*

Surveys of patients' satisfaction with treatments: Surveys provide yet another avenue for assessing benefits of therapies. The medical profession tends to consider these research methods of lesser value, due to the biased belief that self-assessments will be riddled with Type I errors. Surveys are frequently dismissed as "purely subjective evidence." Yet it is the consumers of health treatments who are increasingly voting with their feet and dollars for the therapies that they find helpful and increasing numbers of people are choosing complementary therapies.

Research in wholistic therapies
All of the above-mentioned types of research on spiritual healing are discussed in *Healing Research* Volume I.

In Volume II we focus on studies of a broad spectrum of additional complementary therapies, with a particular focus on biological energies that may be involved in these therapies. Heavy emphasis will be given to RCTs, to establish as clearly as possible that these modalities produce measurable effects and are not placebos.

Growing numbers of rigorous studies demonstrate that CAM therapies are effective and it is surprising that many conventional doctors and scientists are as yet little aware of them. Without having investigated the available scientific evidence, many criticize CAM as being unsupported by research, compared to conventional medical treatments. In fact, today the situation is quite the opposite. Rupert Sheldrake systematically reviewed a range of conventional scientific papers, to see how many included blinds or double-blinds that would control for experimenter bias. He found none in the physical sciences, 0.8 percent in the biological sciences, 24 percent in conventional medicine, only 5 percent in psychology and animal behavior studies and 85 percent in parapsychological studies. No comparison is available for CAM studies in general. For spiritual healing the studies with blinds comprise more than 25 percent.

While the RCT is viewed by many as the golden standard for examining the efficacy of therapies, it has not proven entirely satisfactory for clinical subjects (where statistics may overlook important qualitative aspects of treatment) and the RCT may not be adequate or appropriate for the study of many aspects of complementary therapies. This is because complementary therapies are individualized to the personalities and circumstances of the individual respant (*responsible participant,* per Siegel 2002) much more than allopathic therapies are.

In conventional medicine, an atherosclerotic heart is seen as a muscle whose blood supply is compromised by clogged arteries. The primary therapy is focused on cleaning out the arteries, preventing blood clots or even replacing the heart. Some attention may be given to dietary factors such as cholesterol and salt intake and to lifestyle factors such as smoking and exercise.

In wholistic integrative care, attention may also be given to various vitamins and minerals that can be of help; to the stresses that may be raising blood pressure; to emotional heartaches that may be manifesting in physical heart symptoms; to biological energies related to the heart and to the rest of the body (addressed through spiritual healing, acupuncture, craniosacral therapy, homeopathy, flower essence or other CAM therapies); and to spiritual issues, such as the will to live and concerns over the possibility that the heart disease may prove fatal.

Randomized controlled studies often do not take these additional factors into consideration. It may in fact be inappropriate to use control groups, because each person is so different from every other person that the treatments indicated in complementary therapies may be completely individualized for every patient, despite the similarity of the medical diagnosis. (There are further discussion of these differences in approaches and of individualized treatments in the final section of this chapter.)

Skeptics suggest that complementary therapies have not been explored through controlled studies and should therefore be viewed with the utmost caution – but here they are applying a double standard. The current high standards for research have evolved over recent decades. Many conventional therapies, as mentioned above, have not passed the rigorous tests that would have been demanded of them had they been discovered today.

Despite all of these cautions and warnings, an impressive and growing body of controlled research on complementary therapies is available, as reviewed in the professional edition version of this chapter.

Although much of the evidence available shows that complementary therapies are effective, some health care professionals remain skeptical. This is mostly a problem of adjusting to new concepts and treatments.

> *New options are always suspected and usually opposed, without any other reason but because they are not already common.*
> – John Locke

Qualitative vs. quantitative assessments

> *Not everything that counts can be counted and not everything that can be counted counts.*
> – Albert Einstein

Rigorous research methods have their limitations. While quantitative studies help to analyze *average reactions* to treatments, many important details are missed when we focus on the abstract picture. Double-blind, randomized, controlled studies may provide precise evidence relating to narrow, general questions but they do not give a complete picture of clinical therapies. The very precision of their focus makes them blind and insensitive to many qualitative aspects of treatment.

> *According to the latest official figures, 47% of all statistics are totally worthless.*
> – Ashleigh Brilliant

As mentioned earlier, observational case reports and qualitative studies provide valuable contributions to our understanding of how various complementary therapies can be of benefit. Though often subject to Type I errors, they flesh out the dry bones of the limited, bare facts that are garnered from controlled studies.

Two quotations highlight these limitations of rigorous research:

> *The scientific picture of the world is inadequate for the simple reason that science deals only with certain aspects of experience in certain contexts. All this is quite clearly understood by the more philosophically-minded men of science. But most others tend to accept the world picture implicit in the theories of science as a complete and exhaustive account of reality.*
> – Aldous Huxley

> *Science strives to reduce our experience of symbols. Experiences are colorful, multi-faceted and fuzzy along the edges; symbols are bland, one-dimensional and precisely-bounded. Real world observations can be bulky and ill-shaped and can have both strong and tenuous ties with a myriad of other real world observations; abstractions are built of simple, smooth-faced elements, uncoupled from other constructs... Scientifically, we give*

up the shifting and elusive mystery of the world, but, in exchange, we gain the standardised and reproducible abstractions from which we can build determinate explanations.
– Michael Katz (p. 85)

Qualitative studies explore the subjective experience of dealing with illness. Single case studies offer in-depth explorations of many dimensions of illness and treatments that are often overlooked by quantitative studies that focus on externally measurable symptoms. With single subjects, however, it is difficult to know how much of the result may be attributed to the individual personality of the subject or other factors. When similar responses are found in groups of people with similar problems, we have greater assurance that we are dealing with subjective experiences that are common to a given illness or treatment.

There are valid points on both sides of this argument. Conventional medicine works hard to research and validate its own therapies. Until recently, most of the complementary therapies did not subject their treatments to such scrutiny and there is therefore a modest body of research to validate their efficacy. On the other side of the argument, complementary therapy practitioners complain that it is impossible to assess many of their interventions within standard Western research designs. Homeopathic remedies, for instance, are prescribed to each person on an individualized basis. People suffering from the same illness or syndrome may express similar symptoms, but their personalities and life experiences will be different and therefore the underlying causes of their illnesses may also differ. A standardized therapy applied to a group of subjects for the purpose of research would not be a fair test of homeopathy because some people would not receive the correct remedy for their constitutional makeup, personalities and life experiences. Despite these challenges, in recent years a substantial body of research on complementary therapies has been coalescing.

Integrative medicine and whole person care

To analyze holism is unholistic.
The whole is more than the sum of its parts.
– Tony Pinchuck and Richard Clark

Integrative care combines the best of conventional medical approaches and wholistic energy medicine, to offer the maximal benefits to patients and therapists. When practiced wholistically, this is *whole-person care*.

An atmosphere of competition has developed between various allopathic and complementary health care practitioners, each claiming that their interventions are better in particular ways than those of other therapists. In some instances sick people have been faced with the dilemma of having to choose between conventional and complementary therapies. some allopathic doctors have refused to treat patients who seek therapies they consider to be of unproven value, and complementary therapy practitioners may feel that their approaches are incompatible with allopathic medicine. Many people who find complementary therapies helpful simply don't tell their doctors that they are receiving these treatments and if they do tell them, they may encounter a very mixed reception.

How can I prove I'm not crazy to people who are?
– Ashleigh Brilliant

Conventional, allopathic medicine has for many decades enjoyed a monopoly over the practice of health care in the West. In the eyes of the public, the presumed superiority of this approach had the appearance of legitimate, established fact. This viewpoint has been supported by legislation that is heavily influenced by medical lobbying. But while legislation is necessary to protect the public from unethical practices and practitioners, many feel that such laws have served to restrict the access of the public to therapies that are outside the realm of mainstream medicine. For example, homeopathy was very widely practiced in the US at the end of the 19th Century, but medical doctors successfully lobbied to enact laws restricting homeopathic practice. Such restrictive lobbying continues today. Medical practitioners who refer patients to CAM practitioners or who practice CAM methods are censured by some state medical societies for diverging from conventional medical practice. Were such laws to be rigidly enforced, there could never be any new developments or progress in medical care. The public has responded to these restrictive measures by lobbying for enactment of *access to treatment laws*.

The main strengths of conventional medicine lie in its rigorous research methodology; its precision in diagnosis; its effective treatment of infections and of other illnesses that respond well to medications, hormones and surgery; and the promise of medically indicated genetic manipulations.

Nevertheless, there remain vast numbers of sick people for whom conventional medicine offers only limited understanding and treatment options. In some cases, as in cancer chemotherapies, side effects of conventional treatments may diminish quality of life even more than the illnesses they are intended to treat. Side effects of tranquilizers, antidepressants, painkillers and sleeping pills, among many other frequently prescribed medications, may also be unpleasant or even dangerous – individually and in combination.

A very sobering summary of the dangers of conventional medications is presented by J. Lazarou and colleagues. They reviewed 39 prospective studies from U.S. hospitals between 1966 and 1996 and summarized the incidence of negative drug reactions leading to hospital admissions, or occurring while people were hospitalized – many of which were serious enough to be permanently disabling or fatal. They did not include errors in medication administration, or incidences of overdose, abuse, or allergic reaction.

The person who takes medicine must recover twice, once from the disease and once from the medicine.
- Sir William Osler, MD

Lazarou and colleagues found an incidence of 6.7 percent serious adverse reactions and 0.32 per cent fatal reactions in hospitalized patients. They estimated that in 1994 there were 2,216,000 serious adverse drug reactions in hospitalized patients, with 106,000 deaths. This places adverse drug reactions between the fourth and sixth most common cause of death.[89]

This is not a problem restricted to the US. In New Zealand, a study carried out by Harvard School of Medicine showed that one in four people with serious health problems suffered effects of medical errors. This was particularly likely to occur when several physicians were involved in treating the same person.

Medical errors may also contribute to negative effects and fatalities, for an estimated 44,000 to 98,000 additional annual casualties due to negligent medical care, as reported by the Institute of Medicine.[90] These numbers exceed the annual fatalities from highway accidents, breast cancer and AIDS. It is a sobering statistic that we are 9,000 times more likely to die under medical care than from wounds inflicted by firearms. Len Horowitz, a biting critic of the dangers of medical treatments, calls this *iatrogenocide*.

In contrast, the anticipated annual death rates from consumption of vitamins, herbal products, homeopathic remedies and flower essences are near zero.

This is not to say we should be complacent and ignore the few serious side effects that have been reported, nor that we shouldn't be on the alert and searching for any further serious side effects of these approaches. For instance, improper use of acupuncture needles and inappropriate use of force in spinal manipulations can cause injuries. Kava is an herb which has been used successfully for treatment of anxiety. Recently, it has been discovered that Kava can cause liver damage, which is sometimes fatal. We are also just beginning to learn that there are also herb and supplement interactions with conventional medications.[91] Adverse effects, where apparent, are listed under each therapy. Nevertheless, the CAM therapies remain indisputably safer by far than medical treatments.

Confirmation of the fatal dangers involved in medical practice comes from the statistics of mortuaries in Israel during periodic doctors' strikes. There were 15 to 50 percent fewer deaths during these periods.[92]

> *It may seem a strange principle to enunciate as the very first requirement in a Hospital that it should do the sick no harm.*
> – Florence Nightingale

A further problem associated with allopathic medical practice is the enormous cost of medical treatments, which is of growing national concern in every country in the world.

Likewise of great concern are the costs of days lost from work due to health problems that have not responded to medical care are.

Complementary therapies can help with many of the chronic health problems for which conventional medicine offers limited benefits, such as back pain[93] and other chronic pains; arthritis; neurological disorders (from accidental injury or cerebral palsy,[94] or from diseases such as multiple sclerosis (Gardener), myopathies, etc.); emotional disorders; chronic fatigue syndrome; and many more. These are ailments that cost the health care system enormous sums because they require multiple consultations, expensive diagnostic tests, costly medications and other interventions – and in many cases they are incurable. Health care authorities have responded to the mounting costs with bureaucratic legislation that addresses only the time/ wages and therapy cost factors, leaving both health caregivers and patients dissatisfied. These problems are not new. William Shakespeare quipped: "[You] can get no remedy against this consumption[95] of the purse."

CAM therapists address the whole person rather than just a set of symptoms. This is appreciated by many people who complain that conventional doctors don't take the time to speak with them beyond inquiring about their immediate complaints. To some extent this has been due to the narrow focus of medical practitioners on *physical* aspects of illness. In addition, managed care has steadily lowered the fees of doctors, who have responded by abbreviating the amount of time spent per patient visit, in order to compensate for the drastic reductions in their income.

> *I am not a mechanism, an assembly of various sections.*
> *And it is not because the mechanism is working wrongly that I am ill.*
> *I am ill because of wounds to the soul, to the deep emotional self.*
> *And the wounds to the soul take a long, long time, only time can help*
> *And patience and a certain difficult repentance.*
> *Long, difficult repentance, realization of life's mistake and the freeing*
> *   of oneself*
> *From the endless repetition of the mistake*
> *Which mankind at large has chosen to sanctify.*
>   – D. H. Lawrence

On the other hand, the weaknesses of complementary therapies include a limited appreciation of precision in diagnosis and research; lack of follow-up to determine why some patients treated do not improve; and lower standards of peer supervision and review.

Both allopathic and complementary therapists may have limited appreciation of psychological factors that can contribute to the development of illness and limited training in dealing with them. Most conventional therapists and many CAM therapists may likewise be lacking in spiritual awareness. But for increasing numbers of complementary therapists, particularly spiritual healers, the spiritual aspects of awareness are the most important in assessing health and illness.[96]

There is also a growing appreciation that complementary therapies can be cost-effective. The fact that complementary therapists charge less than allopathic physicians is only one contributing factor in this regard. Their primary cost-effectiveness derives from successfully treating illnesses and getting people better more quickly.

Despite the difficulties involved, complementary and allopathic therapists are learning to understand each other and to interweave their therapeutic modalities so that people who need help can receive the best combinations of therapies. This is not to deny that there are still significant differences in philosophies and practices between the various approaches. We are learning to cooperate and collaborate across these professional divides, respecting that each approach has its strengths and weaknesses, its successes and failures. Each has a piece of the puzzle to contribute to our comprehension of the human condition. If we work together, our understanding will become more complete. It is in this spirit that the discussions of various therapies are presented in this volume of *Healing Research*.

Wholistic care

Wholistic care seeks to bring people to a state of wholeness in body, emotions, mind, relationships and spirit. The main tenets of this approach are as follows:

- It is important to address the people who have the illness rather than merely treating their problems.
- Psychological dis-ease must be addressed as well as disease.
- Caring is at least as important as curing and often moreso.
- The therapist is as important as the therapeutic modality used in the treatment.
- The recipients of care are full participants in their own care and treatment.
- Spiritual dimensions are important aspects of healthy adjustment in the world.

Wholistic medicine is a growing, humanizing movement in the health field. It emphasizes treatment of the person who has the illness rather than of the illness the person has. This is not an innovation so much as a return to the bedside manner that doctors today have too little time to cultivate – under increasing pressures to provide "efficient" medical care.

The focus of wholistic medicine on philosophies and theories of practice rather than on methodologies, discussed at the start of this chapter, is clearly relevant here as well.

Some integrative clinics address various aspects of each patient separately, with a physician treating the body, a counselor or psychotherapist addressing psychological issues, a social worker dealing with relational problems, and a clergy team member attending to spiritual matters. The advantage of this approach is that each of the therapists can gain a more thorough knowledge of the patient according to their area of particular expertise. The doctors, who are paid very high wages, are encouraged to be as efficient as possible with their diagnoses, prescriptions and therapeutic interventions. They usually feel that they cannot spend the hour or more per visit that the other practitioners will routinely give.

While such a subdivision of labor may have economic advantages, it may at the same time leave patients feeling that they are being parceled out in bits, without being fully heard or understood by any one of their therapists – very much in the model of conventional medicine. The therapists may also be dissatisfied if there is little time or opportunity to communicate with each other. When the members of the team that is hitched to a patient's wagon all pull in different directions, even if only by a narrow angle of deviation, it does not serve the patient or the team as well as when there is a fully integrated effort.

Other integrative, wholistic practitioners address illness as an expression of the whole self – the body expressing through symptoms the stress and distress experienced in emotions, thoughts, relationships and spirit. This is not a new concept in health care – though it may be unfamiliar to many Western practitioners. Brooke Medicine Eagle explains:

> ... We now understand our own health as something created through the patterns of our lives; and are beginning to understand disease not as something bad or evil that "comes to get us", but as a symptom of an imbalanced way in which we walk on Mother Earth. With this understanding we can begin the process of healing ourselves through proper nutrition, physical exercise, new beliefs and a more healthy environment, as well as through the balancing of energies and the right use of medicines that stimulate the body's innate healing capacities. (p. 61)

Personal responsibility and prevention are major aspects of wholistic treatment. The respant is encouraged to participate in the treatment, especially with regular exercise, proper diet, avoidance of substances injurious to health (tobacco, alcohol, commonly allergenic foods that we tend to crave – such as chocolate, etc.) and application of active stress-reduction techniques (meditation, biofeedback, relaxation exercises, etc.). In essence, wholistic medicine advocates self-healing.

Since wholistic medicine views the person as a unity of body, emotions, mind, relationships and spirit, disease is seen not as something to be fought or extirpated, but as a problem to be understood. Illness is a dis-ease or disharmony of people within themselves, in their relationships with significant others, or in their interaction with their environment. While this is easy to say, it may be difficult to conceptualize – particularly when a patient has complex problems on several or all of these levels. Figures II-6 and II-7 illustrate this kind of complexity.

Richard Moss (1986), a wholistic, spiritual doctor, states:

> ... If we want to understand the disease, we must understand it as part of life itself seeking expression through a system that is unable to contain or conduct that life except in a diseased mode. To try and label the disease as the problem misses this fundamental point.
> [W]hat we call disease cannot be separated from the total consciousness of the individual. The healthy person isn't someone without the disease; the disease is not some abnormal addition to be eliminated. On the contrary, disease is a part of our wholeness. No matter how miserable we appear from a humanistically biased perspective, all individuals are already whole – now and always. Each of us is a complete system and the energies of being take a particular form of expression in each of us in accordance with our own unique dynamics.

Wholistic care for dis-eased people involves exploration of the roots of the disharmonies in their lives. Moss adds, "[F]ar from being some dark and terrible force, diseases such as cancer are the transformational impulses seeking expression in us... "

Figure II-6. Four aspects of health[97]

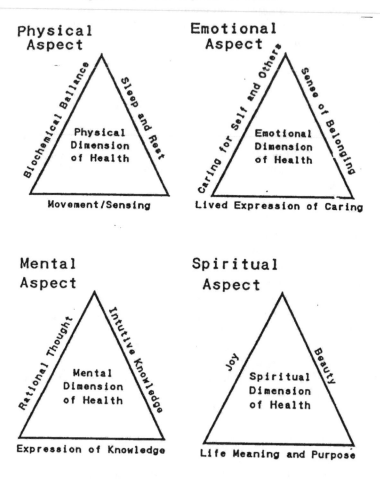

This approach can require major changes in the general attitudes of health practitioners as well as their clients. In a wholistic practice, people will no longer bring their bodies into the doctor's office for repairs, leaving the responsibility for the cure to the health practitioner and waiting patiently for something to happen through agencies beyond themselves.

> [I]llness and loss of inner strength appear together so frequently one could say that they are really different aspects of the same thing.
>
> Consequently, then, any medicine which does not assist us to recover our inner strength and fails to teach us how to look after ourselves in the end only creates a self-serving dependency – or to be frank, a co-dependency. Though we may seem to get well from such treatment, in fact the root imbalance will remain and we will configure new illnesses, one after another, until either death or true healing occurs. In this way, our present system of medicine actually betrays us while appearing to help.
>
> – Michael Greenwood (1998, p. 47)

Figure II-7. Interpenetrating process of healing[98]

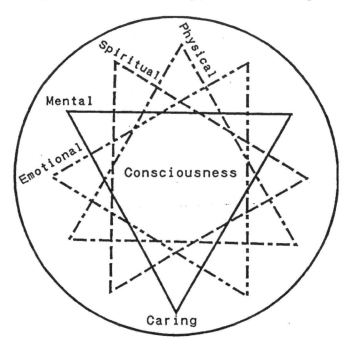

The wholistic practitioner becomes a counselor and midwife during the gestation of healing strategies and in the birthing of a new way for people to relate to their illnesses. In its truest essence, wholistic medicine is about helping people to grow more whole and to take greater responsibility for creating and maintaining their health.

Wholistic approaches are growing in popularity – within an atmosphere of general agreement that health care in the US and in many other countries is in serious need of reform. Medical administrators, legislators and insurance companies are unhappy with the high costs of medical care. Doctors are unhappy with the pressures put upon them to economize, when these pressures are often applied under bureaucratic regulations that are insensitive to the needs of individual patients and practitioners.

The remedies being applied address economic and administrative issues but tend to overlook many of the relevant human issues. Administrators regulate the types and durations of treatments allowable under insurance programs. Doctors are forced to shorten their interventions to work within these limitations and at the same time they are faced with inordinate burdens of paperwork, not to mention endless telephone arguments with bureaucratic administrators over regulations, to justify treatments that are essential for the welfare of their patients.

The public is unhappy with medical services that address bits and pieces of their bodies separately but often ignore them as people, and with a medical administration and insurance companies that view their problems as costs to be minimized and fail to address them individually.

Growing numbers of doctors and nurses are exploring ways to humanize this system and many of them have shifted to treating patients within wholistic frameworks. Holistic Medical Associations and Holistic Nursing Associations can be found in the US, Canada and several other countries around the world.[99] Training and certification in Holistic Medicine[100] and Nursing[101] are now available in the US. The public has been seeking help from a wide variety of practitioners outside the conventional medical system and people are now pressing doctors and insurance companies to include these treatments and attitudes within their medical treatment options. These trends are encouraging, although the overall picture in health care still seems rather bleak – for both practitioners and patients.

> ... The predominant style of medicine too often runs counter to the patient's own healing requirements: They need to develop autonomy, but are instead infantilized, kept in the dark; they need to actively affirm their uniqueness, but are reduced to passive recipients of normative "protocols"; they need time, but are rushed onto a virtual conveyer belt; they need to build up their immune system, but are given therapies that may debilitate it; they may crave life's messy vitality, but are instead sequestered in a sterile ward; they need a helpful vision of the future and are instead provided with often pessimistic ("realistic") prognoses; they may need to reacquaint themselves with their bodies (particularly the diseased parts, where emotional issues may be "somaticized"), but instead receive drugs that block function and sensation, or surgeries which may remove these parts altogether.
> – Marc Ian Barasch (p. 202)

The *how* of treatments may be as important, or even more important, than the *what*. A physician giving conventional treatment can be just as wholistic in his approach as any complementary therapist, when the treatment is given from the heart, with caring and compassion. Conversely, a CAM therapist can be just as un-wholistic as the crustiest allopathic practitioner, if the therapist mechanistically treats the presenting symptoms without attending to the whole person.

> *The utterances of the heart – unlike those of the discriminatory*
> *intellect – always relate to the whole. The heartstrings sing like*
> *an Aeolian harp only to the gentle breath of the premonitory mood,*
> *which does not drown the song but listens. What the heart hears are*
> *the great things that span our whole lives, the experiences which we*
> *do nothing to arrange but which we ourselves suffer.*
> – Carl Jung (1977)

One of my favorite New Yorker cartoons features a patient at the receptionist's desk, asking: "Does the doctor hug?"

Complementary therapies can be vehicles for wholistic care

Acupuncture, homeopathy, spiritual healing and other CAM approaches, when practiced in the fullness of their traditions, address the person who has the disease as a unitary, whole organism – not focusing merely on the presenting symptoms.

Chinese medicine, Native American medicine and medical practices in many other cultures go even further, considering individual people as elements of their communities and their environments, and many even view individuals as parts of the entire cosmos. Collective consciousness and spiritual awareness are integral aspects of wholistic care in traditional cultures.

In contrast with wholistic practices, conventional medicine is particularly poor at dealing with death and dying – and much less so at dealing with spiritual aspects of health and illness. Allopathic medicine is oriented toward fighting disease. I was taught as a medical student that if a person under my care died, I was probably to blame because I hadn't diagnosed her problem correctly or hadn't prescribed the correct treatment. I was not taught to help people deal with impending death. There should be no *blame* imposed on caregivers when people under their care reaches the end of their life, though there is clearly an ethical and moral obligation to ask whether treatments given or not given could have contributed to their demise.

To anyone not aware of the death-avoiding habits of western medicine, the above may be difficult to appreciate. Let me point out how this fear of death impacts the medical care of people who are in the hospital and nearing their time to die. In most of the hospitals where I worked, people who were beyond the benefits of medical interventions were placed in the rooms farthest from the nurses' stations – ostensibly with the intention of sparing them the disturbance of the noise and bustle of the nursing station. However, I believe an even stronger motivation was to spare the nurses and doctors the discomfort of constantly facing what they view as their failure.

Medicolegal issues also contribute to our anxieties and difficulties in dealing with the realities of death. Doctors are afraid of being sued by relatives for not having done absolutely everything possible to preserve and prolong life. Therefore, people who are in the terminal stages of their illnesses may be given cardiac resuscitation and other heroic interventions when they are actually ready (and sometimes even eager – due to the discomforts of their illnesses and of hospital treatments) to make their transition out of their physical bodies.

> [W]hen should health care end? It is no secret that as much as 30 to 60 percent of our health care dollar is spent in the last few days of a person's life. The dirty little secret is that most of it is spent in irrational procedures that do nothing significant to prolong life. In short, we are doing all we can do, not all that we should do.
>
> Listening to death-related visions has the potential to dramatically reduce wasteful medical procedures that are often painful to the patient. These procedures are often used on dying patients without their consent and without any hope of prolonging life. The purpose of much of this last-minute medicine is only to make us doctors feel as though everything possible has been done to prevent death, even when death is imminent. The result, writes Dr. William Knaus, of George Washington University, is "to give treatment of no benefit and tremendous cost, depriving others of treatment while dignity disappears."
>
> – Melvin Morse (p. 136)

Spiritual healing and various other CAM approaches may be of great help to respants and also to caregivers in dealing with death. Within the philosophies that guide these approaches, death is perceived as a natural part of life. Within many of these traditions, death is not the end of one's personal existence. The spirit survives the death of the physical body, continues its path of lessons and may return to the physical world in another incarnation.[102] Helping a person to die a good death is every bit as much a healing as helping them overcome an illness.

Integrative care brings together conventional and CAM therapies
Some allopathic physicians work together with CAM therapists. In other cases the doctors themselves administer acupuncture, homeopathy, or other complementary therapies. CAM therapists are critical of some of the doctors who do this, pointing out that it takes 1-2 hours to properly complete an initial acupuncture evaluation, and can take 2-4 hours or more for a full homeopathic interview – a time investment few physicians are willing or able to make. CAM practitioners also criticize doctors who claim that they can practice a new therapy after attending only a weekend course – when complementary therapists may study for months and years to learn the basic theories and practices of these approaches. Complementary therapists point out that it is not just methodology that must be mastered (such as where to insert acupuncture needles). Practitioners must also develop an understanding of energetic patterns of illness and vast complexes of interventions (e.g. acupuncture points for different types of pain; the indications for herbal and homeopathic remedies; chakra interventions; etc.), as well as an appreciation for the unique individuals who will be treated.

In addition, CAM therapies often rely on the practitioner as an instrument for the treatment – a channel and catalyst for the bioenergy interventions. This is most clearly seen in spiritual healing and bioenergy therapies, but is equally important in acupuncture and other CAM therapies. Practitioner will work on 'clearing the vessel through which the healing is channeled,' practicing meditation and receiving healing for their own issues so that these do not obstruct or distort their treatments.

Psychotherapy acknowledges the importance of self-healing for the therapist – to minimize perceptual distortions and inappropriate responses by the therapist to issues raised in therapy by clients. This is similar to the clearing of bioenergies that CAM practitioners advocate.

Ideally, the doctor will take a comprehensive course in the treatment philosophy and method and will arrange to practice the modality to its fullest potential, allowing adequate session time in which to do so.

It is impossible for any one person to master all of the CAM therapies, but to maximize integrative care it is helpful for doctors to know *about* as many of these therapies as possible, in order to refer patients to appropriate therapists.

The successful marriage of medical and complementary therapies requires close collaboration between the various practitioners. Like other marriages, these relationships may require a fair amount of effort to make them work well. A number of experiments are being developed to investigate these collaborations.[103]

Complementary/ Alternative Medicine Therapies

The greatest good you can do for another is not just share your riches, but reveal to them their own.

— Benjamin Disraeli

Conventional medicine is increasingly responsive to public demand for complementary therapies, and centers providing CAM therapies are becoming more widely available. American medical schools are also introducing courses and graduate programs on complementary therapies[104] in the wake of surveys showing that since 1990 almost as many billions of dollars have been paid to complementary therapists as to medical doctors (Eisenberg et al. 1993; 1998). The British Medical Association (1993) has acknowledged that many doctors are including acupuncture, homeopathy, osteopathy, chiropractic and herbalism in their practices and has recommended that more collaborative research be undertaken.[105] Long-term trends show a growing use of CAM over the last 50 years (Kessler et al). Above all, consumer satisfaction appears to be the most influential factor in the increased CAM use in the West (Eisenberg 1993; 1998).[106]

Figure II-8. Witch Doctor?

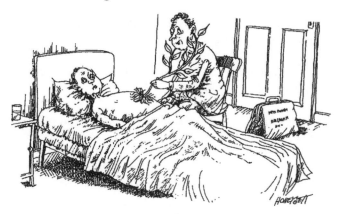

By Martin Honeysett (with permission of Century Publishing, London)

There are many instances in which CAM therapies may be sufficient in and of themselves to treat disease states. Some therapists advocate that these methods be employed routinely as *alternatives* to conventional medicine, when conventional doctors are not open to including them in their practices or are actually opposed their utilization. A few CAM therapists feel that *alternative medicine* should in fact be the label for these therapies, because their therapeutic philosophies differ substantially from Western medical views.[107]

Though the term *alternative* might serve to emphasize differences in attitudes and approaches, I feel it reflects an unfortunate polarization that can only be detrimental to respants' care in the long run. There is also the danger that an alternative therapist who is untrained in medical diagnosis could unwittingly cause harm by overlooking problems in interactions between treatments or serious problems for which allopathic medicine might provide relief or even a cure.

The prevalent view in the West has been that conventional, allopathic medicine is the only reliable method for addressing illness.[108] However, this view is changing as professionals and the public learn more about CAM therapies. Many of these, such as acupuncture, Ayurvedic medicine, Native American medicine and yoga, have been practiced for many hundreds of years in their cultures of origin. These systems of medicinal practice have evolved with worldviews that differ substantially from those of allopathic medicine (Krippner 1999).

The West has much to learn from other cultures and their medical practices. While some of these may seem alien, such as using acupuncture needles for pain management, others may appear sensible when transposed into Western medical cosmologies. For example, Ken Bearhawk Cohen describes a Native American tradition concerning the activation of inner healing abilities:

> When personal gifts ('medicine' in Native terminology) are not used, they rot inside, causing sickness. "Healing," says... Seneca elder Twylah... Nitch, "is sometimes not a matter of taking something in – an herb or other medication, but of letting something out, having the confidence to express yourself". (K. Cohen 1999, p. 237).

Doctors have lobbied state and Federal governments to enact legislation that would limit or outlaw many complementary therapies, but it seems clear that such restrictions would not be in the best interests of the public. This is apparently not a new problem – Benjamin Rush, U.S. Surgeon General and signer of the Declaration of Independence recommended:

> The Constitution of this Republic should make special provision for Medical Freedom as well as Religious Freedom. To restrict the art of healing to one class of men and deny equal privileges to others will constitute the Bastille of medical science. All such laws are un-American and despotic. They are fragments of a monarchy and have no place in a Republic.

The National Health Freedom Coalition is promoting State laws that permit the practice of unlicensed CAM therapies without danger of prosecution for "practicing medicine without a license."[109] Minnesota and California have passed such laws and other states are considering them.

There are many knotty issues involved in health laws.

One obstacle to the acceptance of complementary therapies is related to issues of training and certification of practitioners. For some complementary therapies there are professional boards that set varying levels of standards for training and certification (for example osteopathy, chiropractic, acupuncture, naturopathy, homeopathy, Therapeutic Touch and Healing Touch). For others, there may be a wide variation of training and practice standards. Some states license some but not all practitioners and this is a growing trend. Licensure ensures that CAM therapists have studied a certain number of months or years, that they have mastered a certain body of knowledge and that they uphold certain standards of practice.

In many complementary therapies, however, the *person of the therapist* is a vital aspect of the therapy. This is particularly true of the practices that involve adjustments of biological energies (such as acupuncture, craniosacral therapy and spiritual healing). While training and certification in these methods can assure the public that practitioners know *about* their modality and its ethical applications, these standards do not guarantee that the therapist is a *good* or a *potent* practitioner. Herein lies a major, serious challenge for those of us who want to protect the public on the one hand and to assure full availability of integrative care on the other.

Bioenergies and CAM

> *In general, healing involves the conscious, full engagement of the healer's own energies, plus other universal energies to whish she has access, in the compassionate interest of helping those who are in need. Therefore, healing can be said to be a humanization of energy in the interest of helping or healing another person."*
>
> – Dolores Kreiger, (2002, p. 18)

Subtle biological energies are essential elements of many complementary therapies. They are particularly important in spiritual healing and also function in the meridians of acupuncture, the subtle manipulations of craniosacral osteopathy, the energy patterning of water in homeopathy and so on. Spiritual healers rely directly upon energy medicine interventions, but many Western scientists investigating complementary therapies (other than healing) and indeed many CAM practitioners themselves, de-emphasize the energy aspects of these treatments. It is less challenging to Western worldviews to attribute the efficacy of complementary therapies to mechanical interventions (e.g. insertion of acupuncture needles, or osteopathic manipulations of bones and joints) or chemical agents (e.g. homeopathic preparations) than to invoke explanations involving subtle energies that cannot be measured on conventional instruments.

Spiritual healing is viewed by conventional science as one of the "fringe" modalities of complementary medicine, operating at the extreme limit of credibility, because there isn't even a partial explanation to make spiritual healing comprehensible and acceptable within conventional scientific frameworks. Nevertheless, the numerous studies reviewed in Volume I of *Healing Research* reveal that the opposite is in fact the case. With the exceptions of hypnosis and psychoneuroimmunology, there have been more controlled studies of spiritual healing than of any other complementary therapy.

Spiritual healing is emphasized in this volume for two reasons. First, it appears to be a common denominator in all of the complementary therapies. Not only are subtle energies involved in these therapies, but there are also therapeutic factors including subtle energies inherent in the persons who administer them. Many complementary therapists who are particularly sensitive can detect subtle energies with their hands or through mental imagery. They may also be able to administer subtle energies through their hands. I have heard many grateful recipients of massage and reflexology treatments report to me that their therapist had warm, tingly hands. Many such therapists are totally unaware that they are channeling subtle energies during their treatments.

The second reason for focusing on spiritual healing in this volume is to frame it within the context of a multitude of subtle energy therapies. Each therapy contributes another facet of understanding to the mystery of healing and similarly, spiritual healing helps us to understand aspects of various complementary therapies.[110]

Another criticism of complementary therapies is that their professional standards are not on a par with those of medical practice. Not all of these therapies have profession-wide (rather than school-specific) standards for training and practice and only a few are licensed by various states.

Spiritual healers in Britain who were registered with the *Confederation of Healing Organisations* worked under a unified Code of Conduct. This Code required healers to recommend that healees see their allopathic doctors prior to having healing.

Healers and other complementary therapists generally are untrained in medical diagnosis and allopathic medicine. Likewise, most medical doctors are unaware of energy medicine. Nevertheless, practitioners of both modalities are gradually learning to work with each other – and the greatest beneficiaries will be the respants in their care.

Each complementary therapy offers treatments that can help with some problems some of the time. While each therapy has its own methodologies and theories of health and illness, there are common denominators across the various approaches that will be discussed at the end of this chapter.

Let us begin with a review of CAM therapies.

I have ordered the therapies alphabetically. A more logical order might have grouped various therapies by their derivations (as with acupuncture, applied kinesiology, reflexology and shiatsu), or according to similarities in practice (as with homeopathy and flower essences). However, this would make it more difficult for readers to locate discussions of individual therapies. I have indicated the related therapies at the end of each discussion, so that the associations are clear.

Though some of these have not yet been well researched, I prefer to consider a broad spectrum of practices in order to gather as much evidence as possible from the information available at this time – to help us begin to understand these approaches, both individually and collectively. These clinical methodologies and anecdotal reports of efficacy, along with their explanatory theories, may help us understand how self-healing and energy medicine can bring about improvements in health.

A brief discussion of some of the problems that are effectively addressed by CAM therapies follows the descriptions of the various modalities.

ACUPUNCTURE

> *Now for some words about the theory of acupuncture. But bear in mind that one must not mistake an explanation for the reality. And this is where we are very often uptight. We want things explained. Then we think we can behave as though that explanation is the reality. The explanation of anything is nothing more than a technique or a system that is used to make it comprehensible within the circumference of our own understanding and when your understanding grows and is enlarged then we find that there is a need for new explanations. And this is where the American medical man is going to have difficulty, trying to understand how acupuncture works.*
>
> *... To understand acupuncture we must empty ourselves of all of our theoretical scientific concepts. The American medical man will say, "This is an unreasonable thing. He must make it understandable to me in my terms." And yet he would think that the Oriental acupuncturist was terribly unreasonable if he asked him to explain Western medicine in terms of five elements, yin and yang and Tao.*
>
> *[I]f we are going to understand or try to understand something new, we must be able and willing to learn the language in which it is written. I'm talking about the vocabulary, not national language itself. In the Tao it says, this is the important key: that we must learn to unlearn our learning. And that's the secret to understanding acupuncture.*
>
> – Khigh Alx Diegh

Acupuncture is based on ancient Chinese observations of subtle energy lines called *meridians* that run from the head to the fingers and toes. This energy is called *qi* (pronounced *kee* or *chee*).[111] Each meridian is related to one or more of the organ systems, and diseases are caused by excesses or deficits of energy, or blockage of energy flow in the meridians. Points of special sensitivity exist along the entire length of each energy line. Stimulation of these acupuncture points can influence the related organ systems by altering energy flow in the meridians. The therapist can stimulate the acupuncture points in several ways: by inserting needles, applying finger pressure, burning *moxa* herbs with the stalks held against the acupuncture points, applying mild electrical current, laser rays, or through mental projection of healing to the points.

Some meridians correspond to physical organs (e.g. heart, lungs), while others are correlated with functions for which allopathic medicine has no exact parallels (e.g. the *triple warmer).* The *triple warmer* is a body system that is named but poorly defined. It is that aspect of the body which controls the water-regulating organs (kidney, stomach, small and large intestine, spleen and bladder). The *upper warmer* governs the head and chest; the *middle warmer* the spleen and stomach; and the *lower warmer* the liver and kidneys.

Even where a physical organ corresponds to a specific line, the meridian reference is to energy functions of the line more than to its body functions (per

Western physiology). For instance, a Chinese acupuncturist who speaks of the kidney meridian may be referring to its role in storing life energy (*jing*); its influence on development, maturation and or reproduction; its effects on marrow, bones and teeth; or its interactions with respiration.

The various meridians have specific times of day when they are more and less active. Treatments may therefore be given for specific problems at particular times, even at unusual hours of the night.

For many years, allopathic medicine maintained a very skeptical or even dismissive attitude towards Eastern explanations of acupuncture because no anatomical structures were known that support Eastern theories of energy lines traversing the body. The meridians do not correspond in any way to the well-mapped peripheral or autonomic nervous system and until recently no other communication network in the body had been demonstrated that could support such theories. It seemed patently ridiculous to Westerners that needles inserted at acupuncture points on the foot or arm could influence lungs or heart or other organs at considerable distances from the sites of treatment. It was presumed that acupuncture treatments were effective purely on the basis of placebo responses or other aspects of suggestion. Yet some acupuncturists claim that they can sense acupuncture points with their fingers and others claim that they can manually detect when the meridians have a proper flow of Qi or are blocked. A few sensitives who see auras also claim that they can see acupuncture meridians and acupuncture points.

In addition to treatment by acupuncture, Chinese medicine also recommends self-healing through various movement and imagery exercises focused on facilitating bioenergy flow. Roger Jahnke explains that there are three states of Qi: *jing*, related to earth energies; *Qi*, related to life energies; and *shen*, related to spiritual dimensions. People are seen to be an intimate part of the world around them. Energies within the body interact with and resonate with those of the environment and of the worlds of spirit.

Western explorations of acupuncture

Traditional acupuncture identifies the acupuncture points in relation to anatomical maps. A point will be over a bony prominence such as the end of the clavicle, or measured in finger-width distances from such anatomical landmarks.

Recently, Western science has found several ways of confirming the existence of acupuncture points and meridians. Numerous studies have shown that acupuncture points have a much lower electrical resistance than surrounding areas of the skin. This difference is on the order of a few thousand ohms at acupuncture points, compared to millions of ohms anywhere else on the skin. Simple resistance meters are now in common use to confirm the locations of acupuncture points. These measurements are variable within short periods of time, particularly in respect to the width of individual points, but also to some extend in their locations. It seems that this variability reflects shifting organismic energetic states rather than inherent inaccuracies in the measurements.

Clinical studies have demonstrated correlations between predicted changes on various meridians and the activity of the organs traditionally associated with those meridians. For instance, conductance measured nearly 20 times higher at the Liver 8 acupuncture point (located at the knee) in people with demonstrated liver disease (acute hepatitis or cirrhosis), as compared with a control group with no liver disease. People with lung disease that had been verified with chest X-rays demonstrated 30% lower electrical conductance at acupuncture lung points.

New scientific methods have also been developed to demonstrate the existence of the meridians. Jean-Claude Darras, a physician and president of the *World Union of Acupuncture* and P. de Vernejoul, a physician who heads the Department of Biophysics of Neckar Hospital in Paris, injected radioactive chemicals at acupuncture points and followed the course of distribution of these materials with a Geiger counter at the body surface. They demonstrated that connections exist between acupuncture points, along lines identical with the meridians described by acupuncturists. Similar research completed decades earlier had been rejected due to difficulties in verifying the findings.

Kirlian photography, an electrophotographic technique, reveals an enhanced Kirlian aura at acupuncture points.

Instruments for clinical use that assess electrical potentials at various acupuncture points and through which electrical stimulation of acupuncture points may be applied, are growing in popularity. One of these is the Voll instrument, on which a reading of "50" indicates a healthy state, while lower readings point to degenerative diseases and higher readings are associated with injury or inflammation. I agree with William Tiller (1997), Professor Emeritus at Stanford University, suggests that the intuitive perceptions of the instrument operator may be crucial to the success of readings taken with such devices. The amount of pressure exerted by the operator's hand in touching the acupuncture point can influence the reading, so there is room for the operator's intuitive awareness to find expression in the process of taking the measurements. This effect is often completely unconscious on the part of the operator, who leaves it to the instrument to apparently do the work.

Hiroshi Motoyama, a Japanese biologist trained in Buddhist traditions, developed a different instrument for quantitative measurements of the electrical currents along acupuncture meridians. He calls this an "apparatus for measuring the function of the meridians and corresponding internal organs," or "AMI" for short. Using the AMI he can diagnose illness, sometimes even before the disease is otherwise perceptible. Western scientists are now beginning to confirm Motoyama's findings, using the AMI.

Electroacupuncture assessments are being used to identify remedies for the treatment of physical and psychological problems. Baseline measurements are made of skin resistance at acupuncture points associated with a given problem. The person being tested is then given various remedies or nutrients to hold. It is assumed that the therapeutic substances interact with the bioenergy field. Repeat measurements are made. Healthier readings indicate treatments that are likely to be helpful. The use of these devices has not been adequately researched.

Lively explorations of acupressure techniques are likewise proceeding in the US, especially in the treatment of psychological problems. These methods are rapidly effective for the relief of pains, anxiety and negative self-beliefs. They can also enhance athletic performance.

Other energy centers in the body that have been identified by Chinese medicine are called *chakras* (Sanskrit for *wheels*).[112] There are many chakras around the body, but the seven major ones that are along the central axis of the body are the most important. They project as vortices of energy to the front and back of the body, as well as upwards and downwards. (See Table II-7.)

Table II-7. The Chakras

Name	Location of chakra	Level *Endocrine gland* NERVE PLEXUS	Influence on
Crown *Sahasrara*		Apex of skull *Pineal*	Higher brain centers, spiritual connection
Brow/Third Eye *Ajna*		Brow *Pituitary* DEEP BRAIN CENTERS	Deeper brain centers, eyes, ears, nose, nervous system, visualization
Throat *Visuddha*		3rd cervical *Thyroid* PHARYNGEAL	Voice, breathing, digestive tract, expression, clairsentience
Heart *Anahata*		4th thoracic *Thymus* CARDIAC	Heart, blood, autonomic nervous system, circulation, closeness of relationship
Solar Plexus *Manipura*		8th thoracic *Spleen/pancreas* SOLAR PLEXUS	Stomach, liver, gall bladder, awareness of place in cosmos
Sacral *Svadhisthana*		1st lumbar *Gonads* SPLENC	Reproduction, relating on sexual levels
Base/Root *Muladhara*		Base of spine *Adrenals* COCCYGEAL	Spine, kidneys, levels of energy

The chakras are said to be regions of the body where energies from other dimensions are transformed into forms that are suitable for vitalizing the physical body.

Motoyama also developed an electronic device that verifies the existence of chakras. He associates the seven major chakras with nerve plexuses in the autonomic nervous system. Others associate the major chakras with the hormone-secreting endocrine glands, suggesting that one function of hormones may be to convey information recorded as energy patterns imprinted from sources outside the body to distant parts of the body – in addition to their known biochemical functions.

Elaborate images are used in Eastern teachings about the chakras, associated with the different levels of psychospiritual development that are attributed to each chakra. Some are simple petals in floral designs, with increasing numbers of petals from the base to the crown chakra. Others include Sanskrit characters with animal and human figures from Eastern religious cosmologies.

Frances Vaughan reports that Carl Jung found correspondences between the archetypal images that his patients reported as they individuated in psychotherapy and symbolic images that are found in classical representations of the stages of psychological development associated with the chakras.

Some healers instruct healees in personal awareness of their chakras as a way of initiating self-healing. I have learned to do this, but I found at first that it was quite difficult to learn to trust my subjective sensations, because there was no direct feedback to confirm that I was on target. Over the years, with various meditative practices and life experiences, I have come to a greater trust in my chakra perceptions.

Acupuncture Theories

Most of the acupuncture practiced in the West is mechanistic, as. it has been difficult for allopathic medicine to acknowledge that therapeutic concepts developed outside the realm of Western science might provide a valid method for dealing with disease. Limited numbers of acupuncture points are used, for instance, to address pains in various parts of the body.

Ted Kaptchuk (1984) provides an excellent discussion on aspects of health that allopathic medicine seems helpless to treat, but which respond well to Traditional Chinese Medicine (acupuncture combined with herbal therapies). He also expands on the comments of Khigh Alx Diegh (quoted at the beginning of this section), explaining Chinese views of health and illness.

> For instance, the Chinese do not ask what causes a particular illness. They ask, "Which patterns within the individual and his environment are in harmony and which are in conflict?" Therapy is not aimed at correcting symptoms so much as at bringing the person to greater harmony with the cosmos.
> ... The Chinese description of reality does not penetrate to a truth, it can only be a poetic description of a truth that cannot be grasped. The Heart, Lung and Kidneys... are not a physical heart, lung or kidneys; instead they are personae in a descriptive drama of health and illness. For the Chinese, this description of the eternal process of Yin and Yang is the only way to try to explain either the workings of the universe or the workings of the human body. And it is enough, because the process is all there is; no underlying truth is ever within reach. The truth is immanent in everything and is the process itself...

Chinese medicine also views the body holographically, assuming that a part will reflect the whole.[113] Thus the tongue, teeth, upper palate, face, ear, hand, foot, or pulse may be used to diagnose or treat disorders anywhere in the body. For example, a beefy, red tongue may indicate generalized congestion or blockage of energy, and a pale tongue can mean a lack of energy – not necessarily in the vicinity of the tongue but in other specific parts of the body, or everywhere in the body. Tenderness in points on the foot, hand or ear may likewise indicate disorders in distant body parts or in organs related to these points.

Stimulation of the indicated points may bring symptomatic relief. The stimulation is to release blocks, to enhance energy flows or to decrease excessive energy activity.

It is not recorded how the meridians and *chakras* were identified in some distant millennium. From reports of sensitives (such as Motoyama and others) who state that they can see auras and from practitioners who report that they can sense these energy points by touch, one may readily postulate that it must have been one or more aura-seeing sensitives who originally mapped out these systems.

My own experience of learning elementary touch healing techniques confirms that it is possible to sense gross energy changes in the body via touch. Therefore it does not seem to me far-fetched that people with more highly developed sensitivities could have a more refined ability to sense these energies. I can also personally verify – from my personal and professional experiences – that it is possible to use awareness of one's own *chakras* to influence them for self-healing. Other healers echo these observations.[114] There are some who claim that in modern times the meridians and acupuncture points that most require attention may differ from those that were codified in past centuries. That is to say, there may have been a collective, evolutionary shift in human acupuncture energies.

Whether the visual chakra phenomena are objectively or consensually verifiable has yet to be determined. A survey of the literature reveals variations in descriptions of the chakras by individual sensitives. Perhaps the variations relate to different physical or energy states in the various people observed, or perhaps the differences are due to individual factors in the observers. Most likely, all of the descriptions are affected by the difficulties in translating inner intuitive perceptions of energies and/ or other realities into images and words of our outer-world, sensory reality. Because the chakra and meridian energies that are sensed clairsentiently differ so entirely from anything familiar to Western science, it is quite likely that all the related descriptions are, at best, rough analogies – when put into words that are used to describe our material world.

Here is an example of the challenges in translating these concepts into Western language. Within the cosmology of Chinese medicine and acupuncture, *Yin* and *yang* are polar opposites that must be balanced in order for life to proceed in harmony. The term *yin* denotes the shady side of the slope and may be associated with qualities of femininity, openness, passivity, receptivity, introversion, diminution, repose, weakness and coolness. *Yang* is the sunny side of the slope and may be associated with the sun, masculinity, strength, brightness, assertiveness, movement, extroversion, growth and excitation.

In the body, the front is yin relative to the back; the upper portions of the body are yang relative to the lower parts; the inner organs are more yin than the outer aspects such as hair and skin. Yang disorders are characterized by fever, hyperactivity, heat and strong movements; yin illnesses include weakness, slowing down, feeling cold and lethargy.

Yin and yang complement each other. If yang is excessive, then yin will be too weak and conversely.

In Chinese cosmology, causality is unimportant. It is the *pattern* of relationships which defines reality and all reality is relative to the context which is under consideration.

> The philosopher Zou Yen... describes this idea this way: "Heaven is high, the earth is low and thus [Heaven and Earth] are fixed. As the high and low are thus made clear, the honorable and humble have their place accordingly. As activity and tranquillity have their constancy, the strong and

the weak are thus differentiated... Cold and hot season take their turn[Heaven] knows the great beginning and [Earth] acts to bring things to completion[Heaven] is Yang and [Earth] is Yin."
     Any Yin or Yang aspect can be further divided into Yin and Yang...
                                                    – Ted Kaptchuk (p. 9)

Chinese cosmology also explains health and illness according to the balance of five elements in a person's life, each associated with a set of body organs

- Fire – heart, small intestine, triple heater, master of heart; blood vessels, tongue, complexion;
- Earth – stomach, spleen, mucous membranes, mouth;
- Metal – lung, colon, skin, nose;
- Water – kidney, bladder; back, bones, ears;
- Wood – liver, gallbladder, muscles, tendons, eyes.

These can be better understood as five processes or phases. Each phase controls another and is in turn controlled by yet another. These can be more descriptively characterized, as follows:

- Wood – windy, shouting, anger, sour, goatish;
- Earth – damp, singing, pensiveness, sweet, fragrant;
- Water – cold, groaning, fear, salty, rotten;
- Fire – hot, laughing, joy, bitter;
- Metal – dry, weeping, grief, pungent, rank.

Causality derives from the ways in which each of these five element processes relates to the others, in extremely complex relationships. Opinions vary widely on these interrelationships and they have not stood up to systematic scrutiny, even within Chinese historical traditions. Nevertheless, they continue to be part of Chinese medical tradition (Kaptchuk).
     Environmental influences on health are addressed in the Oriental system of *Feng Shui,* which will be discussed later in the sections on environmental medicine.

Meridians, chakras and spiritual healing
Observations from the tradition and practice of acupuncture may explain various aspects of spiritual healing.
     Some healers focus assessments and treatments on specific *chakras* during healings. These reports make sense in the light of Chinese explanations regarding the functions of the chakras in regulating energies in adjacent organs and not only in the nerves or glands immediately next to each chakra.
     Waxing and waning of activity along particular meridians over the course of each day may be correlated with positive and/ or negative responses to spiritual healing and other medical treatments. It may be that at particular hours of the day, certain organ systems have greater or lesser sensitivity to healing and other therapies.
     Supporting this speculation, Yefim Shubentsov, an ex-Soviet healer living in

Boston,[115] reports that healers may have more potent abilities at particular hours of the day or night. Further support may be found in reports by Western scientists from several decades ago. Harold Burr and Leonard Ravitz found that direct current fields on the body surface varied according to time of day, lunar phase and solar flares. This area of research has not been well explored.

Motoyama's electrophysiological verification of the meridian and chakra systems are relevant to the study and understanding of healing. The energy systems thus elucidated could possibly revolutionize our understanding of the functions of the body. If energy levels and flows within the body can be objectively measured, we can verify whether they are effected via bioenergy inputs associated with healing. This would then give us objective, measurable readouts for the changes brought about by healing, which could in turn provide a biofeedback mechanism whereby healing might be more precisely and effectively taught for the promotion of self-healing and healer-healing. This approach might also facilitate spiritual development through awareness of bioenergetic connections with higher aspects of oneself.

The human body can be conceptualized in ways that differ even more radically from traditional Western cosmologies. For example, the concept of *yin* and *yang* and the linking of human illness with man's place in the cosmos may prove to be useful approaches for understanding and promoting health care.

The theory of acupuncture assumes the body is a sort of hologram. In a holographic picture, one can cut away any part of the negative and this section of the negative will still contain the whole picture. Each part of the picture, therefore, contains the whole picture. If the physical and/ or energetic body function as holograms, this would help to explain how acupuncture diagnosis can be based on the appearance of the tongue or condition of the teeth and how treatments may be applied to points on the ear, hand, or foot that correspond to each of the various organs of the body.[116]

Allopathic medicine practitioners believe that this is the best system of treatment. Yet allopathic medicine is helpless when confronted with many illnesses. Sufferers from allergies, arthritis, cancer, multiple sclerosis, strokes, addictions and other health problems bear ample testimony to these limitations. There is much to be gained by exploring the alternatives that acupuncture and Chinese medicine offer. Furthermore, acupuncture has far fewer side effects than many of the treatments used in allopathic medicine.

If allopathic medicine wishes to include the full benefits of a Chinese system of treatment, it must study the related concepts and traditions. It cannot demand that the approaches of acupuncture be made to conform to Western systems.

Research:[117] It was difficult at first to design acupuncture studies that conform to Western research protocols because Eastern methods of diagnosis and treatment differ substantially from those used in the West. Traditional acupuncture individualizes treatments to each person and therefore does not lend itself to randomized controlled studies that require a standard treatment for each member of a group of subjects with the same diagnosis. Another challenge is in providing a control group. Some studies have accommodated the requirement for applying a standard treatment to subjects who share a Western medical diagnosis and have used control subjects who receive *sham* acupuncture, with needles inserted at points that are not known to produce beneficial effects.

One of the best known uses of acupuncture is in the treatment of pain. Research shows acupuncture can help: tension headaches; migraines; facial pain; dental pain; neck pain; angina, lumbar disk protrusion; tennis; osteoarthritis; renal colic; dysmenorrhea; fibromyalgia; peripheral nerve pain; knee injuries from chronic trauma; and chronic pains of many sorts.

While individual studies may produce only modest results, a series of studies analyzed as a group provides more substantial proof. Meta-analyses of acupuncture studies confirm that it is an effective treatment for chronic pain. More critical meta-analyses questioned the quality of many of these studies

Another well-publicized use of acupuncture is for anesthesia during medical and surgical procedures. Studies have shown significant benefits from acupuncture in controlling the pain and discomforts of gastroscopy and colonoscopy (fiber optic tubes used to examine the stomach and colon) and for postoperative pain.

The way in which acupuncture produces analgesia has not yet been identified. It is strongly suspected that acupuncture stimulates the production of natural opiates (endorphins) in the body, because the effects of acupuncture analgesia are decreased when a chemical antagonist to opiates (naloxone) is injected prior to acupuncture treatments for pain.

Studies have shown significant relief of nausea and vomiting with acupuncture after surgical anesthesia, chemotherapy, morning sickness during pregnancy, and motion sickness.

One extraordinary though little recognized contribution of acupuncture is in the treatment of strokes. Significant effects have been reported in improving muscle strength in leg and arm paralysis. Walking and balancing abilities were improved, activities of daily living (ADL) scores were higher and days in hospital and nursing homes were halved, with estimated savings of $26,000 per patient. Significant recovery of muscle functions and ADL scores were noted in another study, but with no decrease in hospital stay. When treatment was started within 36 hours of the onset of the strokes, those whose condition was poorer at the start of the study showed significant improvements in neurological functions and ADL scores, while those with better initial conditions showed no significant benefits from acupuncture. This would appear to contradict the evidence from another study, which showed that with more severe strokes there was less improvement. A study using 6 weeks of therapy for strokes and a one-year follow-up showed clear benefits. Further research is definitely warranted.

Acupuncture is well known for treating respiratory diseases. Traditional acupuncture has been used widely for asthma, although careful research has shown mixed results. Chronic obstructive pulmonary disease (COPD) is a horrible illness in which lung tissues are destroyed by chronic infections. This reduces sufferers to being unable to move more than a little distance due to oxygen starvation, which leaves them out of breath with the least exertion. COPD has no effective conventional treatment – short of lung transplants. Acupuncture demonstrated improvements in ADL and well-being for people with COPD, with longer walk distances, even thought there were no objective changes in pulmonary functions.

Acupuncture works well as a complement to allopathic treatment for a variety of pulmonary diseases. Not only can it help the lung diseases directly, it can also enhance the effects of medication so that lower doses can be used.

German-language research showed acupuncture is helpful for ear, nose and throat (ENT) problems, allergic rhinitis, sinusitis (especially in children), Menière's disease (middle ear problems), trigeminal neuralgia, facial paralysis and susceptibility to recurrent infections. Benefits were noted in reduction of pain, less need for medications and in more rapid recovery.

Other applications of acupuncture showing significant effects include: facilitating labor and delivery; relief of menopausal symptoms; treatment of depression; enhancement of physical performance; treatment of daytime and nighttime enuresis and of frequent, urgent and painful urination; and tinnitus (ringing in the ears); weight reduction; and chronically dry mouth.

Acupuncture is finding varied applications in the treatment of addictions, including alcohol, nicotine and heroin, although research evidence for efficacy is spotty.

Acupuncture is also used in animals, such as in the treatment of diarrhea of bacterial origin in pigs.

Several studies have shown that acupuncture is cost-effective in the following contexts: in general practice in reducing requirements for laboratory examinations, use of prescription medications and hospitalizations; in a managed care setting in reducing clinic visits, physical therapy, phone consultations and prescription medicines for 6 months following a brief course of treatment; and in reducing anti-inflammatory medication use and recourse to surgery in prospective patients for elective knee replacement operations.

There are thousands of clinical reports on the efficacy of acupuncture for various problems, but these are too numerous to summarize and assess here.

Adverse effects: Both mechanical and infectious adverse effects may occur with acupuncture but most of the serious complications are due to the improper use of needles. Re-use of needles that have not been properly sterilized may introduce bacterial infections, hepatitis B and AIDS. All such infections are preventable by the use of disposable needles. Puncture of the lung and of the heart have been reported – both of which can be fatal. Spinal cord injuries have occurred and minor injuries from broken needles have also been reported. Electroacupuncture can also interfere with cardiac pacemakers.

To put this into perspective, there are about 9,000 licensed acupuncturists in the US, performing millions of treatments every year. In a review of the literature over the past 33 years, about 200 adverse effects, including seven deaths, were reported in the English medical literature of 27 countries, according to Lixing Lao, a licensed acupuncturist and Professor of Complementary Medicine at the University of Maryland Medical School.

Less serious problems may also result from acupuncture treatments. Drowsiness may be produced when a relaxation response is too strong. Light-headedness, fainting (possibly due to extreme relaxation), nausea, vomiting and psychological reactions may occur. As with many complementary therapies (notably homeopathy and spiritual healing) there may be exacerbations of some symptoms, such as pain, prior to the lessening of these symptoms. Occasionally convulsions have occurred and one instance of death due to a severe asthma attack has been reported.

Eastern cosmologies

Here are a few summarizing observations on aspects of the cosmologies that are associated with Eastern systems of medical belief and practice. Any or all of these may be relevant to the success or failure of acupuncture (and other CAM) treatments. These include the concept of *yin* and *yang*, which sees special relationships between mind and body, between subtle biological energies of the patient and the manipulations of the acupuncturist and between mankind and the greater universe beyond the individual and collective that is humanity.

1. The physical body is intimately associated with several non-material bodies. An *etheric double* connects it to the *astral* body. The astral body is concerned with desires and emotions. Motoyama likens this to the Western concept of soul. The Eastern *causal* body is compared to the spirit, which is the non-physical portion of man linking him to God. While many acupuncturists focus primarily on the physical body, much as their Western counterparts do, it is fascinating to find the observations above on Eastern spiritual awareness that closely correspond to those in the West.

2. The chakras are the points of connection and interaction between the various energy bodies and the physical body.

3. Many clairsentient people report that they see the glowing, wheel-like portions of the aura that correspond precisely to the *chakras* described by the Indians and Chinese. A few of the more gifted clairsentients report that they can see lines corresponding to the meridians, with bright spots at the acupuncture points. Some sensitives report they see many more meridians and acupuncture points than are described in classical Chinese teachings.

4. A variant of acupressure, *Shen Tao,* attributes its efficacy to visualizations of energy flows from the acupuncturist to the patient when the acupuncture points are touched with the therapist's finger.

5. There is a diurnal waxing and waning of energy movements in each meridian, as well as monthly and seasonal ebbs and flows of energies. There are thus optimal as well as unfavorable times for treatments of given illnesses. Unless this diurnal variability is taken into account, it may be difficult for Western science to obtain fully consistent measurements of acupuncture energies and valid assessments of the efficacy of acupuncture treatments.

6. Acupuncture cosmology of a holographic aspect to it, not only within the individual, but also between the individual and the entire cosmos. Each person is a microcosmic parallel to the universe and is in constant resonance with it. In this respect, we also become aware of a potential for external factors, such as environmental energies, to enhance or block treatments..[118]

7. All objects have a balance of *yin* (receptive, passive, feminine, empty, small, relaxed, mysterious, etc.) and *yang* (forceful, active, masculine, full, large, excited, revealed, etc.) aspects. Health and harmony require a balance of yin and yang, and full awareness of one polarity requires an awareness of its opposite. An

196 Vol. II Chapter 2 – Wholistic Energy Medicine

object or action may be yin in relation to one thing but yang in relation to another. This Oriental relativity of everything to everything else promotes acceptance and harmonizing of theories and practices as *both-and*, rather than contrasting and rejecting theories and practices – as in the Western *either-or*, dichotomizing approach.

8. There are basic elements that form the building blocks for all matter: wood, fire, earth, metal and water. Each object and living thing is composed of its own unique balance of these elements. The elements are interrelated and imbalances in one element can produce imbalances in associated elements, causing disease. Treatments are prescribed according to the elements that are diagnosed to be out of balance.

9. Acupuncture can be of help in a wide variety of illnesses. Some of these diseases are familiar to us, including the entire range of Western diagnoses such as asthma and cancer, but others are alien to Western cosmologies – such as *energy blocks, excess dampness, deficits or excesses of internal heat*, etc.. Psychological disorders also respond well to acupuncture and acupressure treatments. Animals can be treated with acupuncture too.

10. Various herbal remedies are recommended in treatments of illnesses. Allopathic medicine seeks to understand these substances in terms of their chemical ingredients, which might have effects similar to Western medications. There may be additional energy medicine aspects to herbal remedies, similar to those of homeopathy.

11. Prevention of illness is achieved by maintaining balance and harmony within ourselves and with the cosmos.

12. Indirectly related to acupuncture, it is worth noting that Chinese healers use a method of healing called *Qigong*. Qigong masters instruct healees in self-healing meditations and physical exercises, identified as *internal qigong*. Qigong masters also project healing through elaborate movements of their own bodies and limbs, called *external qigong* (*waiqi*). Qigong healing combined with acupuncture may enhance the effects of the acupuncture.

In summary, we can say that Chinese medicine has been effective in treating many millions of people over many centuries. It draws its theories and practices from a culture that gives greater weight to patterns and relationships than to linear, causal explanations.

> *Chinese medicine is not less logical than the Western system, just less analytical.*
> – Charles Krebs (p. 46)

Acceptance of acupuncture in the West

Over 50 schools in the US teach acupuncture and Oriental medicine and there is a National Accreditation Commission for Schools and Colleges of Acupuncture and Oriental Medicine (NACSCAOM). Its standards include a master's degree following a three-year course in acupuncture (1,700 hours) and a four-year course in Oriental Medicine (2,100 hours) which includes both acupuncture and herbalism. There are briefer postgraduate courses (220-400 hours) in medical acupuncture for physicians. The American Academy of Medical Acupuncture (AAMA), which is the professional organization for medical and osteopathic doctors who practice acupuncture, has developed a proficiency examination and is working towards board certification. NACSCAOM accredits 30 schools in the US and has a licensing exam that is recognized in most states that license acupuncturists.

Currently, 36 states and the District of Columbia regulate the practice of non-physician acupuncturists, with widely varying standards and legislation pending in about a dozen more states. Another estimated 7,000 US physicians have trained in acupuncture.

The National Institute of Health (NIH) acknowledged that "The data in support of acupuncture are as strong as those for many accepted Western medical therapies. One of the advantages of acupuncture is that the incidence of adverse effects is substantially lower than that of many drugs and other accepted medical procedures used for the same conditions."[119]

Clinical efficacy: Positive effects appear most likely when the diagnosis in the Traditional Chinese Medicine system of assessment is clear and distinct. Acupuncture is of proven benefit for treatment of pain in primary illness – such as rheumatoid arthritis, migraine and tension headaches – as well as for pain and discomforts from trauma and surgical procedures, and pains that arise from chronic tensions. It can alleviate nausea and vomiting from morning sickness during pregnancy, motion sickness and chemotherapy, can be useful in treating lung infections, addictions, and in recuperation from strokes. Many other problems may be helped, such as slowing muscle wasting due to disuse (as when a person is bed-ridden or in a cast), diminishing post-surgical scarring, and hastening labor and delivery, but these benefits have yet to be substantiated by research.

Acupuncture therapists must administer most treatments, but self-healing with acupressure is commonly used, for example in reducing cravings for cigarettes and other habituating substances, and in the meridian based therapies.

See also derivatives of acupuncture: Applied Kinesiology, Meridian Based Therapies (under massage); Reflexology; and Shiatsu.

ALEXANDER TECHNIQUE

Give me a lever and a firm place to stand and I will move the earth.
– Archimedes

The Alexander Technique is a series of exercises that people practice under careful supervision of a teacher to correct injuries as well as damage from habitual misuse and abuse of their musculoskeletal systems. The benefits are derived from learning new ways of using one's muscles and correcting one's posture. Pupils are guided through prescribed movements while standing, seated or lying down. The teacher may apply light pressure to guide the body towards healthier movements, as well as to enhance kinesthetic awareness (awareness of the position and action of muscles and joints).

The Alexander technique has been particularly helpful with neck and back pain of postural or traumatic origins, breathing disorders, arthritis, repetitive strain injury and a variety of stress related disorders.

Tricia Hemingway, a British Alexander technique teacher, shared the following:

> Although the impression generally given is that the Alexander technique is primarily mechanistic, the most important aspect of the technique is *direction. Direction* is the intent of the teacher to allow the life force within the teacher to be available to the life force within the student. Direction is best grounded by being still and doing nothing, letting the hands sense what might come through intuitively to the teacher and letting the hands rest lightly on the student's body at whatever locations they are guided to intuitively. Then, only the lightest of touch and the conscious and of course intuitive guidance, of the teacher can facilitate response and generate change in a student. No physical manipulation is used, simply guided movement.
>
> During lessons the hands of the teacher may become very hot or vibrate and students often experience releases of emotions during the lessons. Students commonly report a sense of well being during and after sessions and improvement in whatever dysfunctions brought them for Alexander training.

The similarities between this approach and spiritual healing are broadly obvious. Not all Alexander teachers use direction, which is taught by only one school in England.

Alexander teachers who learn the methods of direction are expected to do so by undergoing the lessons themselves. They spend at least three years in a training course learning to release their own body and emotional blocks before they are ready to sense, handle and guide the direction as teachers. Not to be forgotten are the mechanical skills more commonly associated with the Alexander technique, which teachers are required to polish to a high proficiency as well.

Research: I know of no research that supports the efficacy of this method, though clinical anecdotes suggest it is very helpful – when students take responsibility for doing the exercises regularly. This can be challenging, as many people come for treatments expecting the therapist to "fix" them.

Adverse effects: No harmful effects have been reported See discussion of potential general negative effects from rapid improvements under Spiritual Healing.

Training and licensing: There are no established standards for practice or licensing of Alexander Technique in the US.

Clinical applications: The Alexander Technique can help with musculoskeletal and joint pains; post-injury and post-surgical rehabilitation; enhancing athletic and artistic performance; asthma; headaches; irritable bowel syndromes; depression; and boosting poor self-esteem and self-confidence.

A teacher is required for assessment and instruction in the various exercises, which are then practiced as self-healing.

See also: the *Feldenkrais Method* later in this chapter.

ANIMAL HEALINGS
See: Pet Therapy.

ANTHROPOSOPHIC MEDICINE

Healing is not a matter of mechanism but a work of the spirit.
— Rachel Naomi Remen

Rudolf Steiner, an Austrian philosopher and scientist (1861-1925), devised a spiritually oriented scientific model for psychological development. He applied scientific principles to spirituality in agriculture (biodynamics), social theories (threefold social order), education (Steiner Schools) and the creative arts. Together with Ita Wegman, Steiner developed a training course for physicians, which is intended to develop and preserve healing as an art rather than just as a technology.

His model, known as anthroposophical medicine, combines naturopathy, homeopathy and conventional medicine. Doctors who use these approaches are found particularly in Holland, Germany, Switzerland and Sweden, with a few practicing in other countries as well. They have developed some of their own homeopathic remedies. Spiritual awareness is a major aspect of interventions used in this method.[120]

An important contribution to wholistic medicine are the Steiner schools, which seek to promote children's intuitive and creative capacities. This is truly preventive medicine.

There is no separate licensing for medical or osteopathic doctors practicing Anthroposophic Medicine.

Adverse effects: See under each component therapy.

Research: There are studies supporting some of the claims regarding the efficacy of Anthroposophic medicine. This discipline must be assessed according to its individual components, including the very broad spectrum included under naturopathy.[121]

Clinical applications: Anthroposophical medicine is a very broad approach that can be helpful with most health problems.

The doctor makes assessments and may prescribe various medications, as well as self-healing exercises.

See also: Naturopathic Medicine.

APPLIED KINESIOLOGY (AK)

> *Where is the wisdom we have lost in knowledge*
> *and where is the knowledge we have lost in information*
> – T.S. Eliot

Applied Kinesiology (AK) was developed by a chiropractor named George Goodheart, Jr. AK is based on the principle that certain muscles reflect conditions of internal organ systems because they share the same acupuncture meridian lines. If a given muscle system is weak it indicates that the associated parts of the body also need a rebalancing of energy. Thus, internal conditions may be assessed through muscle tone and strength and the balance of strength between particular muscles. Shifts in muscle strength will then also provide feedback on the degree of success of treatment for the meridian imbalances.

Treatment for disorders identified by AK is applied to acupuncture points and meridians by touch and massage, along with movements of the hands near the body. Chiropractors using AK also recommend spinal manipulations.

CASE: Victor suffered from frequent headaches, abdominal bloating, tiredness and irritability. He had seen his physician, who could not identify any organic problems. He was reluctant to take pain-killers for his headaches and frustrated that no remedy was available for his other symptoms. The AK examiner first showed Victor a method of testing muscle strength with one arm. Next, the examiner placed in Victor's other hand a series of substances (foods and chemicals) that might have been causing his symptoms through toxicity or allergy and again tested the muscle strength in his arm with each substance. When Victor's body sensed that the substance was toxic or allergenic, there was an immediate response of weakening in his arm against the pressure of the examiner. Conversely, food and medicinal substances that his body sensed are salutary produced a strengthening in his arm. Victor discovered he had a wheat intolerance, and his symptoms cleared when he avoided bread and other wheat foods.

Similar techniques may be used to detect conscious and unconscious emotional conflicts. These methods were developed by psychiatrist John Diamond (1996), and they are collectively known as *Behavioral Kinesiology*. After establishing the client's "baseline strength" (described below), the examiner will ask a question. If there is anxiety about the question, the client's arm becomes weak. This acts as a sort of bioenergetic meter that provides immediate feedback about physical and psychological states.

You can try this yourself with the help of a friend or on your own. See the exercises in Chapter 5.

Muscle testing can also be used to explore emotional conflicts and early psychological experiences, with muscle strength or weakness indicating *yes* and *no* answers to questions posed by the therapist. You can do this yourself without the help of a friend, using muscles in your hand, as described in Chapter 5. (Mental imagery can also be used to identify *yes* and *no* responses.)

This process of inner exploration is similar to the hypnotic technique of ideo-motor responses, which have been recognized for at least 100 years. The hypnotist might say, "Your unconscious mind can communicate through gestures. Rest your hands on your knees. Your right index finger will rise if the answer to a question is 'Yes,' and your left index finger will rise if the answer is 'No.'

AK muscle testing provides access to the 95 percent of the brain that is outside of conscious awareness and to the vastness of our transpersonal selves. The great advantage of kinesiology is that it does not require hypnotic induction and can be used by people for their own problems.

One must be cautious in interpreting the results of kinesiology. As with any diagnostic procedure (intuitive or physical), there will always be a percentage of false positive and false negative findings. Several ways to reduce the risk of error include:

1. Use common sense and reasoning to analyze information;
2. Examine your introspective, emotional and intuitive responses to the information provided through kinesiology;
3. Record the precise words used in asking the questions, so they can be re-evaluated in the light of later analysis; and
4. When there are questions about results obtained with AK, use multiple readings and supplement them with readings by others, preferably by clinicians who are experienced and expert in the use of these methods.

The help of a knowledgeable clinician can be invaluable. Clinicians trained in kinesiology know the ways in which innate characteristics and learned patterns of behavior tend to cluster and manifest – both physically and psychologically. Clinicians may identify psychological issues that we ourselves are blind to – particularly around traumatic experiences that we have buried in our unconscious mind. They may recognize blocks or overactivities in various meridians that would not be apparent or even suspected by anyone who is unfamiliar with these patterns, and good therapists will know ways to help unravel the complex structures of defenses built up over a lifetime of human interactions.

Addressing meridian problems may shortcut the process of therapy. For instance, Thomas Altaffer suggests that overactivity in a meridian produces active responses under certain emotional conditions and conversely, underactivity in the meridian produces passivity when you are faced with similar emotional problems. If "John" has a problem in his Governing Vessel meridian, it may incline him towards embarrassment, while overactivity may color his behavior with a sense of superiority and a tendency to judge others negatively. If his meridian is underactive, he will tend to feel inferior and to withdraw from social interactions.

Kinesiologists report consistency in their own clinical assessments of these meridian activity diagnoses, but the research in this area shows very mixed results.

Where there is any doubt or question you must proceed with the greatest caution when using these techniques. Your unconscious expectations, hopes, wishes and fears may all influence your self-explorations. The same may apply for therapists, whose own unresolved issues may make them blind to particular problems their clients may have.

Skeptics will question whether AK could represent anything more accurate than guessing or chance and research is beginning to address this issue. Kenneth Sancier and Effie Chow used sophisticated measuring devices to confirm that AK produces significant changes in muscle strength under stringent testing conditions.

Ray Hyman, a skeptic, reviews selected research and suggests that kinesiology is strictly a variation of *ideomotor response*, based on unconscious movements of muscles, guided solely by the unconscious beliefs of the subject. While this is true, it is only part of the picture. Unconscious awareness may include psychic and healing information that can be of great benefit.

AK is proving enormously helpful in diagnosing and treating children and adults with learning, hyperactivity, attention deficit and traumatic neurological disorders. This is particularly impressive in light of the relatively limited improvements in these disorders achieved through conventional medical and psychotherapeutic approaches.

Charles Krebs is an inspiring example of the benefits of AK. Krebs was an athletic marine biologist who enjoyed deep sea diving. In 1982 he suffered a severe case of *the bends* (cerebrospinal damage from too rapid decompression after a deep-sea dive) and ended up a paraplegic. By dint of enormous willpower and persistence he regained almost full use of his legs, but he still had poor coordination, as well as frequent urinary and bowel incontinence. Residual brain damage also left him unable to cope with the intellectual demands of marine biology. Though he could read and remember facts, he could not organize them into patterns in his mind, so he had to abandon his career. Meditation and emotional releases of rage and frustration helped Krebs to bring back most of his lost functions, but his legs remained poorly coordinated even two years after his accident. A single session of AK produced remarkable improvement in the coordination of his legs, as it helped to identify previously unidentified and unresolved emotions that were influencing his physical condition.

Meanwhile, Krebs shifted careers and began working with students who had learning disabilities. He went on to study AK and to develop techniques for reducing learning disabilities. Today there are an impressive variety of AK approaches that can help to overcome learning disabilities. Krebs describes many cases of people who have been helped through these methods, some of them demonstrating significant changes after many other methods had not helped.

Krebs theorizes that many learning disabilities derive from poor communication between the right and left brain hemispheres across the *corpus callosum* (nerve pathways connecting the right and left brain hemispheres). The vast majority of these blocks are due to emotional traumas but some may also be due to organic brain problems. AK diagnoses and treatments of learning disabilities are directed toward re-establishing the blocked connections across the corpus callosum.

Following are two typical cases in which Krebs found AK helpful in diagnosis and treatment of learning disorders.

CASES: Julie, aged 15, "could not abstract arithmetical concepts that a primary school student could manage easily." In tenth grade "she could not add up numbers greater than 10. She did not know how to carry a digit and couldn't add, subtract, or do fractions." She had nevertheless been allowed to advance with her peers through school, mostly because of her charming personality. Krebs was able to help Julie with a total of 10 hours of exercises that connected up her logical thinking functions to the point where she could understand the concept of carrying numbers in doing addition. With a further five weeks of remedial tutoring during her summer holiday, Julie caught up with her class in school, mastering all of her subjects including algebra.

Steven was nine when he came to Krebs for help with spelling problems. Krebs noted:

> [T]he alphabet was little more comprehensible than alphabet soup.
> I took him through the alphabet to see what letters caused him stress and found the letter K was enormously loaded for him. I did an [AK] emotional stress correction and took him through the age recession procedure to find out why, when he saw the letter K, he would get so stressed. A major emotional stress was revealed at age five. His mother confirmed our findings, saying, "Oh, I remember. When Steven was five, K was the first letter that he learned and he scratched it into the side of his grandmother's cedar wardrobe."
> You can bet that grandma didn't congratulate Steven on mastering one letter in the alphabet. She justifiably hit the roof and the whole emotional context of the event had been locked into that letter for Steven ever since. And since there are Ks in many words and scattered through even elementary reading material, was it any wonder that this boy had been having all sorts of problems with reading and spelling tasks? (p. 256-258)

Theories: I suspect that some of these dramatic improvements may be produced through suggestion via subtle cues provided by practitioners and by the beliefs and expectations of the persons tested – which combine to bring about self-healing. Beyond the effects of suggestion, however, there are interactions of the therapist and respant on intuitive and bioenergetic levels. Both information and energetic patterns that can facilitate healing may be interchanged during the AK therapeutic encounter. Kinesiology provides feedback to the respant and therapist via the body movements of the respant and this makes it possible to explore the causes and potential treatments for problems. These theories would lend themselves readily to further controlled studies.

I believe that Krebs' theory that benefits from AK may derive from enhanced right and left brain communications may have merit. This is more clearly evidenced in other therapies, such as EMDR and WHEE.[122]

Krebs proposes that AK interventions are based on subtle energies. He believes that there are subtle energetic "circuit breakers" that can be switched off due to emotional and physical traumas. AK provides the methods to identify these broken circuits and to reconnect them.

AK also appears to provide a method for identifying foods and medicinal substances that might be harmful or helpful to an individual person.   AK effects appear to represent another energy medicine phenomenon, relating to interactions of organismic and substance energy fields. There is also some speculation about neurological mechanisms for kinesiology.

Research: Clinical controlled studies of these methods have produced mixed results, with some studies confirming AK is helpful (for identifying allergens, diagnosing phobias, and identifying thyroid abnormalities).

Electroencephalographic (EEG) changes in the brain have been correlated with strong and weak kinesiology muscle test responses.

Though the use of AK has many anecdotal reports in its support, we await further controlled studies to rule out alternative explanations such as chance results, suggestion effects and clinical intuition on the part of the practitioner.[123]

Dowsing is clearly related to kinesiology, and impressive early research is reviewed in Chapter II-4.

AK awareness can also extend into the bioenergetic, transpersonal and spiritual realms. Here one may have to take greater leaps of faith, with less solid feedback to verify the answers to questions asked, although formal experimentation is still feasible. For instance, intuitive therapists are increasingly using AK on themselves (not on the client) to aid in diagnosing problems and suggesting remedies. This relies on the therapists' intuitive and psychic abilities. A therapist may use AK to check whether a therapy intervention is appropriate, by posing questions such as, "Is Tom ready to deal with his addiction to alcohol at this time?" This method will tap the resources of the therapist's training and clinical acumen and it can bring various intuitive processes into conscious awareness.[124] Intuitive therapists supplement their own AK responses with parallel responses of clients. However, even greater caution is warranted here, because it is easy to digress on tangents that are purely the creations of fantasy, or mental projections of the client or therapist, or caused by other psychological defense mechanisms.

I have personally found AK techniques clinically useful in helping clients to explore their unconscious beliefs and conflicts, and helpful for myself both personally and professionally..

Cautions: While AK may help the unconscious mind speak about its problems and conflicts, the messages may not be clear or may be misinterpreted. Information from the unconscious mind often rises to consciousness through the vehicle of imagery and this is often far less than entirely clear. Even gifted intuitives are not accurate in their analyses all of the time. Furthermore, if the patient has fears, ambivalence, or a habit of avoidance of issues that are related to the focus of the AK work, these may color the responses. In other words, the AK response may come from a place of psychological defense, rather than from a place that is seeking the changes required for healing. The unconscious mind may continue to resist releasing whatever feelings it has buried, to avoid re-experiencing the initial discomforts that led to the defensive habit.

In using AK for transpersonal explorations, one must be even more cautious. Our ordinary consciousness is limited in its ability to communicate with these realms and there are often distortions in the communications that get through – which adds another potential layer of error to those that may be introduced by the unconscious mind.

Adverse effects: No direct negative effects are known, but the cautions are warranted, as mentioned above, regarding interpretation of intuitive readings.

Training and licensing: There are no general standards for training and no licensing requirements for Applied Kinesiology.

Clinical applications: Applied Kinesiology is limited in its applications only by the inventiveness of the clinician and the client. It is helpful as a primary approach in exploring physical and psychological problems. It can help to identify traumatic psychological roots that may be contributing to states of dis-ease and disease. It can suggest whether clients are ready for particular therapeutic approaches and remedies. It can sharpen the focus of affirmations or other therapeutic interventions, with a query such as, "Is this the best focus for treatment at this time?" Common-sense cautions against false positives and negatives must be applied in intuitive work, as in any diagnostic system.

A therapist is required for assessment and treatment, but individualized self-exploration and self-healing approaches are commonly used.

See also: Medical dowsing; Medical intuition.

AROMATHERAPY

> *When the lotus opened,*
> *I didn't notice and went away empty-handed.*
> *Only now and again do I suddenly sit up from my dreams*
> *to smell a strange fragrance.*
> *It comes on the south wind,*
> *a vague hint that makes me ache with longing,*
> *like the eager breath of summer wanting to be completed.*
> *I didn't know what was so near,*
> *or that it was mine.*
> *This perfect sweetness blossoming in the depths of my heart.*
> — Rabindranath Tagore

Aromatherapists report that the effects of aromatic oils containing any of a wide variety of essences (*essential oils*) can be quite potent and specifically beneficial for a range of ailments. For instance, lavender is used to soothe and calm; lemongrass and rosemary to uplift and refresh; eucalyptus and tea tree are antiseptic; and orange is soporific. Studies have shown absorption of essential oils through inhalation and through the skin. Some therapists also recommend oral use.

Aromatherapy is often combined with massage.

Some claim that in addition to inducing relaxation, essential oils can also contribute to spiritual awareness. The burning of incense and the use of aromatic oils in religious rituals is a common practice in many cultures.

Research: While it is still early days in aromatherapy research, many studies

suggest benefits for a variety of problems. Sadly, the quality of these studies varies widely, with many lacking in details of reporting or statistical analyses.
Aromatherapy has been shown to help in treatment of pains, anxiety, emotional
distress, depression, problems of premature infants, enhancing antimicrobial and
antifungal activity, baldness *(alopecia areata)* and eliminating head lice.

  Bruce Berkowsky describes spiritual aromatherapy, which seeks to release deep
patterns underlying physical and emotional problems..

Theory: Our olfactory sense connects to the deeper, more primitive parts of the
brain, associated with the brain's emotional centers. By stimulating these portions
of the brain it may be possible to alter various mind-body connections, much as
psychoneuroimmunology does.

Adverse effects: Several cautions are advised in the use of essential oils. Stock
solutions are very concentrated and only a few drops are used, diluted in many
times the quantity of water. Stock solutions can even be caustic to the skin. There
have also been toxic, allergic and photosensitive reactions in smelling the oils,
and taken internally some can be toxic to the liver. The manufacture of oils is not
standardized or regulated and various companies may include preservatives or
extenders that can produce allergic or other reactions. Interactive effects of essential oils with some medications are also possible.

Training and licensing: Training is given through workshops and apprentice-
ships. Use of aromatherapy is not licensed, but aromatherapy as massage is
regulated under laws governing massage.

See also: Aromatherapy as massage.

AUTOGENIC TRAINING (AT)

>   *It breathes me.*
>   – Wolfgang Luthe and J. H. Schultz

Wolfgang Luthe and J. H. Schultz developed a form of self-healing that involves
relaxation and acquiring control over various physiological processes. This is a
profoundly potent self-healing method, where clients repeat to themselves six key
phrases addressing various somatic functions: "My hands and arms are heavy;"
"My hands and arms are warm;" "My heartbeat is regular;" "It breathes me;" "My
stomach is warm;" and "My forehead is cool." These sentences can be recited a
number of times until, for instance, one's hands actually become warm.

  Popular especially in Europe, autogenic training has been used for years in the
treatment of anxiety, hypertension and other stress-related states. Many physical
conditions have also been reported to respond to this method. Autogenic training
shades into transpersonal therapy, in the state of passive observation that is at the
core of this approach and in the phrase, "It breathes me," which is recited mentally while breathing.

I am impressed that the combination of meditative concentration with focus on the body is more potent than either method used alone.

Theory: AT phrases are a form of auto-suggestion that may directly influence the body, for example by reducing hypertension or releasing the spasm in peripheral arterioles in cases of Raynaud's disease or migraine. It is possible that the primary relaxation and reduction in anxiety states secondarily produce the perceived and/ or actual improvements that are seen with AT in physical conditions.

Research: Extensive early research conducted in Europe (without control groups) suggests there are significant effects of AT on psychological stress and depression. Combined with the cathartic model of Luthe (taught in Europe but not in the US), controlled studies have modest positive effects for physical problems such as angina, asthma, childbirth, headaches (including migraines), hypertension, infertility, recovery from myocardial infarction and Raynaud's disease and for psychological problems such as pain, stress/ anxiety and eczema. Substantial effects were shown for insomnia.

Preliminary evidence from Kirlian photography indicates that AT may also affect energy states.

Adverse effects: Emotional releases are possible during AT exercises. These may cause fear or could be retraumatizing if one is not alerted to anticipate this possibility and does not have therapeutic support to deal with the surfacing materials.

Training and licensing: The UK has a professional organization for AT but there are no professional standards for practice or licensing of Autogenic Training in the US. AT is not a licensed or regulated therapy.

Clinical applications: Autogenic Training can be profoundly helpful with stress and stress related illnesses, including (but not restricted to) asthma, irritable bowel syndrome, hypertension, migraines and muscular pains. When practiced to its full potential, it provides an excellent entry into psychotherapy.

A teacher is required, to instruct in the techniques and to provide guidance and support. Most of the practice is in the form of self-healing, which continues after the basic course of instruction (usually 8 weekly sessions) is completed. This may become a lifelong practice that leads to ever-deepening benefits.

See also: Biofeedback; Meditation; Relaxation; Self-Hypnosis; Yoga.

AYURVEDIC MEDICINE

> Ayus *means life and* veda *means knowledge/ science in Sanskrit, combining as "a science of life."*

Ayurveda is the natural medicine system of India, which has been practiced for at least five millennia. Ayurveda assumes that health and illness depend upon proper balances in consciousness and lifestyles. Its practices include yoga, specialized diets and herbal remedies. Several hundred American doctors incorporate Ayurvedic methods in their practices.

Theories: Ayurvedic medicine teaches that illness is caused by imbalances in three *doshas* (physiological principles) that govern the body's functions. *Vata*, composed of air and ether elements in air energy, moves one towards change. *Pitta*, or fire energy, gives strength, intelligence and direction. *Kapha*, composed of water and earth elements in water energy, contributes steadiness, calmness and reliability.

Ayurveda identifies three body types, each associated with a dosha and each associated with particular metabolic and personality characteristics, along with susceptibilities to certain illnesses. The *vata* type is slender of build and changeable in moods and activities, intuitive and creative but not good with practical applications. Vata people tend to have constipation, premenstrual symptoms and anxieties. The *pitta* type is of medium build, fair-skinned, steady and regular in routines and generally predictable. Pitta people are intelligent and quick-witted, but they are perfectionists and have short tempers. They are susceptible to stomach problems such as ulcers and may also have hemorrhoids. The *kapha* type is solidly built and strong. Kaphas are laid-back, relaxed, slow to anger and affectionate. They are prone to allergies and tend to be overweight.

Every person has varying ratios of the three *doshas*, each of which is concentrated in a certain part of the body. *Vata* is energy that enlivens the physical body, facilitating breath and circulation of blood. Vata predominates in the pelvis, particularly in the large intestine, as well as in the bones, thighs, ears and skin. *Pitta* encourages the metabolism of food, water and air and energizes the body's enzymes. Pitta resides in the stomach and small intestine, blood, eyes and sweat glands. *Kapha* is contained in the structural elements of the body – the bones, muscles and fat – providing form and protection for the various organs. It is prominent in the chest, lungs and spinal fluid.

When people of these body types have balanced doshas that are harmonious with their constitutional characters, they are healthy. Illness is the result of imbalances in the doshas. Physical and emotional stresses, poor diet, injudicious lifestyles, seasons and time of day can all influence health.

Classical Ayurvedic diagnosis relies on palpation of the radial (wrist) pulse, with assessment of the appearance of the tongue, eyes and nails. Ayurvedic doctors recognize an enormous range of subtle variations in pulses that reveal the relative strengths and weakness in the doshas, as well as suggesting therapeutic interventions. Treatments can include herbal remedies, lifestyle changes (diet, sleep, exercise programs and outdoor exposure time under the sun), meditations and mental/ spiritual healing. It is assumed that harmful waste products accumulate in the body and may contribute to ill health. These can be reduced through massage, herbal remedies, heat treatments and enhancemed elimination through various forms of internal cleansing.

Research supports the benefits of many of these approaches, particularly meditation and yoga exercises. Ayurvedic methods have been effective in promoting healthier blood pressure, cholesterol and reactions to stress, factors that are predictors of cardiac risk. They are also useful in preventing and treating cancers of the breast, lung and colon; for enhancing mental health; and for slowing the effects of aging.

Mentalin, an herbal combination of ginger, bacoba and gotu kola, has been shown to help in the treatment of Attention Deficit Hyperactivity Disorder.

Adverse effects: Side effects of herbs or interactive effects of herbs with conventional medications are possible.

Training and licensing: In India there are about 200 schools that teach Ayurvedic medicine. A five-year course leads to a Bachelor of Ayurvedic Medicine and Surgery (BAMS) and a two-year internship is required prior to commencing practice. Graduate studies that include research are rewarded with a Master of Ayurvedic Science (MASc) degree, recently changed to Doctor of Medicine in Ayurveda (MD in Ayurveda).

In the West, there are no established standards for Ayurvedic education or licensing. For the most part, Western Ayurvedic practitioners are health caregivers who have taken courses of various durations and depth (often very brief and superficial).

Clinical applications: Ayurvedic medicine is a complete system of treatment. It can be particularly helpful in treating problems of digestion, allergies, chronic infections (e.g. acne), obesity, hypertension, emotional imbalance, fatigue and addictions.

Integrative use of Ayurvedic medicine can be helpful with chronic illnesses. It may reduce the need for some allopathic medications and it may also predict that certain medicines are better than others for treating the various characterological types. For instance, a *pitta* type is likely to be extra-sensitive to aspirin, so alternative treatments for pain management might be advised. There is potential for conflict here with conventional medical practices, so dialogue between practitioners is needed as well as further research. One report indicates that preventive use of Ayurvedic medicine can reduce the costs of conventional medical care.

Most Ayurvedic practice is performed under the care of a doctor, though some self-healing exercises may be included.

See also: Naturopathic Medicine; Tibetan Medicine.

BARBARA BRENNAN HEALING

Barbara Brennan was an astrophysicist who left her job with NASA in the mid-70s to work on strengthening her clairsentient and healing gifts, which had been present since childhood. She founded a now prestigious school of healing that has been attended by many doctors and other caregivers The Brennan school has a strong emphasis on psychological and energy approaches, including intuitive assessments of energy field abnormalities based upon the theory and practice of bioenergetics.

Adverse effects: No harmful effects have been reported See discussion of potential general negative effects from rapid improvements under Spiritual Healing.

Training and licensing: The training is modular, over four years, with a major focus on self-healing for the healer. This method is not licensed.

See also: Spiritual Healing, Volume I of *Healing Research.*

BIOFEEDBACK

> *[H]umankind has more talents and more potential for self-regulation than we usually use or take credit for... Mind over body, inside the skin, is a special case of mind over nature.*
> – Elmer Green and Alyce Green (p. 62)

Biofeedback was discussed as a form of self-healing in Chapter II-1. It deserves separate mention here as one of the important complementary therapies.

Some parts of our bodies have no sensory connections, so we are unaware of their state and therefore cannot control them. However, when we use instruments to tell us what is going on in these parts of our body, we can gain some measure of control over them. For instance, if an instrument attached to electrodes on our skin shows us on a dial, or lets us hear by the pitch or loudness of an auditory tone how tense our muscles are, we can then consciously direct our muscles to relax. If we monitor our skin temperature with an electrode taped to one hand, we can relax and dilate the blood vessels in our skin, thereby warming the hand. Another window for feedback is through the electrical resistance of our skin, which changes with our states of physical and emotional tension. Likewise, if we can monitor our own brainwaves, we can learn to enter a state of deeper relaxation by adopting the mental state that produces alpha or theta brainwaves.

Research has shown biofeedback to be effective in the treatment of hypertension, asthma, migraines, Raynaud's disease (spasms of small arteries in the hands when they get cold), irritable bowel syndrome, urinary and fecal incontinence, epilepsy, chronic pain, anxiety, attention deficit disorder and more. Peavey et al. showed that biofeedback-induced relaxation could enhance the phagocytic (germ-destroying) activity of white blood cells.

Adverse effects: None are known.

Training and licensing: Many biofeedback practitioners are health caregivers who hold other professional licenses (psychologists, counselors, etc.). The Biofeedback Certification Institute of America (BCIA) requires 200 training hours at an approved institution for those with no primary certification and 30 supervised clinical hours for licensed clinicians. Written and practical exams are required. Most states classify biofeedback as a subcategory of mental health treatment, though it is not separately licensed.

Clinical applications: Biofeedback helps with problems for which self-regulation of the body can be achieved, such as disorders of the musculoskeletal, digestive and nervous systems, and for cardiovascular problems. While its most common uses are for muscle relaxation, hypertension and migraines, it can also be used for irritable bowel syndromes and ulcers, Raynaud's disease, incontinence, irregular heartbeats, epilepsy and hyperactivity in children. Brainwave biofeedback has been widely used for deepening meditation.

Biofeedback is a helpful primary treatment or adjunct to conventional medical treatments for the above-mentioned problems. Biofeedback adds an important dimension to conventional treatments, empowering people to feel that they can help themselves – both in curing their illness and in a much broader, general sense of enhanced self-confidence.

Biofeedback is initiated and supervised under the treatment of a therapist, but the practice is performed as self-healing.

See also: Autogenic Training; Meditation; Relaxation.

BODYMIND THERAPIES

The most important question to ask in addressing a person's illness is "What do you think your body is saying?"
– D.B.

Many complementary therapies integrate work on the body with work on psychological issues. The body stores memories of events and emotions – as muscle tensions, pains, neurohormonal problems and various diseases. Massage, spinal manipulation or biological energy interventions can access these memories, often resulting in emotional releases. Let me share several examples from my personal practice of psychotherapy combined with spiritual healing.

CASE 1: I observed "Greta," a healee with arthritis receiving spiritual healing at a healing center in England. She had had several treatments over a period of weeks with modest, temporary relief but the pains in her hands kept returning. As she spoke with the healer about her experiences during the previous week, I noticed that her fists were clenched.

I asked Greta, "What do you think your hands might be saying?"

Unclenching her fists and looking at her palms, Greta indicated that she didn't know what I meant. I shrugged and she continued speaking with the healer. In less than a minute her hands were again balled into fists. I repeated my question, getting a similar response.

The third time I asked the question, Greta held up her fists, looked at them and asked in an angry tone, "Are you trying to say that I'm angry?" The incongruity of her tone was obvious to the three of us and we all laughed.

This incident led Greta to explore several chronic, frustrating situations in her life that she was angry about. The discussion, the emotional release and the healing combined to relieve her of all symptoms of arthritis within a few weeks.

CASE 2: I used healing with "Jean," a middle-aged woman who came to me with back pains and fatigue that had been bothering her for several years. Within two sessions, as I was giving a laying-on of hands treatment, she spontaneously re-called incidents of sexual abuse in childhood which she had completely forgotten.

The healing, combined with psychotherapy, helped her work through her anger, hurt and (unjustified) guilt over the sexual abuse. In the course of the treatment, her back ceased to hurt and she gradually regained her energy.

I am impressed that therapies which include touch and manipulation of the body work exceedingly well in combination with psychotherapy. In my experience, the two taken together are more potent than either approach used alone.

Bodymind therapies and psychotherapy
While most reviewers focus on the *body* side of bodymind therapies, several highly effective bodymind approaches that focus on the *mind* are rapidly growing in popularity.

1. *Eye Movement Desensitization and Reprocessing* (EMDR) is a very potent method that helps people deal with severe emotional distress and with crippling patterns of belief (e.g. "I am unlovable," "I can't handle social situations," etc.). Healees focus upon their problems while repeatedly moving their eyes from right to left and back under the guidance of a therapist. Even severe, debilitating emo-tional traumas such as post-traumatic stress disorders (PTSDs) from wartime experiences, auto accidents or rape may be released and the person can be re-stored to normal psychological functioning with a relatively brief course of treatment. People with PTSD who have been crippled with panic attacks and nightmares for decades have been restored to normal functioning using this method.

Although the name of this therapy implies that eye movements are the effective healing process, people may respond equally well to alternating stimulation by sound or tapping on the right and left sides of the body. It is therefore speculated that right-left brain integration may be the underlying process in this therapy.

2. Various acupressure approaches facilitate profound psychological transforma-tions. See under Meridian Based therapies.

3. Neurolinguistic Programming (NLP) *anchors* positive and negative feelings in separate points in the body through touch, then cancels the negative feelings through touching both spots simultaneously.[125]

4. Bioenergetics and related therapies are enormously helpful in releasing buried emotional traumas.

Research: An extensive body of research confirms that EMDR is helpful in treating stress, particularly Post-Traumatic Stress Disorder (PTSD).

Adverse effects: Emotional releases are possible during bodymind therapies. These may cause fear or could be retraumatizing if the person is not alerted to anticipate this possibility and does not have therapeutic support to deal with the surfacing materials.

Clinical applications: Bodymind therapies are particularly helpful for treating problems of emotional stress, musculoskeletal disorders, clarifying emotional factors that may underlie or complicate physical problems of all sorts and in enhancing self-confidence.

A therapist is essential for instruction and guidance in bodymind exercises. Some self-healing exercises are usually included.

See also: Alexander Technique; Bioenergetics; EMDR; Feldenkrais Method; Massage; Meridian Based Therapies; Rubenfeld therapy.

BREATHWORK

Make time as the long march of this day unfolds to pause...
breathe...
collect and focus yourself...
Wake up from the cultural trance that you have been hypnotized into...
　　　　　　　　　　　　　　　　　　　– Michelle Levey and Joel Levey

Ordinary breathing may be shallow and less than fully effective. Yoga and other bodywork therapies often recommend expanding one's breathing capacity to provide better oxygenation of body tissues. Lung volume is increased by exercises for expanding the chest and lowering the diaphragm.

The breath is often used as a focus for meditation, with myriads of variations in techniques.[126] Some therapists recommend chest breathing over diaphragmatic breathing, while others recommend the reverse.

Mental focus on breathing can be a basis for meditation, as this natural metronome is always available to us and is an excellent focus for concentration.

When we shut down our awareness of our feelings, the body may tense up in various places, particularly in the chest. If we expand the chest and breathe deeply, we open up our awareness of the feelings that were inhibited in this way.

Eastern teachings suggest that we inhale cosmic energies (*prana*) along with the air that enters our lungs. Various techniques and practices encourage and facilitate these energy flows.

Therapeutic breathwork is a separate category of therapy. Rapid breathing may induce alternative states of consciousness, which can be used to facilitate and deepen psychotherapies and bodywork therapies such as *holonomic* therapy (Grof/ Halifax) and *rebirthing* (Orr/ Ray). These techniques help people to retrieve very early memories, often related to traumas suffered around the time of birth and while still in the womb.

It is fascinating that in the framework of breathing therapies it is uncommon to find subjects suffering from hyperventilation symptoms (dizziness, tingling and numbness of hands, abdominal pains and panics).

Adverse effects: Intense feelings that have been long buried and forgotten may surface with breathwork. It is advisable to have an experienced therapist for this form of healing.

Training and licensing: Breathwork is a technique often used by various therapists in addition to their other approaches, but some specialize in breathwork alone. There are no standards for practice or certification of breathwork therapies. This is not a licensed modality.

Clinical applications: Therapeutic breathwork provides a potent, rapid opening into deep, early memories of emotional traumas. It can bring about rapid changes in emotional problems.

Breathwork is done under the supervision of a therapist, both for guidance with the technique and for support with emotional releases.

CHELATION THERAPY
See: EDTA Chelation

CHIROPRACTIC AND OSTEOPATHIC MANIPULATIONS

> *The new emphasis on outcomes research is changing the ground rules. There is less interest in theories. Today the bottom line: Is the treatment effective? Is it reproducible? What is the cost?*
> – Robert Mootz, DC

Chiropractic
D. D. Palmer, a "magnetic healer" who practiced at the turn of the century, developed a system of chiropractic therapy based on the thesis that the nervous system controls the body and therefore that any malfunction must be due to blockage of the nerves involved in that part of the body. Treatments are based on spinal adjustments, with the presumption that misalignments of the vertebral column (subluxations) cause pinching of the nerves and thus block their control of the body. Diagnosis is accomplished with manual palpation of the body and exploration of musculoskeletal movement, along with x-rays of the spine. Manipulations are described as *high-velocity, short-amplitude* manual interventions. Chiropractic has split into many and varied schools, some following a *straight* focus upon spinal manipulation and others adopting a *mixed* program that may include kinesiology, nutritional counseling and other such techniques (Schaefer/ Fay).

An estimated 12 million Americans receive spinal manipulative therapy annually.

Theory: Release of the pressure on the nerves pinched in a misaligned spinal cord restores normal functioning to the body. The potential applications of chiropractic for the treatment of musculoskeletal disorders are obvious.

Conventional medicine treats pinched nerves with surgery. This is different from the subluxations treated by chiropractors, as nerves can also be pinched by "slipped" disks (cartilage that protrudes from between the vertebral joints and impinges on the spinal cord or nerve roots).

Many chiropractors also claim to be able to treat various body organ diseases through spinal manipulations, but few have demonstrated causal connections between their interventions and the claimed results. The new and promising specialty of chiropractic neurology may begin to fill in some of these gaps. There is speculation that chronic irritation of peripheral nerves can produce changes in the biochemistry of the peripheral nerves, the spinal cord and the brain, which in turn send abnormal messages to the body, thereby causing disease processes.

Bruce Lipton suggests that the true theories of D. D. Palmer were altered in order to conform to prevailing medical and cultural paradigms and that the original conceptualization of D. D. Palmer was one that focuses on spirit and body consciousness:

> D. D. Palmer was very sensitive to scientists' displeasure concerning concepts related to spirit and vital forces. In formulating the original science of Chiropractic, he coined the terms Universal Intelligence and Innate Intelligence to refer to the inherent organizing intelligence of the Universe and of life...
>
>   In the early years of Chiropractic I used the terms Innate (Spirit), Innate Intelligence (Spiritual Intellect), Universal Intelligence (God) because they were comprehensive and the world was not prepared to receive the latter terms just mentioned in parentheses. It may be even now premature to use them. (Palmer, p. 542).
>
>   ... the basic philosophy of Chiropractic, as defined by D. D. Palmer (before its modification by B. J. Palmer), perceives the flow of information from an externalized source, Universal Intelligence. An eternal "metamerized" portion of that intelligence, referred to as Innate, is needed by each individualized being (pages 494 and 496, The Science, Art and Philosophy of Chiropractic). Although Innate is not localized, its seat of control is the brain. From the brain, Innate's intelligence travels down the spinal cord and from the spinal cord outward to the periphery, a pathway referred to as Above>Down>Inside>Out (A-D-I-O).
>   – Bruce Lipton

Research: See under Osteopathy in the next section.

Training and licensing: The Council for Chiropractic Education sets criteria for training. Chiropractic colleges in the US have entry requirements including a minimum of 60 semester or 90 quarter hours towards a BA or BS degree at a recognized accredited institution. The usual chiropractic course of training is five years. Exams are administered by the National Board of Chiropractic Examiners, with each state setting its own licensing requirements. Postgraduate education is available, with two-year residencies in orthopedics, radiology, neurology, pediatrics, family practice, sports medicine, rehabilitation, meridian/ acupuncture and research.

As of 1993 over 45,000 chiropractors were licensed in the US. Practitioners are trained in 17 chiropractic colleges that produce a total of 2,000 graduates every year. There are also chiropractic colleges in Australia, Canada, England, France and Japan.

It is instructive to consider the efforts of the medical profession in the US to limit the licensing and practice of chiropractic. For many years doctors were warned by their medical societies not to associate with or refer patients to chiropractors. However, a successful lawsuit by chiropractors charging the American Medical Association (AMA) and other medical associations with restraint of trade brought about a dramatic change in 1987. Chiropractors are now working much more closely with doctors.

The benefits of chiropractic (compared to medication and other conventional treatments) for back, neck and other pains include: avoidance of habituation to drugs, addressing (presumed) causes rather than just the symptoms, and cost effectiveness.

Research: No studies have been published on the clinical efficacy of Network Spinal Analysis. However, a British study of Light Touch Manipulative Technique, a method that closely resembles Network Spinal Analysis,[127] showed significant effects for back pain.

Osteopathy

Osteopathy was developed by Andrew Taylor Still (1828-1917), an allopathic doctor who served in the American Civil War. Still was motivated by the death of several of his children from spinal meningitis to seek methods that went beyond symptomatic relief, which at the time was all that medical practice could offer. In 1874 he launched the system he had spent many years developing through diligent study of human anatomy and physiology. Though he had intended osteopathy to be an extension of medical practice, it developed over the years into a separate system – largely due to the fact that conventional doctors opposed and ridiculed his system and actually drove him out of his home state of Kansas. He founded the American School of Osteopathy in Kirksville, Missouri in 1892.

Osteopathy involves techniques of spinal assessment and manipulation that address the body as a functioning unity. This method focuses on posture, respiration and the status of the skeleton and connective tissues. While the primary tool of osteopathy has been seen to be manipulation (and this continues to be the case in the UK), in the US this discipline also incorporates many other approaches. These include physical and occupational therapy, orthotic and prosthetic devices, fitness, pharmacology, surgery, biofeedback, psychotherapy and the whole range of conventional medical treatments. In essence, the practice of most osteopathic physicians trained today is almost identical with the practice of conventional medical doctors.

The remainder of this discussion will focus on the manipulative aspects of osteopathy and chiropractic. Cranial osteopathy and craniosacral therapy, which represent distinct and largely separate advances over conventional osteopathy, are discussed below.

The goal of osteopathy is to remove pressure on nerves that are presumed to be pinched by spinal deformities and to release other tensions in the musculoskeletal system and fascia (connective tissues), thus restoring the body to its natural state of healthy functioning. Doctors of Osteopathy (DOs) have treated many health problems through spinal manipulations.

Classical osteopaths use a variety of manual manipulative approaches, individually or in combination with each other or with allopathic medical interventions:

1. *Soft tissue massage* – relaxes muscles and enhances circulation of blood and lymph.
2. *Isometric and isotonic methods* – relaxes and restores of normal joint mobility.
3. *Articulatory methods*, or manipulation without impulse improves joint mobility.
4. *High-velocity, low-amplitude methods*, or manipulation with impulse - realigns vertebral joints.
5. *Myofascial release methods* address muscles and fascia through direct and indirect techniques.
6. *Functional methods* - address dysfunctions diagnosed by the manual assessments of the practitioner.
7. *Strain and counterstrain methods* – identify sore spots that are related to specific abnormalities in joint mobility or muscle spasm. These *trigger points* are soothed by positioning the body in specific ways for brief periods.
8. *Craniosacral (*also called *Cranial) methods* - are described later in this chapter.

Research in Chiropractic and Osteopathic Manipulations
Controlled studies confirm that spinal compression of nerves does bring about changes in the nerves.

Chiropractic studies: In controlled studies, chiropractic has been found to be: helpful in treatment of back pain of mechanical origin; and better in these problems than a placebo for pain, though no better than physiotherapy for decreasing disability or duration of disorders; effective in treating headaches (compared to antidepressants); thoracic pain; tension headaches; migraines; muscle soreness following exercise; infant colic; dysmenorrhea; and hypertension. Reviews of research series produced mixed impressions, due to faulty research design and reporting.

The limited scope of the existing research is at first glance surprising, in view of the vast popularity of chiropractic over the past century. Because studies of the efficacy of these manipulations have not been published until recently and because until recent years, training in chiropractic in some schools was very brief and insubstantial, conventional medicine has held a generally negative view of this discipline. This has been something of a Catch-22. Because of this skepticism, conventional medicine has not invested in the study of this modality, which medicine then criticizes because it lacks a basis in research.

Osteopathic studies: Studies addressing the mechanisms of action in osteopathy have begun to provide theoretical support for this treatment. Research supports the theory that compression of nerve roots near the spine may cause blockages; that experimentally compressed nerves produce toxic protein substances; that nerve cells near spinal dislocations (*subluxations*) are irritable (*facilitated segments*) and tend to stimulate muscles and viscera excessively; that muscles and joints may reflect the conditions of visceral organs and therefore can provide a basis for manual diagnosis; and that manual manipulations can restore balance in neuromuscular and visceral function.

Inter-rater reliability in diagnosis has been demonstrated in several studies.

A limited number of rigorous studies show that osteopathic diagnoses are consistent between practitioners and that osteopathy actually produces beneficial effects beyond those of a placebo. Studies of clinical efficacy are modestly impressive with back pain, carpal tunnel syndrome (wrist pain due to irritation of tendons), paresthesias (unusual sensations) due to peripheral nerve dysfunctions, burning pain in an extremity, postoperative recovery, postoperative collapsed lungs and hypertension. One controlled study showed significant relief of back pain with reduced need for pain medicine, while other studies showed osteopathic manipulations were no better than short-wave diathermy or placebo for relieving back pain.

Of historical interest are reports that osteopathic treatments were beneficial during the influenza epidemic of 1918.

It is unclear to what extent chiropractic and osteopathic manipulations resemble or differ from each other. Many of the studies do not include controls for suggestion and touch, so there may be a considerable measure of suggestion involved in the benefits attributed to both of these treatments.

Spiritual healing, chiropractic and osteopathy
The reported effects of chiropractic and osteopathic manipulations may also be augmented (without the awareness of the therapists) by spiritual healing in the form of laying-on of hands. Numbers of chiropractors and osteopaths have told me that their hands get warm during manipulations, which is typical of spiritual healing. In fact, some of the reported benefits of manipulations may be due to spiritual healing effects. The study by Dressler of *Light Touch Manipulative Technique,* and the benefits described by Network Spinal Analysis illustrate that this is possible.

Deliberately bioenergy interventions or spiritual healing may be a helpful complement to chiropractic and osteopathy, as with many other manual therapies. Edgar Cayce, an extraordinarily gifted clairsentient diagnostician and a prescriber of unusual, but highly effective treatments, included chiropractic among his recommended therapies. The late Bruce MacManaway, a gifted natural spiritual healer from Scotland, also based much of his healing technique on spinal manipulations.

Some chiropractors include applied kinesiology in their repertoires. This is another biological energy intervention.

Chiropractor Donald Epstein has developed a technique of treatment called *Network Spinal Analysis.* This involves very light touch and it is clearly a form of spiritual healing. More conventional chiropractic manipulations may be used after the initial course of light touch treatments. A retrospective survey of 2,818 people treated at 156 Network treatment centers in the US, Canada, Australia and Puerto Rico showed a 67-71% positive response rate. Significant improvements in physical and mental/ emotional states, stress levels and life enjoyment were reported by the majority of the respondents.

Adverse effects: There are significant risks associated with manipulative therapy (mostly with chiropractic), although the incidence of serious negative effects is low. These have included spinal injuries, with some fatalities and strokes. The percentage of negative effects from spinal manipulations is lower than the percentage of side effects from medications used to treat the same problems. Excessive use of x-rays is a potential long-term hazard that has not been adequately evaluated. Contraindications that might predispose patients to injuries include congenitally absent odontoid process (the bone that stabilizes the skull on the top of the spine), anticoagulant therapy, spinal disc lesions, cancers and osteoporosis. Another potential danger is misdiagnosis, particularly of early neurological diseases.

Training and licensing: Doctors of Osteopathy (DOs) in the US have now joined the mainstream of allopathic medicine and have incorporated medicine and surgery in their training and practices. In the US they are licensed along with Medical Doctors (MDs) under similar, if not identical medical examinations.

The National Board of Osteopathic Medical Examiners follows the criteria of allopathic medical examinations in the US. There were over 32,000 DOs in the US in 1993, with 16 schools graduating another 1,500 each year. Today there are 19 osteopathic schools in the country, with 129 hospitals accredited by the American Osteopathic Association (AOA). The AOA is also the professional body that represents osteopaths and promotes research. The American Academy of Osteopathy promotes the exploration and teaching of manipulative techniques.

Though for several decades osteopaths in the US tended towards conventional medical practice, in the past few years there has been a revival of interest in osteopathic manipulations amongst students of osteopathy.

In the UK, osteopathic practitioners do not have conventional medical training. UK osteopaths have remained focused on physical manipulation and cranial osteopathy in their therapy and do not study medicine. Osteopathy has been acknowledged by the British Medical Association as an accepted therapy.

Clinical applications: Chiropractic and osteopathic manipulations can help with many musculoskeletal disorders, sciatica and other spinal nerve root problems, particularly back and neck aches.

The early evidence suggests that these interventions, when applied by competent practitioners, might be the treatments of first choice for such conditions. These treatments could well be combined with the pain management techniques of relaxation, imagery, hypnotherapy and spiritual healing, plus conventional pain medications and muscle relaxants.

See also: Craniosacral Therapy.

COLONIC IRRIGATION

Irrigation of the colon is recommended for detoxification in Eastern medicine and also by the gifted clairsentient healer Edgar Cayce. It is believed that particles of feces that cling to the walls of the colon (large bowel) may putrefy and produce toxins that are then absorbed into the body. Irrigation of the colon with water inserted in the rectum removes these particles. Irrigation may similarly help to reduce overgrowths of yeasts (*Candida*) in the large bowel.

It is widely believed in the CAM community that toxins are released by the body through the gut, kidneys, sweat, breath and biological energies as a part of various natural healing processes, as well as through holistic therapies such as fasting. Colonic irrigation is believed to facilitate this process by enhancing cleansing of the body's wastes. Colonic irrigation also may be of use in treating liver or kidney disease, by relieving the body of toxins that these organs might otherwise have to process.

Adding nutrients to the enema water is believed to help in healing the intestinal wall if it is irritated.

Colonic irrigation is often offered by chiropractic and naturopathic practitioners.

I have seen no research to validate this treatment method and there are no standards for practice or certification for this therapy.

Adverse effects: Several deaths have been reported from excessive use of coffee enemas.

Training and licensing: Colonic irrigation is practiced by various health care practitioners without any licensing requirement.

Clinical applications: Conditions that may benefit from colonic irrigation include intestinal disorders (particularly sluggish bowel function); toxins in the body; infections; illnesses such as arthritis, chronic fatigue syndrome and other ailments with an allergic component; and skin problems.

Colonic irrigation can be given by a therapist, usually using sophisticated modern equipment. Water enemas can be taken without supervision, though introductory instruction and careful technique are important.

CRANIOSACRAL THERAPY/ CRANIAL OSTEOPATHY

> *... I use intrusive techniques only when I know more subtle diagnostic techniques won't be needed later during that session...*
> *... I have admitted to myself that these are intuitive phenomena which I can not explain scientifically. I am not afraid of them and I trust myself, which is probably the most important part of the whole process.*
> – John E. Upledger

> *Work in the cranial field is largely perceptual. The heart of clinical practice is listening. This demands both stillness and humility on the part of the practitioner. In this inquiry all one can do is to enter into a stillness and see what our journey brings.*
> – Franklyn Sills (2001, p. 3)

A variant of osteopathic therapy using craniosacral manipulation was developed by William G. Sutherland in the early 20th century. Though slow to be accepted, this method has recently become more popular. It is based on the observation of a palpable, rhythmic bioenergy pulsation around the head and body, with a normal frequency of 6-12 cycles per minute, which is unrelated to breathing or heart rate. (This is not to be confused with brain waves, some of which pulse at 3-30 cycles per *second.)* The rate of craniosacral pulsation can be slower or faster than normal due to various malfunctions of the body, though it is rarely faster than 60 beats per minute.

Therapists correct abnormalities in this rhythm through light touch applied with their hands on the patients' head and/ or sacrum, combined with visualizations of the integrity of each bone of the skull and of its proper interdigitation with neighboring cranial bones. Therapists may also visualize the bones flexing across the sutures between them. Further visualizations can achieve temporary cessation of craniosacral pulsation through the mental intent of the osteopath.

Craniosacral manipulation is used for common ailments but its special contribution lies in its purported ability to alleviate problems for which conventional medicine may offer limited treatment options. These include pains in the back and neck; fibromyalgia; frozen shoulder and carpal tunnel syndromes; arthritis; scoliosis; chronic ear infections: hormonal abnormalities; migraines; post-injury/ illness symptoms of head injury; meningitis and encephalitis; behavioral, developmental and learning disorders in children (sometimes attributed to cranial birth injury); and sacral injuries. Craniosacral therapy can also be helpful in treating chronic neuralgia syndrome; hypertension; temporo-mandibular joint (TMJ) pain; strabismus (crossed eyes); amblyopia (lazy eye); migraine headaches; cluster headaches; trigeminal neuralgia; chronic fatigue syndrome; tinnitis; vertigo; asthma; lymphedema (swelling due to blocked lymph vessels); plantar faciitis (inflammation of the tissues on the bottom of the foot); shin splints; tennis elbow; and golfer's elbow.

Craniosacral therapists rest their hands lightly upon the healee's skull and visualize that the bones of the skull can flex and move with the vis*ualized* movements of their hands and that the meningeal coverings of the brain stretch out as their (visualized) hands rise many inches in the air away from the head. These interventions, most of which are not physical manipulations, produce distinct subjective sensations within the head and spinal cord that are difficult to describe, including heat and tingling. At times the therapist will place a hand on the sacrum to sense the biological energies at the base of the spine and to facilitate the energy flow in the lower part of the body.

I attended a basic course in craniosacral therapy in England, where I learned, both as therapist and healee, to perceive the sensations that these practitioners describe. Many subjective sensations were similar to those I experience when giving and receiving healing, yet some of the sensations were uniquely characteristic of craniosacral manipulations. For example, with manipulations of my cranium involving very light touch or with the therapist's hands near to but not touching my head, it felt as if something within my head were being stretched.

I have had numerous conversations with craniosacral osteopaths in England and Americ and I am bemused by their firm insistence that they are engaging in a mechanical manipulation rather than an energy field intervention. The prevailing hypotheses among craniosacral therapists suggest that the brain causes fluctuations of pressure in the cerebrospinal fluid, though no mechanism for the production of such fluctuations has been reasonably postulated. It is claimed that the pressure passes through the dura (tissue layer covering the brain) to cause palpable expansions and contractions of the cranial bones across their sutures and then passes down the spinal canal to the sacrum, influencing the spinal nerves along the way. The fascia (connective tissues between muscles and organs) are proposed as the medium for transmission of these pulsations out to the extremities.

Evidence has been found to support only limited aspects of these mechanistic hypotheses, based on measurable motions of cranial bones.

A growing number of craniosacral therapists are combining manipulations with psychotherapeutic work, as *somatoemotional release.*

Sadly, most of the younger US osteopaths are no longer practicing craniosacral manipulations, having transformed their profession to copy the conventional medical model. Here and there one can find an older osteopath who still uses these helpful manipulations. I find it hopeful that numbers of osteopathic students are again showing interest in this aspect of their studies.

Theories of John E. Upledger
John E. Upledger is a strong proponent of craniosacral therapy,[128] who theorizes that physical and/ or emotional trauma can create an *energy cyst* within the body.[129] He hypothesizes that ordinarily a blow to the body produces heat that is dissipated by the body. (This is similar to the heat produced by a hammer pounding nails.) If the body is unable to dissipate the heat, it may be encapsulated as a localized concentration of energy. This *energy cyst* can obstruct normal body energy flows (of bioelectricity and acupuncture Qi); produce or exacerbate abnormal energy flows; compromise mobility of tissues, especially fascial layers; and produce energy interference waves. Energy cysts can create dysfunction or pain and drain the body's energy. Upledger can palpate a "fullness" on the "upstream" side of acupuncture meridians where they are blocked by a cyst and an "emptiness" beyond the block. Working with acupuncturists, he also found that pulse diagnosis abnormalities were restored to normal after treatments that released the cysts.

Infections or gross physiological malfunctions such as heart attacks can also leave energy cysts in the body. Upledger believes that several factors may determine whether or not a cyst is formed in response to a traumatizing energy. The trauma may be of such magnitude as to overwhelm the body's ability to dissipate it; previous trauma may compromise the ability of that part of the body to dissipate it; and intensely negative emotional states may hinder its dissipation.

Upledger believes that local bioenergy regions of the body (as well as energy cysts) may function autonomously, with associated memory, intelligence and emotion.

> *God will forgive you, but your nervous system will not.*
> – Hans Selye

The *facilitated segment* of the spinal cord is another concept from osteopathy, which describes an excessive sensitivity of nerves at particular spinal cord levels.

A spinal cord segment with a low threshold for excitation may act as a *neuronal lens,* concentrating and focusing energy from the whole nervous system into particular areas of the body. This may keep the muscles and organs of that area in an excessively stimulated state. Hyperactive organs then become more susceptible to irritants and they may malfunction and cause pain, as with ulcers. Such hyperactivity can readily be identified by rubbing the skin of the back along the spine. Facilitated regions will redden more quickly and more intensely than normal ones. This has been termed the *red reflex.*

Upledger describes how to release the tensions in facilitated segments:

> Once you have located a facilitated segment... sit the patient up and examine for tissue change, mobility loss and "red reflex." Place a finger on each side of the spinous process at the affected level. Place the flattened palm and fingers of the other hand lightly over the front of the body at the same level and follow the motion that occurs. The tissues will begin to move back and forth. Gradually you will feel the restricted vertebrae mobilize. It will feel as though you are rolling a barrel hoop around the patient's body. Eventually you will feel a release... At this point, reevaluate for the presence of the facilitated segment; it may be gone. If it is still present, repeat the process... You take away the secondary effects first and then the underlying cause... (Upledger/ Vrederoogd).

Upledger finds that if he positions the body in such a way that the craniosacral rhythm halts abruptly, he can establish the precise position that is most appropriate for the release of an energy cyst. This is done through a process of deduction and intuition. When the rhythm stops, the therapist keeps his hands immobile until it resumes. When the body position is exactly correct for the release of an energy cyst or for somatoemotional release, the craniosacral rhythm suddenly stops. The rhythm also stops abruptly when subjects speak of or think about an issue that is emotionally significant. The pulsations can thus function as "significance detectors," when combined with particular body positions of patients that are associated with their problems.[130]

A dissipation of heat accompanies the release of a cyst. Upledger finds that he must hold the limb still until processes such as the release of heat are completed and the craniosacral rhythm resumes its normal rate and amplitude. Occasionally the limb may move ever so slightly after the release and then the craniosacral rhythm ceases again. The process is then repeated. When the treatment is finished, the patient's entire body relaxes and she reports a sense of completion, often mirrored in the intuitive awareness of the practitioner.

CASE: A skier had had a shoulder injury five years prior to treatment. She suffered from chronic pain and had not responded to numerous conventional medical treatments. Upledger moved her arm till he found a position where the craniosacral rhythm stopped. He then performed the steps described above. She released anger which she had felt at another skier who had caused her to fall. After the cyst was released she discussed the incident and her craniosacral rhythm halted till she got in touch with her anger, which had remained undis-

charged for five years. Once she released the anger and forgave the other skier, the encysted energy remnants of the accident dissipated and she was pain-free.

Upledger proposes that this sort of pathological process in the body can set up interference waves of energy. A therapist aware of such processes can palpate the interference waves to localize them, since they emanate as arcs from the focus of disturbance. This is true for active pathological processes, but not for older ones.

Biological energy processes may evolve in ways that are unique to each organismic system. Upledger (1995a) suggests:

> [W]ithin each of us is the program for a natural process that, once begun, must be completed or it remains incomplete in a sort of frustrated state of suspended animation. This may occur when a fetus does not go through a normal vaginal delivery, such as during a Cesarean section delivery, or in a situation wherein the newborn is not allowed to bond with the mother. It may occur when, although the female has ovulated many times, there are no offspring. Now age 40 is here and the supply of ova is running low, panic for pregnancy ensues. It may occur when an abortion is performed and the pregnancy does not go to completion. (p. 159)

Upledger observes that such frustrated biological processes may cause energetic imbalances that can become symptomatic. One way to clear these is to have the healee use guided imagery to picture the processes continuing to their natural completion, as they would have done if they had not been interrupted.

Of particular relevance to spiritual healing are Upledger's observations that he can intuitively know things about the patient and can deliberately apply his mind to obtain a diagnosis. He holds specific questions in his mind and the information needed to clarify a diagnosis comes to him.[131]

Upledger finds that a group of therapists working together may be more able to facilitate somatoemotional release than individual therapists working alone. He recommends that a team leader be designated to direct this process. The emotional releasees connected with the dissipation of energy cysts may occur immediately or over the following hours or days. Upledger advises against interrupting treatment when the rhythm is stopped (which can produce discomfort) and against scheduling sessions more than two weeks apart (which may lead to regression).

Upledger comes close to calling himself a healer, as is evidenced by his statement at the beginning of this section and by some of his more recent observations as well. Upledger (1995a) reports that experienced craniosacral practitioners can identify obstructions in chakras and acupuncture meridians and can use energy release techniques to correct them. He also notes that people can project negative emotional energies (such as fear, anger, guilt or frustration) into other people. This is of particular concern for both allopathic and complementary therapists of all modalities. This is also a caution for therapists to clear themselves on all psychological and energetic levels in order to avoid harming healees unintentionally.

Here are some of the major overlaps between craniosacral therapy and spiritual healing.

... The use of CranioSacral Therapy, at its most advanced levels, requires the suspension of therapist ego and personal judgments. The therapist cannot take sides, he/ she should only observe, blend, connect with inner wisdom and facilitate and support the therapeutic process as the patient/ client's inner wisdom navigates through the complexities of denials, suppressions and rationalizations.

... It would appear, from clinical observations and experiences, that every cell and every tissue in the body has its own consciousness and its own memory. Therefore, a liver or a muscle or a bone or any other tissue or cell can retain the energy of a past experience. This energy can compromise the functional vitality of that tissue or cell, to some degree and in so doing may create symptoms and/ or disease. The patient's inner wisdom knows of all of these retained tissue memories. It also knows which ones are causing the most difficulty, which ones are requiring the most adaptive energy expenditure and which ones are the most desirable to discharge at any given time. When the therapist blends and connects with the patient/ client's inner wisdom, the inner wisdom first assesses the therapist's skills and particular talents and then presents to the therapist those retained memories that, in the inner wisdom's judgment, this therapist might best be able to work with and clear. It is very frequent that craniosacral therapists feel tested by "inner wisdoms." (Upledger 1986, p. 154)

The healee's inner wisdom can be accessed through the cranial subtle energy rhythm. A suggestion is given to the healee that her cranial rhythm will stop its pulsations as an indication of a "yes" response to a question from the therapist. This allows the therapist to use the cranial rhythm response for questioning the healee's unconscious mind. Some unusual applications include exploring questions even when the healee is in a coma, is an infant, or for some other reason is unable to respond verbally.

Craniosacral therapy patients may sometimes move spontaneously into unpredictable, unusual body positions. At such times their cranial rhythms cease to pulsate. If their body position is supported and held, they may then experience somatoemotional releases of long-buried and forgotten memories that had been repressed in their unconscious minds.[132]

Lessons from Craniosacral Therapy

Very few osteopaths go as far as Upledger in acknowledging that there is a biological energy component to craniosacral therapy. This method was developed from a branch of osteopathy, with a tradition of mechanical adjustment of joints and realigning of posture. This mechanistic background inculcates a mechanistic mode of thinking in many practitioners. The fact that cranial bones do move rhythmically suggests that a mechanical explanation for some of these observed phenomena may one day be confirmed. However, the following points appear problematic:

1. The movements of cranial bones appear to me inadequate to explain the observed clinical phenomena:

2. It is physically impossible for flexion to occur across the frontal bones in adults, after these bones have fused across the suture that was open in childhood, or in the occipital bone, which never had a suture - yet cranial osteopathy claims that there is flexion across these sutures.

3. Craniosacral rhythms palpated on the limbs seem unlikely to be transmitted physically from the spinal cord, across the body by fascia.

4. The sensations of heat, tingling, etc. experienced by patients during soma-toemotional releases are postulated by Upledger to represent the *from* release of bioenergy stored in energy cysts in the healee's body. Healers interpret similar sensations as energies passing from or through the healer *to* the healee.

5. The therapists mentally influencing craniosacral pulsations in the healee and correcting physical misalignments of bony joints, merely by holding their hands lightly on or near the body, appear to be yet further spiritual healing interventions.

My personal experience in learning this technique was that the sensations in my hands were very similar to those I experience in healing, though there are distinctions that I would find hard to convey to anyone who hasn't had similar training. I am puzzled that neither I nor other healers sense *pulsations* of biological energies during spiritual healings, while these are regularly reported by craniosacral osteo-paths. I, too, felt them when I was studying this method, but not when I have subsequently engaged in spiritual healing.

Upledger's assertions that the heat sensed during his treatments originates in the patient rather than in the therapist deserve further comment. I question this also because clients in psychotherapy who release pent-up emotions do not report a focalized sensation of heat at the time of their abreactions. This would bear more careful investigation, however, before one could rule out Upledger's hypothesis with greater certainty. It may be that his observations are valid for emotions linked with physical trauma, or that psychotherapists (including myself) simply have not queried patients about such sensations in the context of psychotherapy.

At present it would seem that the best theory to explain craniosacral therapy involves an energy field within and around the body, which is palpable and which interacts with the minds of the healee and the therapist. In other words, this would seem to be a variant of spiritual healing.

My intuitive impression is that craniosacral therapists' visualizations of manipulations of individual cranial bones facilitate their resonance with the energy field(s) of the healee. This may enable them to resonate with parts and/ or functions of the body in order to diagnose and treat problems through energy interactions. Parallel reports (from Autogenic Training, biofeedback, therapies involving imagery and yoga) of the efficacy of visualization combined with physical activity suggest that this is likely. Visualization may serve as a meditative focus and/ or as a way for the therapists to manipulate bioenergies.

Research: I have found no published research on the clinical efficacy of cranio-sacral manipulations. David Dressler, a therapist who practices the *Light Touch Manipulative Technique,* somewhat similar to osteopathy, showed that this method was an effective treatment for back pain. Dressler also observes that his work might be labeled as healing.

Cranial manipulations and spiritual awareness

The writings of Franklyn Sills (2001) are, in my opinion, among the finest in the literature on spiritual healing. His concise, clear descriptions of what he does and how he does it are an inspiration to practitioners to strive for the highest levels of wholistic healing. Here are a few examples:

> Work in the cranial field is largely perceptual. The heart of clinical practice is listening. This demands both stillness and humility on the part of the practitioner. In this inquiry all one can do is to enter into a stillness and see what our journey brings. The foundation of this endeavor is the experience of our own perceptual and inner process. An appreciation of our inner world is crucial for efficient clinical practice. This awareness of our own interior world is critical in the creation of a safe and efficient healing relationship. In this process, we will come directly into relationship to our own human condition and our own suffering. This is a huge undertaking. It means truly inquiring into who we are. The ground of this exploration is a commitment to learn about ourselves... (p. 3)

Cranial field therapy requires the therapist to focus completely in the present moment, to join with the field of the healee. Sills acknowledges the wisdom of The Buddha in reaching towards and into the stillness that facilitates healing.

> He simply and profoundly stated that *there is suffering and it must be understood*. This simple statement is the ground of therapeutic inquiry. (p. 4)

Sills continues with a discussion on dealing with suffering:

> ... if we hold onto things, onto fixed positions, onto self-construct, self-view and past history, there will be suffering... Most of us, most of the time, tend to see the present through the filters of the past. But if we can find a way to truly live in the present, in the present time-ness of things, then there is the possibility of not suffering. There may be pain, but there needn't be suffering. Within the cranial context, it is seen that suffering is relinquished when the system truly aligns with the present time-ness of things. It is an alignment to something else beyond the fear that seems to hold our sense of selfhood together. It is a realignment to a universal, an Intelligence much greater than our human mentality. To something still, yet potently present. This occurs when the oppositional forces of our past experience are reconciled within us, in states of balance and stillness. Within the Stillness, known only in this present moment, something else can occur beyond the suffering held. It is as simple as that. (p. 8-9)

Adverse effects: None are known.

Training and licensing: There are various schools of craniosacral therapy. Training has not been standardized between them and this therapy is not licensed in the US or elsewhere.

Clinical applications: While research has yet to confirm many of the claimed benefits of craniosacral therapy, clinical reports indicate it can help in treating hormonal problems; migraines; post-traumatic symptoms of head injury; meningitis and encephalitis; behavioral, developmental and learning disorders in children (sometimes attributed to birth injury); and sacral injuries. A therapist is essential for this treatment. This appears to be a form of spiritual healing. The personal qualities of the therapist may be as important as the technique.

CREATIVE ARTS THERAPIES AS HEALING

> *Today, like every other day*
> *We wake up empty and scared.*
> *Don't open the door of your study*
> *And begin reading.*
> *Take down a musical instrument.*
> *Let the beauty we love be what we do.*
> *There are hundreds of ways to kneel*
> *And kiss the earth*
>
> – Jelaluddin Rumi

The creative arts have provided avenues to healing throughout recorded history. Through storytelling, metaphor, poetry, myth, drama, dance, humor and art we can access wellsprings of self-healing energy that lies within all of us.

Music Therapy uses melody, instrumental music, singing, toning, chanting and drumming to restore emotional and spiritual balance and to stir healing energies. Music can be soothing or energizing, commonly attributed to the associations and moods that it evokes. A variety of music that is conducive to relaxation and meditation, as well as to invoke various moods is available at most record shops.

Playing music adds dimensions to its healing potentials. Drumming, chanting and singing can usher us into alternative states of consciousness in which pains may be relieved and healing can occur. Participating in a group that uses any of these musical modalities can enhance their potency. Many traditional cultures make extensive use of music for healing, both individually and collectively.

Alfred Tomatis developed a complex system for using sound to treat children with auditory processing problems, dyslexia, learning disabilities, attention deficit disorders, autism and difficulties in sensory integration and motor-skills. In adults this has been helpful for treating depression, improving communication skills, speeding the learning of foreign languages and enhancing creativity and job performance. It can also be used in a more general way to improve self-confidence, raise levels of energy and motivation and produce a sense of well-being.

> *Words make you think a thought.*
> *Music makes you feel a feeling.*
> *A song makes you feel a thought.*
>
> – E. Y. Harburg

Ilana Rubenfeld, trained as an orchestra conductor, clarifies the links of music to therapy:

> ... As the conductor/ bridge, I was making the music happen, but also stepping aside from it, letting it happen on its own, listening to it happen, *hearing* it happen. I became an insignificant part of the music's energy and also essential to it. I had re-created it, but it had also re-created me.
>
> The same state to ego and egolessness, or insignificance and essence, is true in regard to cosmic energy, of which music is a magnificent expression, for we are all insignificant, essential parts of the cosmic sphere, part of the ascending spiral. And it is true in regard to my therapeutic work with people.
>
> When I'm with clients, I feel that I am in that egoless state. I am still Ilana, yet different: nonjudgmental, totally accepting, loving. I can be both a partner in the therapeutic experience and step aside from it. You sing your own song. I am a vital guide to help you hear and understand it and to accept your body as your musical score.
>
> The tools I use for my therapeutic work – to let you hear your authentic self – are my brain and my hands...   (p. 5-6)

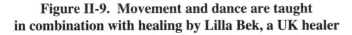

**Figure II-9. Movement and dance are taught
in combination with healing by Lilla Bek, a UK healer**

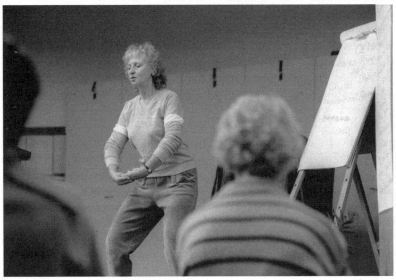

Photograph by Tony Sleep

Some healers use vocal tones or particular music in conjunction with their healings. They feel that the tones and/ or rhythms help healees alter their body and/ or energy field vibrations in healthy ways. For instance, it is said that Tibetan music and chants are tuned to particular healing frequencies, perhaps related to the vibrational levels of the chakras.

[T]he person is instructed to follow the tone of the gong down into the void itself, into the nothingness. When it reaches that void and nothingness from which all things arise – the creative void – they completely let go of whatever they are envisioning. The way we do it, you are lying on your back and you hold your left hand up over your abdomen as long as you can hear the sound. If you can no longer hear the sound, drop it. Say, "I give up." What we have found – and we can't prove this – is that at the moment of surrender, the mental-material interface somehow clicks in. In other words, what was real in the mental realm, to some small extent becomes real in the material realm. Of all the methods we have tried, focused-surrender has turned out to be our most effective induction.

– George Leonard

While the obvious spiritual aspects of liturgical music are familiar to most of us, a further spiritual use of music has been developed by Therese Schroeder-Sheker in the form of *music thanatology*, which is intended to help people make the transition into dying.

Research is confirming clinical reports of benefits of music on several aspects of health, such as relaxation, enhanced activity of white cells and antibodies, and increased production of melatonin (a neurohormone which facilitates sleep).

Felicitas Goodman found that rhythmic sounds helped to create alternative states of consciousness that were particular to specific body postures.

Dorothy Retallach found that plants grew better when exposed to soft music and grew more slowly with loud, hard-rock music. This suggests negative vibrational effects with loud, hard-rock music which might apply to humans, as well.

It has been found that infrasonic sound emanates from the hands of Qigong healers. Various electronic instruments have been developed that produce infrasonic sound at the same frequencies and Chinese researchers report that these can also bring about healing for many problems.[133]

Clinical applications: Music has been particularly useful in promoting relaxation and relieving pains of many sorts. While broad claims have been made by various healers regarding the benefits of tonal vibrations in spiritual healing, these have yet to be substantiated.

Obviously no therapist is needed to help us simply enjoy ourselves and relax with music, but trained therapists may be able to markedly deepen the beneficial effects of tones, rhythmic beats and music. They can help by selecting appropriate pieces, toning their voices to utilize their essence as healers and convening music therapy groups that can enhance vibrational healings.

Dance and Movement Therapy invite the body to participate in rhythmic movements – soothing or stimulating, according to our needs and moods.

Art Therapy invites participants to draw, paint, sculpt, collage and use other media to express feelings, explore psychological issues and resolve both internal and interpersonal issues and conflicts.

Projecting problems onto artistic media allows people to identify and sort through their issues in new and creative ways. Images given a physical form often have more potency than images that are simply visualized mentally.

Storytelling can be healing in several ways. A therapist may use stories to illustrate or suggest ways in which you might see yourself differently and ways in which changes could occur, or to stimulate creative new ways of framing and dealing with problems. Telling your life story and relating the problems that surround (and may have contributed to) your life issues or illness may relieve your symptoms. Stories (either created by the participant or told by others) offer stages upon which to explore conflicts and play out options for their resolution These elements can also be used to clarify therapists' process (counter-transference).

John McEnulty has a lovely example of storytelling as a transformative process:

> There is a teaching method developed by the Educational Center in St. Louis. It is called the Maieutic Method after Socrates' belief that all he could do was to help someone birth what was already within them, that he himself had nothing to teach. So the teaching was always about finding what was within.
>
> There are three questions to the method: (1) What is the actual story? (2) Where do you find the story in your life? (3) Where do you find the story in the world?
>
> We hear the story and talk about what actually happened in the story, perhaps information about the story, its background, to ground ourselves in the elements of the story itself.
>
> Then we agree that whatever anyone finds within that they feel is connected to the story is valid. There is no criticism, no right or wrong. How you relate to the story, how you find it in your life is your own precious and unique meaning.
>
> Each person shares how they relate to the story. So the life experiences of each participant deepen and enrich others who are revealing who they are.
>
> The final sharing is of where we find the story in the world. The same rule applies. Your vision is yours and is precious and valid, not to be contradicted or criticized by anyone else.
>
> The beauty of this method is the love and tolerance that it creates, the safety for each person to express what is within and to grow in understanding through the opportunity to hear other viewpoints and recognize them as valid.
>
> It goes beyond the moral of the story, or lessons to be learned. It connects with the individual and their special way of seeing. It allows each person to reach within and find their own consciousness, process of awareness.
>
> It leads to individual and group awareness of the rich complexity of the human experience.
>
> Where do you see yourself in this story? (2003)

Poetry adds metaphoric and imagery dimensions to these processes, as discussed below.

Journaling can also be an outlet for our feelings and a great aid to sorting out our problems. Writing out one's story and feelings has a cathartic effect, allows a person to consider the problems at a distance, provides new perspectives through the written word, introduces a sense of greater control through the crafting of descriptions of challenges in words, highlights progress as one reviews journaled materials from the past, and much more.

All of these modalities may speak to us in ways that transcend language and logic.

> *Painting is silent poetry, poetry is eloquent painting.*
> – Simonides

> *Dance is the hidden language of the soul.*
> – Martha Graham

> *A merry heart does good like a medicine, but a broken spirit dries the bones.*
> – Proverbs 17:22

Research: I have not reviewed the research in this area.

Humor can bring healing in even the most difficult situations. Norman Cousins is famous for having cured himself of scleroderma, a serious, progressive illness that has no cure in conventional medicine. The therapy he administered to himself was to watch as many funny movies as he could find. (His particular preference was for the Marx Brothers movies.) He literally laughed himself back to good health.

Humor relieves tensions. Medical personnel, who often work under prolonged stress, are particularly likely to indulge in dark humor.

Humor pokes fun at the rules we live by. It makes us laugh when we appreciate incongruities and inconsistencies in our customary ways of doing things. Humor can thus help to point out our frailties and false pretenses, relieving the related feelings of guilt, frustration or anger. It provides comic relief from tensions, as well as from emotional and physical pains. Humor allows us to explore new possibilities by breaking the rules and taking us outside of our usual frameworks for perceiving situations.

Research: Early research suggests that humor can produce measurable effects on the cardiovascular, respiratory and immune systems, in addition to reducing psychological stress reactions.

Poetry speaks to the heart of our human experiences. It can help people to find words for the feelings and conflicts they are struggling with.

Imagery and metaphors invite us to see new connections between various elements in our lives and to explore creative ways of reweaving the patterns of our relationships with ourselves, with significant others and with the world at large.[134]

And a man said, Speak to us of Self-Knowledge.
And he answered, saying:
Your hearts know in silence the secrets of the days and the nights.
But your ears thirst for the sound of your heart's knowledge.
You would know in words that which you have always known in thought.
You would touch with your fingers the naked body of your dreams.

And it is well you should.
The hidden well-spring of your soul must needs rise and run murmuring to the sea;
And the treasure of your infinite depth would be revealed to your eyes.
But let there be no scales to weigh your unknown treasure;
And seek not the depths of your knowledge with staff or sounding line.
For self is a sea boundless and measureless.

– Khalil Gibran

Discussion: Metaphor, storytelling, myth, drama, humor and poetry have resonated through the ages with human joys, hurts, angers, loneliness, elation, bliss, and despair – in short, with all the permutations of the human condition. While we may have difficulty describing these experiences adequately in words, we can acknowledge their resonations through shared metaphors and myths.

Every society has a creation myth among the roots of its belief system. Classical Greek dramas and tragedies still speak potently across several millennia and national myths guide and inspire us. Today the publishing, media and entertainment industries provide us with enormously varied and often rich expressions of shared understanding through these doorways to our inner being.

The creative arts can be tools and avenues for healing our emotional wounds, both individually and collectively. Consider what the TV series *The Holocaust* and the film *Schindler's List* have done to heal some of our residual wounds from Nazi atrocities and what *Roots* and *Amistad* did to raise awareness about the history and sufferings of African Americans. Consider warnings about dangers of biological engineering suggested by *Jurassic Park,* and encouragements to deal with fears of death offered by stories about surviving spirits through the ages, as well as in modern films like *Ghost* and *Always* and the various angel TV series.

In my psychotherapy practice I often recommend books for clients to read for inspiration and to let them know that they are not alone in facing their life's challenges. I may tell stories and jokes or read poems to illustrate or counterpoint issues that we are discussing. In consulting with couples or families who are in conflict, particularly when the trouble has gone on for a long, bitter time, here is one of my favorite stories (source unknown):

George finds himself at the Pearly Gates after a long life of many adventures and misadventures, having struggled – not always successfully – with difficult moral challenges. St. Peter opens his ledger to see where he must go. He shakes his head, bewildered: "I've never seen anyone like this! Your good deeds and sins are precisely balanced. I cannot see a hair's difference to tell us whether you should be in heaven or in hell. I'm going to have to ask God to decide what we should do." Returning shortly, he tells George that under these unusual circumstances, God suggested that George should be given his choice of where to go.

George asks first to visit hell. He is surprised to see tables piled high with the most sumptuous foods. The people sitting around the tables have large ladles with very long handles tied to their hands. No matter how hard they stretch and turn and twist, they are unable to reach the bowl of the ladle with their mouths.

"What terrible torture!" says George. "I certainly don't want to stay here. Take me to heaven."

Arriving in heaven, he is even more surprised to see the very same tables piled high with the same sumptuous foods and people around the tables holding identical, long ladles... but in heaven they are using them to feed each other.

Others describe similar experiences.

> When I ... discovered that the nightmares and other aspects of my obsessive-compulsive disorder were written of in biblical stories and mythology, I was able to understand and integrate my illness as an experience in soul growth rather than as a meaningless bout with madness. A wound with meaning is much easier to heal than a wound that is meaningless or that, worse, is interpreted as divine punishment of other evidence of personal unworthiness.
>
> – Joan Borysenko (p. 93)

Joy is a common denominator of the effects that the healing arts can have on our lives. Lawrence LeShan (1989), a psychologist who has worked extensively on dealing with cancer, emphasizes that to maximize health and increase chances of survival, people must have joy and passion in their lives. Research is beginning to confirm that joy is a factor in cancer survival. Baseline assessments show that greater joy was a predictor of longer survival in women with breast cancer.

> *I slept and dreamt that life was joy.*
> *I awoke and saw that life was service.*
> *I acted and behold, service was joy.*
> – Rabindranath Tagore

See also: Rituals.

CRYSTALS

> *Fifty-five crystal spheres geared to God's crankshaft is my idea of a satisfying universe.*
> – Tom Stoppard

Healers report that crystals augment or focus their healing powers, either by storing healing energies for later use or by concentrating and magnifying them.

Others believe that the crystals themselves carry vibrations that are therapeutic and some claim that electrical currents augment crystal vibration.

While crystals appear to augment spiritual healing effects, it is difficult in many instances to know whether this is due to anything more than suggestion.

Sensitives who see auras report that crystals have brighter auras than many other objects and that they interact with the energy fields which surround living things

My personal experience is that I can palpate energy fields around some crystals and gemstones with my hands. I must admit that despite my own tactile confirmation of apparent crystal energies, I was skeptical that they had healing effects much beyond those of placebos, until I saw the study described next.

Theories: A basis for the healing powers of crystals is suggested by their use as signal receivers and current rectifiers in crystal radio sets, quartz watches and other devices. It may be that they can serve similar focusing functions for the presumed unconventional energies that appear to be involved in healing.

Crystals may be used to make essences, similar to homeopathic remedies and flower essences. This suggests a vibrational aspect to their healing powers.

Research and clinical applications: C. Norman Shealy, a neurosurgeon who began investigating complementary therapies for use in pain management, demonstrated highly significant effects of quartz crystals on depression. I know of no other research to confirm the use of crystals for particular problems, though they are used by some healers to augment healing for many ailments.

> *Amethyst:* Harmonizes relationships
> *Aquamarine:* Treats arthritis
> *Black tourmaline:* Protects against negativity
> *Fluorite, Black tourmaline:* Neutralize irritating energies
> *Opal (gem quality):* Opens and stimulates chakras to higher functions

Crystals may be used for self-healing, but the selection of particular crystals by a healer may be a great help. Crystals may also carry the healing vibrations of self-healing intent, or of a healer who "programs" them.

Adverse effects: Healers report that it is possible to have negative effects from too strong an exposure to crystals, or to other types of misguided uses of crystals.

Training and licensing: There is no formal training.

CURANDERISMO

> *... Even when a curandero uncovers specific causes of illness he is still likely to focus on sin and the will of God as critical factors which have affected the susceptibility of the patient and predisposed him to illness.*
> – Ari Kiev (1968, p. 34)

Curanderismo originated in Spain and spread to every Latin American country, where it integrated with local healing and herbal lore and practices. With the social mobility of our modern world, Curanderismo is now found wherever Spanish is spoken. Traditions therefore vary in each country.

The spiritual orientation of curanderismo, which was originally Catholic, has blended with local traditions as well. Curanderas (women were the original practitioners) and curanderos therefore may invoke the help of God, Christ, saints, indigenous gods and healing powers of nature – particularly of medicinal herbs. Where economic resources are limited and where there is a distrust of allopathic medicine, curanderismo provides natural healing approaches. This method is also widely practiced in the US, where it is influenced particularly by Mexican and Caribbean traditions. As with clients of other complementary therapy practitioners, people who seek the help of curanderas may hesitate to mention this to their Western physicians, anticipating that these practices will be ridiculed or dismissed as folkloric nonsense.

The are various types of curanderismo practitioners who deal with different aspects of the traditional techniques.

- *Yerberas* prescribe herbal remedies, whose properties are enhanced by the practitioners' knowledge of where and when to gather the plants for maximal potency.

- *Sobardoras* offer massage and laying-on of hands treatments. They treat *empachos* (biological energy blocks) in the body (particularly in the gastrointestinal tract) or in the spirit.

- *Parteras* are midwives who provide pre-natal and post-natal care and may also baptize babies. Prayer is a vital aspect of their practice and herbs may also be used.

- *Consejeras* provide counseling that may cover personal, relational and spiritual issues. The *platica* is a heart-to-heart discussion. The *consejaras* encourage healees to pour out their souls, in a process called *desahogar*, which may go on for many hours, over several days.

Treatment may include *the limpia*, a spiritual cleansing, accomplished by sweeping around the body with a bundle of herbs or a feather to remove negative energies. An egg may also be rubbed over the body to absorb negative energies.

Various levels of competence and natural calling are acknowledged among curanderas. The highest level practitioners offer all of the above-mentioned services. Any practitioner may use herbs, feathers, crystals, chants, rattles and drums in their ministrations. All practitioners are encouraged to heal themselves so that their energies can be as pure and strong as possible.

Curanderismo is thoroughly wholistic, addressing issues related to body, emotions, relationships and soul.

Many of the diagnoses used in this modality may have no precise equivalents in Western terminology or conceptualizations. It may therefore be inadvisable, and in some cases impossible, for Western caregivers to properly diagnose or treat people from cultures where expressions of dis-ease as disease are in symptoms that would respond to Curanderismo but not to Western interventions. Culturally congruent therapists may be essential for addressing these sorts of problems.

- *Bilis* (rage) becomes a problem when angers are not expressed and it is caused by over-secretion of bile.

- *Mal aire* (bad air) causes disease by inhalation of germs. *Mal puesto* (hexing or cursing) can cause severe malaise or even death.

- *Mal ojo* refers to illness caused by staring.[1] This term is used to describe problems caused by giving excess attention, especially to a child.

- *Mala suerte* (bad luck) is a destructive force that people bring into their own lives through negative thinking, poor self-esteem and fears.

- *Susto* (soul loss) occurs with severe emotional traumas, following which people feel that they are not really themselves any more. The process of soul retrieval may restore a person's integrity.

- *Espanto* is a fright received from seeing a ghost or from being severely jarred emotionally, which causes the soul to flee in fear.[2]

Adverse effects: See potentials for negative effects under Herbalism, Spiritual Healing.

Training and licensing: There is no official licensing. Training is traditionally by apprenticeship, with students initiating the process as they sense an inner calling to become a healer, or with experienced curanderos approaching people they intuitively feel have a gift that can be developed. This is a highly individualized process, geared to the individual abilities of the practitioner, and setting of standards would appear inappropriate, as this would destroy the uniqueness of the mentoring/ apprenticeship relationship. For similar reasons, it would be difficult to license such practitioners.

Clinical efficacy: While I have not found controlled studies of curanderismo, anecdotal reports abound on Latin Americans who responded well to these approaches, which resonate with them because they find them *culturally congruent.*

Curanderismo is but one of many shamanistic practices. Every culture has its folk practitioners, and it is impossible to list them all. Curanderismo is given by a healer, but it may include elements of self-healing prescribed by the healer.

It is important, however, for health caregivers to become familiar with local subcultural health practices. As one example, in the Los Angeles area a group of Cambodian child immigrants were found to have bruises on their backs. Physical abuse was suspected and the parents were investigated. However it was found that the bruises resulted from the practice of rubbing the back with a coin to treat viral respiratory illnesses. Both children and parents, however, were traumatized by the child welfare investigations and allegations of possible child abuse.

See also: Shamanism.

DEAN ORNISH THERAPY FOR HEART PROBLEMS
See: Psychoneurocardiology.

EDTA CHELATION

*History records no more gallant struggle that that of humanity
against the truth.*
> – Ashleigh Brilliant

Chelation therapy (*Chele* = Greek for *claw*) relies on molecules that bind positive
ions in the bloodstream, just as the pincers of a crab might grab a pebble.
Chelated molecules found in nature include chlorophyll (binding magnesium) and
hemoglobin (binding iron).

Chelation treatment with intravenous *calcium disodium ethylene diamine tetra-
acetic acid* (EDTA) is used to remove toxic chemicals such as lead from the
body. A broader application is the use of EDTA to treat atherosclerotic cardiovascular disease. EDTA binds calcium from atherosclerotic plaques in the arterial
walls, moving the calcium into the blood stream to be excreted through the
kidneys.

Chelation has not been accepted by conventional medicine as yet, although it has
been approved for treatment of hypercalcemia (excessively high levels of calcium
circulating in the blood) and digitalis toxicity. The manufacturer's patent expired
in 1969 and the cost of obtaining approval from the U.S. Food and Drug Administration (at a conservative minimum estimate of $250,000 or more) is prohibitive.
Chelation is given as an outpatient procedure by intravenous infusion over a three
hour period, once or twice weekly over several months. It has been shown to be
safe if administered slowly under medical supervision.

Doctors and grateful patients have reported dramatic benefits from chelation in
clearing atherosclerotic blockage of arteries in the extremities (found commonly
in diabetes); reducing cholesterol levels; lowering blood pressure; promoting
recovery from strokes; addressing ischemic heart disease (due to blocked arteries); and preventing cancers. Its most common use today is for treating heart
disease and it is often used in wholistic practice as an alternative to cardiac
surgery.

Research: A wealth of anecdotal reports supports the effectiveness of this treatment. Formal research, limited by lack of funding, has shown mixed results.

Adverse effects: A study of 153 subjects found no significant adverse effects in
the treated subjects vs. the control group.

Training and licensing: While legal action has been initiated in several states to
outlaw these uses of EDTA chelation, the courts have for the most part permitted
its use, in view of the evidence and testimony of satisfied patients. Treatment
must be given under the supervision of a physician. The American College for
Advancement in Medicine (ACAM) trains physicians in chelation therapy, promotes its use, and advocates for legislation permitting its use.

Clinical applications: Numerous anecdotal reports suggest that EDTA chelation
can slow or even reverse arteriosclerotic cardiovascular disease.

ELECTROMAGNETIC AND MAGNET THERAPIES

[O]ne can easily understand that man is... penetrated by the two-fold stream of universal fluid and that he must have his poles and his surfaces in the same way as do all other substances of nature which are more or less penetrated, according to their own characteristics, by this same universal fluid.

– Franz Anton Mesmer

Local and general electromagnetic treatments are reported to be effective in resolving a wide range of health problems.

Local applications of simple magnets: Small magnets and weak electromagnetic fields have been reported to relieve musculoskeletal stress responses and soft tissue injuries, chronic pain, arthritis, neurological problems and infections and to enhance the mending of bone fractures. The magnets may be applied locally in bands around their wrists, elbows, ankles, or knees, or used generically in the form of magnetic insoles or mattress pads. Ron Lawrence and Paul Rosch, acknowledged experts on magnet therapy, have been impressed to find that any magnets at all may be helpful, regardless of their strength or degree of sophistication. James Oschman and Candace Pert point out that magnetic fields can help with both soft and hard tissue problems simultaneously, though each may require different pulsation frequencies.

The new medical specialty of *bioelectromagnetics* is developing out of intensifying research on the effects of EM fields when they are applied externally to the body. Several categories of EM therapies are evolving, each with different effects and applications.

Thermal effects of EM radiation are used to create heat, which can be beneficial in treating muscles and tissues that have been damaged by trauma and disease. Laser and radio frequency (RF) surgery are also in this category.

Pulsed electromagnetic fields (PEMFs) have been found to promote healing for a variety of problems. PEMFs can enhance Immune system activity, particularly to increase natural killer cells that are effective in responding to viruses and cancers. PEMFs have been shown to reduce swelling, accelerate wound healing, stimulate nerve regeneration and enhance recovery from injuries. PEMFs also produced significant reductions of pain due to injuries of cartilage, tendons and bone and in osteoarthritis. Early evidence suggests that part of the improvement may have been due to regeneration of damaged cartilage under EM stimulation.

Physical healing of fractures that are slow to mend may be facilitated by PEMFs; by alternating current fields; by DC fields and by combinations of these fields. Some therapeutic devices of these types have been approved by the U.S. Food and Drug Administration. Remarkably, failures in bone healing have been corrected using these methods, with full healing achieved after periods of as long as 40 years with no prior improvement.

Microwave resonance therapy is in wide use in Russia, where it is reported to be beneficial for arthritis, hypertension, pain, neurological problems and cancer chemotherapy side effects. The benefits of this therapy are thought to be mediated by changes in cell membranes or in the chemicals that communicate information within the body. It is speculated that EM therapies work through information that promotes healing and that this information may be transmitted within the total body EM field.

Electromagnetic stimulation of specific nerves can be beneficial for:

1. Pain relief and physical therapy, with FDA approval for a variety of transcutaneous electrical nerve stimulation (TENS) devices;
2. Emotional disorders that respond to transcranial electrostimulation (TCES), including depression, insomnia and anxiety
3. Repair of damaged nerves, particularly in the wrist.

A Swedish radiologist named Björn Nordenström reports dramatic cures of tumors treated with application of DC currents to the tumors and the surrounding tissues via electrodes. Nordenström hypothesizes that tumors create local electrochemical imbalances within the body that function somewhat like an automobile battery. The tumor creates a positive charge due to accumulation of damaged and dead cells at its center. The center of the tumor then becomes acidic, creating an electrochemical gradient relative to the surrounding tissues. By applying external electrical current of opposite polarity Nordenström reports that he can arrest and reverse the cancerous growth. Becker and Marino also discuss applying electrical currents to limit tumor growth.

Soft tissue wound healing can be accelerated using this therapy if wounds are slow to heal, particularly in the case of skin ulcers. Various types of EM stimulation may be used directly, or EM current may be used to drive active metallic ions into tissues. Silver has been particularly effective in promoting healing with minimal scarring.

Low energy emission therapy (LEET), which is applied through an electrode held in the patient's mouth, produced significant improvements in stress and insomnia.

An unpublished report by Valerie Hunt et al. presents another angle of investigation. EM measurements and analyses by a sensitive who sees auras (Rosalind Bruyere) were obtained for volunteers who had structural integration treatment (Rolfing) and for matched controls. Structural integration involves deep massage of muscles and joints, during which old memories, feelings and altered states of consciousness may be evoked. EM and acoustic monitoring of chakras and acupuncture meridians correlated significantly with Bruyere's descriptions of aura changes that occurred during and following the structural integration treatments. Recognizable wave forms were consistently observed when Bruyere reported seeing primary and secondary colors. The sequence of wave frequencies recorded over chakras was almost uniformly correlated with the sequence of colors in the spectrum and with colors traditionally associated with the different chakras. These range from red at the base chakra to violet at the brow.

Hunt also used Kirlian photography to detect significant differences between structural integration subjects and controls, but the meaning of these results is as yet unclear.

Valerie Hunt (1992) also reports a study of telemetry electromyography. Using surface electrodes she recorded high frequency EM activity "... during meditation;

emotional states; pain; energy fields transactions between people; laying-on-hand healing of post polio, brain disturbances and tissue regeneration... "

Hunt found that the patterns in EMG recordings that had previously been assumed to represent only "noise" between large waves actually carry an enormous amount of information about the subject. From her readings, she claims she can identify subjective states, sometimes including mental imagery of the subject.

Brain stimulators: A number of transcranial magnetic stimulators (TMS) are able to produce relaxation and deep, meditative states, which have beneficial physical and psychological effects, particularly for depression. Symptoms of Parkinson's disease responded to TMS. TMS may enhance healing through relaxation – by releasing tensions, encouraging greater openness to healing, or by initiating other health-promoting mechanisms that are inherent in meditative states. They may also activate neurohumoral mechanisms in the brain.

Minute doses of ionizing radiation may significantly increase the survival rate of people with Hodgkin's lymphoma. Of additional interest was the observation that when radiation was directed to only half of the body, tumors outside the irradiated region also disappeared. Enhanced immune system activity was also demonstrated.

A number of helpful reviews of bioelectromagnetic therapy have been published.

Theories: Electromagnetic fields exist within each cell, tissue and organ and within and around the body as a whole. These are viewed by conventional medicine as the products of electrochemical properties and activities of the cells and tissues, which produce radiations of these energies outside the cells and tissues. CAM therapists suggest that the bioelectrical fields may, in addition, have a regulating function upon and within the body.

Oschman and Pert note that possible conventional pathways for action of EM fields in enhancing soft tissue injury repairs may include: "enhancement of capillary formation, decreased necrosis, reduced swelling, diminished pain, faster functional recovery, reduction in depth, area and pain in skin wounds, reduced muscle loss after ligament surgery... and increased tensile strength of ligaments and acceleration of nerve regeneration and function recovery."[137]

Research: Controlled studies are beginning to confirm that static magnets can help treat post-polio pain, musculoskeletal pains and the pains of diabetic neuropathy. All of these conditions are usually difficult to treat with conventional pain management approaches.

Static and pulsed magnetic fields (PEMFs) can enhance bone healing PEMFs enhance healing in damaged musculoskeletal tissues, with reduced inflammation, increased vascularization and greater collagen and bone growth through proliferation of osteoblasts, chondroblasts and fibroblasts. This is helpful in the prevention and treatment of osteoporosis and osteoarthritis. PEMFs can also help with symptoms of multiple sclerosis, Alzheimer's disease and Parkinsonism.

Much broader discussions on electromagnetic effects are presented in Chapter II-3, within a general discussion of the fields and energies that may be present in and around the body.

Adverse effects: I have heard anecdotal reports of negative effects, such as worsening of pains and arthritis with misuse of simple magnets. Though as yet controversial, there is strong suspicion that chronic or excessive exposure to EM radiations can have negative effects. This is discussed in Chapter II-3.

Training and licensing: There is no formal training for electromagnetic or magnet therapies, nor is there any licensing.

Clinical applications: Electromagnetic therapies are particularly helpful in wound healing and relieving chronic pain. Their effectiveness for inducing relaxation and treating stress-related illnesses and depression has yet to be firmly established.

A trained therapist is required for administration and supervision of electromagnetic therapies. Simple magnets may be worn over parts of the body that are in need of healing, but initial guidance of a therapist may also be helpful in applying these as well.

ENVIRONMENTAL MEDICINE (CLINICAL ECOLOGY)

> *The very same skills of separation, analysis and control that gave us the power to shape our environment are producing ecological and social crises in our outer world and psychological and spiritual crises in our inner world. Both these crises grow out of our success in separating ourselves from the larger fabric of life."*
>
> – Fred Kofman and Peter Senge

Foods, chemicals and electrical pollution can be detrimental to your health.

In the 1940s Theron Randolph pioneered the identification of food allergens that can cause many symptoms, including fatigue, headaches, muscle weakness and pains, gastrointestinal upset, emotional lability, depression and irritability. Particular dietary culprits include corn, wheat, milk and eggs. Randolph adopted Herbert Rinkel's elimination diet, which requires that people avoid the suspected allergenic food for 4-10 days and then deliberately ingest it to see whether there is a negative reaction. Illnesses and symptoms for which this approach has been helpful include arthritis, asthma, hay fever, eczema, colitis, migraines, urinary disorders, attention deficit hyperactivity disorder (ADHD), anxiety, depression, irritability, fatigue, distractibility, memory loss, chronic fatigue syndrome and enuresis.

Various common chemicals encountered in the environment may also produce debilitating symptoms. The top culprits include industrial solvents, pesticides, formaldehyde, natural gas, car exhaust fumes, cosmetics and laundry soap. Some people are incredibly sensitive to these substances and may develop problems at exposure levels that most other people would easily tolerate without symptoms. In the case of severe reactions, people may become *universally allergic* to multiple chemicals. These people may even be unable to tolerate being in the same room with anyone using perfume or after-shave lotion, may not be able to travel in certain vehicles because of the exhaust fumes and may even be sensitive to electromagnetic fields. In extreme cases they may have to live in a rural setting without electricity. Testing for such allergies may require environmentally controlled units in which exposure to toxins can be monitored and controlled. It also requires an alert diagnostician to detect the presence of such allergies. It is estimated that only a small percentage of people who suffer from them are ever identified.

Environmental medicine acknowledges that different people may have similar symptoms with widely varying causes, as well as widely differing symptoms from the same cause. Susceptibility varies not only between individuals but also in the same individual over periods of time. One common pattern is an initial *preadapted, nonadapted* or *"O"* (zero) phase, with initial exposure causing a brief bout of symptoms. This may be followed by an *adapted* or *masked* phase in which the body copes with the allergen without expressing symptoms. With continued exposure and other stresses, more severe symptoms may occur in what is called the *exhaustion* phase. Contributing factors may include: genetic predisposition, nutritional factors and general health problems (particularly relating to the immune system, digestive system and emotional stress).

Environmental medicine investigations may also reveal more blatant evidence of chemical poisonings. A striking example is that of sudden infant death syndrome (SIDS), which has been a mystery since 1950. For no apparent reason, babies between one and six months old have been found dead in their cribs and SIDS is the leading cause of death in this age group. Lendon Smith and Joseph Hattersley present strongly suggestive evidence that SIDS may in fact be caused by poisonous gasses emitted from mattresses when chemicals used as fire retardants and plastic softeners are metabolized by fungi. The fungi grow in the mattresses due to sweating, urination and the body heat of the infant. A plastic mattress cover that is impermeable to gasses can prevent these crib deaths. Not a single death has occurred in 100,000 babies sleeping on mattresses that are protected in this way. An inexpensive alternative is to raise the head of the bed by two inches, which leads any gasses to gravitate to the bottom of the crib and away through the bars. A rolled towel can prevent the baby from sliding down the slight incline. (This will not work in a bassinet or baby carriage, which have sides that would block the gasses from escaping.) Having the baby sleep face-up is a further preventive measure.

> *We can't yet cure all diseases, but we're already expert at causing many of them.*
> – Ashleigh Brilliant

Electromagnetic (EM) pollution is one of the more common but less appreciated subjects of environmental medicine research. There is a growing awareness that environmental EM fields may have deleterious effects.

Beyond the negative health effects of electromagnetic pollution, there can be further problems in buildings that have sealed windows and closed ventilation circuits, where toxic chemicals can build up in the air. These can create a *sick building syndrome* in people who work and live in such environments over a pe-

244 Vol. II Chapter 2 – Wholistic Energy Medicine

riod of time. Symptoms can include headaches, allergies, arthritis, anxiety, tensions and emotional lability.

Global ecological healing

Health care workers have mostly focused on treating the *effects* of pollution and environmental toxins, but there is a growing awareness of the need to address these problems *preventively* on a national and planetary level, both directly and through political reforms. This subject diverges too far from the general focus of this book, so I have recommended relevant references in the endnotes.

The spiritual perception of environmental healing is to address our planet as a living ecobiological system, popularly called *Gaia*. Humans are intimately linked with this system, and anything that harms the earth is going to harm its inhabitants.

> We must do what we conceive to be the right thing and not bother our
> heads or burden our souls with whether we will be successful. Because if
> we don't do the right thing, we will be doing the wrong thing and we will
> just be a part of the disease and not a part of the cure.
> – E. F. Schumacher

These systems approaches are comfortably within the accepted frameworks of social psychology and ecology.

If we shine the light of wholistic awareness on these issues, extending into bioenergetic and spiritual dimensions, we open into many further ways for addressing our global ecological problems.

Subtle energy environmental medicine

Subtle energies are palpably present in *places* as well as in living organisms. Most of us have had the experience of entering a church or going to a place of natural beauty where we sensed a positive atmosphere, or *positive vibrations*. Likewise, most of us may have entered a room or a place in nature where we felt *negative vibrations*. Some of these vibrations may be the energetic residues of positive human interventions, such as prayer, meditation and joyous experiences, or of anger, grief and pain that have been suffered in these locations. Other sources of positive and negative vibrations can derive from earth energies. For example, a dowser might identify negative energy lines that run through or under a particular part of a room. People who spend a lot of time over such a point might suffer impairments of their biological energy fields, predisposing them to various illnesses such as arthritis, cancer and emotional upsets.

Feng Shui is a Chinese system for identifying and accommodating subtle environmental energies. It is very close to Chinese Medicine in its principles. Various elements are considered in analyzing the subtle energies of a room or building, such as the position of doorways, windows and stairs; magnetic compass orientation; color schemes; and the dates of birth of the occupants. Analyses are made based on a system of the *five elements* (fire, earth, metal, water and wood) and according to a standard map, or *bagua,* that identifies areas within a room that are associated with aspects of the occupants' lives. (See Figure II-10.)

Figure II-10. The Bagua

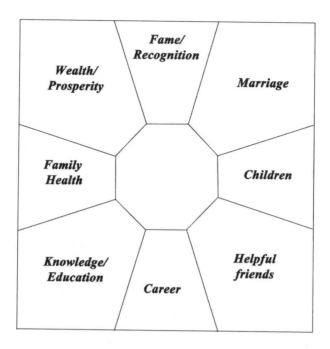

Training and licensing: There is no formal training or licensing in environmental medicine.

Clinical applications: Environmental medicine can be enormously helpful in diagnosing and treating aspects of chronic fatigue syndrome and multiple allergy syndromes. In its more subtle aspects, it can enhance the esthetic and energetic ambience of work, home and play environments. Subtle environmental interventions can improve health and are said to bring good luck as well. In the Far East, no builder would begin construction of a house without consulting an expert in subtle environmental energies. Consultation with a therapist trained in this field can be invaluable in identifying and dealing with environmental irritants. Self-healing is also possible if you have the patience for detective work. Typical methods include carefully watching your diet and exposure to potential allergens.

THE FELDENKRAIS METHOD

> *Learning must be undertaken and is really profitable when the whole frame is held in a state where smiling can turn into laughter without interference, naturally, spontaneously.*
>
> – Moshe Feldenkrais (p. xiii)

Moshe Feldenkrais, an Israeli physicist of Russian origin, developed methods of movement to enhance awareness of how we live in our bodies. I was impressed with how keenly he observed the most minute aspects of posture and movement and how he could detect the smallest misalignments of posture or the tiniest signs of strained motion in his pupils' bodies – simply through visual observation.

In *awareness through movement*, Feldenkrais practitioners guide pupils through sequences of simple motions, such as walking or reaching out with their hands and use these exercises as the basis for teaching body awareness. *Functional integration* adds the light touch of the practitioner to shift pupils' movements towards healthier patterns. Changes in unproductive habits depend upon pupils' altered awareness and actions rather than upon the teachers' manipulations.

Research on the Feldenkrais method has shown improvements in the health of people with chronic rheumatoid arthritis and enhanced physical movements in healthy people. A variety of clinical reports attest to its efficacy for pain management and as a form of physical therapy.

Adverse effects: No harmful effects have been reported See discussion of potential general negative effects from rapid improvements under Spiritual Healing.

Training and licensing: Training lasts 3-4 years. There are Feldenkrais practitioners in many countries, including about 1,000 in the US and Canada. There are no standards for training or licensing in this method.

Clinical applications: The Feldenkrais method is helpful in sports; performing arts; physical therapy; musculoskeletal pain; neurological damage and the like.
A therapist is essential for instruction and guidance in Feldenkrais exercises. Self-healing exercises are usually taught and are essential to the success of the therapy.

See also: Alexander Technique; Bodymind Therapies; Rubenfeld therapy.

FITNESS

> *Walking is man's best medicine.*
> – Hippocrates

Physical fitness is one of the best preventive medicines. It is an aspect of health care that each of us can adapt to our own particular inclinations, abilities, needs and circumstances. Exercise keeps the cardiovascular and musculoskeletal systems in good tone and provides a release for physical and psychological tensions. It is an excellent antidepressant. Perhaps best of all, it is always available in one form or another. You can do isometric exercises, calisthenics, pilates or yoga, take a stroll or a hike, cycle or lift weights.

Particular methods of exercise can promote self-healing, as in Yoga, T'ai Chi Ch'uan and Qigong. Some aspects of these practices appear to incorporate biological energy activations and healing effects that go well beyond the simple exercise of heart and muscles.

Rhythmic exercises can also be a form of meditation, and maintaining an exercise regimen promotes mental and emotional discipline. Hatha yoga and qigong can promote bioenergy and spiritual awareness.

Michael Murphy and Rhea White have a wonderful collection of stories on ways in which exercise can also provide a doorway into spiritual awareness via peak experiences. People who exercise regularly report that at some point they may enter a perceptual space where they are exquisitely aware of every cell and muscle in their body and of their relationship to everything around them. Equestrians report that they become one with their mounts. Time seems to slow down in the flow of peak experiences and you are able to savor every tiny nuance of movement. It is as if you know exactly how everything within and around you works together harmoniously. Having had a peak experience, you may come away knowing that you are an intimate part of something far vaster than your little self.

Research has confirmed that regular exercise is particularly helpful for prevention of cardiovascular problems. Exercise can be a treatment for depression that is equivalent in efficacy to antidepressant medications.

Adverse effects: Muscle, tendon and joint pains and injuries are possible with too vigorous exercises. Consultation with a trainer is advised when beginning a course of fitness training or when developing a strenuous exercise program.

Training and licensing: Sports medicine is practiced by physicians. Fitness education and training is not a licensed profession.

Clinical applications: Graded exercises are advised for building muscle strength and cardiac tone. While this is a self-healing method, the guidance of a fitness instructor may be helpful in developing an exercise program.

See also: Qigong; T'ai Chi Ch'uan; Yoga.

FLOWER ESSENCES

> To see a world in a grain of sand
> And a heaven in a wild flower
> Hold infinity in the palm of your hand
> And eternity in an hour.
>
>   – William Blake

Edward Bach,[138] a Harley Street physician in London, identified flowers whose essences have curative powers. These are prepared in much the same way as homeopathic remedies, except that they are not succussed (shaken) and cannot be diluted more than a few times before they lose their potency.

There are two methods that are used to identify applications for flower essences. The first is through clinical testing on healthy people and on patients with disease/ disease. The second relies on the intuitive perceptions of gifted sensitives who are able to identify medicinal properties of plants clairsentiently.

The flower remedies are intended to correct disharmonies between the personality and the higher self and soul. This method could be likened to a transpersonal homeopathy. Flower essences are widely used and are available over the counter.

Rescue Remedy, a combination of several Bach flower essences, is a popular treatment for stress and trauma and it is available in drops or as a topical cream. This preparation can be a good personal introduction to the efficacy of flower remedies. Taken orally, it calms anxiety and panic, counteracts emotional and physical shock, reduces pain and swelling following injuries and more. Applied topically it reduces the pain, swelling and blistering of burns and other injuries.

Case: A personal experience with our cat, Cuddles, illustrates the effectiveness of this remedy. One day, a stray cat settled into our neighborhood. It bullied Cuddles in our back yard and even came in through the cat-flap at night, got into fights with Cuddles and had the audacity to spray all over our CD rack! Cuddles was traumatized by the intrusions and became very anxious and clinging. For two days she would not separate from us other than to relieve herself in very brief trips outside. She was constantly tripping us up in the kitchen, to the point where she was getting stepped on and we were in danger of falling over her. We decided to give her some Rescue Remedy and after one dose her behavior changed dramatically. She became calmer, stopped clinging to us and went outside in a manner more like her usual behavior. She needed several doses daily over a period of several weeks until the situation with the stray was resolved.

In the past few years many new essences have been developed, based on plants from several continents and on various gems and minerals.[139]

There are books that detail indications for the flower essences. It is often helpful to have clients read the descriptions of the therapeutic indications and anticipated results, in order to develop their cognitive insight about their problems, which can then enhance their responses to the essences.

A recent development is the topical application of flower essences for treatment of various physical and psychological problems. It is hypothesized that the vibrational energies of the flower essences interact with acupuncture points, thereby influencing the body's bioenergies. It may be that the flower energies also interact in a more general way with the bioenergy field, not necessarily through acupressure points. This application opens new ways of studying localized pains and other symptoms. By referring to flower essence topical maps of the body it might be possible to identify psychological conflicts that underlie symptoms at a particular body location.

Flower essences may also be prescribed intuitively in cooperation with the client. The therapist will take a history and recommend essences on the basis of their known therapeutic efficacy, and will also use intuition to select additional essences that feel appropriate. Clients may be encouraged to pick essences for which they sense a particular affinity. While this may seem unusual in terms of conventional practice, several factors recommend this approach. First, there are no negative side effects of these essences – they either are beneficial or produce no apparent effects – so there is no risk involved. Second, there may be subtle reasons for taking certain essences that are not apparent to logic or forethought.

The essences represent far more than just chemicals that interact with the physical body. Their actions, like those of homeopathic remedies, appear to be due to patterning of flower vibrations in the solution used to make them – which, in turn, influence the bioenergy patterns of the person on many levels. In the realms of energy medicine, the flower essences appear to have their effects at the psychological and spiritual ends of the continuum of wholistic interventions.

Steve Johnson, who developed the Alaskan flower essences, observes:

> Flower essences catalyze evolution in consciousness. They help us identify emotional and mental qualities within that need to be awakened or strengthened and stimulate our spiritual growth, which is the ongoing process of grounding our spiritual selves into our physical bodies.
>
> Flower essences are unique in that they are a source of intelligent healing energy that is available to both empower and educate the person taking them. They are empowering because they do not do our healing work for us, but with us – they are powerful catalysts for growth and change but they respect our free will. They are educational because they reveal the causal level of our problems and difficulties. Flower essences illuminate the inner landscape of our psyches and direct our awareness to the conflicting issues and patterns of resistance that are contributing to our disease. They then offer us the precise levels of support we require to resolve our conflicts and release these discordant energies, gently and completely, from our lives. They are like gentle teachers showing us who we really are and reminding us of our oneness with all life.
>
> The gift of the plant kingdom is spiritual consciousness. Flowers are the most evolved part of this kingdom and carry positive, life-affirming patterns of conscious energy. These patterns originate in the higher dimensions and are expressed into our physical world through the specific form of each plant... (p. 5)

Skeptics may question the efficacy of flower essences, saying that the claimed benefits are due to nothing more than suggestion. However, I believe that suggestion is an excellent adjunct to any therapy and can enhance people's responses to treatments of all sorts. The fact that suggestion may be present does not rule out the possibility that a treatment is also effective in and of itself.

Research: Research on flower essences has been very limited. The Bach five-flower essence[140] and Yarrow formula[141] have been shown to alleviate minor stresses in an experimental situation. Electromyograms, used as a measure of stress, showed significant decreases of muscular tension following treatment with the essences, as compared with the placebo. Jeffrey Cram has published several studies showing that flower essences can significantly reduce depression.

Adverse effects: There appear to be no adverse effects from these remedies, other than disappointment if they are not as effective as one had hoped.

Training and licensing: The various flower essence traditions are taught in workshops that are not standardized. Flower essence therapy is not licensed.

Clinical applications: Flower essences may be of benefit in treating most physical and psychological problems, in a manner and range similar to homeopathy. Flower essences lend themselves particularly to treatment of psychological and spiritual aspects of illness. They often appear to open people to spiritual awareness.

While you may take essences as recommended in books and while Rescue Remedy is helpful in dealing with physical and emotional stress, the guidance of a flower essence practitioner can markedly enhance and deepen the effects of essences, through knowledgeable selection and combinations of the remedies. There are also many ranges of essences, so a layperson may not be aware of the particular ones that might be most helpful.

See also: Homeopathy.

HAIR ANALYSIS

Mineral analysis of hair samples is believed by some CAM practitioners to provide an index of states of health. Hair analysis has been fairly well accepted for identifying heavy metal toxicity, but in other applications there have been problems in standardization of measurements.

Research: I am aware of no research to confirm the validity of hair analysis other than in heavy metal poisonings.

Adverse effects: Relying on an unproven method of analysis in assessing problems and making therapy decisions can be dangerous.

HEALING TOUCH (HT)

> *We are teaching how to do the work and nobody owns the work. It is a collective. It is like a focal essay...*
>
>   Janet Mentgen (Wardell, p. 71)

Healing Touch was similar in its basic practice to Therapeutic Touch, but HT healers have diverged from TT to include chakra diagnosis and treatment; the use of pendulums to augment intuitive awareness; spiritual awareness; and a variety of other techniques. Healing energy is perceived as being channeled through the healer from a universal source.

HT practitioners are encouraged to develop their personal healing gifts as well as learning the structured approaches HT teaches.**Research:** HT is the second most researched spiritual healing approach (after TT). HT has been shown to help in treatment of pain, anxiety, depression, enhanced immune function.

Adverse effects: No harmful effects have been reported See discussion of potential general negative effects from rapid improvements under Spiritual Healing.

See also: Spiritual healing; Therapeutic Touch, Volume I of *Healing Research..*

HERBAL REMEDIES
See: Herbal Remedies under Nutrition.

HOMEOPATHY

> *... Hahnemann stumbled upon a phenomenon that is barely beginning to be understood by modern physics, a dynamic that might be likened to spirit, information or meaning in matter...*
> – Edward Whitmont (1993, p. 7)

Samuel Hahnemann (1755-1843), a physician of German origin, developed a system for treating human ills through a sort of immunization process. He believed that the body could learn to deal with symptoms of an illness if it was given minute quantities of substances that produce similar symptoms in a healthy person.

Hahnemann developed this approach after noticing that when he ingested quinine in order to observe its effects on a healthy person, he developed intermittent bouts of fevers, chills and weakness. These symptoms are very similar to those of malaria, for which quinine is a remedy.

A homeopathic evaluation begins with a meticulously detailed listing of symptoms. These are organized according to personality types and diagnostic categories that make little sense in terms of conventional medicine. Remedies are prescribed for *syndromes* rather than for individual symptoms. These include the presenting illness, personality factors, past traumas of a physical and/ or emotional nature, relationships with others (particularly parents), patterns of likes and dislikes, and much more. The syndromes are then organized into *remedy symptom clusters.*

The patient is not placed in a diagnostic box defined by the pathological or psychological causalities that are presumed to produce the illness according to conventional concepts of disease. For instance, symptoms such as inertia or lack of will are viewed in allopathic medicine as defects of character or motivation. In homeopathy, these symptoms are addressed as aspects of disharmony, in addition to other empirically derived symptom clusters for which specific remedies may be effective treatments.

The remedies prescribed are minute doses of substances that would cause similar symptoms to those presented by the patient if these remedies were given to healthy people. Under the stimulus of these substances, the body can learn to handle the symptoms competently instead of being overwhelmed by them as it had been previously. Oddly, this method is successful even when a person is currently suffering from the very same symptoms that are being treated. A clear example is found in the treatment of laboratory rats poisoned with lead. When given homeopathic microdoses of lead, the rats excreted greater amounts of lead in their urine than did untreated rats.

Homeopathic remedies are discovered and developed in two ways. In *conventional homeopathy*, various agents that might be therapeutic are given to healthy people in order to study their clinical effects. This process is termed *proving*. The symptoms produced are then presumed to be treatable in ill people by giving them diluted solutions of these substances. *Intuitive homeopathy* relies on the clairsentient perceptions of highly sensitive individuals who are able to intuitively assess the therapeutic properties of the substances.[142]

Two broad approaches to treatment
Classical homeopaths prescribe of a single remedy, often in one high dose. The remedy is chosen very carefully, considering the personality type of the client. Over a period of several months this may produce major changes in symptoms, underlying illnesses, psychological awareness, and even in personality. A repeat high potency dose, weeks or months later, may be added in some cases. A gentler approach may also be taken within classical homeopathy, prescribing less potent doses of the single remedy, which is then repeated over several weeks or months.

Allopathic-style homeopaths prescribe one or more remedies in repeated doses over periods of days or weeks, with periodic reassessments and adjustments or substitutions of other remedies.

In both approaches, additional remedies are added as the original symptom patterns shift and new patterns arise. The effects of homeopathic remedies can be antidoted (counteracted or stopped) by drinking coffee.

Case: This example will help to illustrate how homeopathy is prescribed for a specific problem in a particular person.[143]

"Patricia" was an intense, loquacious, passionate person who was very jealous and frequently angry and sarcastic with her lover. She had a history of migraines, pharyngitis, tonsillitis and colitis. She hated having anything tight around her throat. She frequently woke with a feeling of being suffocated at night, especially as she was falling asleep. She came for help because her PMS symptoms (irritability, jealousy, depression, headache, hot flushes) had become a major problem and they were threatening her relationship. She also mentioned in passing that she always had diarrhea before her menses.

Patricia's homeopath recognized that this pattern of symptoms points to the remedy Lachesis (a snake venom remedy), which has among its profile of indications the following items that appeared to fit Patricia's profile:[144]

Mental – Passionate, intense people; Jealousy; Loquacity,
    Anger Sarcasm.
Head – Migraine headaches.
Throat – Pharyngitis; tonsillitis; Intolerance to tight collars,
    turtlenecks, necklaces.
Gastrointestinal – Colitis; Diarrhea before menses

Urogenital – Premenstrual syndrome, including irritable,
  jealous, depressed, headache, flushes of heat.
Chest – Wakes with suffocating feeling at night, especially on
  falling asleep.

Patricia was given one dose of 200C Lachesis. When she came back for her next appointment in a month, she reported that her PMS symptoms just didn't happen this month and that oddly she also did not have diarrhea before her menses. Upon inquiry, she also noted that she was waking much less rarely with that old feeling of suffocation and that she just wasn't feeling as jealous anymore.

While such combinations of symptoms as a treatable entity appear strange within conventional medicine, this is not a reason to reject homeopathy. It is, rather, a criticism of the narrowness and exclusivity of conventional medical thinking and practice, and an invitation to broaden our theoretical and therapeutic horizons.

It is of historical interest that the practice of homeopathy originally spread rapidly in Europe, the US, Asia and South America. It was very popular and widely used in the US at the end of the 19th century. It was credited with more than halving the mortality rate from cholera in London in 1854 and from yellow fever during a US epidemic in 1878. There were 22 homeopathic medical schools and over 100 homeopathic hospitals in the US prior to the publication of the Flexner Report in 1910. This report, which was promoted through lobbying by medical doctors, established guidelines for funding allopathic medical schools and led to a rapid decline in the practice of homeopathy, almost to the point of its disappearance in the US. (Naturopathic medical treatment met the same fate.) In Great Britain, the practice of homeopathy was also much reduced but not eliminated. Five homeopathic hospitals remain today and the Royal Family's support of homeopathy has helped to encourage its use.

Recently, research demonstrating the efficacy of homeopathy has helped bring about a resurgence in its popularity in the US, Europe, Asia and Latin America. Several American states have homeopathic licensing boards for physicians.

Homeopathic remedies

Remedies are usually prepared by dissolving small amounts of a medication, mineral or allergen in a mixture of alcohol (generally 87% ethanol) and water. Water may also be used alone, or it is sometimes mixed with other preservatives (especially for alcohol-intolerant patients). Serial dilutions of 1/ 10 or 1/ 100 and greater are prepared and then *potentized* by *succussion* (shaking). The solutions are identified by their degree of dilution. For example the designation of 6c (or C6) means that the substance was diluted by 1/ 10 successively 6 times; 30c is diluted 30 times, etc. Very potent dilutions of as little as one original volume per million (1M) are available. *In contrast with conventional medications, the greater the homeopathic dilution, the greater the potency of the preparation.*[145] (This is very different from conventional medications, where we are used to seeing greater potency with *less* dilute medications.)

Jacques Benveniste and other homeopaths suggest that there is a bioenergetic pattern carried by water which brings about the observed healing effects. For modern commercial purposes, mechanical vortexing is used rather than hand-held succussion, as in earlier days. While it might appear from a Western scientific standpoint that the process of vortexing can improved if it is standardized, and it is certainly more economical to prepare remedies this way, there are sensitive homeopaths who feel that the personal attributes, attitudes and bioenergies of people who succus the remedies manually and of company personnel who manage the vortexing may make a difference in the qualities of the remedies.

Clinical studies and laboratory tests demonstrated that a succussed remedy was effective, whereas an unsuccussed one was not. Ten seconds of succussing suffices to potentize a solution. Heating potentized solutions to 70-80 degrees Centigrade inactivates them. Another unusual observation is that loss of potency in aging solutions can be reversed by repeated succussion.

Potency can be demonstrated in remedies so dilute that they could not contain even a single molecule of the original substance. Studies using nuclear magnetic resonance (NMR) have also shown alterations in homeopathic solutions.

A further odd but consistent phenomenon is that there the efficacy of homeopathic treatments rises and falls repeatedly as the remedies are diluted progressively. An effect observed with initial dilutions disappears with greater dilutions, then reappears when even greater dilutions are applied, etc. This waxing and waning of effectiveness continues in a regular pattern with increasing dilutions.[146]

Another class of homeopathic remedies is prepared from materials associated with disease. These include *nosodes* (from infected tissue), *sarcodes* (from noninfected tissue in an organism that has an infection) and *isopathy* (from infectious agents). Homeopathy was widely used to prevent and treat infections prior to the discovery of antibiotics, and recent studies confirm that homeopathy can indeed prevent infections.

Many homeopaths feel that immunizations are frequent contributors to chronic illness. It is believed that they can lead to later development of neurological diseases, arthritis, chronic fatigue syndrome and more. Conventional medicine does not accept this view. A homeopathic approach to preventing latent side effects of immunizations is to prescribe homeopathic preparations of the immunization substances prior to and following conventional immunizations.

Let's look at two case studies that demonstrate homeopathy in practice.

Case 1: A 9-year old boy was brought to the homeopath by his mother because he was being highly disruptive in school – humming and singing, getting out of his seat, standing on his chair, not paying attention to his teacher and staring out the window over extended periods. He lacked motivation, disliked schoolwork and refused to do homework. At home he was messy and disorganized, never shared toys with others and was unfriendly with his peers. His mother reported that if he read a problem from a book he would be unable to do it, but when he heard the problem spoken by someone he could solve it correctly. Surprisingly, he was still getting good grades at school. The presumptive diagnosis was that he had an attention deficit hyperactivity disorder (ADHD).

The boy was never angry and had no strong food cravings. His mother felt that he was abnormal because nothing seemed to excite him.

In the homeopathic interview, the child was cooperative and pleasant but seemed only partly present. However, when talking about his best friend, he became quite animated. His mother was astounded by this, saying: "Aside from seeing that boy in church, he has played with him only once in the whole year."

His mother had had no problems with the pregnancy or delivery, but she had smoked marijuana for 11 years and had stopped only when she learned that she was pregnant.

Homeopathic Cannabis indica (marijuana) in a single, very potent (1M) dose was prescribed because of the history of cannabis use by the boy's mother in very early pregnancy, combined with his present time-perception distortions and general spaciness. (The basic homeopathic principle holds that the correct homeopathic prescription should be for a substance which produces symptoms similar to those exhibited by the patient.) Within a month the boy's ability to focus improved dramatically; he did homework without reminders and showed enthusiasm for particular foods.

Over the course of a year his behavior remained improved, but then it began slowly to deteriorate. Again, he was not completing his work and seemed less motivated. Another single 1M dose resulted in a renewed remission of his symptoms.[147]

The art of homeopathy is to select out key factors that are amenable to interventions of this sort. Other homeopaths might have prescribed different remedies, addressing different constellations of factors. A good homeopath will have an encyclopedic knowledge of the clusters of effects of various substances, so that the remedies can be matched to the symptom clusters of the patient. Computer programs can be a great help in suggesting remedies, as it is impossible for any one person to know the entire homeopathic pharmacopoeia.

Homeopathy can be a very intricate art, as illustrated in the next case, in which the symptom complex addressed by the remedy, Calcium Carbonate, includes a physical, psychological, biological energies and metaphorical patterns.

Case 2: Edward Whitmont (1993, p., 74) beautifully illustrates the blending of symptom, substance and symbol in the clinical case of a man of about 40, whom I will call "Henry," who suffered from acne.

After taking a detailed history, Whitmont prescribed a single dose of calcium carbonate (extracted from oyster shells) at a dilution of C1,000. This produced temporary spasms of the finger muscles, similar to tetany. This is a typical symptom of parathyroid gland dysfunction, which would produce lower blood calcium levels. The spasms evoked memories from Henry's childhood, when his mother had taped his fingers to his bedside in a position that resembled that of the spasms he experienced from the homeopathic calcium carbonate. His mother had done this to prevent him from masturbating. During the treatment, vivid memories arose in Henry of his anger and shame connected with this experience. As a child he had completely repressed these memories in his unconscious mind. This somehow was translated into his skin condition and a boisterous personality. With the release of these memories, the spasms in his fingers also released and this healing process furthered his progress in psychotherapy.

... Shame, anger, finger spasm, parathyroid hormonal activity, calcium metabolism, the dynamic field of the oyster (in homeopathic practice the "personality of the Calc. Carb. Type" can be likened to an oversensitive but heavily defended person, akin to an oyster without or with too thick a shell) and the functioning of the skin all appear here as different transduction codes of one and the same dynamic field process. (p. 74-75)

As Whitmont eloquently points out, it may be impossible to clarify many of the complexities of linked energetic and imagery components that produce these effects. Every remedy has its particular spectrum of effects – its *personality*. When a person has a cluster of symptoms and personality traits that match those of a particular remedy, then that remedy can effect a clearing of those symptoms and it may also alter the accompanying personality traits. The art and challenge of the practice of homeopathy is to ask the right questions in order to identify the relevant symptom clusters. If the homeopath did not ask the patient about specific related symptoms, many of which might not be at all obvious or likely to be reported spontaneously, the best remedy could easily be missed.

Self-help with homeopathy
Some homeopaths encourage patients to prescribe for themselves (particularly authors of books on homeopathy!), and health food stores carry common remedies in lower potencies as well as books on homeopathy for the layperson. However, while people can benefit from particular over-the-counter remedies for certain problems, these preparations may easily miss the mark with more serious or pervasive problems, as would a prescription from a therapist who does not have thorough training in homeopathy. Computers may be a great help in identifying symptom clusters and potentially relevant remedies.

Intuitive prescription of homeopathic remedies, in which therapists allow their unconscious mind and psi powers to scan for relevant details, may offer distinct advantages in selecting the best remedies from amongst the thousands that are available. Similarly, muscle testing and other intuitive approaches may be used for self-help to identify appropriate remedies. Dowsing and radionics, two other systems of intuitive assessment, are sometimes used for the same purposes.

Research: *Clinical research* on homeopathy is complicated by the fact that remedies are ordinarily prescribed on an individualized basis for each person. Though two people may have the same *medical diagnosis*, such as a streptococcal sore throat, each might receive a different homeopathic medication depending upon their symptoms, personalities and life experiences. In contrast, conventional medicine usually prescribes the same medication for all patients with a given diagnostic problem. Despite these difficulties, some homeopathic research has managed to conform to the requirements of randomized controlled studies.

Most of the reviews of series of controlled homeopathy trials conclude that homeopathic remedies are beneficial, although three critical reviews conclude that there is only limited evidence for clinical efficacy.

The study that is generally acknowledged to be the most carefully designed and executed is that of David Taylor-Reilly et al. (1986), which shows a 50% reduction in the need for antihistamine medication in the treatment of hay fever. Other studies have shown significant effects of homeopathy in treating arthritis; asthma; Attention Deficit Hyperactivity Disorder; fibrositis; influenza; and childhood diarrhea. Other studies confirm that homeopathy can prevent infectious diseases.

Research on treatment using minute doses of homeopathic medications has shown that they do produce observable effects. Within the context of Western scientific practice, it has been hard to accept that serial dilutions of substances can possibly have any medicinal effects, particularly since dilutions beyond C30 cannot contain even a single molecule of the original substance. Skeptics propose that even in double-blind controlled studies there must have been hidden suggestive effects to produce such results. It is therefore reassuring to find studies on cells in laboratory cultures, bacteria, yeasts, plants and animals that also show significant effects.

The principles of homeopathy may also be relevant to other areas of medicine. A rigorous meta-analysis was made of 135 studies on the protection of organisms from poisoning by environmental toxins, using dilutions of C30 or greater (Linde, et al. 1994). This meta-analysis included studies of animals (70%), plants (22%), isolated organs (5%) and cell and embryo cultures (3%). Of the 26 studies that met the reviewers' stringent criteria for design and reporting, 70% showed positive effects.

Even more fascinating and also relevant to the energy medicine thesis of this book, is a study by P. C. Endler of homeopathic dilutions of thyroid hormone that produced significant effects on climbing behavior in frogs. In this study the remedy was entirely encased in a glass tube that was simply held near the frogs. This suggests even more clearly that homeopathy is a subtle energetic intervention.

While clinical effectiveness of intuitively produced remedies has been reported, research to substantiate their efficacy has so far been limited to a single study, which had negative findings.

Basic research shows that the water in very dilute homeopathic solutions differs significantly from plain water and from water with salts dissolved in it.

The above-mentioned research clearly just begins to scratch the surface of the mystery of energy healing – that could transform our understanding of the world when we finally solve it.

Explanatory theories
Homeopaths assert that there are intimate links between the material world, living organisms and consciousness. Particular material substances have clusters of characteristics that become evident when they are used to treat people (animals, plants, etc.). When a group of healthy people ingest a homeopathic substance they will experience a range of symptoms, thus *proving* the characteristics of that substance. These symptoms may be either physical and psychological.

The fact that very high dilutions of treatment substances are potent – even when diluted beyond the point where no single molecule of the original substance could remain in the solution – has been quite challenging to explain.

Much of the theorizing is centered around the nature of water. Water may be a much more complex substance than is generally realized. Two Italian physicians have put together an excellent discussion of this subject. The first is Paolo Bellavita, an Associate Professor of General Pathology at Verona University School of Medicine with postgraduate training in biotechnology at the Cranfield Institute of Technology in England and the second is Andrea Signorini, a medical doctor who also graduated from the Verona Homeopathic School. They propose that water in homeopathic remedies may be imprinted with energies and/ or information which conveys the effects of the remedy, rather than homeopathic remedy effects being due to chemical reactions with the remedy substance. Bellavita and Signorini base their theories on new understanding that is emerging from the study of *complexity theory*. In brief, complexity theory suggests that complex biological systems are more than the sum of their parts. Complex systems, such as those that are modeled on fractal equations, may produce effects that are not predictable on the basis of theories concerning their individual elements. Processes within complex systems may not be reproducible experimentally, as they do not follow linear patterns of interaction. Complex systems may also assume different states, partly depending on the qualities (not just the quantities) of the energies and other components that combine to compose the system.[148]

> *A mind that is stretched by a new idea can never go back to its original dimensions.*
>
> – Oliver Wendell Holmes

David Taylor-Reilly is a physician who completed a Research Fellowship in homeopathy in Glasgow and has personally been a teacher of homeopathy to many physicians in the UK He postulates that homeopathy work by stimulating the immune system (Taylor-Reilly/ Taylor 1987). To support his hypothesis he cites evidence from experiments with minute doses of various substances that are toxic to the immune system in larger doses but which produced stimulation of the immune system in microdoses. To explain the efficacy of solutions in which none of the original substance is present, he suggests that information may be stored within the semicrystalline structure of the water that is used as diluent.

Others hypothesize that it is not the substance itself that produces the effects (even in initial dilutions that still contain molecules of the substance) but rather a field effect or vibration of that substance. William Tiller, a Stanford University Professor Emeritus of Material Sciences and Engineering, suggests that this type of vibration acts upon the etheric body.[149] While his writing is difficult to follow for anyone who has not studied quantum physics, it is nevertheless fascinating that quantum physics may be able to explain bioenergy medicine.

A key postulate is that the condition of health occurs when each type of physical chemical in the *physical* body has a chemical counterpart in the *etheric* body at the appropriate concentration ratio, CE_j/ CP_j, of the j species. Disharmony leading to disease is thought to occur when this ratio is out of balance. Balance may be restored by either increasing or decreasing the j chemical constituent at the physical level; i.e., by manipulating CP_j. Present allopathic medicine utilizes the "increase" mode. The "decrease" mode is not generally possible, although recent studies with blood filtration is a step in the proper direction. Balance may also be restored by increasing or decreasing a chemical constituent at the etheric level; i.e., by manipulating CEj. Homeopathic remedies deal with the increase mode and no apparent method exists at this level for the decrease mode. A potentized remedy is, in fact, the etheric counterpart of the physical constituent that has reached toxic proportions in the body and has produced the specific symptoms. Thus, by combining both allopathic and homeopathic procedures in the increase mode, all values of the ratio CEj/ CPj are possible so that the balanced condition may always be produced.

This can also be looked at from an energy point of view in that each atom is an absorber and radiator of a specific spectrum of energies of the EM or ME variety. Thus, for optimum tuning between the etheric and physical bodies so that energy is most efficiently used, the proper chemical radiators must be available in each body and at a concentration such that the absorption cross-sections for the important specific radiations... are properly impedance matched. (Tiller, 1983)

Although many Western scientists find the theories of homeopathy alien to their conventional medical thinking, Daniel Eskinazi suggests that several aspects of the theories of homeopathy are paralleled by observations that have been made within the context of conventional biomedicine. For instance, several low-dose vs. high-dose responses are well recognized. Very small doses of allergens are used to desensitize people to stronger exposures to the same substances. Therapeutic doses of aspirin lower temperature, while toxic doses can produce hyperthermia, even to a life-threatening degree. An unusual note from China is that exposure to low levels of radiation offers some protection for animals that are subsequently exposed to higher doses of radiation. Another observation is that stimulation of various systems occurs with low doses of some toxic substances, while higher doses of the same substances produce inhibitory effects.

Eskinazi also points out that many of the lower potencies of homeopathic remedies contain active molecules of the medication and have been shown to produce significant clinical effects.

Conversely, in conventional medical research there have been clinical effects with doses so low that no active molecules could have been present. In these studies, serial dilutions of conventional medications are commonly conducted to the endpoint at which no greater effects are noted in experimental subjects as compared to the controls – to establish the lowest possible effective dose. Researchers assume studies of even lower concentrations are pointless and do not continue to explore this possibility. In one study, the lowest concentration of leukotriene (which induces the release of a hormone) produced a stronger effect than a higher dilution. Further dilutions were then tested and a lower peak of activity was identified. Eskinazi also found other studies in which very low dilutions of conventional preparations were effective.

In the worlds of bioenergetic phenomena, there may be types of causality that are completely outside the realm of conventional medical concepts. Homeopathy suggests that there can be energetic predispositions to illness that are hereditary, called *miasms*. It is postulated that certain diseases can cause persons who have that disease, *or their descendents*, to develop particular illness patterns or predispositions to illnesses. Examples of diseases that produce miasms include scabies, syphilis, gonorrhea, tuberculosis, cancer, leprosy, rabies, typhoid, ringworm and malaria. A history of these diseases in patients or their families may be an important element to consider in deciding upon particular homeopathic remedies.

Further metaphysical theories were proposed by the late Edward Whitmont. Whitmont was an amazingly gifted physician, homeopath and Jungian therapist. The breadth and depth of his understanding of the multi-dimensional aspects of healing is truly awe-inspiring. He added enormously to our appreciation of the mechanisms of action of homeopathic remedies.

Whitmont proposes that homeopathy is clearly an energy medicine, as evidenced by the following facts:

1. It is effective in potencies that are beyond the thirtieth dilution (the *ultramolecular* range, where not even a single molecule of the original substance remains).

2. Remedies are imperishable. Whitmont had bottles of remedies that were over a hundred years old and were still potent.

3. Any material with which the remedies come in contact becomes a *vehicle* for their medicinal properties.[150] For instance, if a bottle that contained an ultramolecular dilution of a remedy is refilled with water, it will transmit the medicinal properties to the fresh water.

4. The effects of remedies radiate to distances of over thirty feet and can be confirmed through applied kinesiology muscle testing. For instance, if a person has a particular physical dysfunction, their arm muscles will be weak when they are mentally focused on that dysfunction. If a remedy that is helpful in treating that dysfunction is brought near to the person, their muscle strength will be significantly increased.[151]

5. Whitmont notes that correspondences between remedies and dis-ease or disease (in homeopathy and other therapies) may be metaphoric as well as symptomatic.[152] For instance, part of the potency of metallic gold may lie in the correspondence of gold with the sun. Intuitively, both gold and the sun are associated with the human heart. Homeopathic gold is indicated as a treatment for excesses in expressions of personality traits, as in an over-scrupulous conscience, a tendency to focus on darker sides of issues and problems and in vulnerabilities to burnout and tendencies to black depressions. Homeopathic applications of gold include the treatment of disorders of the heart, circulation, bones and joints.

Whitmont also provides excellent discussions on the collective unconscious, pointing out that if we explore the realms of psychotherapy, in dreams and synchronistic occurrences we will find ample evidence that the mind of man has access to all knowledge, through all time. This capacity enables us to diagnose our own illnesses and to identify the root causes of our problems.

Whitmont wisely notes that many physical problems have their origins in emotional traumas. Memories of these traumas are encoded within specific states of consciousness.[153] Therefore, accessing and releasing these memories may require alternative states of consciousness, often achieved by invoking emotions similar to those which were felt during the original traumas. If these traumas were very severe or occurred during pre-verbal years, and when they have been expressed through the body in physical pathology, homeopathic remedies may be helpful in accessing and releasing them – when they may otherwise be inaccessible.

Whitmont proposes that we can best understand the human condition and homeopathic treatment as manifestations of a holographic universe, in which every living and non-living thing is interconnected with every other thing through subtle and *intricate* dimensions of existence.[154]

Homeopathic remedies, whether based on animate or inanimate matter, restore the innate patterns of people whose physical, psychological or spiritual order has gone awry.

> *... Homeopathy... demonstrates that every possible illness that can affect living organisms has a corollary in some substance that is part of the earth's organism. External substances replicate psychosomatic patterns and are able to induce pathology when foisted upon the organism. However, they are also able to cure when applied in the appropriately diluted or "potentized" form. In a mosaic of unknown scale, the various states of human consciousness and the ingredients of the human drama are encoded in various mineral, plant and animal substances – the unit "particles" of our earth. They slumber in these materials waiting for their unfolding on the human level.*
>
> – Edward Whitmont (p. 22)

Whitmont points out that within a holographic universe, everything in the cosmos may influence a given organism. Conversely, a given organism is an intimate part of everything in the cosmos. Illness and health are therefore seen from perspectives that differ from those of allopathic medicine, which focuses on discrete sub-units of cause and effect. Holographic understanding so of the universe suggest that illness in individuals or groups (such as in epidemics) may serve as challenges that unsettle established orders and make new developments possible. The same may even be true of natural disasters.[155]

Whitmont suggests that life is characterized by *entelechy*, which is an Aristotelian term denoting an *inherent goal-directedness*. Though the ultimate goals are often beyond our appreciation, the influence of entelechy is seen in our avid pursuit of excitement and drama and in our vigorous rebellion against boredom. Illnesses are mechanisms for disrupting stultifying patterns that would otherwise block our personal and collective development. Death – either in miniature (as when we relinquish old patterns of being and behaving) or in major expressions (as when a physical existence on earth comes to an end), is a clearing of the way to invite new patterns and experiences to develop.

This briefest of summaries in no way does justice to the enormous range of wisdom integrated by Whitmont, nor to his style – which is erudite and frequently poetic in its metaphoric richness.

Intuitive and metaphoric applications of homeopathy are being explored by other homeopaths. These are sometimes called the *imponderable* remedies.

Colin Griffiths describes a new intuitive approach that is called *meditative proving*. A group of 13 homeopaths gather for the proving. Only one of them, the

Chair for that session, knows what the remedy is. All the participants except the Chair take the remedy and report their physical, emotional and general states. The Chair then records their observations over a 3-4-hour period of group meditation.

> What became readily apparent was the way a dynamic field seemed to be set up in the group as a whole, as though the provers resonated on a deeper level and were able to spontaneously elicit unique insights into aspects of the remedy that normally would take years of slow and meticulous research. The ensuing empathy created by a group in a state of stillness can create a situation of direct cognition bypassing our normal rational states of awareness and eliciting a far more direct and dynamic identification with the actual object under consideration – the remedy in this case.
>
>   This proving method is tentative in nature but sufficiently germane to excite new explorations in homeopathy. We would therefore request our fellow homeopaths to invoke freedom from prejudice as their first therapeutic ideal and put these proving insights to the test of empirical experience.

Griffiths proceeds to discuss the homeopathic remedy that was developed from a piece of concrete taken from the Berlin Wall when it was torn down. The wall was built of concrete, incorporating bricks and other debris that had been gathered after the bombings of World War II. The piece of the wall that was used to develop the remedy was brought to Britain by a German woman who had lived in the UK since childhood. It was given to Griffiths as a curiosity and it lay in a drawer for about a year till he presented it to a psychic *sensitive* and homeopath for her intuitive impressions.[156] She instantly felt fear, panic and distress, though she was totally unaware of the source of the piece of concrete. This encouraged Griffiths to have a homeopathic company prepare a remedy from the rock. When the sensitive was given a 30c dilution of the preparation she felt it was so extraordinarily potent that she advised it should be kept separate from other remedies because it might mutate them or antidote them.

  The Berlin wall was built in 1961, separating Communist-dominated East Germany from West Berlin, which was a Western enclave buried deep within East Germany. The wall was the product of Communist fears about the infiltration of Western influences and the source of enormous tensions and conflicts between East and West. Thousands died in attempts to escape to the West, hoping for freedom and reunification with families that had been torn asunder by the war and its aftermath. With the coming of *glasnost* the wall was torn down, releasing large floods of people who had been trapped and powerless to oppose the governing authorities.

  Griffiths and other homeopaths have found that the remedy prepared from this highly symbolic material is helpful for treating people who are suffering in various ways from oppression, suppression, depression or repression. An example from Griffith follows.

CASE: A 28 year-old woman had been taking homeopathic remedies for several years for depression and several other complaints. One day she came to the clinic in deep misery, feeling that nothing was right, or had ever been right before, or would ever be right thereafter. She felt deprived in her inner life and her relationships. Iin particular, she felt short-changed by her parents, who had separated when she was a little girl. She complained of always giving and not receiving, of being alienated from loved ones and of marking time to no purpose. She longed to be protected from the world, feeling she had never really wished to grow up and pining for the security of her family and the place of her birth, in Berlin.

The woman was given a single dose of Berlin Wall 30c and after 3 days she reported that she was quite changed.

> ... She had resolved a number of difficult issues with both her boyfriend and her father and, in the case of the latter, felt that she had established the first proper communication for years. She had also been offered a decent job, after years of doing indifferent work. She felt as though a wall had been broken through that had stood between herself and the rest of the world. She has not needed to come since. (Griffiths 1995)

The obvious alternative explanation of suggestion as the causal agent in this case awaits clarification via controlled studies of such metaphoric remedies.[157]

Debate on homeopathy in the scientific community
In 1984 Jacques Benveniste, a scientist at the Université Paris-Sud (INSERM), submitted a paper to the journal *Nature* describing effects of antibodies in homeopathic dilution upon white blood cells. Because the study was performed to adequate standards of scientific rigor and because it came from a respectable laboratory, it could not be ignored. However, because it contradicted the worldview of John Maddox, the editor at that time of the journal (a journalist with expertise in physics), he demanded that the study be independently replicated before publication. Benveniste complied. After four years he submitted successful replications from laboratories in Canada, Israel and Italy, and Maddox had no choice but to publish the combined reports (Davenas, et al. 1988). However, Maddox appended an "editorial reservation" expressing incredulity regarding these observations, which he viewed as being utterly impossible, and promised a prompt investigation of the experiments.

> *Scientists, especially when they leave the particular field in which they have specialised, are just as ordinary, pigheaded and unreasonable as anybody else and their unusually high intelligence only makes their prejudices all the more dangerous...*
> – Hans J. Eysenck (1957, p.108)

Maddox invited Walter Stewart and James Randi (an American stage magician), both confirmed disbelievers and avid debunkers of psi phenomena, to join him in observing replications of Benveniste's work in his Paris laboratory. Three open replications and one with "blinds" were all confirmatory. Three further replications with blinds showed no significant results. Maddox reported that Benveniste had not paid attention to sampling errors and expressed incredulity that Benveniste had previously rejected some biological samples that did not respond to his system of study and had found periods of months at a time when the experiments did not work at all. Benveniste complained that Maddox's investigation had been performed by people who were completely unfamiliar with biological research methods. He claimed they had introduced into the process "a tornado of intense and constant suspicion, fear and psychological and intellectual pressure unfit for scientific work... " Maddox provided no evidence that he had checked with the other laboratories which had replicated the study, nor did he invite the consultation of scientists who were competent in biological research. In July 1988, Maddox rushed to publish his report, which claimed that "'high dilution' experiments (are) a delusion."

The pressure tactics employed by Maddox and his colleagues have been widely decried in the complementary/alternative medical literature, where it has been pointed out that laboratory studies in the field of biology are often subject to variability and that the *Nature* team was no way competent to assess this kind of research.

We would do well to keep in mind the advice of Carl Sagan:

> *It is the responsibility of scientists never to suppress knowledge, no matter how awkward that knowledge is, no matter how much it may bother those in power. We are not smart enough to decide which pieces of knowledge are permissible and which are not.*

Ignoring the hysterical reaction of Maddox, whose "boggle threshold" was obviously exceeded, we may discover in this incident some further hints about aspects of homeopathic effects and energy medicine. Psi phenomena[158] can be inhibited by the presence of negative observers. Fluctuations during laboratory studies of proteins and in industrial experiments on water, were both found to be associated with sunspot activity (Gauquelin 1969). Any of these factors might be influential in homeopathic studies as well.

Subsequent repetitions by Benveniste and others confirm the original reports, demonstrating significant cellular effects of homeopathic remedies.

Lessons from homeopathy
In earlier years the fact that relatively few controlled homeopathic studies had been done led to widely-held suspicions that homeopathy might include a significant proportion of experimenter/ placebo effects. Despite masses of clinical reports claiming successes with homeopathic remedies, even in treating chronic conditions that had not responded to wide varieties of other treatments over months and years, skeptics could always question whether the positive results were due to factors other than the remedies. Today, the growing body of controlled trials demonstrating significant effectiveness of homeopathic therapies is gradually remedying this situation. The effects of homeopathic treatments on non-human subjects provide especially strong evidence against the placebo hypothesis.

Various empirical observations on the behavior of homeopathic remedies suggest that we need to keep our minds open to entirely new ways of conceptualizing energy medicine therapies, even if the evidence runs counter to our every-day experience. The potency demonstrated in solutions that cannot contain even a single molecule of the original substance suggests that the potentizing material either *chemically* patterns the solution in which it is prepared, or patterns an *energy template* onto the solution or onto the solution's energy field. Three facts suggest that the latter explanation is more likely:

1. potency is observed when none of the potentizing substance is present;
2. stale solutions may be revitalized by succussion; and
3. the potency of remedies waxes and wanes with increasing dilutions.

Evidence from other branches of energy medicine which is detailed in this volume also suggests the influence of energy interactions in the treatment of disease.

> *To say... that a man is made up of certain chemical elements is a satisfactory description only for those who intend to use him as a fertilizer.*
> – H. J. Muller

Spiritual healing and homeopathy

Spiritual healing overlaps with homeopathy in several areas.

Spiritual healing can alter the spectrophotometric properties of water – apparently producing an energy effect upon the water.[159] One must wonder whether this is comparable in any ways to the changes in water that occur with homeopathic remedies. The similarity between the laying-on of hands and homeopathy is closer if succussion of remedies is done by hand, but today it is mostly done with automated shaking machines.

Kirlian photographs of water that has been treated by healers, water left in churches and water drawn from "healing" springs produce an altered image as compared to Kirlian photographs of "normal" water.

Mental intent may be involved in preparation of homeopathic remedies, as it is in spiritual healing and in various other CAM therapies. Elsewhere in this chapter I discuss the use of electroacupuncture devices for intuitive assessments and in Chapter II-4 I review the use of *radionics* devices that can project spiritual healing effects. Various dials are set on the machine to attune it to healing bioenergy frequencies. Similar devices have been developed for the preparation of homeopathic remedies. Spiritual healing works through the mental intent of the healer. It is speculated that the operators of the radionics devices may be using their intuitive gifts unconsciously to tune these devices and to project healing.

Radionics may have other overlaps with homeopathy. In India, a system of radionic diagnosis with projection of healing via homeopathic remedies has been practiced for several decades. The operator uses a series of cards with coded homeopathic patterns to imprint tablets with the homeopathic remedy vibrations. While this process may stretch the belief systems of Western science, it is supported by anecdotal reports of excellent responses to these remedies.[160] Later in this chapter we will consider the processes of visualization whereby the mind may influence the body and in Chapter I-3 we reviewed psychokinesis (mind influencing matter) research. These may be further mechanisms or contributing

factors in energy-medication phenomena. It may be that homeopathic preparations are in some part influenced by the intent of those preparing them.

Further clues that energy phenomena may be involved in these processes may be
found in the report of the late Sigrun Seutemann (Stelter) in which she noted
changes in the auras of patients who had been given homeopathic treatments and
similar reports of other sensitives (including Cayce) regarding the efficacy of homeopathic treatments add.

We may also find that in bioenergy treatments involving realities beyond sensory perception, evidence from individual case studies may merit greater credence
due to the *nature of knowing* in other realities.[161] Intuitive perceptions provide
immediate, direct psychic perceptions of people's conditions and of changes in
their conditions. As we gain further experience from intuitive explorations of our
world, we may come to trust intuitive observations as valid evidence for healing
effects. The case is of course stronger when multiple observers participate in intuitive observations so that such explorations can be consensually validated.

Electromagnetic and other analogues of homeopathy

Jacques Benveniste reports that he can record EM analogues of homeopathic and
conventional medications that are clinically effective. Samples of the therapeutic
ingredients are placed between two electrodes, one of which emits white noise
while the other records the signals that are modulated by the substance. The recorded frequencies remain effective after they are transmitted electronically.

Jean Monro and Ray Choy are British doctors who specialize in allergic disorders. They utilize allergens serially diluted in homeopathic doses to diagnose and
treat people with unusual allergies, such as sensitivity to very large numbers of
allergens. They report that if a particular dilution of an allergen produces clinical
symptoms when placed on the skin, even greater dilutions of the same allergen
placed on the skin will cure the same symptoms. Patients keep a vial of the effective therapeutic dilution for use at home and find equally positive effects when
the treatment is applied in their natural environments. They report nearly instantaneous relief of symptoms, suggesting this may in fact be an energy field effect.
Double blind trials are said to have produced the same results, though I have not
seen any confirming reports.

Some people are so highly sensitive to allergens that they develop symptoms if a
vial of allergenic solution is brought into the room without their knowledge.
Aluminum shields around the vials completely inhibit this reaction, while aluminum mesh with smaller than one-centimeter holes provides partial protection.[162]

Cyril Smith, working with Choy and Monro, reported that a variable electrical
oscillator could be tuned to particular frequencies that would produce the same
symptoms and to other frequencies that would relieve them. After applying the
therapeutic electrical frequency to vials of water, this water could be used thera-
peutically as well. Its potency was retained for up to six weeks.

Overlaps of various imprints of healing effects in water

These are fascinating reports, but fuller descriptions are needed for assurance that
we are not being misled by subtle placebo effects. It is unclear from the available
summary of Monro's work whether these types of allergic responses to water that

has been imprinted are seen only in unusually sensitive people or also with more common, less severe allergies. If their results were confirmed, these studies could provide important contributions to our appreciation of some of the mechanisms of energy medicine.

Radionics specialists report that they are able to sense *vibrations* that are typical to specific states of health and illness and that they are able to project corrective vibrations through their radionics devices when illness is found. Radionics treatments appear to function similarly to the electromagnetic imprintings of water. It would be helpful to study whether one could distinguish between mental and electromagnetic imprinting of water by researchers. There are radionics specialists who utilize homeopathic remedies along with radionics treatments to correct the disharmonies that have been identified.

A healer related to me that she once went on holiday and forgot to take along her homeopathic remedy. She visualized to herself that she was holding the actual remedy (though she was actually holding only a glass of mineral water) and she felt that her "treated" water produced the same effects as the actual remedy. Similarly, a world-renowned homeopath (who asked to remain unnamed) reported that he had once been phoned by a friend and colleague from Africa with an urgent request for a remedy to treat an illness. Unable to provide the remedy expeditiously, the homeopath mentally imaged the remedy and his friend reported a rapid, very positive response.

Whether these reported results are valid, are only placebo effects, or are effects of healing intent awaits clarification through further studies.

Adverse effects: Intense emotional releases, accompanied by intense physical reactions are possible, particularly when high doses are given – as in classical homeopathy. Negative effects can be antidoted with coffee.

Training and licensing: There are a variety of homeopathic training programs but training is not standardized in the US. The National Center for Homeopathy in Alexandria, Virginia is a professional training and support organization. The Council for Homeopathic Certification (CHC) is the sole board certifying competency in homeopathy practice without regard to professional training.

In the US until recently, homeopaths were rare and were viewed with extreme skepticism by the medical community. They are now growing in numbers and acceptance, although many health authorities in the US are reluctant to grant licenses to practice homeopathy except to medical doctors. This is ironic, as MDs who have minimal training in homeopathy may be licensed to practice, while homeopathic doctors with years of training and experience may not.

Homeopaths are currently licensed in only three states.[163] In most other states, the practice of homeopathy is restricted to physicians, although unlicensed lay homeopaths may be found practicing in many states. Minnesota and California include homeopaths in their CAM Freedom of Practice Acts.

In the UK, homeopathic practitioners are accredited by their schools, the most prestigious of these being the Royal Society of Homeopaths. Many UK doctors had courses in homeopathic medicine after finishing conventional medical school and there are five homeopathic hospitals around the country. Homeopathic remedies are covered under the National Health Service, and close to half of all general practitioners (primary care physicians) refer patients to homeopaths.

Clinical applications: Homeopathy can be beneficial in treating most physical and psychological problems, including many serious conditions for which conventional medicine has no cures. This is an enormous boon to those who suffer from chronic conditions, often complicated by side effects of conventional medications.

Homeopathic remedies are available in the US and Britain over the counter in lower potencies. While there are self-help books for homeopathic remedies and substances such as arnica are popular and anecdotally effective treatments for stress and other common ailments, a homeopathic therapist can help patients benefit much more extensively and deeply from this treatment.

Many of the patients who respond well to homeopathy are often served poorly by allopathic medicine, which addresses the symptoms of anxiety and depression in a rather heavy-handed way, using tranquilizers and antidepressants to tone down or suppress the symptoms, but not getting to the underlying problems.

Counseling and psychotherapy can help with these problems, but it may take many months and years to bear fruit. Homeopathy offers profoundly transformative changes and often with startlingly rapidity, when a remedy is found that resonates with the person's situation. Conversely, the emotional releases that may be brought about by homeopathy can be worked out through psychotherapy, as may various chronic resistances and entrenched patterns of behavior. The best approach may be to use a combination of the two modalities.

I can certainly testify to the potency of this combination in my private practice of psychotherapy. Clients taking homeopathy and flower essences are able to unearth inner conflicts more rapidly; are better able to tolerate the anxieties of emotional releases; achieve more rapid resolution of their mood disorders; are better able to improve their relationships and more.

See also: Flower Essences.

HYDROTHERAPY
See: Water Therapies.

HYPNOTHERAPY

> *Your unconscious mind can listen*
> *To me without*
> *Your knowledge*
> *And also deal with something else at the same time.*
> – Milton Erickson (Rossi 1976, p. 38)

The basics of hypnotherapy are discussed in detail in Chapter II-1, but this modality deserves separate mention here as one of the important complementary therapies, whose potentials for therapist-interventions and self healing have been vastly under-utilized.

Hypnotherapy has not gained as wide an acceptance as one might expect, considering that it has been used in various forms and applications for 200 years. The greatest obstacle to its use in allopathic medicine is that not all patients respond to hypnosis. While everyone has some measure of hypnotizability, levels range from profoundly deep to almost negligible. For a good hypnotic subject, this treatment offers a spectrum of benefits with virtually no side effects, though it requires an investment of a period of time to learn and to utilize the induction techniques, and may often have to be done under the continued guidance of a therapist.

Various clinical tests (most of which are essentially forms of mini-induction of hypnosis) and a questionnaire are helpful in assessing hypnotic potential.

When people are responsive to hypnotic inductions, the benefits of this treatment can be enormous. Hypnotherapy can help in pain management; migraines; hypertension; irritable bowel syndromes; fibromyalgia; accelerating healing of burn wounds and bone fractures; halting traumatic and surgical bleeding, decreasing bleeding in hemophiliacs, stabilizing diabetes; easing menstrual problems; enhancing breast development; managing children's distress during unpleasant procedures; curing insomnia; and reducing the side effects of chemotherapy. It is also useful in treating warts[164] and allergies; obesity; asthma, and tobacco addiction.

Hypnotherapy can greatly facilitate psychotherapy, opening a quickly accessible window into repressed memories and feelings from traumatic events that have been repressed. I have used hypnotherapy successfully with post-traumatic stress disorders in people traumatized by war and rape.

I have also found it helpful in strengthening people's willpower to apply themselves to constructive and healing tasks.[165] It is not, however, a magical cure-all. It may require therapists who are willing and comfortable in being more directive to be successful.

Training and licensing: There are many and varied courses available in hypnotherapy. Treatment is best provided by therapists competent to treat the given problem through other therapies as well, because responses to hypnotherapy are so variable. Various professional associations provide guidelines for training and practice.[166] Hypnosis is not regulated by law and people who are unlicensed in any other helping profession may advertise that they practice hypnotherapy.

Adverse effects: Hypnotherapy must be used with caution.

A serious risk is that during hypnotherapy a subject may open up repressed feelings too rapidly and be overwhelmed with emotions that they have worked very hard to keep out of their conscious awareness. It is important therefore to have a hypnotherapist who is well trained and experienced for such work.

Stage hypnotists lead people to do silly things that may be embarrassing, which can be damaging to a person's self-confidence and self-image.

Considering the potential risks, one must be cautious in selecting a hypnotherapist. The public is cautioned to check the training, experience and other qualifications of hypnotherapists prior to seeking treatment.

Clinical applications: Hypnotherapy can be of great help in treating pains of every variety. Dentists, surgeons, obstetricians, emergency room physicians, and pediatricians, all of whom regularly deal with pains, have reported great successes with hypnosis. However, in today's world of managed care, constraints on the doctors' time severely limit the use of this modality.

Many illnesses in which a measure of self-regulation is possible respond to hypnotherapy (such as asthma, irritable bowel syndrome, hypertension, fibromyalgia and anxiety), as well as many other problems, including hormonal disorders; addictions; phobias; problems of poor self-image and self-esteem; and more.[167]

A hypnotherapist will help the subject find the best ways to enter hypnotic states and can be of great assistance in exploring contributions to health and illness from the unconscious mind. Once this method has been mastered, self-hypnosis can be of enormous benefit.

See also: Suggestion, Placebo Effects (self-healing) in Chapter II-1.

IMAGERY
See: Visualization; Metaphor (under Creative Therapies).

INTUITIVE ASSESSMENT
See: Medical Intuition.

LEECHES

> *A skilful leech is better far, than half a hundred men of war.*
> – Samuel Butler.

Leeches were used for bleeding over several centuries in Europe in the treatment of many ailments, such as heart disease and infections. American leeches were deemed less effective than the European varieties and this led to a thriving import trade, which at times even depleted European supplies. Leeches suck blood through wounds that they create by biting and the blood flow is maintained with anticoagulants that the animals secrete.

While bleeding is no longer accepted as a treatment for most of these ailments, a few applications have been found in which leeches are still beneficial. For instance, when fingers or toes are sewn back on after they have been accidentally amputated, there is often a residual swelling that can completely cut off the blood supply to the digit. When skin is grafted, when breasts are reconstructed after mastectomies and when there is severe injury with a black eye, there is often swelling that can impede wound healing because the swollen tissues limit the local flow of blood which removes broken down tissues and facilitates reapirs. In these limited applications leeches have been found to be useful adjuncts to conventional care.

Adverse effects: Leeches can invade the body and historical notes caution against letting them enter the vagina, through which they can invade the uterus, or the throat, where they may cut off the airway. There can be prolonged oozing after the leech is removed and if the creature is not removed carefully, parts of its mouth may remain and cause infections. Having a bleeding tendency is a contra-indication for treatment with leeches.

See also: Maggots.

LESHAN HEALING

> *In Type 1 healing, the healer goes into an altered state of consciousness in which he views himself and the healee as one entity. There is no attempt to "do anything" to the healee... but simply to meet him, to be one with him, to unite with him...*
> — Lawrence LeShan (1974a, p. 106)

This method was developed in the late 1960s by Lawrence LeShan, a clinical and research psychologist who specializes in psychotherapy for people with cancer. LeShan was initially a skeptic, as noted earlier, and believed that healing was at best some combination of wishful thinking, suggestion and avoidance of facing up to one's problems. He set out to observe healers in order to expose their charlatanism, but was surprised to find some impressive people with real abilities to bring about unusual arrests or remissions in various diseases, occasionally with such rapidity as to be considered instantaneous or "miraculous."

LeShan has an outstanding gift of pattern recognition, and a clarity of observation and reasoning that make him highly qualified for these tasks he undertook. He carefully observed some of the better healers, noting the following common denominators in their practices:

1. They were able to focus or *center* their minds;
2. They found ways to join with the healees in a profound way; and
3. They felt themselves and the healees to be "one with the All."

LeShan practiced meditation in order to center his own mind and then began offering healing as he had observed it, with very positive results. He subsequently went on to teach others to develop their healing gifts. Part of LeShan's motivation in developing this method was to have a standardized method of healing that would be amenable to research.

For three decades Joyce Goodrich has carried on teaching the LeShan method, while LeShan has continued to focus on self-healing through psychotherapy for people with cancer and other serious illnesses.

LeShan healing focuses primarily on distant/ absent/ *Type 1* healing. Healers are taught a range of meditative and imagery approaches to help them center themselves, focusing on the image that they are one with the healee and one with the All. Healers are encouraged to work in pairs.

Research: Goodrich has been working for years to develop collaborative research on LeShan healing, with modest success. However, there have been no studies that clearly confirm the effects of this method.

Adverse effects: No harmful effects have been reported See discussion of potential general negative effects from rapid improvements under Spiritual Healing.

Training and licensing: Basic and advanced training are offered by Joyce Goodrich, PhD. There is no licensing for healing.

See also: *Spiritual Healing* – Volume I of *Healing Research.*

LIGHT AND COLOR THERAPIES

> *The heavy dark falls back to earth*
> *And the freed air goes wild with light,*
> *The heart fills with fresh, bright breath*
> *And thoughts stir to give birth to colour.*
> > – John O'Donohue

Full-spectrum light can influence the cycles of waking and sleeping, with their associated cycles of hormonal ebbs and flows. Various hormones are secreted in greater and lesser amounts, corresponding with our body's needs at different times of day and night. For instance, melatonin is a hormone secreted by the pineal gland in the brain under stimulation of the body by light This is the body's timing messenger, relaying information to all parts of the body about the circadian (daily) cycle. In response to this message, levels of other hormones such as adrenal steroids are raised and lowered – to help us deal appropriately internally with the external energies that shift as day alternates with night.

Each species has a circadian rhythm that is close to 24 hours long. In the natural cycle, which alternates the light of day and the darkness of night, these rhythms conform to the 24-hour solar day. These rhythms continue even in total darkness.

Light is helpful in healing. Full spectrum light can treat *seasonal affective disorder* (*SAD*), a depression experienced by some people during the short days of winter. Exposures to full spectrum light of 40-60 minutes just after sunrise or before sunset, which in effect extends a person's experience of daylight, can prevent or reverse SAD depression.

Colored light is said to convey healing vibrations, and particular colors are used to treat particular problems. Many of these colors correlate with the basic colors associated with the chakras. As you will recall from the description under acupuncture, there are seven major chakras along the midline of the body. The root chakra, at the base of the spine, is identified with red; the sacral chakra, below the navel, with orange; the solar plexus chakra with yellow; the heart chakra with green; the throat chakra with blue; the "third-eye" chakra, on the forehead above the nose, with violet; and the crown chakra, at the top of the head, with indigo or white.

Various healers recommend different systems of color treatments. For example, healees might be exposed to light of the color associated with the chakra that is in the region of the body that needs healing. Others recommend colors based on the color perceptions of healers who see the biological energy field and the chakras as colors. The different colors indicate a healthy, stressed, or diseased state.

Other systems of color diagnosis and color/ light therapy have been developed through empirical observations of the health benefits of shining particular colors upon specific parts of the body and of shining light into the eyes.

One area of light therapy has a well established physiological mechanism. Blue light has been found to cure neonatal jaundice by facilitating the metabolism of excess bilirubin and this method is widely used in hospitals around the world.

It is also known that ultraviolet light kills bacteria. Niels Finsen was awarded a Nobel Prize in 1903 for treating tuberculosis of the skin with ultraviolet light.

Jacob Liberman extends light, color and vision therapy to effect profound healings on physical, emotional, mental and spiritual levels. Particularly impressive are the summaries of his findings that constricted visual fields in children with learning disabilities are correctable with colored light therapy.

Research: Research has confirmed that full spectrum light is an effective treatment for seasonal affective disorder.

Liberman reviews evidence from controlled studies showing that blue light may help in arthritis and full spectrum light combined with particular colors on the walls may enhance learning and improve children's behavior in schools. Children in these circumstances also had fewer dental cavities, a result supported by further evidence from a study of full spectrum light in hamsters. Liberman adds his clinical observations that red light may relieve migraines.

While these uses of color have no known causal relationship to disease processes, they are reported empirically to have helped many patients. Scientists in Russia and America have found that red light stimulates the sympathetic nervous system, while blue stimulates the parasympathetic system. Maximal increases in blood pressure, pulse and respiration were obtained with yellow light; modest increases with orange; and minimal increases with red. Maximal decreases could be obtained with black; modest decreases with blue; and minimal decreases with green.

The color of bubble-gum pink has a calming effect on violent behavior. While the mechanisms for this effect are unknown, criminals and juvenile delinquents placed in rooms painted pink demonstrate far less aggression and violence.

Healers may recommend that clothing of particular colors be worn to help alleviate particular problems. Colors may also be used in visualizations of subtle energy projection. In Therapeutic Touch, imaging green or yellow light energizes the healee, while blue calms or soothes.

Krieger (1993) suggests a simple experiment you can try for yourself. Picture in your imagination that you are in a church on a sunny day. Sense that your face is bathed in the light coming through a stained-glass window. Sense the feeling of each color in turn as you move from one spot to another. Check with other people what their experiences are with this imagery.

Color therapy appears to be a fertile ground for future research.

Adverse effects: Excessive use of full spectrum lighting can make people uncomfortable, and anecdotal reports indicate it may precipitate manic reactions in people with bipolar disorders.

Training and licensing: There is no formal training or licensing for light and color therapy.

Clinical applications: Light therapy is of proven value in seasonal affective disorder and in neonatal jaundice. Light and color treatments appear to have much broader ranges of applications, but these remain to be substantiated with research.

   Light and color therapies require the guidance of a therapist. Self-healing through the proper use of appropriate lights and colors can then be implemented.

LOVE

> *Love and intimacy are the root of what makes us sick and what makes us well. I am not aware of any other factor in medicine – not diet, not smoking, not exercise... not drugs, not surgery – that has a greater impact on our quality of life, incidence of illness and premature death.*
> – Dean Ornish (1998)

Though discussing love as a therapeutic technique might seem to trivialize this profound and complex emotion, it must be acknowledged that love is one of the most powerful forces for healing.

   Most importantly, Bernie Siegel and other healers feel that respants must love themselves in order to be healed. Much of our dis-ease and disease derives from self-doubt, self-criticism and self-hate. These attitudes and emotions can block the flows of our bioenergies. They create disconnections from nurturing environmental energies and stagnations within the body that can either allow or cause illness to manifest. From this perspective, illness is like an alarm set off by the bodymind to alert us that our energies are not flowing properly. Often this is a direct result of feeling unloved.

   Love as a factor in therapy was never even mentioned in my medical school training. In contrast, it is a word that is heard quite often in discussions at the American Holistic Medical Association, where I once heard Leo Buscaglia speak. Famous for his teachings and books about love, he told of how he had once been invited to speak at a hospital. When he submitted the title of his lecture, "Love," he was contacted by the hospital and was told politely that this probably would not be acceptable as a topic in a medical setting. When he changed the title to "Unconditional Positive Regard," they had no trouble approving it.

   Caregivers are better at promoting healing when they have a loving attitude. My first supervisor in psychiatric residency training, Joe Golden, advised me, "If you cannot find something in your patient that you love, you should not be treating that person." I didn't realize at the time what a profound piece of advice that was. After thirty-five years of psychotherapy and healing practice, I am now more sure than ever that this is true.

Spiritual dimensions of love are powerful adjuncts for healing. People who have near-death experiences often report that they were transformed by being in the presence of a "Being of Light" that was unconditionally accepting (i.e. totally loving). They felt that they were then able to forgive and accept themselves and others, when they had never before been able to do so.

Research: Although research on human love is fraught with difficulties, the effects of love have been studied in laboratory animals. In one study, rabbits were fed a high cholesterol diet for several weeks. One group was also given love (handled, stroked, talked to, played with) and another group was merely given the minimal physical care that is usual for laboratory animals. When the arteries of both groups were examined at the end of the trial period, the rabbits that had received loving attention showed 60% lower levels of atherosclerotic changes.

Love has traditionally been associated with feelings in the heart. It is fascinating to find that research is confirming effects of feelings of love upon heart muscles. Glen Rein and Rollin McCraty found that when people learn to meditate on love their electrocardiograms (EKGs) show a significantly increased coherence in their heartbeats. When they enter this meditative state, they are also able to intentionally alter the winding of DNA in the laboratory. As a demonstration of an intentional effect upon living matter, this is by definition a form of healing.

If two people sit opposite each other a few feet apart while they are both in this state of cardiac coherence and the first projects loving thoughts and feelings toward the other, the electroencephalogram (EEG) recorded in the frontal lobes of the second person will reflect the heartbeat rhythm of the first person. However, some people's EEGs do not become entrained in this way. A further reflection on the power of love is that those who *do* respond in this situation report that their parents demonstrated a caring attitude toward them in their childhood, while those who *do not* respond report that their parents did not demonstrate a caring attitude.

Adverse effects: The English language is lacking in words to distinguish "unconditional positive regard" love from sexual love. This is where love, as in sexual activity between therapists and clients, has given love a bad press. Laws in many states now prohibit psychotherapists and psychiatrists from touching their patients, as a precaution against slipping from one expression of love into another. This is a serious impediment in the conduct of psychotherapy, as touch can be a potent healing intervention.

People who have not known unconditional acceptance as children may have difficulty when they encounter a loving person, be it a therapist, a family member, or a friend. Their automatic pilot may have been programmed in childhood to distrust others and not get close to them, in anticipation that they will be rejected or hurt. It may take counseling or psychotherapy to change and overcome such defensive programming.

Clinical applications: Love is an essential element in care-giving and healing.

See also: Massage, Touch.

MAGGOTS

There are in fact two things, science and opinion; the former begets
knowledge, the latter ignorance.
                                        – Hippocrates

Maggots are fly larvae that eat decaying flesh. They refuse to eat live flesh and
have therefore been helpful in treating infections through many centuries. They
quickly clear out pustular wounds, leaving clean tissues that heal rapidly. Prior to
development of antibiotics, maggots were the primary treatment for pustular
wounds. Ronald Sherman, MD, MSc, professor of surgery at the University of
California at Irvine, has brought back this ancient method, which has proven invaluable in treating chronic infections that have not responded to antibiotics. Flies
are raised in labs and their eggs are sterilized so they will not add new infectious
organisms to wounds. The eggs are packed into the wounds, leaving an open airway so that the hatched maggots can breathe. Maximal benefits are found one to
three days after maggots hatch. Rarely is it necessary to repeat the treatment more
than once for full clearing away of dead flesh in even the most difficult wounds.
The maggots also secrete ammonia, which slows growth of bacteria. It is believed
that they also secrete substances that enhance wound healing, because the results
with maggots are often realized faster than would be anticipated with antibiotics.
   Doctors have been amazed and patients have been delighted with the results.
Treatment produces a rapid decrease in pain and foul odors. Patients who were
candidates for amputations of their limbs due to chronic skin ulcers (common in
diabetes) and bone infections (osteomyelitis) have been spared the surgery and
their legs and arms have been saved. Other applications have included treatment
of bedsores, venous ulcers due to varicose veins, burns, wounds from surgery or
trauma and wounds with bacterial infections that are resistant to antibiotics.

Adverse effects: Patients and medical personnel often have to overcome a revul-
sion at the sight, or even at the thought of using maggots in this way. While it was
initially feared that there might even be psychological trauma from using maggots, patients have almost uniformly been very favorable in their response to the
treatment – especially when they observe the rapid, positive results.

See also: Leeches.

MASSAGE AND MANUAL THERAPIES

The hands of those I meet are dumbly eloquent to me. There are those
whose hands have sunbeams in them so that their grasp warms my heart.
                                        – Helen Keller

Ashley Montagu points out that touch is one of the most potent means of communicating care. It relaxes muscles and releases the tensions that form part of the
familiar vicious circle of tension → spasm → pain → anxiety → tension, etc.

Massage[168] is one of the oldest of all known therapies, with records acknowledging its benefits in China dating to 4,000 years ago and from Hippocrates in the 4th century BC. Two brothers named George and Charles Taylor, both New York physicians who studied in Sweden, introduced massage as a therapy in America in the 1850s. Because of the time constraints of medical practice, massage was initially delegated to physical therapists and nurses. These, in turn, have likewise succumbed to the pressures of time, relinquishing massage to the hands of massage therapists. A move back toward integrating massage with psychotherapy is growing amongst psychotherapists, who are finding that touch markedly enhances therapeutic rapport, relaxation, exploration of bodymind memories and more.[169]

Western massage approaches emphasize mechanical interventions, including gliding strokes (*effleurage*), kneading (*pétrissage*), rubbing/ friction and percussion (*tapotement*), vibration, compression and range of motion. A variety of other therapeutic approaches may also be combined with massage. It is estimated that more than 80 different types of massage are practiced, many of them adapted from other cultures. The following list describes a few of these, ranging from methods that primarily address the body, to those that focus upon subtle energies and others that include psychological components (*bodymind* therapies).

1. *Swedish massage*, the most common variety, directs long, gliding strokes and kneading to superficial layers of the muscles, usually from the periphery towards the heart (Maanum/ Montgomery). It induces relaxation, relief of muscle tensions/ spasms, improved circulation and enhanced range of motion.

2. *Deep-tissue massage* directs pressure across the grain of the muscles with slow strokes and greater pressure than (1), for the same effects and purposes.

3. *Sports massage* combines (1) and (2) to treat athletic strains and injuries.

4 *Manual lymph drainage* uses light strokes to enhance lymph flow when there is edema, inflammation or circulatory problems due to nerve damage. Research has shown that lymphedema massage is superior to mechanical methods in reducing swelling after radical mastectomy and also lowers treatment costs.

5. *Neuromuscular massage, myotherapy* (J. Witt) *and trigger point massage* (Prudden) address specific muscles that may be in spasm due to emotional or physical stress, or may have *trigger points* that initiate pain. Sometimes pressures on nerves from various tissues can also be relieved.

6. *Traditional Chinese massage* has been practiced for 2,000 years. It may include rubbing and tapping with the palms and finger tips, pinching, lifting and/ or twisting pinched flesh and similar techniques. In addition to treating musculoskeletal problems, this massage may be given for headaches, stomach aches, dysmenorrhea, upper respiratory infections, asthma, enuresis, insomnia and more.

The next therapies in the list involve very light pressure or massage at discrete points on the body, rather than deep tissue massage.

**Figure II-11. Healing and other complementary therapies,
such as massage and aromatherapy, work well together.**

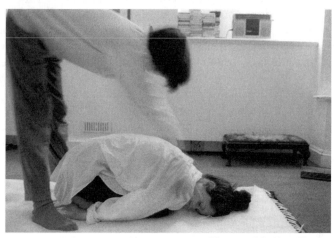

Photograph by Tony Sleep

7. *Aromatherapy* is named after the aromatic oils that are used to lubricate the skin during the massage, which is usually similar in method to (1).

The effects of these oils can be quite potent and specifically beneficial for a variety of ailments, in and of themselves.

8. *Structural Integration* (*Rolfing*) is deep massage directed to fascia (connective tissues) rather than to muscles. The theoretical basis for rolfing is that the fascia hold and maintain the tensions of misalignments in the body that are adopted unconsciously in response to emotional stresses and defenses. Support for this theory is drawn from the architectural model of the Buckminster Fuller's *tensegrity mast*, in which wires under tension hold the solid elements together. It is proposed that in the human body, the fascia parallel the wires and the bones resemble Fuller's solid elements.

Research has shown that rolfing can be helpful in treating cerebral palsy, stress and other symptoms from whiplash, low back pain, and anxiety, and in influencing various other physiological and psychological problems. Deep emotional hurts may be released during rolfing.

Hellerwork and *Aston Patterning* are both offshoots of rolfing that are somewhat less forceful in their physical manipulations of body tissues.

9. *Pressure point therapies/ Meridian-based therapies* act through particularly sensitive pressure points on the body, using the pressure of the practitioner's fingers. The pressure points often correspond to the meridian and acupuncture point systems.[170] These therapies, with the exception of (b) below, often rely on touch rather than massage, although pressure or tapping at the acupressure point may be used. The touch may be quite light or very firm, depending upon the therapy. These therapies rely on subtle energy medicine interventions rather than on massage of muscles, tendons and fascia for their effects.[171]

a. *Acupressure* may be used instead of acupuncture needles at acupuncture points anywhere on the body. There are several types of acupressure. *Shiatsu* and *tsubo* (Japanese) use sequences of pressure from one end of every meridian to the other. As in spiritual healing, these acupressure therapists project Qi energy through their fingers as they apply pressure. *Jin shin jyutsu* and *jin shin do* (Japanese) apply pressure along selected meridians according to the problems being treated.

Several variants of acupressure facilitate profound psychological transformations through treatment applied to specific points on the head, chest and hand.

> *There's an ancient Chinese medical text that names three levels of healing[:] ... Address a person's complaints to diminish her pain, ... understand someone's nature, ... [and] assist a person in fulfilling his or her destiny.*
> – Harriet Beinfield and Efrem Korngold

While these approaches are highly innovative in terms of allopathic medicine, they are simply rediscoveries of long-forgotten, traditional healing lore.

b. *Reflexology* (*zone therapy*) addresses points on the feet that correlate with the rest of the body, including the internal organs. This method is closer to massage, as firm pressure may be used, though the pressure is intended to stimulate healing through the meridian energy lines rather than through relaxation of the specific muscles and tissues that are being touched.

Reflexology can help in treating a broad variety of health problems in a manner similar to that of acupuncture, from which it is derived.

Some reflexologists claim they are able to diagnose problems by assessing tender zones in the feet that correspond to the parts of the body that are diseased.

Recently, awareness has been growing that reflexology can be a potent intervention for emotional problems as well, sometimes inducing strong emotional releases during treatments.

Research: A single, randomized controlled study shows reflexology is effective in treatment of premenstrual syndrome. A study of diagnosis by reflexology demonstrated no success.

c. *Polarity Therapy* was developed by Randolph Stone, a chiropractor, osteopath and naturopath, in the early 19th century. He studied healing methods in China and India and settled in India, where he developed this method. It is based on energy interventions in the patterns of chakras and in the specific directions of flows of energy in and around the body. In this method, particular points on the body are pressed with the fingers. Exercise, diet and psychological states are also addressed, the latter through *positive thinking*.

d. *SHEN Therapy* was developed by Richard Pavek, an American scientist. This method addresses emotional tensions that manifest in physical symptoms, using light touch at particular points on the body. It has been helpful in treating anorexia, bulimia, migraine, pains of all sorts, panic attacks, post-traumatic stress disorder, pre-menstrual symptoms, irritable bowel syndrome and more.

Research: Pavek showed that decreases in white cell count during the course of chemotherapy of four patients could be reversed significantly with *SHEN* treatments to the thymus gland. Pavek also reported that *SHEN* therapy provided long-term relief of premenstrual symptoms in 11 out of 13 women. Although *SHEN* therapy did not significantly shorten the hospitalization time of 6 people with major depression (compared to 6 randomized controls), Pavek found significant changes in emotional expressiveness, dreams and interpersonal relations of the subjects receiving *SHEN* therapy.

e. *The Bowen Technique* is another form of gentle massage with healing. Sharing from my brief introductory course in this method, let me take a moment to flesh out the description of this interesting type of hands-on therapy. The Bowen Technique was developed in the 1950's by Tom Bowen, a gifted Australian intuitive. The methods he developed are claimed to be effective 85-90% of the time with 1-3 treatments. Bowen was able to treat serious problems very rapidly, seeing up to 13,000 people in a year. The Bowen method is available in Australia, England and the US.

This method involves a very gentle rolling of selected muscles under the hands of the therapist. A standard set of manipulations is used to treat most problems. Particularly responsive are musculoskeletal problems, even when they have been present for many years and have been unresponsive to conventional medical treatments and other complementary therapies. For example, frozen shoulders respond so well that Bowen therapists routinely invite people with this problem to receive treatments when they are demonstrating the method at public meetings. Many are permanently cleared of all pain and limitation of motion within minutes. Others may take a few days to demonstrate changes and one or two more treatments often produce further improvements. Numerous other conditions have responded dramatically, including anxiety, asthma, emphysema, irritable bowel syndrome, hiatus hernia, skin conditions, hyperactivity, depression and more. This method helps the patient on organic, emotional and psychological levels simultaneously.

Diagnosis is unnecessary with the Bowen method because the body is allowed to readjust itself and return to health rather than being pushed to change in particular ways. Conditions other than the presenting problem (which often are not even mentioned to the therapist by the client) may improve as well. Here is an example from the experience of my course instructor.

> I treated "David," an elderly man who came in bent over and moaning, obviously suffering with serious back pain. In a thick Yiddish accent he explained that he had been to numbers of other therapists over many months without benefit. I gave him a standard treatment and he went out hobbling just about as much as when he entered, as do many clients of Bowen therapists.
>
> The Bowen method is so simple and quick that it isn't uncommon to have clients feel they have been duped when they are asked to pay for what seems to be of no immediate benefit, involving so light a touch for so brief a period, often not particularly directed to the site of discomfort. We al-

ways book two appointments a week apart, knowing that a second treatment at that interval is often necessary. I reminded him of his second appointment and knew from the look on his face as he departed that he was thinking, "I'm not *that* foolish that I'm going to return and pay you good money again for nothing."

The next week, he returned at the scheduled time, walking normally and beaming. He came in and said, "I'm all better. I have to show you." Whereupon he turned his back, dropped his trousers and underpants and bent over. I could understand his bending over to show me his back was better, but not the rest of his show. He gleefully announced, "My hemorrhoids!" Still bewildered, I told him I didn't see any hemorrhoids. "Of course!" he said. "They're gone! I suffered with them for years. And I didn't even tell you about them! If I was Christian, I'd think you were Jesus returned to help the sick."

– Julian Baker

Unlike other forms of healing, which may be complementary to a wide variety of therapies, the Bowen method is recommended as a complement only with homeopathy, Bach flower remedies and counseling/ psychotherapy.

Lest you think that this is purely a mechanical therapy, the Bowen method has been reported effective with the use of a proxy patient[172] in cases where the person with the illness cannot be treated directly.

Research: A pilot study suggests that the Bowen technique can be helpful in the treatment of frozen shoulders.

I will mention two further therapeutic methods to round out the above list of therapies. These are subtle energy interventions rather than forms of massage, but they may involve light touch.

f. *Therapeutic Touch* (*TT*), Healing Touch (HT) and *Reiki* are sometimes categorized as massage techniques, because they may include touch, though they do not involve physical manipulation of the body. These and other spiritual healing approaches are combined with massage by some practitioners.

See also: Reiki; Therapeutic Touch; Spiritual Healing.[173]

10. *Trager psychophysical integration* involves gentle, rhythmic rocking, bouncing and shaking movements, to free up chronic tensions in muscles and joints. It was developed by a Hawaiian physician named Milton Trager, out of his experience as a trainer for boxers. Trager treatments address emotional patterns that have lodged in body tensions. The principles of *hookup* (a meditative state) and, *mentastics* (physical movements) are also taught to increase enjoyment in movement. Clinical successes have been reported in treating cerebral palsy and many other conditions, including chronic musculoskeletal pains, headaches, temporomandibular joint (TMJ) pain, spinal cord injuries and neurological impairments from spinal cord injuries, polio and strokes.

11. *Bioenergetics*, derived from the work of Wilhelm Reich, uses focused manual pressure by the therapist, various positionings of the body, focused breathing and other physical exercises. These are designed to release emotional tensions and *armoring* (stiffening) of the body that result from emotional traumas and stresses. Emotional releases may be intense, with accompanying emergence of memories of old traumas that were long buried and insights about how the unconscious mind kept these from conscious awareness through body armoring. Variations on bioenergetics have been developed under the names of *Neo-Reichian therapy, Lowenwork* (Lowen)*, Core Energetics* (Pierrakos) *and Radix.*[174]

12. There are other variations on the theme of massage that are less well known and less commonly available in many parts of the world.[175]

Research lags well behind the popular acceptance of these bodymind therapies.

Critices often cite the lack of controlled studies on these manipulative techniques. They ignore the fact that conventional medicine has accepted that physiotherapy is effective for musculoskeletal disorders, but there is little scientific data to support this general agreement in the profession.

Adding a few personal observations: I have had Lowen-type bioenergetics treatments that I found most helpful in getting past my intellectual defenses and releasing long-buried feelings. In stress management workshops I lead for doctors, nurses and others, massage is one of the most appreciated modalities.

Overview of the effective components of massage

Several distinct components contribute to the efficacy of massage.

Touch is one of the most potent means of intervening to offer healing. Because this method of communication is non-verbal it reaches deep into people's awareness, at levels that resonate with nurturing which they may have experienced early in their lives. Touch conveys caring, facilitates rapport and builds trust – all of which help people to relax under the hands of their massage therapist.

In relaxing a patient physically and psychologically, the three modalities of touch, massage and (in aromatherapy) aromatic oils all address the tensions that contribute to the familiar vicious circle of tension ▯ spasm ▯ pain ▯ anxiety ▯ more tension, etc. In addition, some aromatherapists claim that the oils they use can also interact with subjects' biological energy fields. The bienergies of the person giving the massage may also convey spiritual healing effects.

Massage relaxes muscles. When muscles and joints are painful due to tiredness, physical strain or injuries, massage acts directly upon the problem areas to relax the muscles. Sometimes massage can relieve *trigger points* of sensitivity in muscles and tissues that appear to set off more generalized muscle tensions and spasms. There may be emotional traumas that are associated with painful muscles and joints, as the physical body participates in storing emotional memories. Systems of deep massage have been developed to facilitate emotional releases along with releases of physical pains. When there is a general level of physical tension due to emotional stress, massage can relax the overall tension of muscles in the body.

Aromatic oils are used in aromatherapy to smooth the contact between the therapists' hands and the clients' skin. They also have medicinal benefits based on the aromatic and bioenergetic qualities of the substances used in preparing the oils.

Spiritual healing may be an aspect of any complementary therapy, particularly those that include touch.

Research: While abundant testimonials suggest a very high success rate (85-90%) for the various bodywork therapies, with complete resolution of phobias and other problems, little research is available on these modalities and I have found no controlled studies.

Adverse effects: While I have not seen reports of harm from massage or bodymind therapies, common sense cautions apply to applying massage or other physical manipulations too vigorously, with a potential for physical harm from the manipulations. Other potential negative effects may arise from rapid releases of emotional traumas that have been locked into the body.

Training and licensing: In the US, training in massage varies enormously from one school to another, as do licensing standards in various states. A National Certification Exam has been established under the Psychological Corporation.[176]   A Commission on Massage Training Accreditation and Approval recognizes more than 60 training programs.[177]

National organizations have been unable to agree on standards for training and licensing. Massage therapists are licensed in about half of the states.

Massage therapists are lobbying for the licensing of massage in a growing number of states in the US. Healers object to this whereever the laying-on of hands is considered to be a sub-category of massage and would therefore require massage therapy licensing. This would require that healers study manipulative massage for licensing, even though this is outside of their practices of spiritual healing – which in most healing practices involves only light touch and no manipulation.

Some US states prohibit psychotherapists from touching clients (as a firm precaution against sexual temptations), thereby limiting the use of these approaches in some disciplines. A few psychotherapists are acquiring training in hands-on therapies to give them the license to touch clients.

Clinical applications: Massage in its many variants can be enormously helpful in addressing musculoskeletal problems. It is also useful as a relaxation method in treating almost any condition. For instance, it can be enormously beneficial for women during labor and for neonates, particularly in premature births. For infants, touch is actually a necessary element for survival.

In its bodymind applications, massage can facilitate emotional releases and restructuring of the mind as well as the body, thus easing the progress from diseased and diseased states towards health. Anxiety, phobias, panic attacks, depression, sensory deprivation with prolonged illness or hospitalization and lack of self-confidence can all respond well to these methods. Massage is also lovely for inducing relaxation, not only as a treatment but also as a preventive to stressed states and just for the pleasure of physical stimulation.

A therapist is essential for a full massage, though it is possible to massage a limited number of one's own muscles. Once you are familiar with some of the simpler methods of massage, you may share and exchange this pleasurable healing technique with others. Many of the meridian-based therapies and some of the bioenergy healing approaches can be practiced as self-healing.

See also: Bodymind Therapies; Meridian Based Therapies.

MEDICAL INTUITION (Intuitive Assessment)

> *The intuitive mind is a sacred gift and the rational mind is a faithful servant. We have created a society that honors the servant and has forgotten the gift.*
>
>   – Albert Einstein

Intuition is inner knowing that alerts and informs us about things that we would not otherwise know, through ordinary sensory perception, memory or reasoning.

Many health caregivers report that they occasionally intuitively know various bits of information about people who come to them for help. Some who are more sensitive may intuit what a diagnosis is (before completing the examination and laboratory tests), or even identify the underlying physical and psychological causes in the recent and distant past for patients' current physical or emotional problems.[178]

In almost every group of doctors and nurses I have spoken with, many report that they have had inexplicable hunches about patients who needed urgent attention – at times when there were no sensory indications that this might be the case. They report that attending to their intuitive hunches, they have sought out these patients and found that indeed they were in serious and urgent need of help. Such incidents are rare occurrences, but so distinctly odd and impressive that they are clearly recalled. Most health caregivers who have had such experiences are unwilling to discuss them because they anticipate that their colleagues will not believe them – especially if they aren't sure themselves whether this was a real hunch or just an unusual coincidence.

A few caregivers have more highly developed intuitive abilities and find that such experiences are common, though not regular. They simply know that the patient before them has heart disease, kidney disease or whatever – even before she opens her mouth to state her problems. They may also intuit specific medications that could be of help, such as the correct antibiotic for a given infection – prior to receiving the laboratory report on bacterial culture sensitivity to antibiotics.

With very highly developed intuition, it is possible to intuit what is wrong and what will be helpful for almost every patient. Several fascinating books have been published by medical intuitives, some of whom are doctors.

For some, the intuitive knowing comes as an inner feeling, like an itch that urges them to explore what is tickling the edges of their awareness. For others, it comes in the form of words or mental images. Another avenue for intuitive knowledge is through the senses, most commonly perceived as an aura of color around the patient that reveals the state of their body, emotions, mind, relationships and spirit. Some intuitives report smells or tastes that appear when patients have particular physical conditions or emotional problems, and yet others mirror in their own bodies the sensations that are troubling their patients.

Some intuitives can even identify past causes for present-day problems. They may also see into the future, to discover the outcome of treatments.

The more highly gifted intuitives work with only the name of the subject they are diagnosing, sometimes using additional information such as their birth date and city of residence. They can diagnose the condition of anyone in the world, from any distance.

A far more common ability is intuitive diagnosis through sensations in the hands of the healer as they are moved around the body of the subject. Sensations in the hands of intuitives, which are apparently caused by interactions with the biological energy fields of the subjects, can provide information relating to states of health, psychological dis-ease and illness, which the intuitives then interpret.

Medical intuitive abilities are no different from the sensitivities of psychics, which have been thoroughly studied by parapsychologists. Extensive studies, including meta-analyses, show statistically significant results. They confirm that telepathy, clairsentience, psychokinesis (PK), precognition and retrocognition can all be demonstrated. Everyone has a measure of these abilities, as has been shown in extensive studies of ordinary people. However, in most people these abilities are weak and produce effects that can be identified only through statistical studies of large groups. Interestingly, the results obtained in trials of intuition in non-believers are frequently significantly *lower* than chance, suggesting that the subjects' unconscious minds process the psi awarenesses and produce results that are consistent with their beliefs.

Theories: Several varieties of intuition are apparent (Benor 2002d).
Automatic responses from previous experiences and memory

> *In seeking knowledge, the first step is silence, the second listening, the third remembering, the forth practicing, and the fifth is teaching others.*
> – Ibn Gabirol

When we learn a skill such as driving a car, we initially have to practice each component of turning on the engine, releasing the parking brake, putting the car in gear, steering as we step on the gas pedal, scanning for road clearance and hazards, braking, and so on. As we become proficient in all of these maneuvers, they become habitual and we can do them with little thought. Our automatic responses may be so good that we could be lost in thoughts and suddenly realize that we have driven some distance and cannot recall any conscious adjusting of the steering, braking, or other controls of the car. The same processes of automating responses occur as we learn other skills, such as clinical medical and nursing interventions. Going through a medical history and examination is initially a complex process, involving myriads of details of information and procedures. The more experienced we are with these, the more they become automatic.

Clinicians are able to draw from their mental databases of knowledge in order to respond to situations rapidly and efficiently, often with little thought. The surgeon instantly applies a clamp and stops a bleeding vessel. The patient retches, and the nurses' hand is immediately reaching for the nearest handy towel or basin.

This is a basic level of intuition, in the sense of recognizing a problem and knowing what to do without having to consciously analyze the details and respond through conscious, logical deductions in order to respond to a situation.

Cognitive pattern recognition

> *Let us train our minds to desire what the situation demands.*
> – Seneca

Case: A patient presents with depression, gravelly voice and thick hair. The doctor, who hasn't seen a person with hypothyroidism so severe since reading her medical school textbooks many years earlier, instantly recognizes this is a case of hypothyroidism.

Case: A surgeon asked me to see a 23 year-old patient after his appendectomy because he was depressed. His parents reported he had always been a loner. I felt uncomfortable because his eyes would not meet mine. The diagnosis of Asperger's syndrome came to mind, from having seen children 5 to 10 years old with such presentations - particularly the avoidance of gaze. Further questioning confirmed this as likely diagnosis. I hesitated before sharing my impression because it suggests an incurable problem, with the person likely to remain autistic and distant from everyone. The parents, however, were very grateful because at last they understood their son's problems and could plan how to deal with them.

Clinical pattern recognition may be more subtle. Clinical sensitivity often leads doctors, nurses and other caregivers to recognize when something is going wrong or going well. Postoperative nurses will often report a sense of a patient "not being right," although objective signs and symptoms are within normal limits. Often, these sorts of intuitive awarenesses prove correct, and an internal bleed or other problem develops soon after the nurse's intuitive "alarm bells" start to ring. At other times, the nurse will sense that all is well, and the patient will have an uneventful postoperative course (King and Clark 2002).

Studies that consider the use of intuition in nurses with varying levels of experience confirm that this is a valid modality for decision making. These studies note a progressively greater development of trust in intuition - according to levels of experience, from nurses who are beginners, through those who are competent, proficient, and expert.

Pattern recognition appears to be (at least in part) an extension of learned knowledge, honed to a fine, automated instrument. As clinicians learn more and become more experienced, they can perceive increasingly subtle patterns of appearance, behaviors, monitored body data (from sophisticated instruments), and laboratory studies which alert them to unusual changes and dangers in their patients .

This is the art and science of medical and psychiatric practice. It is medical detective work, the gathering of evidence and seeking the underlying pattern that explains the underlying dynamics (physical, psychological, spiritual) that solve the riddle of what caused the problems. Dreyfus and Dreyfus (1986) discuss pattern recognition as a factor in intuitive awareness.

This level of intuition, pattern recognition, is congruent with the prevalent materialist paradigms that guide and inform conventional medical and nursing practice. Intuition, however, can reach far beyond this level.

Inspiration and creativity

> When you are inspired by some great purpose, some extraordinary project, all your thoughts break their bonds; your mind transcends limitations, your consciousness expands in every direction, and you find yourself in a new, great and wonderful world. Dormant forces, faculties and talents become alive, and you discover yourself to be a greater person by far than you ever dreamed yourself to be.
>
> – Patanjali

Poets, writers, actors, painters, sculptors and others in the arts speak of inspiration that sparks their creativity. Inspiration may come as an idea in words. It is as though a voice speaks to them from another dimension, planting a new idea or a new way of perceiving or explaining something they are working on. Many speak of a *muse* that has the feel of a wise entity with a distinct personality, visiting from some other dimension when they are quiet and receptive to its whisper. The muse may show them directly what is helpful or may speak through imagery - sometimes in dreams. Among those acknowledging such inspiration are scientists, including André Ampère, Karl Gauss, Henri Poincaré, Michael Faraday, Lord Kelvin, Albert Einstein, Nikola Tesla and Thomas Edison, as well as poets, authors, actors, musicians and artists.

Where does the muse reside? Various explanations have included psychic abilities, a collective consciousness, spirit guides and Divine inspiration.

Research: Very few controlled studies have been published on intuitive assessments, but numerous workshops and courses in psychic development are advertised for the public. The following studies examined whether one such course, *The Silva Mind Control,* produced any positive results. Robert Brier and colleagues tested several graduates of this course, finding non-significant results overall. However, several children were included among their subjects, and when the individual adult subjects were studied separately, it was found that some achieved modestly significant results. Alan Vaughan, studying a single subject, found no significant results for her intuitive diagnoses.

Several tabulations of distant intuitive impressions (without control groups or statistical analyses) have been published. C. Norman Shealy, a neurosurgeon who has been a pioneer in the study of medical intuition and a past president of the American Holistic Medical Association, published several series of studies on medical intuitives, including the very gifted Carolyn Myss. In one series which required identification of the site of pain on the body, two of the intuitives studied achieved 75 percent accuracy and another reached 70 percent.

Nils Jacobson and Nils Wiklund studied a single subject who had taken a similar course called Swedish Mind Dynamics. He was unable to produce significant results with 10 diagnoses.

A series of 2,005 paired diagnoses by naturally gifted intuitives and doctors was briefly summarized by Karel Mison of Prague, in the Czech Republic. While the overall diagnostic agreement was 29 percent, one subject achieved 85 percent.

There are several controlled studies of energy field diagnosis. Susan Marie Wright's doctoral dissertation studied two healers' energy field diagnoses – to locate the pains in the bodies of 54 subjects. Highly significant results were found. Gary Schwartz and colleagues (1995) studied the abilities of 20 ordinary people to identify when the experimenter's hand was held above their own hand, finding modestly significant success. In a second experiment (Schwartz et al. 1996), 41 subjects were studied, and most of the subjects in the second group were familiar with their experimenter. In this study, highly significant results were obtained.

In contrast with the studies mentioned above, research by Linda Rosa et al, published in the prestigious *Journal of the American Medical Association* showed negative results for energy field diagnosis. This is an extraordinary study in several respects. First, it was a science fair project of a 10-year-old girl. Second, the negative findings of this study were interpreted by the journal editor, George D. Lundlberg, as proof that Therapeutic Touch healing is a worthless method of treatment. These findings and the editor's conclusion were widely publicized in the popular media, and widely criticized in the alternative medicine media. These studies are considered in detail in Chapter II-3.

A caution in research on medical intuition is highlighted by two pilot studies I did with healers who see auras (Benor 1992). The healers simultaneousl observed the same people with known medical diagnoses. Their observations differed substantially from each other. It appeared that each healer was looking at the subjects through a different window of perception. This was a great surprise to the healers, each of whom assumed that she had been seeing *THE way the aura appears*.

Figure II-12. Intuition

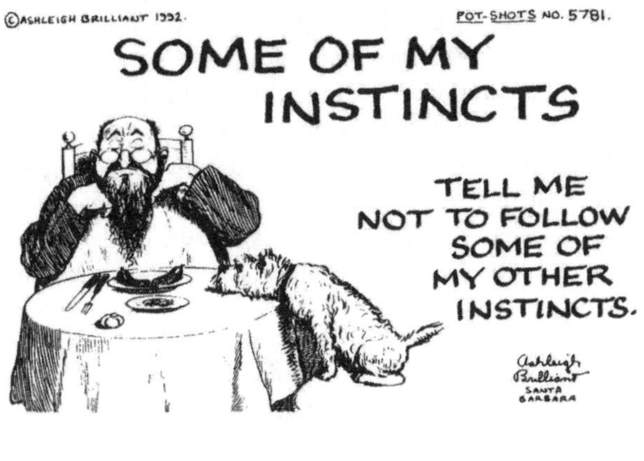

The second surprise came from the people whose auras were being observed. Each acknowledged the accuracy of the perceptions and interpretations of most of the healers. They validated that each of them was perceiving accurately – but only sensing part of the whole picture. One healer, however, apparently was projecting her own imagination on whatever she was perceiving, as there was no correlation with her "readings" with the patients' conditions.

Adverse effects: No harmful effects have been reported, though obvious cautions are needed to assure that the intuitive readings do not mislead us into foolish or dangerous assumptions or actions. See also the discussion of potential general negative effects from rapid release of buried emotional hurts and rapid improvements under Spiritual Healing.

See also: Pet therapy

Training and Certification: C. Norman Shealy, and Carolyn Myss have developed a certification for medical intuition.[179]

MEDICAL DOWSING

> *... Little appeared to be known of basic and primary causes, and it seemed impossible to diagnose departures from the normal in the very earlies stages. The average doctor was mainly engaged in baling out leaking boats.*
>
> – Aubrey Westlake (p. 3)

Dowsers are known for using intuition to locate water and other materials underground, and some develop medical intuitive diagnostic and healing gifts as well.

Dowsers use rods and pendulums to allow their unconscious minds to speak through unconscious movements of their hands and arms. This is very similar to the ideomotor movements of hypnosis and applied kinesiology. A dowser will hold a question in his mind and allow the instrument to answer it with movements that indicate a "yes" or a "no." Dowsers will walk across a field, focusing on the question, "Where is there water?" The dowsing rod will move in a distinct way to indicate when they are standing over an underground water supply. Dowsers can also get intuitive information from a distance, using a map to locate water or other substances.

I am impressed that the feedback derived from field and map dowsing provides an excellent way for many people to develop their intuitive gifts.

Many healers in other traditions, such as Healing Touch, use pendulums to get in touch with intuitive knowledge for diagnosis and healing.

In Britain there are also practitioners of *radiesthesia* and *radionics* who are essentially dowsers using instruments with dials, affectionately called *black boxes*, for dowsing and distant healing. These practices have been outlawed in America by the Food and Drug Administration, which has been very vigilant and at times merciless in prosecuting people who promote the use of these instruments.

Research: While no controlled studies on medical dowsing have been published, there is a promising body of research on field and map dowsing, reviewed in Chapter II-4.

Discussion: While genuine intuitive abilities can be of great help to therapists and people seeking diagnosis and treatment, one must be cautious in interpreting intuitive impressions. There is a distinct margin of error in this practice, as with all physical, psychological, and laboratory-based examinations. Also, intuitive impressions bear a strong imprint of the intuitive diagnostician. That is, different medical intuitives will perceive different impressions, even when examining the same subject at the same time (Benor 1992). While skeptics would view this as proof that medical intuition is faulty, I believe the truth is that it is simply more individualized – both to the particular medical intuitive and to the subject. Each intuitive appears to look into the being of the subject through a different window, providing a unique perspective on their condition.

Medical intuition is a vital element in numerous complementary therapies, often moreso for experienced therapists than for beginners. For instance, acupuncturists may learn to identify where acupuncture points are through their fingertips. Craniosacral therapists sense the rhythms of craniosacral biological energies, and may diagnose specific problems anywhere in the body through this process. Homeopathic and Flower essence practitioners and herbalists may intuitively identify which remedies are needed, and very advanced practitioners may intuit the specific problems that a new plant or other element can treat. Any therapist may intuitively think to ask a particular question or suggest a particular avenue for understanding or dealing with a problem that may be unusual, but which nevertheless precisely hits the mark and brings about new awareness of or changes in physical or psychological conditions (Benor 2001a).

Various approaches for self-assessment of health problems are growing in popularity. These include a spectrum of muscle-testing methods and imagery techniques. In the late 18th Century, hypnotherapists were able to induce profound trances called *somnambulism, or plenary hypnosis,* an altered state of consciousness in which people were able to diagnose their own physical and spiritual problems (Ellenberger). Medical dowsing is a sub-category of medical intuition. While these approaches may provide useful information, we must be cautious in interpreting and relying on these materials, as they can be distorted by our wishes, fears, beliefs or particular life experiences (Hayman). In addition, each intuive may perceive different aspects of a person's problems (Benor 1992).

Theories to explain intuitive awareness of problems that exist outside oneself include collective consciousness,[180] psychic perceptions, energetic resonations, a holographic universe, and spiritual awareness.[181] These overlap broadly with various theories that seek to explain aspects of healing.[182] Intuitive self-awareness is is well described in the literature on hypnosis.

Training, certification and licensing: It is possible to develop and enhance medical intuitive abilities. Intuition grows naturally through the practice of laying-on of hands healing. Meditation and imagery exercises can enhance it as well, and these approaches can also improve distant diagnostic abilities.

There is no general standardization of training or practice for medical intuition or dowsing, though several methods of healing, such as Therapeutic Touch, Healing Touch, and Barbara Brennan Healing, teach specific techniques. C. Norman Shealy, MD has developed standards for certification.[183]

Clinical efficacy: Medical intuition can be an enormously helpful supplement to integrative care - in clarifying problems and identifying issues of body, emotions, mind, relationships (with others and with the environment – and in selecting and guiding treatments.

While conventional wisdom recommends consulting a highly gifted intuitive to help in identifying causes of mysterious medical symptoms, developing our own intuitive capacities to identify the roots of our problems is also enormously helpful. In fact, this is one of the most effective of the self-healing approaches. It helps us connect with deep sources of inner wisdom – not just in our unconscious mind, but also through a deeper, spiritual awareness of the world beyond.

See also: Applied Kinesiology; Medical dowsing; Radionics and Radiesthesia; Remote viewing[184]

MEDITATION

> *... Question put to a Zen monk, while walking down a busy street. I was amazed by the way he took up the shock and the repercussions of the traffic and of the shoving crowds. After a while I said to him, "How do you get this way – self-controlled, orderly, integrated?" Because in those days I was searching for these qualities within myself.*
> *He said, "Well, if I'm different from anyone else, I must lay credit to one thing."*
> *"What is that?" I asked.*
> *He replied, "I never leave my place of meditation."*
> – Marcus Bach

Meditation appears to be a gateway to *alternative states of consciousness (ASCs)* in which self-healing and spiritual healing may occur.

How to meditate, and the experience of meditation
Meditation is not a way of mentally focusing upon a task as in ordinary states of consciousness, where the will is engaged in order to achieve a particular end. It is an opening up to allow a process to happen. The process is simply given a space or channel through which to occur.

There is an intentionality associated with meditation for healing, but it is passive rather than active. As one would not push a river to flow, so the healer does not *push* the energy to flow for the healing, nor does he push healees to improve faster than they are ready to be healed. It is as though a stream of energy is invited to flow through the meditator, and meditation clears away obstructions to this flow – gradually and thoroughly.

The effect of meditation has been likened to looking at the stars at night and at noon. During the daylight hours the competing stimuli of the sun's rays block the weaker light of the stars, making them invisible. At night, as in the meditative state, the process of turning off the overwhelming stimuli occurs and the stars are clearly visible.

– Marianne Borelli

For many of us, Meditation is hard work, because we do not know how to let go of our thinking in order to experience *being*. Though this sounds like a simple thing to do, many people find it requires practice. There are numerous ways to mediate, and I will discuss just a few of the better known approaches here.

Figure II-13. Stephen spends his morning on a snowy mountain peak in silent meditative communion with the rising sun

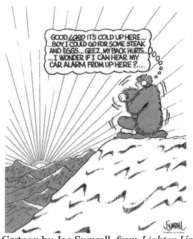

Cartoon by Joe Sumrall, from *Lighten Up*

Lawrence LeShan (1974b) summarizes practical aspects of meditation, ranging from the why and how of this practice to the social significance of its use. These are relevant to healing in many ways. LeShan identifies several paths and varieties of meditation:

1. *Intellect:* meditation "uses the intellect to go beyond the intellect, the will and directed thought processes to transcend themselves." (p. 33)
2. *Emotions:* there are "meditations that loosen the feelings and expand the ability to relate to others, to care and to love... some meditational schools concentrate on learning to love the self, some on learning to love others, some... to love God. Ultimately all arrive at the same place, loving all three." (p. 35)
3. *Body:* "... one learns to be aware of one's body and bodily movements and to heighten this awareness through practice, until, during... meditation, this awareness completely fills the field of consciousness to the exclusion of anything else." (p.36)
4. *Action:* meditation "consists of learning how to 'be' and to perceive and relate to the world during the performance of a particular skill... Various skills have been

used: archery, flower arrangement, Aikido and karate (two methods of unarmed combat) in the Zen tradition and rug weaving in the Sufi tradition. Singing and prayer have been used in the Christian tradition." (p. 37)

5. *Structured:* meditation "carefully and precisely defines what the inner activity is that you are working toward... Any straying... is corrected as soon as you become aware of your wandering." (p. 41)

6. *Unstructured.* "... you think about a subject and simply stay with the subject and your own feelings about it." (p. 42)

LeShan suggests specific meditations for each of the above-mentioned categories, recommending graded series and ways of varying meditations to suit individual needs. It is possible to do much of this on a self-taught basis, though the guidance of an expert may be desired with some types or in some stages of meditation. LeShan also details several distinct states of inner consciousness.[185]

Patricia Carrington reviews studies of meditation and related states. She has many practical suggestions on how to meditate, emphasizing the use of *mantras* (words repeated mentally). She discusses many functions and benefits of meditation, focusing most heavily on aspects of personal growth and psychotherapy. She summarizes her views:

> Meditation... is a time when the organism shifts gears from the active to the receptive mode; from a state of ego dominance to a state where the ego is subordinate and can be partially dispensed with; from a state of automatization to one of deautomatization. It may also be a time when the organism experiences a shift from the dominance of one cerebral hemisphere to a state of concordance or harmony between both hemispheres of the brain; and perhaps a time when it experiences a shift from limited contact with some as yet unidentified energy source toward a more deep fundamental contact, or 'flowing with', that source. (p. 315)

Arthur Dykeman has a lovely experiment demonstrating how simple it is to enter another reality through meditation. You simply stare for a while at a blue vase to get a sense of "being one with the vase." Many subjects report marked experiences of alternative states of consciousness within a short while.

Research: Benefits of meditation include reductions in pain; improvements in stress responses, diminished levels of substance abuse, and other behavioral parameters;[186] reduced pulse and blood pressure; changes in respiration rate, oxygen consumption and carbon dioxide elimination; reduced muscle tension and blood lactate levels (associated with anxiety and hypertension); subjective experiences of "feeling better" in various ways; lower cholesterol; reduced blood cortisol levels, when these are elevated due to stress; and reduced prostate specific antigen (PSA) with prostatic cancers. Extensive overviews of meditation research have been published.

Because meditation influences mental activities, its effects have been studied with electroencephalograms (EEGs) and brain imaging devices. These confirm that there are measurable changes in brain activity with meditation, but the interpretations of the findings are as yet far from clear. The brain is an extremely complex organ, whose capacity exceeds that of the best computers in the world.

In its subjective effects, meditation is a clearing of all extraneous preoccupations from the mind, and as such it can be of great benefit to healees because it allows them to focus exclusively upon the task of self-healing. It also facilitates release of worries, anxieties and fears related to serious illness – which can become self-perpetuating vicious circles. Meditation in and of itself also appears to convey benefits on physical, mental, emotional and spiritual levels.

For healers, meditation appears to provide a gateway to states of being in which spiritual healing can be facilitated. Quiet meditation by the healee appears to facilitate distant healing, especially when it coincides with the sending of healing.

The practice of meditation has been found to be cost effective, in that those who meditate regularly have significantly reduced health care use.

I have mentioned only a few of numerous teachers who discuss meditation and its benefits. A fuller knowledge of this important branch of human exploration can be of benefit not only in developing greater self-knowledge and awareness but also in learning to heal ourselves and others of the ills that can mark or accompany our progress along the paths of our existence.

Lessons from meditation
The improvements in physical conditions that result from meditation may be explained as relaxation effects that reduce physical and emotional tensions. These changes then bring about neurophysiological and neurohormonal changes that improve physical problems.

If we allow that bioenergies may be shaped by consciousness, we can see how these can provide pathways for relaxation effects to influence the body. Meditation can alter our energy fields, which in turn can improve body functions. Furthermore, in helping us to connect with our higher selves, meditation may strengthen our abilities to access those energetic aspects of ourselves which can facilitate healing.

The subjective experiences of meditation have far-reaching effects and implications. Meditation can open the mind into awarenesses that transcend the individual self. Our ordinary states of consciousness rely on our outer senses and thought processes, which are grounded in the experiences of physical existence. Inner experiences of emotions are tied to our physical being and our relationships with others in our physical environment.

In meditative states we can become aware of transpersonal realms that extend beyond the individual self. These may be explained as:

1. Fantasies, wishful thinking, denial of death, or other mental projections;
2. Awarenesses of realms of experience that legitimately extend beyond our perceptions of the ordinary, physical and psychological world (These are extensively discussed in Chapter II-1 and Volume III); or
3. The result of activity within particular parts of the brain, which create the subjective experience of unusual experiences.

The first hypothesis is difficult to support, in view of the similar reports of transpersonal experiences from cultures all around the world.

A logical argument can be made for the third hypothesis. The similarities of meditative experiences and other altered states of consciousness in cultures around the world could be an indication that these are simply products of the biochemical and bioelectrical processes of the brain.

However, an argument can equally well be made for the second point of view. The similarities of meditative experiences and other altered states of consciousness in cultures around the world could be an indication that these are consensual perceptions of realities in other dimensions.

I believe that there are other dimensions of reality which we can reach through spontaneous psi experiences and alternative states of consciousness, such as those achieved through meditation and prayer. My subjective experiences, particularly in spiritual healing interactions, is that these intuitively perceived realities feel more valid and real on deeper levels than the outer realities in my life. I will discuss these issues in much greater depth in Volume III.

Meditation offers profound healings in and of itself, and can enhance and deepen the effects of spiritual healing.

Effects of meditation on healees

1. Meditation may act directly to normalize respiration, blood pressure and other neurohormonal concomitants of anxiety. These effects alone may be beneficial, regardless of which disease processes may be present. Reduced anxiety and relaxation may also lead to subjective relief from pain.

2. Meditation may powerfully sharpen the focus of inner energies – as a single-minded activation of self-healing – to deal with whatever disease processes are present or to correct hormonal and/or energy imbalances or disharmonies. In ordinary consciousness the mind may be distracted, so mental energies may be scattered and therefore less than optimally focused on healing. With meditation, all of the healee's mental energies can be directed towards healing, thereby achieving more potent effects. This may be analogous to karate, where physical energies are narrowly focused on a target along with mental intent, maximizing the effect of the applied energies. The mental intent is vital to the success of the karate. Meditation may be a mental karate, enhancing internal applications of healing energies.

As self-healing, this enhanced focus may be similar to the increased control over body processes achieved under hypnosis. There are many points of similarity between meditation and hypnosis, such as concentrating on one subject to the exclusion of all others; focusing on rhythmic, repetitive stimuli; and relinquishing investment in outwardly-directed thought. In the context of spiritual healing there is the further similarity of placing one's self in the hands of a skilled therapist.

3. Meditation may teach healees to focus mentally and to visualize themselves free of disease, in the process of self-healing. This could be a form of positive thinking, de-emphasizing the illeness aspects and enhancing the awareness of the healthy aspects of one's life.

4. Meditation may enable healees to tap healing resources from other levels of reality. Healees may achieve this on their own, or may be aided in linking through meditation with a healer who can facilitate connections with other dimensions. The realms of higher self/ spirit and angelic guides/ Divine inspiration become available through meditative practices.

Effects of meditation on healees

For many healers, the meditative state facilitates healing, and may even be a prerequisite for activation of healing. Important components of this state include:

1. Reduction or elimination of sensory and mental distractions may permit a more efficient, forceful utilization of healing powers or energies. This could permit activation of portions of the healer's mind that are ordinarily unused, by shutting off the constant noise of observing, thinking and emotional activities. Perhaps this involves shifts from left-brain to right-brain functions, or a more balanced coordination of the right and left brain hemispheres.[187] It may also involve the activation of deeper, less conscious portions of the mind.

2. Mental concentration may facilitate a greater ability to focus the transfer of energies from within the healers or through them to the healees. The analogy to karate is again applicable.

3. (1) may lead healers into a mode of *being* rather than *doing,* in which they can set aside preconceptions, associations and thoughts, and just commune with their healees. It may facilitate an unconditional acceptance of the healees, which is the sine qua non of psychotherapy..

4. (1) may enable healers to be more in contact with and to deliberately utilize forces and energies in the realms of realities that are otherwise not available to them. Healers may then channel these cosmic forces of nature through themselves to the healees.

5. (1) and (3) may help to release of perceptions of a disease-reality and may permit the establishment of a health-reality via (2-4). This process, which may include visualization, may lead to a restructuring of healees' bodies so that they can relinquish disease processes and begin to be healed, or, in special cases, be instantaneously transformed to a state of health.

> *When the mind is still, tranquil, not seeking any answer or solution even, neither resisting nor avoiding, it is only then that there can be a regeneration, because then the mind is capable of perceiving what its true and it is the truth that liberates, not our effort to be free.*
>
> – Krishnamurti

It is fascinating to me that some healers do not seem to require a state of meditation for successful healings to occur. They are able to invoke a healing state automatically. Many healers report that the frequent releases of conscious focus that they practice during healing also carries over into everyday life. It is particularly common for healers to be easily distractible and to have memory problems. Some of these healers easily enter an alternative state of consciousness in which they can even converse freely without disturbing the healing process. These healers seem open to healing awareness most of the time, so that they don't have to shift out of ordinary awareness to enter a healing state.

I know one strong healer who finds that her long-term memory does not record much of the data processed in conversations that take place during healings, although she is able to discuss any normal topic intelligently and coherently while she is healing.

Subjective and psychotherapeutic benefits of meditation
The mechanisms for self-healing effects of meditation require further research. It is clear, however, that meditation can be used in practical ways to address focal problems. For instance, if you are stuck with an issue that you can't resolve, using a creative imagery meditation can open up possibilities that you have overlooked.[188]

It is common to practice meditation while focusing upon an external object, such as a lit candle, a plant, or some other aspect of nature. With even a modest meditation period of 30-60 minutes you may find yourself so strongly identifying with the object that you feel you *are* the object, and can sense many aspects of its essence. You can equally well focus on some inner part of yourself, such as an ache or pain, an illness, or a psychological conflict. With the support and guidance of a therapist (you are strongly advised not to do this on your own), you may immerse yourself totally in a symptom or issue. By totally connecting with a problem, rather than avoiding its unpleasantness, you may find that its negativity is rapidly and markedly diminished. A variety of meditations can be helpful in this way.[189]

Going deeper, you can invite your pain, illness, or other problem to speak to you, and to tell you what it wants to say in words – rather than just in symptoms. Symptoms may often be messengers from your unconscious mind, inviting you to explore or release old issues.[190]

> *It is only with the heart that one can see rightly; what is essential is invisible to the eye.*
> – Antoine de Saint-Exupéry

These are very different sorts of meditations than those associated with more prolonged traditional meditative practice. These are deliberate forms of therapy, intended to help particular problems.

Deep therapeutic changes are also often reported with regular meditation that is practiced for spiritual development. Meditators frequently claim that with prolonged practice they find that very profound positive changes occur in their personalities, their outlooks, their interpersonal relationships, their physical health and in other aspects of their life.

> *He who looks outwardly, dreams. But he who looks within, awakes.*
> – Carl Jung

These changes often resemble the results achieved through successful transpersonal psychotherapy.

For many years I was puzzled by this spontaneous resolution of problems during meditation that did not deliberately focus on the problems – but in fact seemed designed to focus the mind *away* from these, along with the avoidance of all other intrusions on the meditative focus.

In psychotherapy the goal is usually to uncover conflicts and emotions that have been buried in the unconscious mind and then to deal with them. The repressed problems reveal themselves though troublesome reactions and behaviors that are disproportionate to the stresses in one's present life. The work of psychotherapy is often long and arduous, requiring meticulous conscious analysis of associations from conflictual material and projections of feelings upon others, tracing back to the roots of these problems in the depths of well defended repressions. Alternatively, behavioral approaches seek to restructure cognitive responses and reactions to inner and outer stimuli that are troublesome.

Newer techniques permit the rapid release of symptoms and hurts – even when we have carried them with us for years. As mentioned above, you may immerse yourself totally in a symptom or issue (with the support of a therapist) and surprisingly, this often leads to release of suffering – rather than to greater suffering (that logic suggests might result from focusing on the problems). [191]

In meditation one does not follow associations, or look for repressed material, or push to release emotions that have not been expressed in times past. In fact, it would seem that meditation seeks to teach the exact antithesis of such endeavors – which is to set aside all associations and feelings and not to invest them with attention or importance. This appears at first glance to be similar to, if not identical with pathological processes such as denial and repression that produce so many of the psychological problems that I work very hard to get clients (and myself) to overcome.

I finally realized that this puzzle is only an apparent paradox, and is related to the questions that are asked about meditative practices and processes. It appears problematic only as long as one focuses on what occurs in *psychopathology*. If we ask instead what is occuring in psychotherapy and meditation that is *positive*, the similarities begin to emerge and the apparent contradictions disappear. Both meditation and psychotherapy teach people to let go of their attachments to prior belief systems and unhealthy habits of self-criticism and doubt. Psychopathology can be seen as a dis-ease engendered by a disparity between an individual's present situation and the way she believes her situation to be (based on experiences from the past), or the way she wishes it to be (based on hopes, aspirations, anxieties or fears regarding the future). In this context, the task of psychotherapy is either to help her identify and release her rigidly maintained guidelines from the past or relinquish her unrequited wishes or worries about the future. Similarly, meditation helps people to let go of all of their conflicts that do not exist in the immediate here and now.

Newer psychotherapy techniques also permit the rapid release of symptoms and hurts – even when we have carried them with us for years. You may immerse yourself totally in a symptom or issue, and surprisingly, this often leads to release of suffering – rather than to greater suffering.

Meditation may take one even deeper, opening into transcendent awareness in which everything is in the eternal *Now* and physical existence is but a moment in a vaster awareness.

> *Now is the only time over which we have dominion.*
> – Leo Tolstoy

Some holistic therapists believe that meditation alone is sufficient as a way of dealing with stresses and emotional problems. While this may be true in some cases, psychotherapy may be necessary in others. Jack Kornfield (1993, p. 249) observes, "Just as deep meditation requires a skilled teacher, at times our spiritual path also requires a skilled therapist. Only a deep attention to the whole of our life can bring us to the capacity to love well and to live freely."

While meditation may be practiced purely for its spiritual benefits, Kornfield suggests other benefits:

> The purpose of spiritual life is not to create some special state of mind. A state of mind is always temporary. The purpose is to work directly with the most primary elements of our body and our mind, to see the ways we get trapped by our fears, desires, and anger, and to learn directly our capacity for freedom. As we work with them, the demons will enrich our lives. They have been called "manure for enlightenment" or "mind weeds," which we pull up or bury near the plant to give it nourishment.
>
> To practice [meditation] is to use all that arises within us for the growth of understanding, compassion, and freedom. Thomas Merton wrote, "True love and prayer are learned in the hour when love becomes impossible and the heart has turned to stone." When we remember this, the difficulties we encounter in practice can become part of the fullness of meditation, a place to learn and to open our heart. (p. 99-100)

Meditation may involve different practices and processes and have different effects for people in Eastern and Western cultures. In Western culture we emphasize individuation, while in the East people are expected to function primarily as a part of their family and social group. As Joseph Campbell (1972) points out:

> The word 'I'... suggests to the Oriental philosopher only wishing, wanting, desiring, fearing, and possessing, i.e., the impulses of what Freud has termed the id operating under pressure of the pleasure principle...
>
> The virtue of the Oriental is comparable, then, to that of the good soldier, obedient to orders, personally responsible not for his acts but only for their execution. And since all the laws to which he is adhering will have been handed down from an infinite past, there will be no one anywhere personally responsible for the things that he is doing...

In a related observation, Kornfield reports:

> ... When I worked in Asian monasteries there was very little attention to what might be called personal, or psychological problems. In fact, upon returning from America, one of the great masters commented that he had seen a kind of suffering over here that he wasn't so familiar with – "they call it psychological suffering, whatever that is."

It would be fascinating if sensitives who perceive mental and emotional layers of the aura would observe meditators from the East and the West, and report on any differences they note in the energy fields of meditators – over the immediate and the long term practice of meditation.

Some may use meditation as a means of avoidance or escape, rather than as a form of cleansing, which is sometimes termed a *meditational bypass.*. Jack Kornfield calls these meditators *skippers*. I know many who have reached very refined levels of development on spiritual dimensions, but who have neglected to work through or release much of the dross in their physical/ psychological/ emotional levels.

Meditation offers additional psychotherapeutic elements. These include encouraging an appreciation of one's place in the cosmos; placing psychological conflicts in a new and more healthy perspective; and introducing an inner peace that appears to derive from the deeply satisfying, spiritual, noetic experience of being one with the All.[192]

It is conceivable that practicing meditation from childhood, or in other ways learning the art of being in the present, may help one avoid unnecessary conflicts caused by self-imposed, unsatisfying comparisons between conditions in time-present and other temporal contexts, wishes or fears. It is unclear whether the ideal of total self-differentiation without conflicts is attainable. Satprem leads us to believe this is possible in gifted individuals. Kornfield and Irina Tweedie provide excellent descriptions of the processes and challenges encountered on such paths.

The subject of potential negative reactions to meditation deserves further study. It is my impression that people who are emotionally unstable, or whose personal boundaries between themselves and the rest of the world are not very firm, may find the experience of meditation frightening. The impairments in psychological boundaries in their ordinary states of consciousness, due to their emotional instability, is often troubling to them and to others around them. The loss of conscious awareness during meditation may arouse further anxieties.

This sort of anxiety may lead people to become anxious about being anxious, which I term *meta-anxiety.*[193] Unchecked, this can escalate to panic proportions. It is possible that some of the negative reactions to meditation are due to meta-anxiety around fears of losing control rather than to effects of the meditation in and of itself.

For all of the discussion *about* meditation, it is impossible to appreciate its nature and benefits without trying it for yourself. I highly recommend this practice to anyone interested in self-healing and spiritual development.

Adverse effects: Though it is a rare occurrence, there have been occasional reports of serious negative experiences with meditation. People who are prone to emotional instability are advised to use meditation only under professional supervision. Meditation may intensify obsessiveness; produce insomnia and depression; elicit psychosomatic symptoms; precipitate psychotic decompensation; and bring about withdrawal from engagement with normal life activities and relationships.

Short of such severe effects, which are not very common, simple *emotional releases* are common and mild negative experiences are not uncommon during meditation. It appears that as people relax, their psychological defenses also relax. Long-buried emotional hurts may then surface to consciousness, with accompany-ing releases of buried feelings. At times this brings recognition of the earlier precipitating traumas, but it may also occur as a release of feelings without attached memories.

These potential problems are best dealt with by experienced meditation teachers.

It is worth mentioning here that teachers are human and all of them are still learning the challenging lessons of life. None is perfect. In fact, some are so far from perfection that one may wonder how they presume to teach others. One is cautioned, therefore, not to assume that everyone who claims to be a teacher of meditation is competent to do so with people who may have serious life issues to deal with. Meditation instructors, as with any therapist, should be screened by prospective students – as is suggested at the end of this chapter. This is not to say that because of their imperfections, we cannot learn from flawed teachers. Brugh Joy (1990, p.102) reminds us, "You are not there to verify facts about the teacher. You are there to experience some aspect of your Self."

There is no general credentialing and no standard training in the teaching of meditation. Eastern religions and Transcendental Meditation specify clear requirements for instructors. Several stress management programs at universities have developed courses for the therapeutic use of meditation.[194]

Clinical applications: Meditation is an excellent avenue to relaxation, and it can contribute to prevention and treatment of most stress-related illnesses. It is great for development of spiritual awareness.

See also: Chapter II-1 on self-healing and on meditation as a transpersonal therapy; Chapter I-1 on healer and healee reports of subjective experiences of healing; Volume III of *Healing Research* on research in spiritual dimensions; Chapters IV-2 and IV-3 on dissections of the spiritual healing experience.

MERIDIAN BASED THERAPIES (MERIDIAN PSYCHOTHERAPY)

> *There is only one corner of the universe you can be certain of improving...*
> *and that's your own self.*
>
> – Aldous Huxley

Included among these approaches are *Thought Field Therapy* (*TFT*),[195] and its many derivatives.[196] Healees focus on their psychological problems while to applying pressure to acupuncture points on their head, chest, and/ or hand with their fingers. Within minutes they usually find that irrational fears or the hurts of old emotional traumas are released, and long-held disbeliefs and negative beliefs are transformed. These approaches can markedly alleviate and sometimes even cure chronic pains and allergies.[197] Positive beliefs and feelings can then be instilled through the same techniques, to replace whatever negativity has been released.

Muscle testing of applied kinesiology can be used to guide clients to the roots of their problems, and to set up the mental focus for pressure point treatment.[198]

Often, mental processing of the roots of their problems is not necessary, although in many cases people do spontaneously come to understand how their problems developed and how they were maintained by choice or through psychological and relational reinforcements. This contradicts the teachings of many varieties of mainstream psychotherapy, which insist that without cognitive awareness and understanding of the roots of our problems we cannot achieve true healing.

CASE: Joe was afraid of heights, which interfered with his life in a variety of ways. If an elevator was not working, he could not climb the stairs if there was an open stairwell where he could see the stairs below him, and he couldn't go down a flight of stairs without suffering a panic attack. He had to take tranquilizers to travel by plane, and this made him groggy when he landed, necessitating extra days' stay during business trips to clear his mind. Repairing anything in his home that required standing on a chair or ladder was something he avoided at all costs.

At a stress reduction workshop, I introduced WHEE, which is rapidly and potently effective in dealing with stresses of all sorts. WHEE differs from other meridian based therapies because it includes major components of EMDR.[199] Joe, who wanted to work on his fear of heights, participated skeptically, not really expecting to have any response. He alternated tapping on his right and left eyebrows, while repeating an affirmation, "Even though I'm afraid of heights, I love and accept myself wholly and completely, and God loves and accepts me wholly, completely and unconditionally."

Before starting to tap, Joe estimated his initial level of anxiety when thinking about heights was 15 on a scale of zero to ten. Within 5 minutes, after four rounds of tapping, he was down to zero – much to his amazement. Next, using the same technique, he installed a positive affirmation: "I can look down from a height and feel comfortable." After several rounds of tapping he brought this from a zero to an eight. He just couldn't believe this would really work, so we had him go out and climb the stairs. He reported back in amazement that he felt only mild anxiety going down the stairs, and none going up – even though it was an open stairwell. With repeated tapping, he strengthened the positive affirmation to a level ten.

He subsequently used this technique himself to overcome his fear of flying as well. I had a grateful note from him several months later, reporting that WHEE had transformed his life in many ways.

One of the greatest benefits of these approaches is that they can be practiced by the client for self-healing. Once people know the methods, they can proceed, if they wish, to do a systematic house-cleaning of old emotional and habitual debris that they may have carried around for years.

> *'Tis not enough to help the feeble up,*
> *But to support them after.*
>
> – William Shakespeare (*Timon of Athens*)

My personal experiences with these Meridian Based Therapies is that they are profoundly effective in releasing old hurts and in relieving many of the accompanying chronic physical problems, and in installing positive beliefs. EMDR may also spontaneously bring people into a deep state of spiritual awareness. I was at first skeptical that these results could be more than superficial or temporary improvements because I had been biased by my conventional psychotherapy training to believe that psychological insight and conscious understanding of problems are required for full healing. The astounding results achieved with these therapies testifies that one can release old hurts and move on to healthier psychological functioning without conscious understanding of the roots or develop-mental processes of the problems.

Research: While there is a solid database of research for EMDR, there are only a few studies demonstrating effectiveness of the meridian based therapies.

Clinical applications: I am personally impressed that this the meridian based therapies are among the best and most potent of self-haling interventions – helpful with emotional stress and distress, limiting beliefs, self-defeating attitudes, addictions (food, smoking, drugs), acute and chronic physical pains, and allergies.

See also: EMDR, Applied Kinesiology.

NATIVE AMERICAN MEDICINE

> *... When we come into the Earthwalk, we come in with truth encoded in us. But we can lose sight of that. The only ones who do not know who they are are the two-leggeds. So sometimes we have to open up and receive messages from the Spirit to remember...*
> – Grandmother Twylah Nitch

It is difficult to speak of Native American medicine generically when there are about 500 distinct Nations or tribes, each with its own traditions and practices that date back over an estimated 12,000 to 40,000 years. There is also the universal Native American tradition of honoring individual innovations, which are derived in varied clinical situations according to the intuition of each individual healer.

Common denominators in Native American medicine include a belief in a *life force* (called *ni* in Lakota) or *divine breath,* and a concept of disease seen "in terms of morality, balance, and the action of spiritual power rather than specific, measurable causes." Illnesses are felt to occur when individuals are not in harmony with themselves, their relationships with other people, and with the natural world. Diagnosis may be derived by speaking with the person and their family and community, or through divination, prayer, and consultation with nature guides and spirit guides. Treatments may include counseling to identify internal problems (such as negative thinking); dream interpretation; herbal medicines; chanting or other rituals (drumming, dances, fasts, sweat lodge ceremonies, laying-on of hands); and asking the help of spirits of the natural world, or of the Great Spirit. Diagnosis and treatment is a highly individualized art, so it is impossible for outsiders simply to copy rituals and expect that they will work for anyone but the original practitioner.

Native American medicine is not exclusive of other practices, and it can be used in harmony with Western treatments.

Adverse effects: No harmful effects have been reported. See discussions under Spiritual Healing and Shamanism.

Training and certification: There are no standards for practice or certification. Training is by calling and apprenticeship and highly individualized to the gifts of the individual medicine man or woman.

Clinical applications: Native American medicine is a complete therapy system. While it is particularly helpful for Native Americans, it has also been effective in treatment of many disorders in people who are not native to this tradition.

A medicine man will guide and lead the healee through appropriate ceremonies, and can recommend various practices and herbs for healing. Self-healing exercises and practices may be prescribed.

See also: Shamanism.

NATUROPATHIC MEDICINE

Medicine may be good or bad according to the intent with which we use it or how it affects people. A kind word is good medicine, and an insulting or a discouraging word is bad medicine. A natural herb received from a compassionate healer is good medicine. The same herb, offered by an angry person, is bad medicine. A stethoscope is good medicine when used by a caring and wise physician. A stethoscope is an instrument of evil if the physician is demeaning to the patient.
                                                  – Ken Cohen (2003)

Naturopathic medicine has been practiced in the US since the early 1900s. At the height of its popularity, there were over 20 naturopathic medical schools. In 1910, the Flexner Report established guidelines for the funding of medical schools. This was a political coup for allopathic doctors, as the Flexner recommendations gave preference to schools approved by the American Medical Association. This led to a rapid decline in the practice of naturopathy, almost to the point of its disappearance in the US. In the past 20 years naturopathy has seen a marked revival. There are 3 naturopathic medicine schools and about 1,000 naturopathic doctors (NDs) practicing in the US today.

Naturopathy includes nutrition and life-style counseling, herbal remedies, homeopathy, flower remedies, acupuncture, traditional Chinese medicine, various manipulative therapies and other CAM approaches. The major focus is on supporting, stimulating and strengthening the self-healing potentials within the body. Treatments are directed at causes rather than at symptoms. The doctor is a teacher who promotes and maintains optimal health in the whole person.

Research: Rigorous research in naturopathic treatments is in its infancy. For instance, a study of naturopathy for treatment of abnormal cells in the cervix showed a return to normalcy in 38 out of 43 women with abnormal Pap smears.

Adverse effects: See under specific therapeutic modality.

Training and licensing: Naturopathic training in the US involves a four-year, 4,100-hour course at a recognized school. Naturopathic physicians (ND or NMD) are licensed in a dozen states after passing a nationally standardized formal examination[200] for provision of primary health care,[201] and in most of the Canadian provinces. In other states, anyone may claim to be a naturopathic practitioner, even with minimal training. There are also Naturopathic doctorate programs at several universities.[202]

The Council on Naturopathic Medical Education (CNME) accredits schools and training programs and is recognized by the US Department of Education. The American Association of Naturopathic Physicians (AANP) is the US professional association.

In the UK, the General Council and Register of Naturopaths (GCRN) is the professional organization for Naturopaths, who are not covered by statutory regulation. Training also varies, with some Naturopaths graduating from 4-year courses and others with far less training.

Growing numbers of medical and osteopathic physicians and nurses in the US and UK are incorporating many naturopathic approaches in their practices. The American Holistic Medical Association (AHMA) promotes these approaches and the American Board of Holistic Medicine (ABHM) offers Board examinations in Holisitc Medicine. The American Holistic Nurses Association (AHNA) similarly promotes naturopathic practices integrated with conventional nursing.

Clinical applications: Naturopathy encourages a healthy lifestyle and is certainly helpful in promoting and maintaining health and preventing disease. As naturopathy may include a very broad range of treatments, one must assess its efficacy according the successes of the individual treatments applied.

Integrative care is developing gradually, with naturopathy complementing conventional medicine particularly in herbal and nutritional interventions,[203] as well as in other CAM approaches.

A naturopathic doctor can be helpful in prescribing and recommending therapies for most illnesses. Self-healing practices may also be recommended.

See also: Anthroposophic Medicine, Ayurvedic Medicine, individual CAM therapies.

NUTRITIONAL AND HERBAL THERAPIES

> *2000 BC: Here, eat this root.*
> *1000 AD: That root is heathen. Here, say this prayer.*
> *1850 AD: That prayer is superstition. Here, drink this potion.*
> *1940 AD: That potion is snake oil. Here, swallow this pill.*
> *1985 AD: That pill is ineffective. Here, take this antibiotic.*
> *2000 AD: That antibiotic is no longer effective. Here, eat this root.*
> — Anonymous

Diets

Numerous specialized diets have been recommended by various types of practitioners for health maintenance and for treatment of illnesses. These range from
trendy fads to well-studied regimens of inclusion and exclusion of particular nutritional elements.

One obvious recommendation is to eat organically grown fruits and vegetables
that do not contain pesticides or preservatives, and meat from animals that have
not been given growth hormones, antibiotics or other chemicals. Such chemicals
could be toxic – if not immediately, then on a cumulative basis.

Other cautions include avoiding irradiated and genetically modified foods, foods
cooked in Teflon (over 600 degrees) or in aluminum cookware, and foods stored
in plastics. Water from municipal supplies is often recycled without clearing out
the metabolized products of myriads of drugs taken by people who excrete these
into the sewage system – providing those who drink this water with a cocktail of
unknown chemicals. Bottled water alone may be unhealthy over the long run.
Another suggestion is to avoid foods that have been cooked in Teflon (at over 600
degrees) or aluminum cookware, as these may be unhealthy.

The general field of nutrition is too vast to summarize adequately here. I can
only discuss a few salient problems and studies.

Elimination diets can help to identify food allergies. An initial restriction of intake to non-allergenic foods such as rice for a week may allow the body to clear
itself of allergens and of the various related symptoms. Specific allergies can then
be identified through serial additions of single food items, spaced over several
days. Avoidance of the offending foods, and implementation of various desensitization procedures can then be instituted. Desensitization may include meridian-
based therapies, which involve a self-healing acupressure technique.

We commonly think of allergic reactions as direct responses of our digestive
systems to something we eat or drink. Sometimes other organs may also respond
with allergic reactions, such as our skin (with hives and other rashes); airways
and lungs (wheezing, asthma, or even complete shutting off of our breath from
sever swelling of the airways); eyes (itching, redness); muscles (weakness, fatigue, fibromyalgia); and brain/ mind (confusion, memory problems, tiredness,
attention and hyperactivity disorders).

Elimination of allergens and/or toxins may help in treating many of these problems. For instance, there are numerous anecdotal reports that mercury in dental
amalgam may produce signs of toxicity, which can be relieved by removal of the
offending fillings. In Attention Deficit Hyperactivity Disorder, elimination of
allergenic foods may reduce symptomatology.

Fasting is helpful in several ways. It can clear toxins, as in the initial phase of an
elimination diet. Fasting is in itself a discipline, and it can produce alternative
states of consciousness that are conducive to meditative and spiritual experiences.

Vegetarian diets can promote better health in several ways. Especially today,
when pesticides and other chemical pollutants are accumulating in our environment, this may be very wise advice. Many of the synthetic chemical pollutants are
not metabolized by plants or excreted by animals. Animals who eat chemically

polluted vegetation accumulate these substances in their bodies, and the levels in their flesh may be much more concentrated than those found in the environment. When we eat the flesh of these animals, the toxins accumulate in our bodies as well.

Organically grown vegetable, poultry, fish and meat products are a precaution against ingesting pollutants and toxic chemicals. Healers sensitive to bioenergetic vibrations report that organic foods have far greater vitality than those grown with chemical fertilizers, pesticides and hormones.

Specific benefits of vegetarian diets have been observed. They can reduce our fat and cholesterol intake, which is helpful in treating cardiovascular disease.

Significant improvements in rheumatoid arthritis were demonstrated with four months on a vegetarian diet, followed by gradual reintroduction of non-vegetable foods, with careful observation to see whether they caused any reactions over the course of a year. In the field of cancer there are promising studies suggesting the efficacy of some diets. The most common recommendation is to avoid red meat.

Vitamins: Ordinary (rational) doses of vitamins prevent vitamin deficiency diseases. They may also be helpful in treating certain conditions, such as learning disabilities in children.

Recommended dietary allowances (RDAs) for vitamins were established in 1943 by the US National Research Council. These standards represent the minimal doses required to prevent vitamin deficiency syndromes such as scurvy and rickets. Since 1945, food manufacturers have been required by 22 states to enrich certain foods with vitamins.

In recent decades there has been a growing awareness that various supplements can alleviate and prevent many more diseases than was previously appreciated. Now, various governmental agencies are in the process of updating and replacing RDAs with Dietary Reference Intakes (DRIs). These will include Estimated Average Requirements (EARs) and Tolerable Upper Intake Levels (ULs). Where recommended doses have not been established, Adequate Intake levels (AIs) are provided, based on the best available estimates.

Megavitamin therapy has been recommended for many problems. It is speculated that some people are less efficient at absorbing some vitamins, so they may require larger doses to achieve normal metabolic function. Megavitamin doses may also be recommended for specific problems. For instance, doses of 4-6,000 units of vitamin C are anecdotally reported to prevent and to hasten recovery from viral upper respiratory infections.

Other supplements: Coenzyme Q_{10} (CoQ$_{10}$) may prevent and help treat cardiac problems because it facilitates metabolism, particularly in heart muscle. In cardiac disease, heart muscle is often deficient in this enzyme. Significant improvement in cardiac function and survival time were achieved when 100 mg/day of CoQ_{10} was given. In another study, there was less fluid accumulation in the lungs and fewer hospitalizations were required for people with congestive heart failure when CoQ_{10} was given.

Galantamine, derived from the snowdrop plant *(Galanthus nivalis)* and related species appears to enhance intelligent, purposive consciousness, and it is being explored as a treatment in early Alzheimer's.

Orthomolecular medicine is a growing specialty in the spectrum of megavitamin and mineral supplement therapies, focused on preventon and treatment of disease through optimal doses of natural substances..

A sample of problems treated with vitamins, minerals and enzymes

Osteoarthritis, which most of us suffer as our bones and joints degenerate with age and wear, has responded to treatment with several natural substances. In clinical studies, 900-4,000 mg. of niacinamide taken daily increased the range of motion in joints and decreased pain and stiffness within four weeks of starting treatment, with further improvements as the therapy was continued. Niacinamide has been shown to produce better pain reduction than the pain medicine ibuprofen. It appears that glucosamine not only reverses symptoms but also stimulates repair of arthritic joints. Glucosamine sulfate at doses of 500 mg. three times a day produced significant relief of pain, swelling, and joint tenderness.

Allergies: Various nutritional and herbal therapies help in treating allergies; reducing incidence of kidney stones; treating digestive disorders; addressing women's endocrine problems, diabetes, cancer, gingivitis, anxiety, depression, and schizophrenia. This area of research is blossoming rapidly, and only a few of many examples of the potentials of orthomolecular medicine are given here.

Fatigue is a classical symptom suggesting a need for vitamins. Vitamin B_{12} (5 mg. twice a week) significantly enhances overall well-being and happiness, and suggestive results were found for fatigue and appetite loss as well.

Theories: One of the theories behind some of the megavitamin therapies is that oxidants in the body may predispose certain people to cancers. Some vitamins and minerals are anti-oxidants. While anti-oxidants may help prevent cancers, there has also been speculation that they might interfere with chemotherapy or radiotherapy. A review of research on this subject has not confirmed these fears.

Conventional medicine has been skeptical about nutritional approaches, and most medical schools provide little or no education in nutrition and nutritional therapies. Hospital diets are notoriously unhealthy, in some cases not even providing the minimum daily requirements of nutrients and vitamins to sustain health, much less to assist in recuperation from illness and surgery.

This is too vast a subject to even touch upon adequately in this book, and further reading is highly recommended.

Herbal remedies

In Europe, herbal medicine *(phytotherapy)* has been extensively researched over the past decade. For instance, milk thistle *(Siloybum marianum)* helps alcoholic cirrhosis of the liver. Bilberry *(Vaccinium myrtillus)* alleviates veinous insufficiency in the legs; relieves cramps from varicose veins; and reduces pain and itching of hemorrhoids due to venous insufficiency after pregnancy. Valerian (*Valeriana officinalis*) helps people to fall asleep and also deepens sleep.

St. John's Wort (*hypericum perforatum*) is the most widely used antidepressant in several countries in Europe because it is both effective and has almost no side effects. A meta-analysis of 23 studies of *hypericum* for mild to moderate depression showed that 61 percent of users improved on a low dose, while 75 percent improved with a higher dose. Another meta-analysis, with more rigorous criteria, also concluded that St. John's Wort was superior to a placebo. People with decreased activity, fatigue and sleep disorders, as well as people with seasonal affective disorder (SAD), were particularly likely to benefit. An extract of St. John's Wort called *hyperforin* proved as effective as Elavil (an antidepressant medication) in mild to moderate depression, witrh fewer side effects. Compared to Tofranil and Prozac, *hyperforin* had equal efficacy and fewer side effects in treating mild to moderate depression. These studies focused on short-term effects, as have most of the studies of conventional antidepressants. Further work remains to be done in order to establish the efficacy of *hypericum* in long-term treatment of depression. St. John's Wort is not recommended for severe depression.

St. John's Wort combined with valerian produced better effects than diazepam[204] in treatment of anxiety.

Ginkgo biloba has been shown to slow the progress of dementia in Alzheimer's disease. Ginkgo is an ornamental as well as a medicinal tree, which was domesticated in China thousands of years ago and now grows only under cultivation. A meta-analysis of 40 studies of *ginkgo biloba* found 8 that conformed to high standards, and confirmed that mild to moderate memory impairment was improved. Egb 761, an extract of *Ginkgo biloba*, stabilized and improved the cognitive and social functions of demented patients over 6-12 months.

Green tea is widely touted as a tonic and remedy in the East. Research suggests it may lower serum cholesterol and triglycerides; lower rates of strokes and cerebral hemorrhage; and lower rates of recurrence of stage 1 and stage 2 breast cancer. Meta-analyses of series of cancer studies were less conclusive.

Boxwood (*Buxus sempervirens*) extract, in doses of 990 mg daily, slowed the progression of HIV+ disease in a double-blind controlled study that was terminated before its 18-month planned duration because the researchers considered it unethical to deny the control group the benefits of the active treatment.

Ginger (*Zingiber officinale*) is used as a medicine as well as a spice. It has antiemetic properties in motion sickness, seasickness, postoperative vomiting, and vomiting in pregnancy.

Echinacea or the purple coneflower, was introduced by Native Americans to the European settlers as a tonic for many ills. A meta-analysis of 26 clinical studies showed that for 22 out of 34 measured factors echinacea proved better than a placebo in enhancing immune functions, and other studies confirm its efficacy in the treatment of upper respiratory infections. Animal and laboratory studies also confirm that it can enhance immune system activity.

Garlic (*Allium sativum*) has been used for several millennia in Mediterranean countries and China as a seasoning and a medicine, and it has many popular medicinal uses today. Over a thousand studies have explored its efficacy in treating various ailments. In Europe it has been approved as a preventive treatment for atherosclerosis and for elevated serum lipids. Meta-analyses confirm its efficacy for hyperlipidemia, and for hypertension.

PC-SPES a combination of eight Chinese herbs (PC indicating prostate cancer; *spes* = Latin, *hope*) has been helpful in treating prostate cancer in men who had undergone no hormone treatment or were resistant to hormone treatment. The blood level of PSA (prostate-specific antigen), which is used as a measure of the development of prostatic cancer, decreased by over 50 percent in 9 out of 12 subjects of both types studied. Estrogenic side effects included gynecomastia (breast enlargement), loss of libido, and nausea. These appear to be less serious than the side effects of androgen therapy (one of the standard conventional medical treatments), which also produces decreased bone density, muscle degeneration, and depression.

Mentalin, an Ayurvedic combination of ginger, bacoba, and gotu kola, has been shown to help in treating Attention Deficit Hyperactivity Disorder.

Extensive studies have been made of the use of herbal remedies in China, Japan, and Korea (the more rigorous ones using animal subjects), and of Ayurvedic herbal remedies in India, and a few studies have been done on North American Indian herbal remedies. Searches for the active pharmaceutical ingredients in herbal remedies have been initiated, and integration of herbal remedies with conventional medical practice is well on its way.

This is an area of growing interest in wholistic medicine. There have been many other studies of herbal remedies, but these are beyond the scope of this book.

Regulation of herbal remedies
Until recently, US laws used to discriminate against herbal remedies by requiring applications of such complexity, with so much supporting research and clinical data, that the costs for approval of a new medication could run between $140-500 million. Botanicals are not patentable, and therefore no manufacturer can possibly afford this sort of outlay. Research on medications in the US is primarily funded by pharmaceutical companies, so there are very few laboratories where scientists investigate herbal remedies. To remedy this problem, the Food and Drug Administration reclassified herbal remedies as food supplements. The Dietary Supplement and Health Education Act of 1994 permits claims regarding compound structure and function, but outlaws claims regarding diagnostic and therapeutic specificity. While this facilitates access to herbal remedies, the lack of standards and regulation has spawned a bewildering number of varieties of commercial products. The prohibition against stating a therapeutic indication creates an awkward situation wherein people buy products that are not labeled for their target symptoms and illnesses. Quality control is also often lacking in production. Many producers do not standardize the potencies or the remedies, and some do not standardize doses of their products. Many suggest that their products are of benefit for physical and psychological problems, but provide no research to substantiate their claims.

The European community is also developing regulations for herbal products.

Education and Training: There are no standards as yet for herbal education or licensing in the US. Training courses may last from one weekend to 400 hours.

Most conventional physicians are inadequately trained in nutritional medicine.[205] Naturopathic doctors and a few medical physicians specialize in this area. Nutritional medicine is so vast and complex that there is little agreement within conventional or CAM groups as to what constitutes adequate standards of training and clinical competency. The American Herbalists Guild is the leading professional organization. There are standards for Registered Dieticians and Licensed Dieticians under the Commission on Dietetic Registration of the American Dietetic Association. These practitioners advise about specialized diets, for instance for patients with hypertension or diabetes, but they will not diagnose illnesses.

Theories: Traditional healers relate to herbal remedies in a wholistic fashion. They do not consider that they are simply giving a chemical preparation. The remedy is part of a ceremonial and ritual healing process addressing body, heart, community, harmonization with nature, and spirit. A traditional herbalist once suggested, "It's not just the herb that helps, it's what you tell the herb to do!"

> *The Rebbe used to say that it is not the medicine that heals but faith in God's loving-kindness.*
>
> – Rabbi Kolonymus Kalman Shapira (p. xv)

Conventional medicine and the pharmaceutical companies seek to extract active ingredients from herbal remedies that can be patented. While this may open doors to development of new pharmaceuticals, and may standardize doses of remedies, it may also miss the unique combinations of ingredients and the bioenergetic essence in herbal remedies that make them effective.

In my personal and clinical experience, adding healing and prayer to medications of any sorts, whether herbal or allopathic, enhances their effectiveness and diminishes side effects. While many would see this simply as evidence of the power of suggestion, I believe healing actually enhances medication potency.

Adverse effects: While generally much safer than conventional medications, side effects may also be caused by nutritional supplements, megavitamin therapy, and herbal remedies. Some of these are dose-related. For instance, very high doses of vitamin E can greatly increase the body's requirements for vitamin K. If sufficient vitamin K is not available, blood clotting disorders may result. Patients may also have allergic reactions to any substance, even if it is a natural product.

Adverse effects may occur if natural remedies are used with conventional medicines: additive effects may be toxic; one remedy may interfere in the effects of the other; and one may interfere in absorption or elimination of the other.

The evidence is overwhelmingly clear that herbal remedies have fewer side effects and produce far fewer fatalities than conventional medicines. I would anticipate that spiritual healing could potentiate the effects of herbal remedies and reduce their side effects. Witness to the fact that spiritual healing can lessen side effects of conventional medication is the report of a nurse working in a hospital cancer unit where she wasn't allowed to use her spiritual healing gifts. She gave healing to the IV bottles that carry the chemotherapy. Her patients had noticeably fewer side effects such as headaches, nausea, and vomiting.

Clinical applications: Nutritional and herbal therapies can be of enormous benefit for health promotion and weight adjustments, as well as an adjunct to treatment of most illnesses. They can help people build up resistance to illness, provide building blocks for repair and recuperation, and enhance general wellbeing. Specific vitamins, minerals and other food elements can be curative for particular illnesses. We are only beginning to appreciate the enormous benefits of these remedies. The interested reader is highly encouraged to pursue further readings in this area, through the many recommendations in the endnotes.

While many people recommend diets that have helped them and others they know, a nutritional or herbal consultant can suggest special diets, vitamins, minerals, and herbal remedies that may be unfamiliar to the non-specialist.

Dieting for weight loss
My experience as a therapist is that controlling intake by whatever diet is only a small part of weight management. A rounded program will include exercise plus individual and/or group counseling/ support.

The last word on our understanding of nutrition
Here's the final word on nutrition and health. It's a relief to know the truth after all the many conflicting medical studies.

1. The Japanese eat very little fat and suffer fewer heart attacks than the British or the Americans.
2. The French eat a lot of fat and also suffer fewer heart attacks than the British the Americans.
3. The Japanese drink very little red wine and suffer fewer heart attacks than the British or Americans.
4. The Italians drink excessive amounts of red wine and also suffer fewer heart attacks than the British or Americans.
5. The Germans drink a lot of beer and eat lots of sausages and fats and suffer fewer heart attacks than the British or Americans.
CONCLUSION: Eat and drink what you like – speaking English is apparently what kills you.

See also: Naturopathic Medicine, Ayurvedic Medicine.

PET THERAPY AND ANIMAL HEALINGS

Pets heal as well as heel.
— Anonymous

Anecdotes and case studies abound on the benefits of having pets. Research is beginning to confirm that there are psychological and physical benefits to pet ownership. One longitudinal study showed that dogs and cats enhanced wellbeing indices on assessments of the activities of daily living (Raina et al.). However, the mere presence of a pet is not a guarantee of enhanced health. The level of bonding with the owner appears to be the crucial factor. Benefits include decreased anxiety and loneliness, lowered blood pressure, increased survival following heart attacks, and more. In the UK, pets are allowed in many hospice care wards, and in the US pets who are trained for therapy interventions are allowed in hospitals.

Anecdotal reports indicate that dolphins may be able to participate actively in healing, contributing as very gifted and potent healers for psychological and physical problems. People who swim with dolphins have also reported that they feel a deep joy and spiritual uplifting.

Case: Gladys was bereaved inconsolably when her husband died, after 35 years of marriage. She withdrew from her active social life, stopped taking care of herself, and refused antidepressants. She seemed ready to die. A stray cat who appeared on her doorstep was her healer, bringing her out of depression within two months.

Of note are books and therapists who can help with bereavement over the loss of a pet – an often neglected aspect of counseling (McElroy; Traisman/ Nieburg).

Wholistic healing *for* pets is another healing. There are now CAM therapists who offer acupuncture, homeopathy and other complementary therapies for pets.

Intuitive medical assessments for pets can provide information that is helpful in wholistic ways as well as in clarifying symptoms and identifying underlying diseases. It is very common to find that stress in the home is an issue in pet illnesses, and that addressing the owners' psychological issues relieves pet illnesses.

Research: I know of no controlled pet therapy studies. Most people find a pet that is intuitively compatible with their needs.

OSTEOPATHY
See: Chiropractic and Osteopathic Manipulation; Craniosacral Manipulation.

POLARITY THERAPY

Polarity Therapy was developed by Randolph Stone, an osteopath, naturopath and chiropractor. This form of healing balances energies between various points on the body. It addresses positive (top/ head, right) and negative (bottom/ feet, left) polarities of energies in the body. Massage, light touch, and near-the body healing are also used. As with other spiritual healing modalities, treatment is often guided by intuitive and bioenergetic assessments.

Research: I have found no research on polarity therapy.

Clinical applications: See Spiritual Healing.

See also: Spiritual Healing; Chapter I-1

PROBIOTICS

Probiotics is the deliberate application of bacteria to achieve positive effects in the body.

Countless bacteria and yeasts live harmlessly in our gut, as well as on our skin and mucous membranes. Some of these have been found to be very helpful, repaying us, so to speak, for being their hosts.[206] The intestinal tract contains bacteria and yeasts that participate in digesting food, producing B3 and B6 vitamins; lactase for digesting milk; and recycle estrogen. In breast milk, helpful microbes contribute to food absorption and immunity in babies. Our normal microbial population produces antibacterial chemicals that can deactivate or kill pathogenic bacteria.

We are usually unaware of these harmless residents on and in our bodies until something happens to upset our relationship with them. The most frequent cause of such problems is treatment with a course of antibiotics, which kills off many of these harmless and helpful organisms along with the pathogenic organismss that are causing the disease. The void left by the absence of the ordinary inhabitants of the gut, vagina or other parts of the body can leave a fertile ground for overgrowth of survivors or of new invaders. A common problem following treatment with antibiotics is *candidiasis*, an overgrowth of *candida* yeast in the gut and vagina.

Research: Probiotics is still in its infancy. Early research shows promise in the treatment of antibiotic-induced diarrhea and diarrhea in children.

Adverse effects: None known

Clinical applications: Probiotics, or replacement of friendly bacteria that have been killed off with antibiotics, has been shown to be helpful in treating colitis, irritable bowel syndrome, allergies, migraine, rheumatic and arthritic problems, candidiasis, cystitis, acne, eczema and psoriasis. Probiotics may prevent diarrhea in children following courses of antibiotics. There is even a suggestion that certain cancers may respond to probiotic treatment, and that the side effects of radiation therapy may be alleviated or prevented.

See also: Chronic fatigue syndrome.

PSYCHONEUROCARDIOLOGY

> *The best doctors in the world are Doctor Diet, Doctor Quiet, and*
> *Doctor Merryman.*
> > – Jonathan Swift

The practice of psychoneurocardiology involves relaxation, meditation, imagery, group support/ therapy, dietary, and exercise programs. Developed by Dean Ornish, this method has been shown to enhance cardiovascular functions and to provide an effective treatment for some cardiovascular conditions – even when they are severe.

A measure of the success of this method is the fact that insurance companies are willing to pay for it, having found that it can often alleviate cardiac symptoms and sometimes makes cadiac surgery unnecessary.

I find it sad that this method has been so slow to be adopted by physicians, who are so wedded to the conventional medical model of prescribing medications and performing surgery that they find self-healing exercises to be alien to their ways of offering healing. The slow acceptance of these methods is also a reflection of the Type A personality – prone to heart disease.

The other problem, here as in other wholistic approaches, is that they require more investment of therapist time than most physicians will invest, and certainly more than most insurance companies will compensate. An obvious way around this is to train physicians' assistants and nurses to manage such programs. They often lend themselves readily to group interventions, so they can definitely be cost-effective.

See: Discussion of psychoneurocardiology in Chapter II-1.

PSYCHONEUROIMMUNOLOGY (PNI)

> *[L]ist the five major stresses that were going on in your life in the six months preceding the onset of the disease[E]xamine how you partici-pated in that stress, either by creating the stressful situation or by the manner in which you responded to it...*
>   – O. Carl Simonton, Stephanie Matthews-Simonton,
>   and James Creighton (p. 112-113)

The practice of PNI includes relaxation, meditation, imagery, and group support/therapy.

Research: An enormous body of research, spanning more than two decades, con-firms that the mind can influence the immune system. Some even speculate that the immune system is a part of the mind. This hypothesis is consistent with the fact that many chemicals found in the nerve cells of the brain, serving as chemical messengers between nerve cells, are also found in immune cells. This suggests that these chemical messengers serve as well to communicate between the nerv-ous system and the immune system, and may also explain the memory inherent in the success of immunizations.

Clinical applications: PNI appears to prolong life and sometimes to lead to re-missions of cancers. It may also be helpful in treating various allergy problems, such as multiple allergy syndromes.

See also: Detailed discussion of PNI in Chapter II-1, Relaxation, Meditation, Visualization, Psychoneurocardiology.

PSYCHOTHERAPY

> *The Unconscious is not unconscious, only the Conscious is uncon-*
> *scious of what the Unconscious is conscious of.*
> – Francis Jeffrey

Psychotherapy is an essential aspect of every wholistic therapy; it is the part of
each treatment modality that addresses the person who has the illness. Sadly,
many medical schools do not prepare doctors to deal with this aspect of treatment,
and even psychiatrists today may have no training in psychotherapy.

Psychotherapy is a deeper form of counseling, which relies not only on cognitive
counseling but also makes extensive use of the relationship between the therapist
and the client as an instrument for healing. *Transference*, the projection of anticipated responses by the client onto the therapist, and *counter-transference*, the
emotional responses of the therapist towards the client are also a major focus in
psychotherapy.

Research: Enormous bodies of research confirm the benefits of a broad spectrum
of psychotherapies – from behavioral, throiugh rational emotive, psychosomatic,
and into psychodynamic variations on this theme. Quantitative and qualitative
studies have shown significant benefits of various forms of psychotherapy in
treatment of anxiety, panic, obsessive compulstive disorders, depression, marital
and family issues, schizophrenia and more. I am not aware of studies of efficacy
of transpersonal psychotherapy.

Clinical applications: While many of us grow and mature with age and experience, psychotherapy can add many dimensions to our personal growth.
Psychotherapy provides support, insight regarding intrapsychic (within the careseeker) and interpersonal issues, education for new ways to understand issues,
and opportunities for restructuring and repatterning one's ways of perceiving and
relating to the worlds within and without. It is particularly helpful in identifying
and dealng with blind spots and shadow issues – areas in our lives that we tend to
avoid noticing and would often rather ignore.

Psychotherapy can help with problems in areas such as emotions, relationships
(with spouses/ partners, parenting) and psychosomatic disorders. Transpersonal
psychotherapy helps with spiritual issues.

Psychotherapy is second only to healing in its dependence on the person who is
the caregiver as much as it relies on whatever methodologies and approaches used
in the therapy.

Once we acknowledge that the body is intimately related to the emotions, mind,
relationships and spirit, then it is clear that psychotherapy can help people to deal
with any physical problem. Psychotherapy can help in the following crucial areas
of the proactive management of disease:

- accepting the illness;
- adapting to living with the illness;

- dealing with the illness, through relaxation techniques, meditation, imagery, psychoneuroimmunology;
- exploring and dealing with psychological contributors to the illness;
- exploring and dealing with relational aspects of the illness;
- dealing with secondary gains;
- exploring transpersonal and spiritual issues.

Training and licensing: Psychotherapy may be offered by social workers, psychologists, nurses, physicians, clergy and other caregivers. Psychotherapy is usually defined as involving more training and promoting therapy in greater depth than counseling, although some use these terms interchangeably. The person who is the therapist is often more important than the label or the training, as discussed in greater detail at the end of this chapter.

Psychotherapy and counseling are defined and licensed differently in different states, and in some cases is not a licensed modality. In addition to a degree or certificate, many hundreds of hours of supervised therapy with careseekers are usually required. In some branches of psychotherapy, therapists are also required to undergo their own therapy – to clear themselves as much as possible of blind spots and shadow issues that could intrude in their ministrations to clients. Ethical practice also suggests it is wise to have ongoing supervision.

See also: Psychotherapy in greater detail in Chapter II-1; brief summaries of varieties of psychotherapy in Appendix A; self-healing exercises in Chapter II-5.

QIGONG

> *Qigong is a wholistic system of self-healing exercise and meditation, an ancient, evolving practice that includes healing posture, movement, self-massage, breathing techniques, and meditation.*
> – Ken Cohen (2000, p. 4)

The *Qigong* (pronounced *chee-gong*) system of physical exercises and bioenergy healing was developed in China some time prior to the 6th Century BC, to address the flows of biological energies in the body and to exert a calming effect on the mind through meditative focus. *Qi* means "life energy" and *gong* means "work" and "the benefits acquired through perseverance and practice" (K. Cohen 1997). Qigong self-healing is excellent for treating many physical problems, and anecdotal reports claim dramatic improvements in chronic diseases, including cancer.

Roger Jahnke has a lovely and thorough discussion of various forms of qi, with advice on how to enhance their flow and potency, and a spectrum of exercises for self-healing. Qigong exercises are used frequently as a complement to the qigong healings (*waiqi, external qigong*) that are given by trained masters. External qigong healing is similar to the many forms of spiritual healing detailed in *Healing Research*, Volume I.

There are thousands of different styles of qigong. A few rough categories can be delineated (K. Cohen 2000):

By form: *Jing gong* – Tranquil qigong, without movement
                  Dong gong – Active qigong, with movement
                  Ruan gong – Soft qigong
                  Ying gong – Hard qigong

By application: *Yi gong* – Medical or healing qigong
                  Wu gong – Martial or sports qigong
                  Fo gong – Buddhist qigong
                  Dao gong – Daoist qigong

Qigong is a practice of self-healing. Exercises are done daily, much as are yoga or other fitness practices, but both meditative and bioenergy aspects are included in most varieties qigong. There may be a focus on visualizing energies flowing into the body, through the meridians and other bioenergy pathways, and connecting with other dimensions.

Research: A wealth of research, almost entirely from China, is summarized by Kenneth Sancier, in his monumental *Qigong Database.*[207] Unfortunately, the quality of this research is questionable.

Adverse effects: No harmful effects have been reported.

Training and licensing: There are no standards for training or licensing in. Qigong is a healing art, rather than a system of treatment. Because there are so many styles of qigong, it is difficult to see how standards could be established.

Clinical applications: Qigong practices can improve relaxation, muscle tone and breathing. It can contribute to improvements in stress-related illnesses such as hypertension and musculoskeletal pains. By enhancing biological energy flows it can strengthen the body's abilities to deal with many other illnesses – in ways that cannot be explained within Western medical theories. Even some cures of cancers have been reported anecdotally. It can also facilitate the development of spiritual discipline and improved sense awareness.

   Qigong can be integrated with conventional care in many applications. External qi, projected by qigong masters for healing, can also complement any therapy. T'ai Chi Ch'uan and Qigong exercises are excellent as preventive medicine and for maintaining muscle tone and normal flows of bioenergies. They may also be helpful in rehabilitation following injuries or illnesses.

   While initial instruction is usually necessary in these techniques, their practice is self-healing.

See also: T'ai Chi Ch'uan; Yoga.; research on infrasonic sound emitted by qigong masters (Chapter II-3).

REFLEXOLOGY
See: Massage.

REIKI

The process of attunement or initiation is what sets Reiki apart from every other form of laying on of hands or touch healing. The attunement is not a healing session, it creates the healer...
                                                    – Diane Stein (p. 17)

Developed in Japan by Dr. Mikao Usui in the mid-nineteenth century, this system is one of the most popular and widely used healing methods in the Western world.

Usui trained twenty-two Reiki masters. It appears that each of these masters was empowered with individualized gifts and healing symbols, which could differ from those of the other masters in subtle or substantial ways.

Reiki is growing in popularity, with many thousands of healers now practicing around the world. Graduated levels of instruction are offered. Reiki-I teaches beginners a pattern of laying-on of hands on the head and torso. Reiki healers initially adhere to this pattern in each healing treatment, to assure that they will not overlook aspects of healees' problems, or introduce energy imbalances by addressing only the symptomatic sites on the body of the healee. A pain in the head, for example, might be due to local muscle spasms from fatigue, but it might also be due to poor posture, emotional imbalances such as anger or depression, systemic dysfunctions such as hypertension, hormonal shifts such as in premenstrual tension and more. An essential part of level one teaching involves an *attunement, induction* or *empowering* of healing abilities in the healer by the Master.

Reiki II teaches distant healing, and Reiki-III is an induction to Master level. Japanese ideograms are used as power symbols that embody and transmit healing.

Various Reiki traditions use different symbols for healing. Originally, masters were carefully selected by teachers. Nowadays there is generally less and less selectivity in most traditions, and in some cases masters have very limited innate healing ability, training, or experience.

Modest fees are charged for Reiki I and II courses, and fees of several hundred to several thousand dollars may be charged for Reiki III training.

Research: Very limited research has been done on Reiki, with only a few of these studies suggesting healing benefits.

Training and licensing: Training is by weekend workshops. There are numerous different schools, each with its own variations of practices. Originally, masters were carefully selected by teachers but in recent years a person can attend three weekend workshops and become a master. In some cases masters have very limited innate healing ability, training, and experience.

Modest fees are charged for Reiki I and II courses, and fees of several hundred to several thousand dollars may be charged for Reiki III training.

Reiki is not a licensed therapy.

Adverse effects: No harmful effects have been reported See discussion of potential general negative effects from rapid improvements under Spiritual Healing.

Because there is very brief training for Reiki healers, one is cautioned to seek references if healing is needed for serious problems.

Clinical applications: See spiritual healing.

See also: Rituals; Spiritual Healing, Volume I of *Healing Research.*

RITUALS

> *Rituals are formalized patterns which, like classical dance steps, require particular behaviors but may also allow for individual interpretations and variations of the practitioners.*
> – D.B.

Rituals create windows of drama through which we can draw support, enact our conflicts, explore intuitive and creative solutions to challenges, seek inner inspiration and guidance from our higher selves (from collective consciousness and spirit), celebrate our progress – and offer our thanks. In traditional societies, community involvement, prayers and religious elements may be included in healing rituals, as these all lend power to the healing experience. Modern society has distanced itself from much of the healing available in rituals, as we have distanced ourselves from religious practices and from the wise habit of living in proximity to several generations of family. We tend to limit this healing modality to the doctor's white coat and stethoscope hanging out of her pocket or around her neck.

These creative approaches may facilitate healing, in and of themselves or as aspects of other therapies. They may seem to share more with the artist's palette and the tones of the lute than they do with the needles of the acupuncturist or the remedies of the herbalist, but their healing power has been recognized and respected since earliest times.

In traditional societies, shamans make extensive use of healing rituals. These may include meditations, prayers, chanting, drumming, dancing, feasts, ingestion of ritual drugs, smoking, libations, fasting, feats of endurance, sacred art, sweat lodges, pilgrimages to traditional sacred sites, vision quests, and invitations to spirits and the Divine to participate. While many Western caregivers view these as magical beliefs that are more in the realm of wishful thinking than anything resembling an effective treatment, there are many reports of successful, even dramatic healings through these rituals.

Complex sets of rituals may be used in ceremonies that serve to ground people in the traditions of their cultures and to facilitate communal healing.

In and of themselves, particular rituals may be used as potent spiritual healing interventions. Whether it is the ritual or whether it is the person conducting the ritual that is the agent for healing is unclear.

See also: Creative art therapies as healing; Qigong; Reiki; Shamanism; T'ai Chi Ch'uan; Yoga.

SHAMANISM

[S]hamans were the world's first physicians, first diagnosticians, first psychotherapists, first religious functionaries, first magicians, first performing artists, and first story-tellers...
– Stanley Krippner and Patrick Welch (1992, p. 27)

Shamanism is practiced in every known culture. The shaman acts as a counselor, physician, spiritual healer, community authority and priest. Shamans call upon psi powers for diagnosing and treating illness, counseling, predicting the future, and guiding their society in spiritual matters. Technically speaking, shamans are more diverse in their skills, training, and interventions than *medicine men*, who are specialists in diagnosing and treating illness. [208]

A rich literature is available on healing in indigenous, non-industrial cultures, which is usually practiced under the hands of shamans. The most comprehensive discussion on shamanism and healing is by Krippner and Welch. They point out that although Western scientists have been eager to borrow herbal knowledge from shamans, they have ignored teachings in diagnosis and treatment for physical and psychological problems. The presentation by Krippner and Welch is enormously helpful in increasing our appreciation of the spectrum of healing practices and beliefs around the world.

Shamans may use herbs, rituals (dancing, chanting, and painting), divination, spiritual healing, prayer, and alternative states of consciousness. They often invite participation of the entire family of the person who is sick, and may even involve a broader segment of their community in the healing ceremony. Conversely, healings for individuals are often viewed as healings for the community as well. Their healing ceremonies may last for many hours or even for several days.

Traditional shamanic education consists of three parts: expansion of one's ability to see beyond the ordinary five senses; destabilization of mind and body habit of being bound to one plane of reality; and encouragement of the ability to voyage into "otherworldly" dimensions and return with spirit guidance for individual and community healings, advice on dealing with serious challenges and predictions about the future..

It is refreshing today to see Western scientists seeking the wisdom of so-called "primitives." These ancient cultures may be less advanced than ours in technology, but they are far more advanced in application of psi skills, especially intuitive awareness and healing. They are attuned to spiritual dimensions of awareness, which include the participation of all living things in the ecobiological system of our planet (commonly called *Gaia*), and in the cosmos beyond. We may learn new ways of healing from them that complement our modern medical approaches. The shamans, in turn, may learn from us to distinguish between the essential elements of their teachings and superstitious beliefs that may have little therapeutic benefit. Thus we may all gain insight into how healing works and be better able to help people in need.

Much of the literature on shamanism (e.g. Eliade; Harner) and eastern medicine (e.g. Kaptchuk) elaborates worldviews in which human beings constitute a small part of the cosmos, linked with nature via a vast web of psi and spiritual interactions. Descriptions of these interconnections vary widely, and to Western eyes they may seem so alien as to constitute mere superstitious beliefs. Nevertheless, people living in each culture believe wholeheartedly in their cosmologies and respond to elements within them. A shaman draws upon imagery and beliefs from her or his culture in order to facilitate spiritual healings. In fact, it may be impossible for a healer from one culture to heal some patients from another, because of their dissimilar frames of reference. The converse is likewise true. Healers from a different culture from those of the healee may bring about dramatic healings, partly because of the charisma that is attributed to healers from distant places.

> *Jesus said, "No prophet is accepted in his own village; no physician heals those who know him."*
> — Gospel of Thomas (31)

We may take profound lessons from cross-cultural studies that are relevant to our own systems of medical care.

> There are shamanic healing methods that closely parallel contemporary behavior therapy, chemotherapy, dream interpretation, family therapy, hypnotherapy, milieu therapy, and psychodrama. It is clear that shamans, psychotherapists, and physicians have more in common than is generally suspected...
> — Stanley Krippner and Patrick Welch (p. 37)

If we allow that healing in various cultures may appear entirely different from healing in modern Western society, we may then be in a better position to re-examine the attitudes of patients toward their healings in our own culture. Western investigators tend to discount patients' beliefs as unimportant or inessential to the actual processes of healing. If we can agree that alternative views may apply to healing in other cultures, should we not consider the possibility that the perspectives of patients in our own culture are relevant to their success in healing, even if this view differs from that of our scientist subculture?[209]

Research: I have found no research on shamanic healings.

Adverse effects: No harmful effects have been reported. Where herbs are used, see cautions under herbal and nutritional remedies. See also discussion of potential general negative effects from interactive effects with herbs (under Nutritional Therapies) and rapid improvements (under Spiritual Healing).

Training and licensing: Training is by apprenticeship in traditional cultures. Michael Harner has developed a school for shamanic healing, translating shamanism into Western culture. Growing numbers of healthcare professionals are participating in these courses and integrating shamanic practices in their work.

There is no licensing specifically for shamans as such, but they are generally regarded as religious leaders and accorded the same authority and protection under the law as other religious priests and ministers.

Clinical applications: Shamanism can address all psychological and physical problems. Many shamans recognize that allopathic medicine has much to offer, particularly in the treatment of infectious diseases and trauma. Shamanic treatments can be complementary to conventional medical care – or perhaps in this case I would say that conventional care may complement shamanism..

See also: Spiritual Healing; Rituals.

SHEN HEALING

SHEN therapy was developed by Richard Pavek, an American scientist. This method addresses emotional tensions which manifest in physical symptoms, using light touch at particular points on the body. While this method is relatively unknown, I am impressed with the integrity of the training, which requires therapists to undergo their own therapy to "clear the channels" so that they can be as effective as possible in their own practice.

Clinical applications: SHEN healing has been specifically helpful in treating anorexia, bulimia, migraine, pains of all sorts, panic attacks, post-traumatic stress disorder, pre-menstrual and irritable bowel syndrome.

See also: Spiritual Healing,

SPIRITUAL HEALING

Healing is not a matter of mechanism but a work of the spirit.
— Rachel Naomi Remen

Spiritual healing (often called simply *healing*) is any sort of purposeful intervention by one or more persons wishing to help another living thing to change via the sole processes of focused intention or the laying-on of hands. Healers may invoke outside agents such as God, Christ, other "higher powers," spirits, universal or Cosmic forces or energies; special healing energies or forces emanating from themselves; psychokinesis (mind over matter); and self-healing powers or energies latently present in the healees.

The laying-on of hands may involve light touch or holding the hands near to but not touching the body. It may also be given through a wish, simple intent, meditation, or prayer for the healing of the subjects. Healing may be sent from any distance, with no direct contact between healer and healee.[210]

Spiritual healing is a natural gift, much like playing the piano. Everyone has some ability, but only a few are truly gifted. A mother kissing away a child's hurt is probably giving healing along with her physical and emotional comforting. Most of us can learn to improve our healing gifts with diligent practice. Some are better off (or their potential healees are better off!) if they don't engage in healing, because they lack the sensitivity, emotional balance or the required discerning judgment to engage in what can be an unsettling experience of trans-formation.

While healing may be given specifically as spiritual healing, it is also a component of most other therapies – though it may be an unmentioned or even unconscious part of the therapeutic interaction (Benor 1995a).

Historically, shamans and medicine men have practiced healing in every known culture throughout the ages. Shamans are not only healers. In their wider social and spiritual roles they mediate between the natural world and the worlds of spirits. A variety of popular forms of healing are practiced today.[211]

Research: This is one of the most thoroughly researched forms of CAM, with numerous studies (including several hundred doctoral dissertations) showing effects on hemoglobin, skin wounds, hypertension, immune system function, pain, and anxiety.[212]

Clinical applications: Spiritual healing can be used alone or as a complement to all other therapies. It may, in fact, be a component of many other therapies – even without the conscious awareness of therapists or their clients. It is usually given by a healer, though self-healing is also possible.

Adverse effects: No harmful effects have been reported from spiritual healing. There may be emotional releases during treatments, as with many of the other CAM therapies. These are often experienced as less traumatic with healing treatments, since spiritual healing is also excellent for treatment of physical and emotional stress and pain and helps to deal with the stress of emotional releases.

Physical pain may increase briefly following the initial healing treatments, but this is generally viewed by healers as a positive response, a sign that there is a shift in the bioenergetic pattern of the pain. With further healing treatments the pain then reduces below the initial levels of intensity.

Relief of pain and other symptoms may sometimes be rapid and experienced by the healee as a dramatic shift. While to many this is pure relief, to others it may be a challenge, as they have to adjust their lives to being without their symptoms. Healers who are not sensitive to psychological issues may not know how to counsel careseekers who are too rapidly relieved of their symptoms.

Training and Licensing: There are no generally accepted standards for training or licensing in spiritual healing. This may be a gift from birth or developed at any time later in life, and can be enhanced through training. There are widely varying courses in the several types of healing reviewed in this book, with Reiki offering weekend courses; Barbara Brennan School of Healing requiring four years of training; and other modalities ranging in between.

In Britain, the organization of healers into self-regulating and certifying bodies was a major contribution to the acceptance of healing. [213]

See also: Barbara Brennan Healing, Healing Touch, LeShan Healing, Native American Healing, Network Spinal Analysis, Polarity Therapy, Qigong, Reiki, Shamanism, SHEN Healing, Therapeutic Touch, Volume I of *Healing Research.*

T'AI CHI CH'UAN

... Focus your eye on every detail, every expression, every movement, and do not look away until you have seen the Divine. This is the vision, the awareness that will heal our wounds, repair our brokenness, and safeguard this world for those to come.
  This and nothing else.
                                                                    – Jan Phillips

T'ai Chi Ch'uan is a ritualized series of movements developed from martial arts practices in China. Unlike the combative martial arts, this is like a slow dance.

Research: No controlled studies are available. Anecdotal reports, case studies, and clinical observations indicate that T'ai Chi is excellent for developing and maintaining muscle tone and enhances the flow of biological energies. It can help with problems of balance, cardiovascular system, immune system, mood, relaxation, respiration, stress hormones, and weight bearing ability (Krapu).

Training and Licensing: There are no Western standards for training or licensing. It is essentially a healing art. In China there are established standards.

Adverse effects: None known.

Clinical applications: T'ai Chi practices can improve relaxation, muscle toning and breathing. They can contribute to improvements in stress-related illnesses such as hypertension and musculoskeletal pains. By enhancing biological energy flows, they can strengthen the body's abilities to deal with many other illnesses – in ways that cannot be explained within the context of Western medical theories. T'ai Chi can also facilitate spiritual discipline and higher sense awareness.

  T'ai Chi Ch'uan exercises are excellent as preventive medicine, because they maintain muscle tone and normal flows of biological energies. They may also be helpful in rehabilitation following injuries or illnesses.

  While initial instruction in these techniques is usually necessary, their practice is effective as self-healing.

See also: Qigong; Rituals; Yoga.

THERAPEUTIC TOUCH (TT)

[I]n the final analysis, it is the healee (client) who heals her- or himself. The healer or therapist... acts as a human energy support system until the healee's own... system is robust enough to take over.
                                                        – Dolores Krieger (1993, p. 7)

TT was developed by Dolores Krieger, PhD, RN, a professor of nursing at New York University, and Dora van Gelder Kunz, a gifted clairsentient and healer. It has been taught to a conservatively estimated 80,000 nurses and other health practitioners in America and around the world, and it is now taught in more than 90 nursing schools in America. TT has generated the largest number of research studies of any spiritual healing modality.

TT teaches people to *center* themselves and to develop their awareness of bio-fields around the body. Students learn to scan the body, passing their hands a few inches away from the body from head to toe, front to back. They note any asymmetries or abnormal energy sensations and address these energetically, by holding their hands above, or lightly touching these parts of the body. They may image that they are conveying energy to the healee if energy depletions are noted, or that they drawing energy from the healee if excesses of energy are found. Healers may project images of particular colors to correct or counteract energy imbalances. The aura may be *combed* or *smoothed* if negative energies are to be removed.

The source for the healing energy may be imaged as coming from the healer or from a universal source of energy. In some of her more recent writings, Krieger is suggesting that TT can open healers and healees into greater transpersonal awareness (Krieger 2002).

Research: TT is the most thoroughly researched of the spiritual healing methods.[214]

Adverse effects: No harmful effects have been reported See also discussion of potential general negative effects from rapid improvements under Spiritual Healing. Kunz warned that only the most advanced healers should give treatments to the head, as they may inadvertently cause sever energy imbalances.

Training and licensing: Training and certification is available through the Nurse Healers Professional Associates, Inc. Weekend introductions to TT are also offered, and relatives of ailing people may be taught to offer TT. As with other forms of spiritual healing, there is no licensing.

Clinical applications: See under Spiritual Healing.

See also: Spiritual Healing, Volume I of *Healing Research.*

TIBETAN MEDICINE

The tradition of Tibetan medicine dates back fifteen hundred years. It was influenced by Chinese and Indian traditions but it has a distinct character of its own. It was also practiced extensively in Mongolia and parts of Russia. There are many variations within the Tibetan tradition, which are passed down through the lineages of the ancient practitioners.

Tibetan medicine is based on a cosmology of *Chi* (space, air),[215] *Schara* (subtle energy, bile), and *Badahan* (the material world, phlegm). Ten essential elements influence all of existence: awareness, willpower, compassion, structure/ temperature, gas/ liquid/ solid, plants, gender, animals, man, and mind. The basic triad and the ten elements combine in various proportions to determine the nature of everything in the world.[216]

Every individual is responsible for maintaining his or her own health and preventing illness. Each person must achieve this through an understanding of their relationships within their family, community, society and the cosmos, and through proper nutrition, lifestyles, adaptation to seasonal changes, and awareness of their characterological predispositions. For example, different foods and food combinations are recommended for each season. Emotional and mental "digestion" are also stressed, and spiritual awareness is considered of great importance.

Diagnosis is made according to the triadic types. *Chi* people are tall and lean, with dry skin and thin hair. They tend to be intelligent but not practical, anxious and changeable, and they may lack perseverance. They are not comfortable in parenting roles. They prefer sweet, light, hot foods. They are susceptible to illnesses but tolerate and adapt well to being ill. They tend to have psychological and neurological disorders, as well as arthritis. They have strong desires but low energy. Illness occurs more in fall and winter, and later in life.

Schara people are of medium build and strong, with a pink complexion but tend to have freckles, moles and acne. Hair grays and thins early. They tend to be intelligent and critical thinkers, strong-willed, and gravitating toward leadership positions, where they may focus more on programs than on the people they are meant to serve. In family life they are passionate, demanding, authoritative, and dominating. They prefer sweet and bitter foods. They are prone to infections, ulcers, liver and pancreatic diseases, skin allergies, rashes and infections, and cancers. Illnesses tend to occur in late spring or summer, more often during early and middle adulthood.

Badahan people are heavy-set and tend toward obesity, with pale moist skin and thick hair. They are stable, loving, and compassionate but tend not to assume leadership positions. They are pleasant, quiet, good listeners, slow to react, and unimaginative. They are very devoted to their partners and like to have a comfortable marital nest. They favor sour, strong tastes. Their resistance to illness is high, but when sick they have low endurance. They are particularly sensitive to emotional stresses from deprivations, metabolic disorders, asthma, cardiovascular problems, diabetes, pulmonary disorders, and tumors. Their susceptibility to illness is higher in late winter or early spring, and they tend to suffer illnesses early in life.

Mixtures of these three types are more common than pure types. In addition to reading the physical types, practitioners place great emphasis on reading the pulses at the wrists. Various pulses reveal the entire state of health and illness of the person (not only their cardiovascular condition). Three fingers are used to sense the pulses, each finger applied with a different pressure. I have heard reports of amazing diagnostic assessments with this method, relating to physical and psychological problems.

In addition to recommending nutritional and lifestyle changes, herbal remedies, and massage, the physician must approach healees with compassion. Mental focus and concentration are essential to proper practice – in healees and practitioners. The goal is to awaken the healee's self-healing abilities, which are further enhanced with breathing exercises that facilitate the flows of biological energies through the body. Spiritual teachings may be included in the treatment when the physician is also a lama or priest, but only after physical and emotional problems have been addressed.

Adverse effects: No harmful effects have been reported Where herbs are used, see cautions under herbal and nutritional remedies. See also discussion of potential general negative effects from rapid improvements under Spiritual Healing.

Training and Licensing: There are no professional organizations or certifications for Tibetan Medicine practitioners. There is no licensing for Tibetan Medicine.

Research: A few studies suggest that a standardized combination of 25 herbal and mineral ingredients may be helpful in treating peripheral vascular diseases as well as in arresting the progress of dementia.

Clinical applications: Tibetan medicine is a complete system of treatment that is applicable to most illnesses. It has been used as integrative care in parts of the West since the 1930s.
   A therapist is required for the practice of Tibetan medicine.

See also: Ayurvedic medicine.

VISUALIZATION/ IMAGERY

> *Mind no longer appears as an accidental intruder into the realm of matter; we are beginning to suspect that we ought rather to hail it as the creator and governor of the realm of matter.*
> – Sir James Jeans

Visualization is the deliberate holding of images in the mind's eye with the intent of imprinting these images upon one's own mental and physical states or upon those of others. Visualization is an important element in self-healing. Many healers also emphasize this method as a part of centering and treatment in spiritual healing.
   Advanced practitioners of meditation tell us that all of what we experience in life is brought into being through our expectations, wishes and needs.

> *But to the eye of the man of imagination Nature is imagination itself.*
> *As a man is, so he sees.*
> – William Blake

William Blake and other visionaries have been called *mystics*. They say that if we release our everyday expectations and wishes we may experience the world very differently.[217] The word *mystic* derives from the same root as *mystery*, harking back to the Greek mystery cults in which esoteric knowledge was kept as a secret of the priesthood.

Visualization is a component of so many healing approaches that it deserves special consideration and emphasis here.

Westerners would like to define visualization and related healing processes in a scientific manner. Robert Jahn and Brenda Dunne observe:

> [W]e find ourselves fishing in a metaphysical sea with a scientific net far better matched to other purposes. Inevitably, much of the anomalous information we seek will slip through this net, leaving us only skeletal evidence to retrieve, but it is on that alone that we can base systematic analysis and scientific claim.

It is in this spirit that we approach these areas of healing, such as visualization, that are more difficult to define. We must continue personal and clinical explorations of these elements that could slip through our more rigorously constructed net of scientific study and elude our observation, while striving to develop new nets that may retain them for closer scrutiny.[218]

Numerous self-healing books present a variety of applications for visualization. They all point out that visualizing yourself in a new state of being or in a new activity, and mentally practicing the experience of being in that state can vastly enhance your actual ability to achieve these altered physical states. Visualizing yourself practicing a sport can produce marked gains in skills and ability in that sport (Murphy/ White). Visualizing one's body improving from illness to health seems to be in another realm because it involves physiological and structural changes rather than alterations of behavioral patterns and athletic achievements. Research is beginning to confirm that imaging physical changes can actually alter many conditions in our bodies.

The simplest use of imagery is for reducing tensions. You may find it relaxing to picture yourself on a holiday, enjoying fresh surroundings and pleasurable activities. You might image yourself on a beach or by a pool, savoring a cool drink after a refreshing swim. You'll find that your body will relax as you relax psychologically.

Figure II-14. Visioning happiness

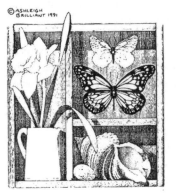

© ASHLEIGH BRILLIANT 1991

POT-SHOTS NO. 5551.

THE MEMORY OF A HAPPINESS

CAN LAST MUCH LONGER THAN THE HAPPINESS ITSELF.

More complex imagery approaches might involve problem-solving exercises focused on issues that are causing you tension. You could allow yourself to imagine as many ways as possible of dealing with someone whom you find oppressive or abusive. Your visualizations could take the form of vengeful interactions, or – more constructively – of successful confrontations and problem resolution. You might bring up memories of pleasant and satisfying experiences with that person, to remind you during times of stress and distress that good things are still possible. Such visualizations may also introduce hope in situations where you feel despair, provide immediate emotional satisfaction, and suggest creative solutions that you might not have considered previously.

Imagery can provide healing for various physical problems. Pain responds particularly well to this method. If you have a headache or other pain and you image that a compress of exactly the right temperature is being gently applied to the painful spot, the pain may diminish. Picturing the pain as a color (often an angry red or a dark black), you might think of lighter colors and find that the pain lightens along with the shifting mental picture.

Multiple mechanisms may contribute to pain reduction through visualizations. The psychological effects of suggestion may reduce pain perception or emotional responses to pain. Muscle spasms may be reduced through muscle relaxation. Further effects may be possible through shifts in physiological conditions that are facilitated by the imagery – for example through hormonal mechanisms or possibly through alterations in biological energy fields that influence physical conditions or pain perception.

Many find that self-generated imagery is the most potent, as it holds the structure and associations that are most suitable for the individual person's specific needs. Others find that imagery suggested by a therapist may be more helpful to them, as it can introduce new elements that they may not have considered themselves. Even better, a therapist may suggest new approaches that people can then individualize to meet their own needs.

Research: Visualizations can be effective for severe illnesses. For example, visualization is used in self-healing for cancer. Healees picture their bodies fighting off their disease in every way possible. Classical examples include: seeing their white cells as white knights attacking cancer cells, imaging the blood vessels that feed the cancer as pipes with spigots that the healee shuts off; and so on. Conversely, respants can picture themselves as being healthy (in particular organs and in general) and doing things they like (such as sports; visiting with family and friends; working). Each respant must find the specific images that work for her. Intensive practice has often produced improvement in quality of life and occasionally has brought about arrests or even complete remissions of cancer.

Jean Bolen's summary of Simonton's results shows that when patients applied themselves diligently to the visualization exercises their improvement was more marked. If they discontinued the exercises, symptoms tended to worsen; if they resumed them, symptoms again improved.

Similar methods have been helpful in improving quality of life and length of survival with AIDS (Solomon) and with heart disease.

Critics have pointed out that this research may represent a circular, self-validating system, in that people with a better prognosis may tend to volunteer for these new therapies. They may have more energy, better spirits, more willpower or other factors that permit them to apply themselves more vigorously or successfully to these methods.

One measure of the validity of a method is its predictive value. Therapists working with imagery report it is possible to determine the status of people's illnesses from their visualizations, and even to predict the course of an illness. The unconscious mind reveals a person's physical condition via the imagery in their fantasy visualizations and drawings. Jean Achterberg (1985, p. 188) presents scales for scoring these visualizations in dealing with cancer. Fourteen critical factors include: "... vividness, activity and strength of the cancer cell; vividness and activity of the white blood cells; relative comparison of size and number of cancer and white blood cells; strength of the white blood cells; vividness and effectiveness of medical treatment; choice of symbolism; the integration of the whole imagery process; the regularity with which they imaged a positive outcome; and a ventured clinical opinion on the prognosis, given the previously listed thirteen factors."

These factors were derived from a study of about 200 cancer patients, predicting "...with 100% certainty which patients would have died or shown evidence of significant deterioration during the two-month period, and to predict with 93% certainty which patients would be in remission." (Achterberg, 1985, p. 189)

While it was initially proposed that the mechanism for the effectiveness of visualization in slowing the development of cancer could be through influencing the immune system, this was only a conjecture. Researchers showed that visualizations could alter immune globulin A (IgA) in saliva, which was a step in confirming this hypothesis. Other studies of self-healing have confirmed changes in this and other immune markers as a result of imagery exercises\.

Clinical applications: Gerald Epstein, a psychiatrist in private practice, helps people to self-heal a wide range of illnesses with imagery exercises. His approaches are very direct and mechanistic. For instance, a patient may have an enlarged prostate, which is the gland between the bladder and the penis that produces seminal fluid. This can constrict the urethra, making it difficult to start and stop urinating, causing dribbling, etc. Epstein might prescribe the practice of mental imagery, such as picturing the prostate encased in a net that the patient draws tight, constricting the swollen gland to encourage it to shrink. At the same time, the person could visualize that he is massaging his prostate, encouraging the flow of urine and semen through the urethra. Though there is no known spontaneous mechanism whereby an enlarged prostate will shrink, Epstein's patients have had success with such exercises.

In another example, a pregnant woman whose baby is lying with its feet towards the cervix in the last month of pregnancy is in danger of delivering the baby feet-first. This can be dangerous because the umbilical cord is at risk of being constricted by the head as it descends through the birth canal. Because of this danger, caesarian delivery is often recommended. Epstein might suggest to the woman that she image herself entering her own body, going to the baby through the cervix, and helping it to turn to the more common and safer head-down position.

Epstein does not emphasize sleuthing for psychological causes underlying physical conditions, although he does accept that emotional and social factors may become apparent in the course of treatment. He feels that if illness is present it should be addressed directly, and the rest will follow as required by the individual.

My own preference tends strongly toward exploring underlying psychological causes behind physical problems. Before assuming that a symptom, however troublesome, should be encouraged to diminish or disappear, I recommend to my respants that they ask their symptoms what lessons they might be offering. A neck pain may be a metaphor for someone in your life who is "a pain in the neck." A cough, stomach ache or indigestion may be the unconscious mind's way of bringing to your attention that you are having to "swallow down" feelings which you are uncomfortable with or fearful of expressing. I believe that if underlying causes are not addressed then there is an increased likelihood that the same problem will return, or that other symptoms will develop in its place.

However, not everyone is open to such psychological explorations. For some it may be enough to be relieved of their symptoms and illnesses. It is always possible that a symptom may have outlived its psychological utility and may be hanging on as an old habit. It is also possible that respants' unconscious mind may be inviting them to engage in the process of mastering their physical problems as a pathway to greater personal or spiritual awareness.

These beliefs are not supported as yet by research. I would be delighted to see studies on whether the treatment of symptoms brings about as much long-lasting relief as the search for underlying causes in combination with symptomatic treatments.

How do they do that?
It has been known for decades that the mind may influence the body through the nervous system and the endocrine system, and in the past decade it has been found that the mind may also influence the immune system. Visualizations have been shown to enhance the functioning of neurohormonal, antibody, white cell and other body defense mechanisms. Dozens of proteins called neuropeptides are found in the brain. These are presumed to serve as chemical messengers between brain cells. Interestingly enough, all of these very same neuropeptides are also found in the immune system. The immune system therefore appears to be far more closely integrated with the mind than we had formerly realized, and they may even function as a unit. We are thus beginning to find more links that will help us understand the interactions of mind and body, as well as pathways by which the mind can influence the body through visualizations.

Clinical applications: Visualization can help with pains, allergies, and musculoskeletal and gastrointestinal disorders. Sports performance can be enhanced.

Visualizations in spiritual healing
Visualization by the healee is reported by many healers to be an essential element for spiritual healing. Helpful imagery may include inhaling healing energies along with the air that fills the lungs; picturing a colored light connecting one's

own heart with the healer's heart; imaging healing energies surrounding the whole body and focusing on the parts that are in need of healing, and so on.

Healers may visualize healees as whole and well in order to bring them to that state. A number of gifted natural healers suggest that this is truly a mind-over-matter effect in which the picture of wellness in the healer's mind imposes itself on the energy field and/ or on the body of the healee, restructuring the aspects of the healee's being that need healing.

While conventional medicine views the physical body as a structure that can only change with physical interventions, CAM practitioners believe the body can respond to psychological and bioenergy inputs. Many CAM therapies assume that there is a bioenergetic "template" or guiding plan that organizes and maintains body form and functions. By changing the bioenergy structure of the template, it is possible to remove disease patterns and insert healthy ones.

Oszkar Estebany reported that he visualized himself giving laying-on-of-hands treatment to healees during distant healing. He did not project images or "push" the healees to change.

Vladimir Safonov visualizes the healee sitting in a chair in his presence during distant healings. He passes his hands around the imagined body of the healee, obtaining the same sensations in his hands as though the healee were present.[219]

Suzanne Padfield visualizes the healee in perfect health (Herbert 1975). She images herself beside the healee's bed, telling the healee that he is getting well. She projects this image and this thought into the healee's mind. When she receives an image of cloudiness, she projects an image of clearness to counteract it. Padfield warns that it is important for healers to let go of the picture of illness that they observe diagnostically, so that they will not experience similar symptoms.

Dean Kraft says that he likes to understand the physiological mechanisms of disease processes in order to bring about healing more effectively. For instance, he visualizes increased blood flow to the affected skin in cases of shingles; cellular disintegration of tumors; and so forth.

Philippine psychic surgeon Tony Agpaoa frequently saw a murkiness within the healee at the place where he was ill (Stelter). He would then visualize this murkiness moving out of the body via one of the orifices. If the murkiness did not come out he would perform psychic surgery to heal the sick parts.[220]

Many healers report spontaneous visual perceptions of white or colored light surrounding the healee during a successful touch or distant healing. This has led to the common healing practice of deliberately visualizing light around the healee. Some healers, such as Dolores Krieger and Therapeutic Touch healers she has trained, visualize particular colors for particular effects.

Lawrence LeShan (1974a) made a careful study of common denominators amongst gifted healers. He found that they tend to visualize that they are united in some way with the healee, and that both healer and healee are united with the "All." By using these visualizations and studying meditation, LeShan learned to be a healer himself, and he has been able to teach others to develop their healing gifts in a similar way. An alternative state of consciousness is the third common denominator LeShan defined. This comes without effort to most gifted, natural healers, and is attained through mental concentration by healers who study in order to develop their gifts.

Healers may also visualize themselves sending or channeling energy to the healee, trusting that the healee will utilize the energy as needed for healing.

Vladimir Safonov also suggests that people may achieve rejuvenation by visualizing themselves in scenes from their earlier years. [221]

The use of words, and particularly metaphors, in healing is well known from studies of suggestion and hypnosis. Words can create images and expectations that become templates for change. [222]

V. P. Zlokazov et al. hypothesize that psychokinesis (PK) may be more prevalent in people with a "high level of generated images" (proficiency in visualization).

Tony Agpaoa (Stelter) and F. W. Knowles (1954; 1956) reported that a positive attitude is required for the healee to maintain the gains achieved with the help of the healer. Conversely, if a healee sees himself in a negative light, this may impede healing.

Osteopath John Upledger and biofeedback specialist Elmer Green have shown that traumatic physical and emotional experiences may leave their imprints in the body, in the apparent form of energy cysts that can cause a host of chronic symptoms. Upledger reports that he can visualize these cysts within the body during craniosacral therapy, and can bring about cures through their release.

Craniosacral therapy employs visualizations of the therapist manipulating the bones of the skull and the meninges lining the skull and spinal cord to clear away scars and facilitate the flow of cerebrospinal fluid. Physical manipulations are not used. The osteopath's hands are held lightly on the patient's body while they visualize the desired motions of the bones and tissues. Visualizations are also used to alter the subtle energy pulsation of the craniosacral rhythms.

Visualizations are also sometimes helpful in working with plants. Luther Burbank, an American nurseryman in the early 1900s, was able to get a cactus to grow without spines by using various processes including visualization.

Machaele Small Wright (1997) suggests that we can visualize ourselves as garden projects, inviting nature spirits to help us grow spiritually.

Imagery exercises
All of the words in the world will not convey the power of visualization, just as it is impossible to know the taste of cactus fruit from words that describe this uniquely delicious morsel. Only by actually tasting that fruit can we truly know the essence of its taste. In Chapter II-5 I suggest some experiential exercises that you can do to sense how potent visualization can be. Pick a time to do these when you feel confident that you can give this your full attention.

Research on visualization with spiritual healing is scanty. William Braud and colleagues report a laboratory experiment in which Matthew Manning, a famous British healer, was challenged to protect red blood cells from the harmful influence of a dilute saline solution, which ordinarily causes them to burst. He visualized a white light surrounding the cells, and thus helped them to survive significantly better than cells that did not receive his treatment.

S. Wilson/ Barber describe people with a "fantasy-prone personality," who also are very strong visualizers and who often have psi abilities.

Discussion: Visualization appears to be a powerful method for self-healing and spiritual healing. Visualizations are important aspects of several of the spiritual healing modalities. I am impressed that those modalities which include visualizations may offer certain advantages to the healing process.

Craniosacral therapy appears to be a very effective introduction for therapists to energy medicine practices. The craniosacral therapist visualizes the bones of the skull flexing and moving at their sutures, and projects the bioenergy image of halting the craniosacral rhythm pulsations for a brief period and then allowing them to restart.

In Therapeutic Touch, healers may visualize various colors being projected to the healee, in accordance with their perceptions of the healee's needs for enhancing, reducing or unblocking bioenergy flows.

Imagery may also help healers focus on or resonate with healees. In other words, the visualizations in these modalities may facilitate a linking between the healers and healees.

Self-healing techniques may utilize ritualized movements combined with self-healing thoughts or meditations. In *Qigong, T'ai Chi* and *Yoga* there is a focus on very specific, ritualized movements of the body. These represent another form of connection with the body that can help to bring about healing. In *Autogenic Training,* general phrases are recited that focus attention on the body, as in "My right hand is warm." In psychoneuroimmunology and psychoneurocardiology, there is a meditative focus on images of aspects of the body – such as white cells or antibodies – while holding an intent for a change in the body. I believe that the potency of these treatments derives in some measure from their focus on visualizing the body while being in a meditative state.

It appears that consciousness can focus and direct the therapists' healing through intent, as supported by the many studies of spritual healing, and as reported anecdotally by many CAM bioenergy therapists. It seems reasonable to speculate that intent can shape the actions of bioenergies – both in the process of a healer manipulating these energies and .in their effects as templates for physiological processes in healees.

Perhaps it is not visualization alone that is effective in self-healing, and it may be that any meditative and sensory connection with the body will have the same self-healing effect. We have much to clarify yet in this fascinating modality.

Studies of group visualizations

How we see the world is to some extent shaped and even determined by what our family and culture tell us to perceive. Consensual validation serves to maintain beliefs about reality. There are strong processes of indoctrination within each culture that imprint upon children the prevalent beliefs about the world, so they will *see things in ways that are congruent with their society.* In Western culture the prevalent beliefs are materialistic. They condition us to believe that the body is independent of the influence of the mind, and that it is primarily through physical and biochemical treatments that a person may be healed.[223] These beliefs may actually create the reality that they propound.[224]

Consensual validation may also be used to alter our everyday reality. Charles Tart (1969) describes experiments involving mutual hypnosis between two subjects. In his study, one person hypnotized another and then instructed that person to hypnotize him. Under these conditions both parties were able to share identical visualizations that appeared real to them. In one instance a third person entered the room and was also able to participate in the consensually visualized experiences. This supports the view that it is possible to create a separate reality via visualization.

An unusual series of consensual imaging was explored by Iris Owen and Margaret Sparrow in *Conjuring up Philip*. In this experiment, a group of people explored whether they could produce psychokinetic (PK) effects if they pretended to communicate with an imaginary personality in a seance. They made up details describing a fictitious person named "Philip." They then held regular seances over a period of many months in which they explored communications with this patently imaginary spirit. To their surprise, they began to get mediumistic information in the form of table-rapping which purported to be from that entity.[225] The information obtained was entirely consistent with the fantasy story they had created.

The visualization of Philip took on a very real quality for the participants. It worked best when they were relaxed and when conversation with Philip revolved around topics and questions that were comfortable and familiar to the group. If topics were raised that made members uncomfortable (such as Philip's sex life) then Philip might answer evasively, or not answer at all, or answer with scraping sounds or vibrations in the table instead of distinct raps. All of these responses were consistent with the experimenters' previous experiences of conversation with independent, discarnate entities.

Careful scrutiny of recorded sessions revealed that the personality of Philip varied according to the presence and/ or absence of particular members of the group at the seance. The information he conveyed was limited to the knowledge that was available to those present at any given time.

Communication effects would occur when the above conditions were met and when a jovial spontaneous, unfocused atmosphere prevailed. If deliberate, conscious efforts were made to produce Philip communications, they did not occur.

Communication with Philip proceeded as described *so long as all of those who were present believed in Philip's existence.* If his existence was called into question by a visiting skeptic or if his communication became the focus of conscious awareness and analysis by the participants, few or no communications occured.

Discussion: It seems that three elements in the group members were essential to the production of *Philip effects:* first, an unfocused, relaxed intentionality; second, the visualization or conceptualization of a discarnate entity named Philip; and third, a total belief in the existence of "Philip."[226]

Kenneth Batcheldor and others have obtained communications in this fashion from allegedly real spirits. In the light of the Philip experiments it is unclear whether these other studies represent channeling of discarnate spirits or creations of the fantasies of the experimenters.[227]

Such experimentation may contribute a great deal to our understanding of healing. Observations of this kind may help us understand how the healer may create and consolidate a new vision of a healthier reality with the healee. This may help to explain why it is often more effective to consult a healer than to practice self-healing. People may need an authority figure who gives them permission to relinquish their habitual consensual reality of being ill, and who can help them build a new reality. I will discuss this further below.

I know of no replications of Tart's mutual hypnosis work.

Meditative visualization practices

Eastern meditative practices help to develop independence from everyday, linear, sensory reality.

Alan K. Tillotson studied *Ayurvedic medicine* in Nepal. He reports the following sequence for training of spiritual healers in Nepal, according to the *Chanda Maharosina Tantra,* an ancient book on healing. The initiate, after suitable preparation in *vajrayana* Buddhist meditation and six years training in standard Ayurvedic medicine, embarks on another six-year course of intensive studies. His first year is spent in isolation in a monastery cell. He comes out once daily to bathe and eat and to obtain instruction and guidance, but otherwise remains totally alone.

He sits for long hours before figures of a many-limbed god called Chanda Maharosina (the god of dread and anger) until the student can clearly visualize every part of the god with his eyes closed. Next, he practices visualizing the same figure with his eyes open, to the point where he can see this figure in three-dimensional form in front of him. He then merges the figure's energy field with his own and becomes Chanda Maharosina himself. This figure becomes the symbol for a destroyer of everyday perceptions and realities, and it is capable of channeling *prana* (bioenergy) to the meditative disciple who worships him. This process may take a year to learn, but many are unable to achieve proficiency in this training.

Chanting aimed at stimulating the chakra system is practiced simultaneously with the visualization of the god. A rosary is held in the right hand while the mantras are chanted for hours. The rosary is usually made of human skull bones. All these techniques are used to gain control of prana.

Vajrayana Buddhists do not believe in the reality of the iconographic figure – they see the universe as a mental construct only. They seek to master the power of mind through meditation and visualization, and those who succeed are given further training, with daily meditation and exercises in mobilizing prana for use in healing. With proficiency in these techniques, the initiate can alter the realities of another person's state of health, especially nerve disorders such as paralysis.

These reports suggest that visualization may be a template for ordering and altering physical reality. It would be helpful to have careful observations, and better yet, formal studies of the practitioners of these theories and methods.

Another such report is that of Alexandra David-Neel, who studied Eastern philosophies at the Sorbonne and spent fourteen years in Tibet, where she became a lama. Her attention was first drawn to visualizations when she encountered an apparition of her Master while she was far away from him. Later, upon meeting him in person, he explained that he had deliberately projected himself to where she was in order to see how she was doing.

In response to her query, her Master told her that she could learn to do this, and he instructed her in the prescribed practices. She reports a number of curious phenomena of visualization and/ or materialization that she learned to perform. For example, she visualized a short, fat monk repeatedly over a number of months. Gradually his form came to have the appearance of being real, as though he were a guest living in her apartment. When she went on a trip, the monk accompanied her. He gradually began to perform various actions that she had not commanded, but which were appropriate to the situation he was in. Though the illusion was mostly visual, she also sometimes felt he rubbed against her or touched her. Gradually his appearance changed – he looked leaner, and then also began to appear sly and malignant. These were changes that were beyond David-Neel's control. Another person also was able to see the monk and actually mistook him for a live person. She finally decided that she wanted to be rid of this apparition of her creation. It took her six months to dissolve the phantom.

David-Neel reports:

> ... Tibetans disagree in their explanations of such phenomena: some think a material form is really brought into being; others consider the apparition as a mere case of suggestion, the creator's thought impressing others and causing them to see what he himself sees.

However, Tibetans have reported that such materializations may have physical solidity and may interact in a physical way with physical beings and objects in the world.

David-Neel also reports that she was told the following by another adept:

> [B]y means of certain kinds of concentration of mind, a phenomenon may be prepared in connection with a particular event which is to take place in the future. Once success is obtained with the concentration, the process goes on mechanically, without further cooperation of the man who has projected the energy required to bring about the phenomenon.

She was also told that in some cases, once such a plan had been put into effect, it might be impossible for the originator of the plan to change it.

Discussion: The limits of visualization and materialization are unclear. David-Neel's reports add to the indications that far more may be possible than Western worldviews generally acknowledge. Relevant to healing, her evidence suggests that it may be possible to create new realities – perhaps even materializations of items such as tissues required for healing a wound, or other restructuring of the body. Her last observation on the impossibility of altering certain visualizations may indicate some sort of natural law of imaging realities into existence that could explain why particular disease realities cannot be helped through healing.

Visualizations of being in other realities
It is certain that visualizations can help us to alter our psychological reality. We often assume that our past casts its dark shadow on our present lives, influencing our behaviors through the habits we developed in response to our early experi-

ences. Many also assume that their past experiences are etched in stone, and though they might wear a little smoother with time or might be ignored, they cannot be changed in any substantial manner. Within this belief system, we are burdened with our past errors of commission or omission and can only ask for forgiveness or absolution but cannot change them.

Recent studies show that visualizations can be used to change our relationships with our past experiences. For instance, if an unhappy childhood has left you feeling unloved and unlovable, you might find it hard to believe that anyone in your current life could love you. This is a common problem that keeps people from developing satisfying, close and intimate relationships. One way to heal such crippling childhood scars is to visualize that you are nurturing and loving your *inner child* – that part of each of us which continues to crave cuddling and loving and reassurance – teaching that now all is safe and all will be well. Claudia Black teaches that by engaging in such imagery practices you can alter the feeling-experiences of your inner child so that this part of yourself is more trusting and more open to receiving love in your current life.

Visualizations may also influence our awareness in transpersonal dimensions that extend outside our bodies. D. Scott Rogo suggested that the form people assume during *out-of-body experiences* (OBEs) may be determined by their state of mind. People having OBEs may perceive themselves as ghost-like figures with human forms; as balls of light; or as points of consciousness located in physical space.[228]

The Tibetan Book of the Dead (Rinpoche), an ancient Eastern religious text, emphasizes that the last thoughts in your mind before death influence your fate when you leave your body. Elaborate visualization exercises and prayers for the dying and for their relatives are prescribed to help project the souls of the dying into the higher and purer dimensions.

There appears to be a suggestion here that our state of mind at the time of death can project us into the sort of spiritual reality that corresponds to that state of mind. This might lend a transpersonal reality to the words of John Milton:

> *The mind is its own place, and in itself*
> *Can make a heaven of hell, a hell of heaven.*

People who have had *near-death experiences* (NDEs) report that they encounter a Being of Light who is all-knowing, unconditionally accepting and loving.

In NDEs (Moody; Ring) and in pre-death visions (Osis/ Haraldsson; Morse 1994) people report seeing the spirits of relatives coming to welcome them. In deathbed visions people also report that they see Christ, God or a being of light.

Western sensitives who counsel the dying will often suggest that they should look towards the light as they are breathing their last breaths, so that they may find their way more easily across the barriers between realities and into the next dimension.

Some healers report that they are aided by spirits in giving healing (e.g. H. Edwards; Turner 1970). Paul Beard carried this several steps further, in his investigation of channeled reports. He gathered stories indicating that spirits in the afterlife may create whole environments for themselves through their expectations and visualizations. A person who disbelieves in life after death may, upon entering the world of spirits, congregate with others of similar beliefs. Together they may visualize into existence whole earth-like suburban communities. Such a person may go on for a long time mowing his astral turf before he reaches enlightenment.[229]

Discussion: The consistent reports of healers, mediums, and people close to death suggest that either there is a widespread human need to project a visualization of an afterlife, or that spirit levels of existence are real and perceivable through intuitive senses. I believe that the latter is true because of the consistent, coherent reports of an afterlife from very diverse sources in many cultures around the world.

Visualizations as "thought forms"
In other dimensions of existence visualizations reportedly shape and mold the substance of those realms.

 Annie Besant, the second president of the Theosophical Society[230], and C. W. Leadbeater were gifted clairvoyants. They describe forms that appear in an individual's aura in association with what that person is thinking. Besant and Leadbeater depict a variety of examples of these forms, along with their interpretations of them, though they say it is impossible to render the thought forms from clairvoyant vision accurately in drawings.   Here are some of their explanations:

> What is called the aura of man is the outer part of the cloud-like substance of his higher bodies, interpenetrating each other, and extending beyond the confines of his physical body, the smallest of all. Two of these bodies, the mental and desire bodies, are those chiefly concerned with the appearance of what are called thought forms. Every thought gives rise to a set of correlated vibrations in the matter of this body, accompanied with a marvelous play of color, like that in the spray of a waterfall as the sunlight strikes it, raised to the n-th degree of color and vivid delicacy. The body under this impulse throws off a vibrating portion of itself, shaped by the nature of the vibrations – as figures are made by sand on a disc vibrating to a musical note – and this gathers from the surrounding atmosphere matter like itself in fineness from the elemental essence of the mental world. We have then a thought-form pure and simple, and it is a living entity of intense activity animated by the one idea that generated it. If made of the finer kinds of matter, it will be of great power and energy, and may be used as a most potent agent when directed by a strong and steady will.

> Each definite thought produces a double effect – a radiating vibration and a floating form. The thought itself appears first to clairvoyant sight as a vibration in the mental body... The mental body is composed of matter of several degrees of density...

> There are... many varieties of this mental matter, and it is found that each one of these has its own especial and appropriate rate of vibration, to which it seems most accustomed, so that it very readily

responds to it, and tends to return to it as soon as possible when it has been forced away from it by some strong rush of thought or feeling. When a sudden wave of some emotion sweeps over a man, for example, his astral body is thrown into violent agitation, and its original colors are for the time almost obscured by the flush of carmine, of blue, or of scarlet which corresponds with the rate of vibration of that particular emotion. This change is only temporary; it passes off in a few seconds, and the astral body rapidly resumes its usual condition. Yet every such rush of feeling produces a permanent effect: it always adds a little of its hue to the normal coloring of the astral body, so that every time that the man yields himself to a certain emotion it becomes easier for him to yield himself to it again, because his astral body is getting into the habit of vibrating at that especial rate.

[L]ike all other vibrations, these tend to reproduce themselves whenever opportunity is offered them; and so whenever they strike upon another mental body they tend to provoke in it their own rate of motion. That is – from the point of view of the man whose mental body is touched by these waves – they tend to produce in his mind thoughts of the same type as that which had previously arisen in the mind of the thinker who sent forth the waves. The distance to which such thought-waves penetrate, and the force and persistency with which they impinge upon the mental bodies of others, depend upon the strength and clearness of the original thought. In this way the thinker is in the same position as the speaker.

[T]his radiating vibration conveys the character of the thought, but not its subject.

[E]lemental essence, that strange half intelligent life which surrounds us in all directions, vivifying the matter of the mental and astral planes... thus animated responds very readily to the influence of human thought, and every impulse sent out, either from the mental body or from the astral body of man, immediately clothes itself in a temporary vehicle of this vitalized matter. Such a thought or impulse becomes for the time a kind of living creature, the thought-force being the soul and the vivified matter the body. Instead of using the somewhat clumsy paraphrase, "astral or mental matter ensouled by the monadic essence at the stage of one of the elemental kingdoms," theosophical writers often, for brevity's sake, call this quickened matter simply elemental essence; and sometimes they speak of the thought-form as an "elemental." There may be infinite variety in the color and shape of such elementals or thoughtforms, for each thought draws round it the matter which is appropriate for its expression, and sets that matter into vibration in harmony with its own; so that the character of the thought decides its color, and the study of the variations and combinations is an exceedingly interesting one.

If the man's thought or feeling is directly connected with someone else, the resultant thought-form moves towards that person and discharges itself upon his astral and mental bodies. If the man's thought is about himself, or is based upon a personal feeling, as the vast majority of thoughts are, it hovers round its creator and is always ready to react upon him whenever he is for a moment in a passive condition...

If the thought-form be neither definitely personal nor specially aimed at someone else, it simply floats detached in the atmosphere, all the time radiating vibrations similar to those originally sent forth by its creator. If it does not come into contact with any other mental body, this radiation gradually exhausts its store of energy, and in that case the form falls to pieces; but if it succeeds in awakening sympathetic vibration in any mental body near at hand, an attraction is set up, and the thoughtform is usually absorbed by that mental body.

Franklin Loehr, who studied healing effects on plants, summarizes succinctly what has been repeated by others: "A thought is a thing."

Robert Leichtman (1984), a clairsentient physician in Baltimore, writes about the emotions in parallel with Besant and Leadbeater:

Emotions are a type of subtle, invisible energy, much like electricity or light, although different in quality. The easiest way to visualize them... is as streams of living energy that circulate throughout the planet. This emotional energy is alive, active, and has specific characteristics of shape, size, and color. As a living force, it exists independently of human beings, but of course we are influenced by it, conscious of it, and able to use it.

Together, these living streams of emotional energy form a vast "sea" of emotions that permeates the entire planet... Literally, this sea of emotions is the collective emotional consciousness of all life forms on the planet. Within this sea, there are many grades and types of emotions, all of which can be contacted by human beings for better or for worse.

Leichtman finds that there are positive and negative emotions of many sorts, which appear to be polar opposites of each other. They all have varying elements of intensity, form, magnetism, plasticity and motion. He believes that emotions should be used for *touching* others, i.e. "... to heal conflict and negativity... " Incorrectly used, he believes, emotions are superficially experienced as *feeling*:

[W]e are seeking only the *appearance* of wealth, comfort, and status, not the *qualities* of compassion, peace, and wisdom. Because we are only interested in feeling the surface of life, our life ends up empty.

The "feeling" approach to emotions also commonly leads to the perpetual quest for some kind of ultimate sensation – which of course does not exist.

These observations by Leichtman suggest that one may be able to draw upon or in other ways interact with the energies or aggregates of thought/ feeling forms that either exist naturally in our environment or are collected over periods of time from human (and other?) sources, or both. He seems to corroborate Besant and Leadbeater's observations on thought forms.

Lastly I will mention that there are a number of reports of sensitives who say that they perceive in another dimension some sort of "ring of information" or "*Akashic records*" that contain all knowledge. This might represent a subtle energy repository for thought forms that exists in the aura of the earth, or perhaps may be a linear description for "super-psi," through which all knowledge is available. In other words, if we all possess psychic abilities – which can reach anywhere and anywhen – there may be a realm we can visit psychically, in which all knowledge resides.

Observations on visualization in self-healing and spiritual healing

The evidence regarding visualizations is intrinsically subjective. This area has not yet been sufficiently researched for us to describe with any confidence what might be the intermediary processes between mental/ emotional projections of visualizations and any potentially more objective source for these perceptions.

The most methodical applications of visualization are in self-healing for serious illnesses and in craniosacral therapy. These applications have the convincing weight of numerous reports supporting them, many of them gathered by people familiar with research techniques. The observations of gifted or practiced sensitives, though lacking consensual validation in the individual reports, appear to have sufficiently consistent common denominators to merit modest credence as well.

Let us first analyze visualization from the vantage of the healee. Common experience and the explorations of psychotherapy reveal that habits are hard to change. People tend to see themselves in certain ways, and they act in accordance with these perceptions – which are comfortable to them because of their familiarity. Relatives and friends come to have certain anticipations regarding their behavior, based on previous interactions with them. If they start to change, their own habits of perception and behavior, along with the expectations of others, will often get in their way. It is usually much easier to stick with the familiar and known. Even when change may be for the better, people tend to resist it both in themselves and in others. For instance, a man who has been obese and is dieting may be teased by the rest of his family about his efforts to lose weight. A wife who tends to be habitually late in getting ready to go places with her husband may be on time for once. Instead of complimenting her, he may say, "Well! What on earth happened to you today?"

These are only persistent habits of *behaving* – so how much more difficult must it be to change habits of *being*. This requires alteration of self-perceptions that have become so automatic that they are second nature. A perfect example is when a chronic pain is eliminated and the relieved sufferer feels odd, as if something has been removed from her life, rather than restored to it. After healing relieved her pain, one healee said, "I feel as though I'm walking around without my shoes or skirt." Following successful healings, people have actually managed to retrieve their lost pains by tensing their bodies where they used to hurt, because it is so unfamiliar to have body free of pain.

There are many ways that visualizations can help to shift our self-awareness.

Self-healing visualizations involve *mental* practice of patterns of behaving that anticipate subsequent *physical* changes. Through these auto-suggestions healees may be opened to new elements of behavior that are partial steps in the desired direction of the healing they seek. For example, people suffering from cancer might well feel depressed. Because of debility from the disease itself, combined with the weakening side-effects of chemo- and X-ray therapy, they may become even more depressed. Depression has its own vicious circle of: lack of energy → hopelessness → reduced socializing and weakened attention to daily living routines → fewer satisfactions in social and other aspects of life, weakened PNI and other systems → worsening depression, etc. By visualizing themselves engaging in desired positive activities, these people can prepare themselves to work their way out of such vicious circles. In mechanistic terms, we may see this as "starting to put your mind in gear," or "partializing" the problem into manageable steps. The people may then more readily engage in social or intrapsychic actions that produce positive changes in their lives, creating what I call a *sweetening spiral* – which is the opposite of a vicious circle.[231] Both their inner and outer lives may be transformed. Feeling better, they will then have more energy to do more Æ to feel still better.

We can postulate that healees may use visualizations to open themselves to changes of a more radical nature, which are brought about by healing energies. Visualizations may serve as templates for them to literally restructure themselves by reshaping their bioenergy fields. This postulate is consonant with the visualization practices described above. It is also supported by theories and research on *Life-fields* (Burr) and/or *Thought-fields*, which suggest that the mind may influence the body through biological energy fields that are present in all living things.

Healers appear to be able to help healees to let go of old images or visions of themselves and to insert and adjust to new ones. A number of factors are probably at play, either individually or more likely in concert.

The first of these is the power of suggestion. Healees usually come with the expectation that the healer is going to help them change. Thus, both through a process of selection for those people who are looking for and/or willing to accept changes, and through the build-up of hope associated with a visit to the healer, the stage is set for real change to occur. Sitting in a waiting room or in a crowded revival meeting tent may likewise enhance healees' readiness to relinquish outdated self-images.

Healers may pray, move their hands around healees' bodies, and touch them, or they may engage in more dramatic rituals (especially in revival meetings and shamanistic healings). All of these procedures will enhance the healees' anticipation of and readiness for a lasting change, which they will accomplish in part by letting go of their old visualizations of themselves.[232]

The second important factor in healing is the belief that another person can bring about the desired changes. "Placing themselves in a healer's hands" may permit healees to relinquish their mental grip on their sick self-images, allowing new, healthy, restructuring images to take hold.

It requires a major act of faith to dare to hope for success through such techniques. Even though this is difficult, our mind is capable of such shifts, as was waggishly pointed out by Franklin Loehr:

> One day I sat upon a chair.
> Of course the bottom wasn't there.
> Nor legs, nor back. But I just sat,
> Ignoring little things like that.

The healer may hold the image of a new state of being for the healee in her mind's eye, as with Loehr's chair, until the healee is ready and able to hold it himself. Visualization may be one of the key factors in bringing about healing. It may be that the visualization is transmitted by the healer to the healee telepathically as a *template* for change. It may be easier for the healee to accept a new template transmitted by a healer than to build one from scratch.

Healers often attribute their healing gift to agencies beyond themselves. These may include God, Christ, angels, spirits, the "higher self" of the healer or healee, or cosmic forces and energies. Many healers engage in healing rituals. These may aid the healer to let go of the image of the sick patient sitting before him, and to visualize an image of the healee in a healed state. This is obviously a parallel to the healee's reliance on the healer or on the healer's external aids as agents of change. Without such adjuncts, both the healer and healee may be too bound to the self-perpetuating "reality" of their senses and memories of past experiences.

The introduction of higher powers into the process of healing may also encourage the healee to relinquish his sick *templates*, by invoking an authority higher than the societal teachers who created his disbelief in his own ability to change himself.

With the support of these external aids, healers and healees may be able to put their minds, their beings and their healing energies to work through mechanisms that function in other dimensions but which influence our everyday reality. Rituals and beliefs may be mental "keys" or release mechanisms on the doors that lead to such alternative realities.

The degree of success in visualization achieved by the healer and healee may be one factor that accounts for part of the spectrum of success and failure observed in healings, which can range from mild, partial and slow changes to radical, total and sometimes near-instantaneous transformations. This theory predicts that a class of potent healers may be identified whose greatest strength lies in their powers of visualization. With healees, either an ability to visualize or a pronounced suggestibility would be complementary characteristics.[233]

The whole-and-well visualization might also act as an effective mechanism for releasing images of sickness that retard self-healing.

Although many healers visualize their healees as whole and well, they often do not do this as a focused, volitional act. It is more commonly a "wishing the healee well" and "leaving her in the hands of a higher power." Healers report that they can achieve surprisingly potent healing through visualizations of sending energy in a general way like this, without mentally specifying its intended action –saying in effect, "Thy will be done." Quite often the specific condition that brought the healee in for a treatment is not affected. Yet other conditions, which sometimes not even mentioned to the healer or not in the conscious awareness of the healee at the time of the healing, may be the very ones that respond to the treatment. It is not uncommon to hear a healee say, "Though I came to have healing for my heart condition, it was the patch of psoriasis on my elbow that cleared up." This seems at face value to contradict my thesis that visualization is an effective part of healing. However, it may be that visualizing the healee as whole and well allows the healing energies to act where they are most needed, much as an antibiotic injected into the body would. It would be of great interest to study whether such scattered healing responses occur more frequently with healers who use a general rather than a focused approach to healing. It may also be that extraneous factors such as time of day, geomagnetic activity, or other variables interact with healing to influence which ailment responds to the treatment. [234]

Leaving the healing process "in the hands of God" may activate collective unconscious images of the healer's society. Rupert Sheldrake suggests that such images may accrue power with repeated applications, thus building up what he calls *morphogenetic fields*. [235] The collective unconscious of mankind may store the visualized healing images of God from individual healings performed throughout time. This stored imagery may somehow provide access for individual healers to tap into a shared healing force or a healing awareness. Thus, while God could be an external source, the effects attributed to God could be drawn from the collective sum of healing by all healers through all time.

The healers' beliefs in what they do are often sincere and confident – with an inner certainty that transcends linear logic. Trusting in outside agents may strengthen their belief that healing will work, which may in turn enhance the potency of their visualizations.

If mind can influence matter, and if the mind of one person can affect the mind and body of another person, how can this occur? Besant and Leadbeater describe clairsentient perceptions of what appear to be parts of an etheric energy process. Do their observations represent objective, physical world" phenomena? Or could they be mental images constructed in the minds of the perceivers in order to give "substance" of a more familiar sort to clairsentient perceptions that derive from unfamiliar processes that unfold in other dimensions?

At this stage of our knowledge we can only speculate that thoughts and feelings may shape aspects of dimensions of which we are only dimly aware in our conscious minds, and which we must therefore distort when we try to use linear language and concepts to describe them.

Whether there is objective validity to spiritual healers' claims and descriptions of higher sentient beings such as spirit guides and angels is another question that we cannot presume to answer with any certainty at this stage. It is widely felt that there are entities and/or sentiences on other planes of existence who can help us. It could be postulated that these are simply cosmic energies that can be tapped into, which healers and mystics have anthropomorphically transformed into caring entities. In either case, processes of visualization may facilitate the healers' mediation between their healees and the Infinite Source.

I would also reiterate an intuitive observation that visualization combined with some sort of physical intervention is more potent than visualization alone. We see hints of this in *hatha* (exercise) *yoga* and *pranayama* (breath) *yoga;* Chinese

Qigong healing; craniosacral therapy; biofeedback; autogenic training; home-opathy; and the "passes" of touch healing.

Though much of this discussion has focused on spiritual healers, I believe that similar visualizations are utilized by many other complementary and conventional therapists, often without their conscious awareness.

Negative contributions of visualization in healing

Visualizations may also hinder healing. If people cannot or will not relinquish their self-images of being sick, it may be difficult for them to be healed. If they do not believe that they can recover, they may simply remain ill. Doctors and healers can influence these tendencies for better or worse. W. C. Ellerbroek, working with people who had venereal herpes (which has been notoriously resistant to medical treatment) reports: "I refrained from telling patients they were intractable, and they all got well... "

In a broader context, visualizations of a consensual reality may build, maintain, and perpetuate that shared reality. Social evolution may thus depend upon the creation of inspiring images that encourage, create, energize and shape changes into being new realities.

> *"Human nature" is self-validating. Whatever answer we live with will come to approximate the truth.*
> – Gregory Bateson

Many healers feel that healees possess within themselves a healthy template, or a part of themselves that remembers what wellness is. Others go further, saying that our *conscious* mind is only aware of a small portion of the many realities in which we live, and that much of the time we are actually participating in other dimensions of our existence, in a vaster reality. Brugh Joy (1988), the American physician-turned-healer, shared the following:

> My experience with this miracle called being is that there is an or-chestration to it beyond our wildest imaginations, and that you and I are actually beings much different than we think we are. And... when you begin to trust that there is a richer, vaster resource that orches-trates the process of manifest reality you would never think of directing it through the little ego awareness, the one that thinks it un-derstands what's going on. For that would be like the subatomic particle in the molecule in the cell of the hair on the dog wagging the dog. That's what the outer mind is. We are 99.9999% comatose.

If visualization can shape or even create reality, then group consensus can main-tain it. Through self-validating spirals we tend to hold on to our "truths" and to defend them against those who may question, alter or negate them. Yet with time there is a gradual drift in consensual beliefs. Thus, prevalent beliefs help a par-ticular treatment be effective, and over time the efficacy of this treatment may grow with the strength of collective belief in its potency. With negative beliefs, the efficacy of the very same treatment may fade and not work as well, if at all.

Modern science is reluctant to relinquish its view of the world, and this is one reason why spiritual healing has not enjoyed wider acceptance in the West. Spiritual healing suggests that the material world is not as solid or stable as we are told to believe. It feels threatening to us to be challenged to alter our view of reality. Many would prefer to deny the challenging evidence that is rapidly accruing for the potency of healing than to re-examine their cherished beliefs.[236]

Group visualizations may create *local, temporary* consensus realities. These can make it difficult to conduct repeatable studies of bioenergy medicine. Heraclitus observed, "We cannot step into the same river twice," and this may be a more basic truth than we ever realized. Differing consensus realities shared among different groups of people may explain part of the difficulty in replicating psi and healing effects. It may be impossible to reproduce a given reality when it is shaped by multitudes of factors in the diverse participants in the creation of local consensus realities – many of them outside of our conscious awareness. A replication of an experiment, even when procedural protocols are identical, can never be completely identical to the original as far as subtle biological energies are concerned. There will be differences in the energies of the experimenters and subjects as well as in the laboratories; in geomagnetic and sunspot activity; in the times of day at which interventions are instituted; in the extensions of all of these factors into geobiological interactions; and probably in hundreds of other variables that are impossible to control.

> You are led
> through your lifetime
> by the inner learning creature,
> the playful spiritual being
> that is your real self.
> Don't turn away
> from possible futures
> before you're certain you don't have
> anything to learn from them.
> You're always free
> to change your mind
> and choose a different future,
> or a different
> past.
>   – *Richard Bach*

Adverse effects: No harmful effects have been reported.

Training and certification: Imagery work is taught in workshops and has no certification or licensing.

Clinical applications: The best research on visualization has focused on its uses in the treatment of cancer and atherosclerotic cardiovascular disease.[237] Less rigorous studies suggest that it can improve quality of life when people are seriously ill, can enhance sports performance, and facilitates many of the processes of psychotherapy. Its applications seem limited only by the clinical vision of therapists and respants. There seem to be no physical or psychological problems that cannot be aided to some extent through imagery work.

In my own clinical work I have been able to help clients with anxieties and fears, old emotional traumas and severe allergies to make significant changes in their lives by using imagery. Severe emotional traumas can be cleared very rapidly using imagery (Benor/ Stumpfeldt/ Benor).

Imagery techniques are readily learned and used as self-healing. A skilled, experienced therapist can markedly broaden the range and scope of possible techniques and applications of visualization for careseekers to consider.

See also: Discussions in Chapter 1.

VITAMINS
See: Vitamins, under Nutrition.

WATER THERAPIES (HYDROTHERAPY)

> *Water at research establishments concerned with probing its characteristics should never be so intensively analysed and measured. The "water corpse" brought in for investigation can in no circumstances reveal the natural laws of water. It is only with natural free-flowing water that conclusions can be drawn and ideas formulated. The more profound laws are, however, hidden within the organism of earth.*
> — Viktor Schauberg (Alexandersson, p. 52)

Water has been used throughout recorded time in a variety of ways to treat an enormous range of problems.

Drinking water in large quantities is advocated as an element of some therapies to detoxify the body. It is assumed that some therapeutic procedures release toxins that are bound up in the body, and that flushing them out with quantities of water facilitates recovery.

Hot baths, showers, and saunas may be used to detoxify the body through sweating, in a similar fashion.

Colonic irrigation with water (Donovan) is widely practiced to clear the colon of wastes that may accumulate due to sluggish bowel function, build-up of toxins in the body, infections, and illnesses.

Ice is used to reduce swelling after injuries, and baths may relax tired and strained muscles.

Swimming supports the body's weight and can therefore provide gentle exercise, particularly for people recuperating from injuries and debilitating illnesses.

Flotation tanks contain water with inert salts that buoy the body up, creating a feeling of weightlessness. Combined with the sensory deprivation of a quiet, dark, enclosed tank, this therapy provides an atmosphere in which meditative states are markedly enhanced, sometimes resulting in peak experiences.

Steam in shamanic ceremonial sweat lodges may contribute to altered states of consciousness that promote spiritual awareness.

Research: No controlled studies support the above-mentioned uses of water in and of itself as a therapy

The body is composed of 65 percent water. There is evidence from homeopathy, flower essences and spiritual healing that healing vibrations can be imprinted in water. There is speculation that the water in our bodies may transmit the healing vibrations of various therapies to whatever parts of the body are in need of treatment.

Research has shown that spiritual healing can alter the UV and IR spectrum of water, and that healing intent and psychological states of people who hold water can alter its effects on the growth of plants.[238] This lends further support to the hypothesis that water may become a vehicle for healing.

Adverse effects: Common sense must apply in drinking water. It is possible to drink so much that necessary body chemicals are washed out of the system, creating dangerous imbalances in the body.

Drinking water may carry infections and toxins. One of modern medicine's greatest contributions to health care has been in the development of water supplies that are safe to drink.

Sadly, most water supplies today are potentially dangerous to our health. They may contain pesticides, fertilizers and countless drugs that are flushed down the toilet. Recycled water is purified of common chemicals such as chlorine and some fertilizers. The cocktail of medicinal drugs and pesticides that find their ways into the water system escapes purification because these are complex and diverse chemicals which would be enormously expensive to detect, much less to eliminate from the water supply.

Clinical applications: Water therapies have been used for relaxation and as adjuncts in treatment of musculoskeletal and psychological problems.

Most water therapies are self-healing in nature.

YOGA

> *The old Yoga teaching was... non-authoritarian[A] person has only to learn to listen within – to become aware of, and finally at-one with, his own "God" – in order to find all the direction he needs for his life on earth[I]n the course of time... every man would recognize some form of its truth as applicable to himself and would begin the journey to his own atonement with God.*
> – Joan Cooper (p. 42)

One of the oldest forms of self-healing is yoga, a series of disciplines which built up through many centuries of Hindu practices. *Yoga* is derived from the same root as *yoke*, applicable here in both senses of the word: to link together and to "place under discipline or training" (H. Smith p. 31). Yoga practices unite one's spirit with God.

Huston Smith presents a beautifully clear and concise description of these approaches, which are more varied than is generally appreciated in the West. He begins with Hinduism, which recognizes that there are four main paths that people may choose for spiritual development, depending on their personality and preferences:

1. *Jnana yoga* is the path of knowledge, which is the most direct but also the most difficult. On this path students first study the texts of past masters. Second, they observe themselves to learn the distinction between the masks of personality they have developed and their deeper Self, which is eternal. Finally, they shift their identification to that deeper, eternal part of their being.

2. *Bhakti yoga* aims "to direct toward God the geyser of love that lies at the base of every heart." This is the most popular variant of yoga in India. First, a student clarifies that the God he loves is not himself.

> [H]is aim will not be to perceive his identity with God but to adore him with every element of his being...
>   All we have to do in this *yoga* is to love God dearly – not just say we love him but love him in fact; love him only (loving other things because of him), and love him for no ulterior reason (not even from the desire for liberation) but for love's sake alone... (p. 37)

The practice of Bhakti yoga includes the constant repetition of God's names; the exploration of the manifold nuances of the student's love for God; and the steadfast worship of God in an idealized image of each student's choice – from among a myriad that have been created and worshipped through the ages. As man is familiar with love towards man, the personification of God in a concrete image is viewed as a helpful intermediary step in developing love and devotion to God the infinite.

3. *Karma yoga* is the path towards God through work, which may be practiced philosophically or through love.

> ... the point of life is to transcend the smallness of the finite self. This can be done either by shifting the center of interest and affection to a personal God experienced as distinct from oneself or by identifying oneself with the impersonal Absolute that resides at the core of one's being. (p. 41)

In *karma yoga,* students must work without any thought of self, in order to move closer to God.

> ... Every act of his diurnal routine is performed without concern for its effect upon himself. Not only is it performed as a service to God; it is

regarded as prompted by God's will, executed for God's sake, and transacted by God's own energy which is being channeled through the devotee. "Thou art the doer, I the instrument." (p. 42)

4. *Raja yoga* brings students closer to God through scientific experiment. They practice mental and physical exercises with the aim of moving toward awareness of the infinite Being that underlies their body, their conscious, and their unconscious. Eight steps are recommended to reduce distractions in daily activities, in the body, in breathing, in the senses and in thinking. Breathing exercises help to channel *prana* (cosmic energy); *hatha yoga* (physical exercises) disciplines the body; and meditation disciplines the mind.

In the West, *hatha yoga* exercises have been popular for the benefits they provide to physical health, such as maintaining fitness, reducing hypertension, improving diabetic control, and the like. Breathing exercises *(pranayama)* have helped in treating asthma and other pulmonary conditions.

The energy aspect of these practices has been largely ignored in modern Western applications, but this was not so in the original Hindu teachings. Breathing exercises are said to increase flows of healing energies into and throughout the body. Hatha yoga exercises and meditations open channels within the body to energy flows that purify the body and spirit, bringing practitioners to states of *samadhi* (enlightenment; union with God).[239]

Eastern traditions point out that particular physical exercises and *kriyas* (postures) help in developing and experiencing specific states of consciousness.

A store of energy *(kundalini)* is said to reside near the base of the spine, coiled like a snake, available but dormant in most people. When the suitable levels of meditation and spiritual development are reached, this energy rises through the spine to the head, bringing with it psychic awarenesses and spiritual enlightenment. If the yoga practitioner is not properly prepared, however, this transformation may bring with it a host of physical and emotional disorders.

The experience of *kundalini* is so powerful that it dramatically and profoundly transforms those who experience it. Christopher Hill observes: "[B]elief in... *kundalini*, whatever it is, must be based on direct experience and not on some teacher's parroting of cultural brainwash."

The *chakras,* or energy centers in the body, were described in Sanskrit writings on yoga. The bioenergies may be channeled by the yoga adept to heal others. It seems likely that these are the same energies that are focused in the Chinese self-healing and healer-healing practices of *Qigong*, which are used to treat numerous illnesses.

Spiritual aspects of health form an integral part of yoga and other Eastern healing systems. For instance, reincarnation is an accepted belief in Hindu religion. This belief provides a framework within which people can cope with some of their difficulties in life and with their fears of death.[240]

Integrative care and Eastern approaches
Medical practice in the West has focused on manipulations of the material world and consequently on the *physical* aspects of disease.

In contrast, the healing arts in the East have focused on *energy medicine* and on harmonizing all aspects of life. One does not negate the other, and both can help to heal.

In *hatha yoga* and *pranayama* we again find a combination of meditative and physical exercises. This combination appears especially effective for self-healing.

Some Christians have hesitated to be involved in yoga because it has religious overtones that are not accepted in their church. Christina Jackson has developed yoga exercises that are harmonized with Christian prayers.

There are also numerous Western methods of exercise for self-help and for developing awareness that involve harmonizing of body, emotions, mind, and spirit. Many of these have considerable overlaps with yoga.

Rebirthing (Orr/ Ray), *Holotroopic Breathwork* (Grof/ Halifax), and other breathing methods have been developed to help people release old memories that are buried in the unconscious mind, and sometimes locked into physical pathology. These methods may also bring out memories of past life traumas.

Bodywork psychotherapy uses physical exercises to promote physical health and facilitate emotional release.

Meditation is widely recommended in the West for health enhancement and spiritual development. Many meditations use the biological metronome of breathing as a focus for concentrating the mind. Variations on the theme of pranayama suggest that meditators visualize healing energies entering their body along with their breath, and then picture the release of tensions and other expressions that they are ready to let go of.

Adverse effects: While generally a gentle and safe practice, there have been injuries reported with exercises that are too vigorous or advanced. The supervision of a trained yoga teacher is advised in developing a program of yoga practice.

Training and certification: There are no Western standards for training, certification or licensing in these practices.

Clinical applications: Yoga practices can improve relaxation, muscle toning and breathing. Hatha yoga exercises are excellent as preventive medicine, and helpful in maintaining muscle tone and normal flows of biological energies. They may also be helpful in rehabilitation following injuries or illnesses. Yoga can contribute to improvements in stress-related illnesses such as hypertension and musculoskeletal pains. By enhancing biological energy flows it can strengthen the body's abilities to deal with many other illnesses, in ways that cannot be explained within Western medical theories. It can also facilitate spiritual discipline and higher sense awareness.

While initial instruction in these techniques is usually necessary, their practice is self-healing.

See also: Qigong; T'ai Chi Ch'uan.

Problems addressed effectively by CAM modalities

In general, CAM therapies have been particularly helpful with chronic illnesses, where conventional medicine has no cures and where conventional treatments may often cause serious side effects that diminish quality of life. This is not to say that there is no place for conventional treatments in chronic illnesses or that CAM therapies cannot help in acute illnesses. The best approach, of course, is through integrative care that includes the best of both approaches.

ALLERGIES

CAM therapists may identify allergies as causal agents in chronic illnesses where conventional medicine would not consider this a possibility. These may include health problems such as anxiety and panic attacks, depression, headaches, attention deficit hyperactivity disorder (ADHD), learning disorders, arthritis, asthma and other respiratory problems, sinusitis, menstrual problems, digestive disorders, and chronic fatigue syndrome. Symptoms that may suggest allergies include rashes, abdominal pains, nausea, vomiting, diarrhea, headaches, irritability, chronic fatigue and even epileptic fits.

Multiple allergy syndrome may occur on its own or in combination with chronic fatigue syndrome and candidiasis. For no apparent reason, people may develop hypersensitivity to numerous chemicals and foods. It seems as though their immune systems are working overtime in response to numerous chemicals which they had previously handled without difficulties.

Treatment begins with identification of allergens and avoidance of these substances for a period of time so that the immune system can recover its normal functions. CAM modalities that may be helpful in identifying allergies include applied kinesiology; medical dowsing and electroacupuncture according to Voll; and in treating allergies meridian based therapies,[241] homeopathy, nutritional counseling, Anthroposophic medicine, and Ayurveda.

ARTHRITIS

Osteoarthritis is degeneration of joints from chronic wear and tear. Rheumatoid arthritis (along with other variations, such as Lupus) appears to be caused by a malfunction of the immune system, where tissues in the joints are misperceived by the body as alien and are then attacked by the immune system. Some forms of arthritis follow particular bacterial infections. The causes for others are unknown.

Conventional preventive treatments are helpful where bacterial infections that can initiate arthritic processes are treated with antibiotics. Surgical interventions to deal with arthritic joints, particularly in late stages where prosthetic replacements are necessary, can give people suffering from arthritis a new lease on life. Conventional medicinal treatments can help to cope with many of the symptoms of arthritis, but are fraught with numerous side effects – up to and including fatal ones.

CAM therapies have an enormous contribution to offer in arthritis.

Several studies support the use of healing for pain. Anecdotal reports indicate that swelling and mobility are also significantly helped by healing (including craniosacral therapy) and that spiritual healing gives promise that it can be curative – especially in early stages of arthritis.

Acupuncture is excellent for pain relief and can have much deeper effects as well. Traditional Chinese Medicine adds herbal remedies that are helpful.

Homeopathy addressed the individual constellations of symptoms in each person and can help with arthritis, as with most other problems.

Diets, including Ayurvedic therapy, nutritional supplements, and elimination diets to remove allergens that precipitate or worsen arthritis may help.

Many other CAM therapies are recommended for arthritis, and have numerous anecdotal reports to recommend them, but still await research to confirm their efficacy.

Environmental medicine, including feng shui and medical dowsing, have identified negative energies that can contribute to arthritis and can advise on ways to relieve this. Included on this list are:

Pulsed Electromagnetic Fields (PEMF) and simple magnets

Light therapy

Movement therapies, such as the Alexander Technique, can improve mobility

CANDIDA YEAST INFECTIONS

The condition of Candidiasis often develops following a course of treatment with antibiotics that kill off the normal bacteria in the gut and allow yeasts to grow there instead, or with steroids that weaken the immune system. This condition may present with any combination of the following symptoms:

- "feeling lousy" without reason, being irritable or easily angered;
- craving yeasty foods (bread, alcohol, fermented cheeses) and sweets;
- eating these foods may provide temporary relief, but this may be followed by a worsening of symptoms,
- symptoms resembling hypoglycemia (fatigue, sharp hunger spells, weakness, trembling, drowsiness, cold sweats, dizziness, headaches, blurred vision, palpitations, rapid pulse, and irritability);
- abdominal pains;
- premenstrual syndrome, menstrual irregularities and pain;
- vaginal infections and local discomfort during intercourse;
- prostatitis or impotence;
- loss of libido;
- persistent fungus infections of the feet, crotch, toenails, or skin;
- fatigue that is worsened when exposed to molds (basements, gardening); and
- heightened sensitivity to tobacco smoke, perfumes, and other chemicals.

Treatment may involve avoidance of foods that promote yeast growth – which are often the very foods that are craved; avoidance (to a reasonable extent) of antibiotics; taking the anti-yeast (prescription) drug nystatin; eating yogurt; taking capsules of lactobacilli to replace the normal flora that are killed off by antibiotics; drinking special herbal teas (taheebo, la pacho, pau d'arco); and having cleansing enemas (Trowbridge/ Walker).

CHRONIC FATIGUE SYNDROME (CFS)

CFS and fibromyalgia both often begin with a viral illness such as a severe flu. Symptoms that persist for weeks and even months, and may include severe weakness, insomnia, headaches, muscle aches and depression. When muscle aches predominate, the usual diagnosis is fibromyalgia, but the dynamics and treatments are similar in either case. Sufferers are doubly and triply afflicted because nothing in conventional treatment tends to help, and malingering is often suspected. The resulting weakness may be so severe that sufferers cannot even get out of bed. Symptoms typically persist for months and years.[242] Candidiasis, fibromyalgia and multiple allergies may be present concurrently.

Helpful treatments include spiritual healing, acupuncture, homeopathy, massage, psychotherapy, meridian based therapies, relaxation, imagery techniques, identifying allergens, whole-food and allergy diets.

Conventional medicine has been slow to acknowledge CFS as a real entity, as no clear cause has been identified, nor is there any definitive diagnostic test for it.

> ...Presently, modern medicine does not proceed on clinical observation and experience alone but relies almost exclusively on objective laboratory data. Where CFS is concerned, it's hard to see the beast. Given the limitations of our present medical technology, we can only follow its footprints.
>
> – Jesse Stoff and Charles Pellegrino (p.60)

Multiple allergy syndrome may occur on its own or in combination with chronic fatigue, fibromyalgia and candidiasis. In these conditions, people develop hypersensitivity to numerous chemicals and foods for no apparent reason. It seems as though their immune systems are overwhelmed and unable to deal with chemical stresses which they had previously handled without any difficulties. (See discussion of allergies, above).

While some wholistic medical doctors are familiar with these syndromes, many who are afflicted with CFS are disappointed to receive little or no help from their conventional family physicians, and find relief only from CAM therapists.

FIBROMYALGIA (FM)

Fibromyalgia often presents with many of the same symptoms as chronic fatigue syndrome and multiple allergy syndrome. It involves chronic pains in muscles all over the body, with weakness and tiredness on exertion. People with FM may be unable to manage more than a bare minimum of self-care without utter exhaustion.

Treatments are similar to those of CFS and multiple allergy syndrome. Careful pacing of exertion, with budgeting of energies allotted to tasks is essential.

CANCER

We treat dogs and cats better than we treat people with terminal illness in our society. When our pets are afflicted with major debilitating and painful terminal illnesses we put an end to their suffering with a merciful sleep into death.

Western medicine has difficulty accepting its limitations to cure human disease. The possibility that cancer will prove fatal leads conventional medicine to treat cancer aggressively – fighting it and waging war against it, cutting it out wherever possible, poisoning it with toxic chemicals and bombarding it with x-rays.

Treatment of the cancer often is the focus rather than treatment of the person who has the cancer. The prolongation of life at all costs becomes the goal of treatment, often carried to extremes, well past the point that the person with cancer might wish. Quality of life is not given as high a priority as fighting off what is viewed as the grim reaper. While some chemotherapy and radiotherapy can be extremely helpful in slowing or reversing the growth of cancers, there are many times that highly unpleasant side effects are produced – seriously diminishing the quality of life.

People with cancer are often frightened and bullied into accepting treatments that produce major side effects which seriously diminish the quality of their remaining months and days on earth. When they elect to refuse these treatments, some doctors may take extreme measures. In some places, if a child has a terminal illness and the parents refuse to accept a doctor's recommendation for toxic therapies, the child may even be removed from the parents' care by the child welfare department at the doctors' insistence and forced to undergo the recommended treatments.

CAM therapies for cancer more often focus on the whole person rather than just on the disease, as with CAM therapies for other illnesses. There are no studies to show which therapy is best. Here is a modest list of CAM therapies commonly used in treatment of cancer: Nutrition; herbs; macrobiotic diet; self-healing for cancer; living and dealing with cancer; exceptional cancer patients; hypnosis; psychoneuroimmunology (PNI); spiritual healing;[243] family involvement in cancer therapy.

NEUROLOGICAL PROBLEMS

Strokes leave people with perceptual, cognitive and motor deficits. Acupuncture can markedly enhance recuperation from strokes. I feel it is verging on malpractice for physicians not to recommend acupuncture for strokes.

Phantom limb pain is pain that is perceived to come from a limb or other body part that has been amputated. This is particularly responsive to spiritual healing.

Multiple sclerosis is a condition in which plaques of white matter proliferate in the nervous system, extending from the myelin sheaths of the nerves, and disrupting nervous system function. The course of the illness is highly variable and unpredictable, with periods of worsening symptoms alternating with periods of quiescence of the disease. Rates of progression are also quite variable.

Conventional Western medicine is limited in the treatments that it has to offer.

CAM therapies have not been well documented in their applications for the treatment of MS. Nevertheless, I have heard several reports of marked improvement, even in severely advanced cases, which have responded well to a combination of spiritual healing (Gardener) and intensive psychotherapy. The new meridian-based therapies appear particularly promising in facilitating the use of psychotherapy in these cases. I am impressed that some of the reports appear to indicate improvements that go well beyond those that occur with the periodic waxing and waning of symptoms typical of MS.

Coma following head trauma and various infections is reported anecdotally to respond well to craniosacral therapy and spiritual healing in some cases.

Complementary/ Alternative Medicine (CAM) Issues

ETHICAL ISSUES IN CAM

Ethics is how we behave when we decide we belong together.
— Brother David Steindl-Rast

Ethical issues may be more complex for CAM practitioners as compared with conventional medical practitioners. The following are some of the key issues that apply to most therapists.[244]

Competence – Some CAM therapies, such as massage, acupuncture, chiropractic, dietary and nutritional supplement therapies, and homeopathy, involve knowledge-based and specific intervention-based treatments. In these cases, objective criteria for competence can be established. In other CAM therapies, such as healing and craniosacral therapy, competence may be more difficult to establish because the energetic interventions are subtle and impossible to measure (as yet), and procedures in the art of therapy may vary enormously between one practitioner and another.

In all of these interventions, the person of the therapist is to a lesser or greater extent a variable in the intervention. For instance, in acupuncture it is not just the insertion of needles that brings about changes, but also *how* the needles are inserted. In other words, the person doing the acupuncture is a part of the physical therapeutic intervention. Herbalists in traditional cultures suggest that it is not just the plant essence that heals, but *what you tell the plant to do*. Intuitive assessments and interventions by sensitive practitioners can lead to much deeper and more effective interventions in all CAM therapies.

To have any semblance of standardization of the subtler dimensions of these treatments it is necessary for given modality practitioners to agree on clinical competencies in their CAM therapies. It is advisable to include an apprenticeship with certified teachers, along with a thorough, formal demonstration of knowledge and technical skills.

Even with the best and tightest of such standardizations, many of these modalities are as much an art as a skill. Subtle factors relating to the peson who is the caregiver and the person who is the careseeker, as well as to the "chemistry" of their relationship may have major impacts on the outcomes of treatments. These may determine to a great degree how people respond to the therapy – regardless of the specific modality interventions.

Negotiating therapy contracts with clients – In CAM therapies it is important that informed consent be established before any procedures begin. With healing and other CAM approaches there is often an expectation that rapid, even miraculous cures can be achieved in a single treatment. Few people coming for their initial assessments know much about these approaches, so appropriate time should be invested to explain how they work and what results to expect from the therapist and the interventions. Expectations of client responsibilities in using these therapies should also be spelled out.

Respect for autonomy and consent – Compared with conventional medicine, CAM clients are often given more autonomy in choosing therapeutic modalities, as well as greater responsibility for their own treatment. CAM therapies may be therapist-generated, as in acupuncture and homeopathy, but they may also rely heavily on client participation, as in nutrition, fitness, Qigong, meditation, relaxation, meridian based therapies, and imagery approaches. Self-assessment and self-healing are essential aspects of many interventions, and their effectiveness may depend on regular self-healing practices.

Records of treatment – Proper record keeping is essential for continuity of care, as well as for legal purposes. This can also provide databases for evaluation and research.

Research – Responsible use of CAM approaches requires that therapists assess the results of their interventions, both to know that what they are doing is effective and to monitor any side effects or adverse effects that may occur. Basic research need not be complicated. Much can be learned from systematic review of records of treatment, case presentations and qualitative studies.

Continuous professional development – There are frequent advances that enhance treatment potentials in most therapies. Therapists should stay current with developments in their own areas of specialization, and to the extent that is possible, in other CAM methodologies as well. In addition to cognitive updates, personal development is particularly important wherever the therapist is an essential component in the treatment. Clearing emotional dross, clarifying blind spots that result from prior emotional traumas, and staying alert to issues of transference and counter-transference will markedly enhance the therapy. This process requires personal psychotherapy and/ or other CAM therapy interventions for the therapist. This is one of the most important aspects of ethical practice.

Collaborations and referrals to other health caregivers – No single therapy is appropriate for every person or every problem. It is important to know the limits of any CAM approach and of one's personal competence in its methodologies, and when to refer to other therapists for treatment. Making appropriate referrals is an art that requires at least a basic knowledge of other therapies, and of the competencies and personalities of specific therapists. Collaborating with other therapists is an even greater challenge. We don't know very much about the range of efficacy of individual CAM therapies, much less about combinations of these modalities. For many problems, such as arthritis, backaches, chronic fatigue syndrome, fibromyalgia and cancer, multimodal approaches seem to be more effective than single therapies. It takes both self-confidence and humility to be able to admit one's own limitations and to work productively with other therapists in helping people faced with complex problems.

Special duties towards children – Children may not be able to articulate or explain their problems, and their judgment usually is not sufficiently mature to allow them full responsibility for making healthcare decisions. However, their cooperation is often vital to the success of treatment. Therapists have to rely to a great extent on parental impressions about their children's problems, and parents will also carry out or supervise treatments at home.

Therapists must also remain alert to the possibilities of children's problems being caused – directly or indirectly – by their parents. On the mild end of the spectrum, tensions in the home may contribute to children's tensions, which may cause or worsen their illnesses. On the severe end of this spectrum, parents may be directly harming their children through emotional, physical, or sexual abuse. CAM therapists should take responsibility for reporting suspected abuse to the appropriate authorities, just as conventional therapists do.

Respecting confidentiality – Clients expect that therapists will maintain confidentiality regarding their problems and treatment records. Written permission should be obtained before releasing information or records to anyone. In the US, confidentiality is now regulated by the Health Informations Privacy Act Administration (HIPAA).

Maintaining professional boundaries – Clients are needy and vulnerable when they come for help. Therapists must not take advantage of clients to satisfy their own ego, emotional or sexual needs.

Professional etiquette, respect for colleagues – Careseekers who come for CAM therapies often have chronic problems and may have seen a series of conventional and CAM therapists already. While clients may have justifiable complaints, their stories often represent just one side of a situation and may be distorted by misperceptions, faulty or selective memory, or psychopathology. While therapists should not totally discount or discredit clients' stories, judgment should be withheld until the other side can be heard.

Availability of effective complaint mechanisms – Responsible professional associations must establish procedures for clients to file complaints, and for review and discipline of therapists' conduct.

The practices of conventional medicine, nursing, psychology, and social work all have established ethical standards. Physicians take the Hippocratic oath, and the principle of "first do no harm" is repeatedly emphasized in their training. CAM therapies would do well to develop similar codes of ethics.

CERTIFICATION AND REGULATION
OF CAM PRACTITIONERS

Regulation of complementary therapy practitioners is a complex issue. Some modalities such as acupuncture, chiropractic, homeopathy, massage, Therapeutic Touch and Healing Touchhave professional organizations that set standards for the education and practice of their members. Many other therapies are represented by no professional organization, and have no generally accepted standards for education or practice or any disciplinary authorities or procedures.

There are three broad forms of regulation for healthcare practitioners:

1. *Licensing* – requiring that practitioners meet standards imposed by the state;
2. *Certification* – protecting the title of people who meet specified standards, but not restricting others from practicing without using the title; and
3. *Registration* – requiring only that practitioners file their names, qualifications, and addresses.

While it is desirable to protect the public from incompetent, unethical, and/or fraudulent health care practitioners, many state laws have been written in language that favors allopathic medicine, stating that no one may practice as a health care professional outside of the norms of local medical practitioners.

State laws governing medical practice have been enacted in consultation with medical doctors over the past 100 years. Medical doctors have actively used these laws to promote the exclusive legal legitimation of allopathic medicine, and have sought to deny practitioners of other therapies the right to practice. In the early 1900s, medical doctors were successful in eliminating competition from homeopathic and naturopathic physicians through such legislation. Since then they have endeavored to limit the practices of other complementary therapists as well. In addition, some local medical societies strongly discourage their member physicians from introducing CAM in their practices, by applying restrictive recommendations based on legal definitions of proper practice. These legal limits state that doctors are judged to be practicing properly or improperly according to the "standard medical practices of their local colleagues or of the school in which they were trained." While this provides the courts with some standard for judging whether a doctor was liable in a malpractice suit, it is not a suitable basis for restricting the use of other methods. Were such standards rigidly applied, there would be very little progress in medical treatment, and what therre was would be very slow.

> *When everyone is wrong, everyone is right.*
> – Nivelle de la Chaussée

These restrictive laws were successfully challenged by chiropractors in 1985. Other complementary therapies have been accepted by several states – often as the result of constitutional challenges of existing laws by practitioners and the public. A restrictive attitude is still prevalent in the majority of states, though this is steadily improving.

It is difficult to find the best balance between protecting the public from harm on the one hand, and excessively restricting complementary therapy practices on the other. Therefore complementary therapists are challenged to improve their own internal professional regulation and to support their claims of efficacy for their modalities with research evidence. Where they have done so, they have often achieved better recognition and acceptance within the existing laws.[245]

Spiritual healing is not yet among the modalities that have professional licensing boards in America. In fact, there is even dissention and schism between healers trained and practicing in different traditions, such as Therapeutic Touch and Healing Touch, and the various Reiki lineages and schools.

Complementary therapists complain that physicians can take weekend courses in CAM methodologies (e.g. acupuncture for pain control) and then be allowed by law to practice these modalities, while CAM practitioners who have years of training and experience are denied this right because they don't have a license to practice medical.

Ironically, in some states restrictions are applied just as vigorously against pioneering physicians who engage in the practice of complementary therapies. Doctors have been hounded by members of their own medical societies on the grounds that they are practicing therapies that are not accepted by their peers – often with no consideration of the evidence for the efficacy and relative safety of these therapies.

> *If a little knowledge is dangerous, where is the man who has so much*
> *as to be out of danger?*
> – T. H. Huxley

INSURANCE AND LEGAL CAM ISSUES

Insurance coverage for CAM treatments
and malpractice coverage for practitioners

With increasing awareness that the public is paying billions of dollars annually out of pocket for CAM therapies (Eisenberg et al. 1993; 1998), a growing number of insurers now include payment for some CAM services in their policies. Several states now have laws requiring health insurers to include CAM benefits (Firsbein). Acupuncture, chiropractic, and massage are the most commonly covered modalities. This is a reflection of the general rate of usage of these modalities, as well as an acknowledgment of the professional membership organizations that their practitioners have formed.

Growing numbers of states mandate insurance coverage for licensed CAM therapies.

The numbers of insurance claims against CAM practitioners is much, much lower than the number of claims against medical practitioners (Studdert/ Eisenberg et al.). This is probably due to the facts that CAM therapies have much lower rates of serious complications and that closer, more personal and trusting relationships often develop between CAM practitioners and their clients – for all of the reasons detailed elsewhere in this book. It may also be that awareness regarding the possibility of litigation has yet to grow in this area to the extent that it has in conventional medical practice. A last factor is that there are far deeper pockets in medical practices that make it worth a lawyer's efforts than in CAM practices.

Malpractice insurance is now available for many CAM practitioners. Again, there are more insurers offering coverage for the more commonly used and accepted modalities, such as acupuncture and chiropractic.[246]

Legal status of CAM therapies

CAM practitioners and the public may have difficulty understanding why the medical profession has been slow to develop programs of integrative care, when so many practitioners and recipients of CAM therapies report that they are beneficial. Several issues are at play here.

Private medicine in the US has viewed CAM therapies as competition for the healthcare dollar. The AMA has lobbied against the acceptance and legal recognition of CAM practitioners, starting with homeopathy and naturopathy in the early 1900s. These discriminatory practices continue today. For instance, the AMA has discouraged hospitals and medical schools form providing Continuing Medical Education credits for conferences on CAM.[247]

*Our ideas are only intellectual instruments that we use to break into phe-
nomena; we must change them when they have served their purpose, as we
change a blunt lancet that we have used long enough.*
                                            – Claude Bernard

Three primary objections to physicians' involvement with CAM have been
proposed:

1. *There is no good evidence for the efficacy of CAM therapies.* This is patently
ridiculous, considering the wealth of evidence summarized in this book.

Critics like to suggest that CAM research is not up to the level of conventional
medical research. This is likewise untrue, as witnessed by the growing involvement
of physicians in publishing research on CAM therapies. To some extent, this claim
is a product of ignorance caused by the limited access conventional doctors have
had to this body of research.

There is a major problem with publication bias against CAM in the conventional
medical literature. This has limited the dissemination of information in the
medical community, thus perpetuating the division between CAM and allopathic
approaches and impeding the development of integrative care. [248]

2. *Use of CAM therapies may delay the application of more effective therapies
beyond the point where these are able to help.* This might be true if people with
medically treatable illnesses used CAM therapies exclusively in place of
conventional therapies. However, this is a spurious argument in cases where CAM
is used within a program of integrative care. It is also far from clear that all
conventional therapies are of proven efficacy. Furthermore, the side effects of many
conventional therapies (particularly with cancer, pain and depression) may diminish
quality of life to such an extent, while offering minimal hope of palliation or cure,
that respants may seek out CAM therapies that can enhance quality of life.

3. A doctor who refers a patient to a CAM practitioner may be liable for
malpractice claims if the patient suffers harm at the hands of the CAM practitioner.
This is a very complex legal issue (Studdert/ Eisenberg et al.).

A doctor could be liable if his referral of a patient to a CAM practitioner is
negligent. For instance, if the doctor knows that an acupuncturist does not sterilize
needles after use or does not use disposable needles, the doctor could be held liable
if the referred patient gets hepatitis B or AIDS as a result of treatment by that
acupuncturist. If the doctor maintains a supervisory relationship with the CAM
practitioner there would be a clear liability, and the same might apply if the doctor
and the CAM practitioner work within the same institution or under the same health
management plan.

A doctor might conceivably be held liable for referring a patient to a particular
type of CAM practitioner when another type of CAM therapy is significantly more
appropriate.

In all of these cases, the injured party would have to demonstrate a causal
relationship between the alleged substandard referral and the injury.

On the whole, the liability rate for physicians referring patients to CAM therapists
is likely to be low, considering the low rate of malpractice claims against CAM
practitioners.

4. The AMA has often objected to physicians' use of CAM on the basis that these therapies are not standard local practices. Because the AMA has successfully lobbied to have many state legal codes reflect this standard for deciding upon the suitability of care, this complaint often carries the force of law. The illogic of the complaint is again patently obvious. If it were rigidly applied, there would be very little progress in the practice of medicine. Few new treatments would ever be discovered or developed.

The AMA has promoted legislation to outlaw the practice of medicine without a license. All states license chiropractors, and growing numbers license acupuncturists, massage therapists, naturopaths, and homeopaths. Most do not license other CAM practitioners. A therapist who offers to diagnose or treat a disease without a license can be subject to prosecution. The law does not consider it an adequate defense if patients testify to the efficacy and benefits of the therapy, or claim that no harm has come from the therapy. Even research evidence supporting the efficacy of the therapy often may not be accepted as a legal defense.

Here is an example of this policy in practice.

> This is the true story of a man who cured himself of a near-fatal cancer after conventional medicine had mutilated and then abandoned him. He spent the next thirty years helping others with the disease. In the struggle to keep hi clinic open, he faced raids and robberies, a near-fatal beating, a kidnapping, and a prison sentence many called justice gone wrong. He is in jail for a second time as this book goes to press in 1998, for the offense of treating cancer patients. The therapies that made up his treatment protocol were an eclectic assortment that covered the gamut and drew from the best of thte available natural cancer remedies. The details of this therapies, and the history and vicissitudes of the non-traditional health care movement that his life personifies, are woven through his story.
>
> Is effective non-toxic cancer treatment being suppressed? Hundreds of people who wrote to the court in Jimmy Keller's defense in 1991 thought so. Many wrote that he had kept their cancers in remission when nothing else would... (E. Brown, book jacket)

True, the therapies used by Keller were not researched. However, there was no evidence that he was causing direct harm, and many reported that he had been helpful to them.

Several CAM therapy groups, aided by grateful recipients of their treatments, are lobbying state governments for changes in such restrictive laws. Minnesota has passed the most progressive legislation, allowing great freedom for CAM practitioners, Followed by California, and other states are considering similar legislation. This seems a far better approach than was used in the case of chiropractors, who had to sue the AMA for restraint of competitive trade in order to obtain governmental approval for their right to practice.

Licensed CAM practitioners are tried by the courts according to the standards of their CAM schools of practice, just as physicians are tried according to the standards of their individual medical schools.

CAM practitioners whose methods of treatment are not licensed are tried according to standards of conventional medical care or lay healthcare standards.

All of the health regulations vary by state. While having 50 different legal systems for health care allows for local practice to influence legislation, it makes it very difficult for CAM practitioners and the public to bring about changes in the laws that govern their health care..

Considering the fact that the general public pays more visits to CAM practitioners than to conventional medical doctors, there are bound to be shifts in the degree of collaboration and in legal status. The current situation finds patients visiting CAM practitioners and not telling their physicians about it – and this is a poor state of affairs.

David Studdert, David Eisenberg and colleagues suggest:

> Physicians who currently refer patients to practitioners of alternative medicine or who are contemplating doing so should not be overly concerned about the malpractice liability implications of their conduct... [I]t may be useful to ask the following questions. First, is there evidence from the medical literature to suggest that the therapies a patient will receive as a result of the referral will offer no benefit or will subject the patient to unreasonable risks? Second, is the practitioner licensed in my state? (Some added comfort can be derived from knowing that the practitioner carries malpractice insurance.) Third, do I have any special knowledge or experience to make me think that this particular practitioner is incompetent? And fourth, will this be the usual kind of referral (i.e. basically at arm's length, without ongoing and intrusive supervision of the patient's management)?
>
> If the answers to the first and third of these questions are no and the answers to the second and fourth questions are yes, then this should remove many of the concerns a physician has that the referral decision itself will be construed as negligent. This conclusion holds even if the patient suffers an injury caused by the alternative medicine practitioner's negligence. That practitioner should be held accountable for his or her autonomous actions and should be judged according to standards set by fellow practitioners.

The legal status of spiritual healing differs in several respects from that of CAM therapies in which herbs or other substances are prescribed or which use physical interventions such as massage or physical manipulation. When healing is given without touch, either with the healer's hands held near to but not touching the body, or through distant healing, it is unlikely that any causal connection could be established between a claimed negative effect and the healing treatment. Even where light touch is used in spiritual healing, the same constraint would apply.

However, this would not provide a defense against charges of delaying treatment that might have been of greater benefit, of sexual misconduct, or of other common-sense damages.

Some spiritual healers protect themselves legally by being ordained as religious ministers, which allows them to practice healing without fear of legal restraints.

INTEGRATIVE CARE: WHICH THERAPY FOR WHICH PROBLEM?

Holistic Medicine – New map, old territory.
— Patrick Pietroni

It is a challenge both to practitioners and to people seeking help to decide which therapy is most appropriate for which health problem. We are barely beginning to understand the spectrum of efficacy of individual therapies, let alone being able to make informed choices between them. The case is a little clearer for the question of allopathic medicine vs. CAM therapies, though the research base is no stronger.

Conventional treatments

Allopathic medicine has a major contribution to make with treatments for certain problems. However, many conventional medical treatments have distinct disadvantages:

1. *Infections* caused by bacteria (e.g. bacterial pneumonia and meningitis), by spirochetes (e.g. syphilis), by rickettsia (e.g. Rocky Mountain spotted fever), and by some other organisms often respond well to treatment with antibiotics. Specific antibiotics must be given in recommended doses for specific periods of time if they are to be effective.

However, if they are taken for too brief a period or in doses that are too low, antibiotics may worsen the problem by selectively killing the weaker infectious organisms, leaving the patient with a *super-infection* of antibiotic-resistant organisms.

Bacteria can develop resistance to antibiotics. Viral illnesses do not respond to antibiotics, yet many people ask their doctors for antibiotics when they have the flu or other viral infections, and many doctors find it easier to give an antibiotic than to argue against these requests. This leads to a very serious public health problem. It is becoming increasingly difficult to deal with infections caused by drug-resistant strains of bacteria. This has become a serious concern with tuberculosis and venereal diseases in particular.

Allergic reactions may limit the use of antibiotics in certain individuals, and can present a danger to health and even to life when the reactions are severe. Severe allergic reactions constitute a significant portion of the many deaths in the US annually caused by medications (which were properly prescribed).

Antibiotics given for an infection in one part of the body may eliminate other useful or apparently harmless bacteria in another part of the body. Gastrointestinal and mucous membrane infections with yeasts and other organisms may result from antibiotics that eliminate the benign organisms that normally dwell on these tissues.

Homeopathic medicine offers an alternative to antibiotic use that has not yet been adequately explored or researched.

2. *Medications* may help in treating many problems such as pain, cardiovascular disease, epilepsy, arthritis, anxiety, depression, schizophrenia, and more. New medications are constantly being developed. In some cases medications can cure problems completely, as in single episodes of depression that are relieved by

368 Vol. II Chapter 2 – Wholistic Energy Medicine

antidepressants and do not recur. In other instances, symptomatic relief can be obtained. For instance, the physical symptoms of viral illnesses can be alleviated – even though the viral infections are not eliminated. Though herpes and AIDS are not cured by taking medication, quality of life can be substantially improved and life may be prolonged.

The downside of medications is that every drug may produce side effects in some people some of the time. When these effects are mild, the benefits of medicinal therapy may outweigh the costs. However when side effects are severe, quality of life may be compromised to the point that the medications cause as much distress as the illnesses for which they are prescribed – or more. This is particularly true of *cancer chemotherapy* (and *radiotherapy*). While these treatments may prolong life, their negative effects must be weighed carefully against their benefits. With some cancers the prolongation of life can be considerable. With others the efficacy of these treatments may be minimal, and the impairment to quality of life is sufficient to raise serious questions as to whether the treatments are of real benefit to the patient. Their use actually could be a symptom of the patient's and the doctor's denial of the fatal nature of the illness.

The annual rate of deaths from serious negative reactions to medications is about 100,000, as was mentioned at the beginning of this chapter.

I remain hopeful that some day CAM therapies such as spiritual healing, relaxation, and imagery will be used to help reduce the side effects of medications (as in chemotherapy, or with drugs used to treat pain, depression, and anxiety). This would be far preferable to the current practice of prescribing further medications to control the side effects of the primary treatment.

3. *Surgically correctable problems* can be addressed by conventional medicine with excellent results, as in: treatment of injuries resulting from physical trauma; draining or excision of localized infections (e.g. lancing boils, appendectomy, gall bladder surgery); removal of localized growths (e.g. cysts, benign and cancerous tumors); orthopedic corrections; corneal replacements; insertion of cardiac pacemakers and bypass surgery; skin grafts and other cosmetic surgery; caesarian sections; joint prostheses; organ transplants; and more.

In some cases, however, there is serious doubt as to whether surgery is even necessary, as in hysterectomies for heavy bleeding or mildly abnormal Pap smears, or with caesarian sections for brief episodes of fetal distress.

Any kind of surgery can be dangerous to one's health. It is estimated that up to 20 percent of people who are hospitalized develop secondary problems during their hospitalization, such as infections, poor results from anesthesia or surgery, allergic reactions to medications, problems due to medical errors, and the like. Because medicine is an art as well as a science, there will always be some errors in diagnosis and treatment, and some of these may prove fatal.

Surprisingly, even serious surgical interventions may become faddish. Numbers of procedures have been developed and used to treat thousands of people, only to be proven over time to be ineffective. Examples include internal mammary artery ligation for pains of angina; radical mastectomy for breast cancer (in which much more than the breast tissue is removed); extracranial-intracranial artery bypass surgery; splenectomy for all ruptured spleens; prostatectomy for all prostate cancers; and recently, arthroscopic knee surgery. Thousands of people have been treated and have been exposed to considerable medical risks with ineffective surgery. Though many reported improvements, these were apparently placebo effects.

The questionable advisability of surgical interventions is particularly relevant where CAM therapies may be helpful, especially considering the low incidence of side effects with these therapies. Examples can be found in CAM treatments that can eliminate the need for cardiac bypass surgery for atherosclerotic cardiovascular disease - such as the Ornish approach (which is well supported by research), and EDTA chelation (which is still considered controversial, but nevertheless carries negligible risks).

4. *Hormone replacement* can be life-enhancing (as in menopause) or life-saving (as in diabetes, hypothyroidism' Addison's disease, and more). Treating hormonal hyperfunctions can also be life-saving (as in hyperthyroidism, Cushing's disease, and others).

Hormone treatments also have side effects, and sometimes they are quite serious. For many years women were encouraged to use hormone replacement therapy during menopause, with the promise that this would slow the processes of aging and reduce the risks of heart attacks and arteriosclerosis. Recently however, it has been shown that hormone replacement therapy does not reduce the risk of heart attacks and that it can increase the incidence of thrombosis of the leg veins (with the risk of pulmonary embolism due to clots from the legs being carried to the lungs). It may also increase the need for biliary surgery.

5. *Genetic manipulations* promise to help with many health problems, as in the tailoring of new antibiotics and other drugs, the correction of inborn errors of metabolism, and more.

However, the potential for negative or even disastrous effects, especially in long-range terms, poses a serious concern. Nature has selected the current pool of genes through many years of trial and error, with the errors weeding themselves out. If we introduce new genetic changes, the complexity of human existence will in many cases exceed our limited abilities to foresee the consequences of our tampering.

6. *Diets* can be helpful in treating various problems, but very few doctors are trained in nutrition. Here too, there have been examples of serious medical errors. For many years, doctors strongly recommended low-fat diets to reduce the risk of cardiovascular disease, but this now proves to have been poor advice (Taubes 2002). Similarly, low fiber diets for chronic diverticulitis have proved to be ineffectual (Nuland).

7. *Prevention of illness* is another major contribution of allopathic medicine.

Improved sanitation to prevent the spread of infectious diseases has probably saved more lives around the world than any other medical intervention.

Immunizations have lowered the incidence of numerous serious illnesses, and in the case of smallpox, have actually eliminated the illness globally.

On the negative side, some people have severe (and occasionally even fatal) immune reactions to immunizations. There is an increasing suspicion voiced by many CAM practitioners that immunizations may have long-term negative effects on the immune system. This has yet to be confirmed by rigorous research, although several surveys are supportive.[249] Perhaps the new generation of cell-free immunizations, which eliminate a major source of allergic reactions, will be better in this regard.

Identification and elimination of insect vectors and animal hosts for illnesses have provided further avenues for prevention.

Another disadvantage of preventive allopathic interventions is that the pesticides used to limit carriers of diseases may produce serious toxic effects and side effects in people and in the environment. Pollution of the planet with pesticides is a particularly serious problem. For example, increasingly toxic levels of DDT are killing enormous numbers of birds and fish, and are working their way up the food chain to human consumption.

8. *A specific diagnosis* is required before treatment can be prescribed. This is a mainstay of what is considered good and ethical medical care. This principle is based on a linear, cause-and-effect analysis of physiology and of disease processes. It is assumed that a person is endowed at conception with specific genetic programs. These are then influenced by nutrition, physical and emotional environments, traumas, infections, toxins, allergies, neoplastic and degenerative processes. The belief and hope of allopathic medicine is that eventually every health problem will be understood in terms of physical and biochemical processes, and that once this has been achieved, then mechanical, biochemical, or genetic interventions will be devised to prevent and/or treat all problems.

Knowing what your own problem is – giving it a name and a focus for addressing it – may provide healing in and of itself. Without a diagnosis, you may worry that anything is possible. Even when you receive a diagnosis of severe illness, there is still the relief of being able to begin to do something about the problem.

> *We are half dead before we understand our disorder, and half cured when we do.*
>
> – Charles Caleb Colton

In allopathic medicine, diagnosis focuses upon symptoms and diseases, with therapies prescribed accordingly. Conventional medicine prides itself on its thoroughness in this regard. Specialists are available to address various elements of the body, diverse disease processes, and an enormous spectrum of treatment interventions. Research is emphasized as a basis for establishing diagnoses and for identifying effective interventions.

While these practices and standards have advanced and refined medical knowledge, they have posed some difficulties in clinical applications. One of the most frequent complaints about medical doctors is that they take little time to listen to people's problems. They focus on the disease the person has, rather than on the person who has the disease. Bearing witness to this dissatisfaction is the high percentage of prescriptions that go unfilled (estimated to be as high as 50 percent), and the enormous number of people who are now utilizing complementary therapies – and are willing to pay billions of dollars annually out of pocket for these treatments. In many cases, conventional medicine is simply missing the target with its mechanistic diagnoses and interventions.

9. Doctors are clothed in a mantle of enormous respect, which has been earned by the profession as a whole through dedicated care provided over many decades.

Doctors take upon themselves a heavy burden of responsibility when they care for patients. Diagnoses and treatments must be accurate – within the limitations of human ability. Care is provided around the clock, every day of every year. No other profession regularly requires and provides 24-hour coverage. Moral and ethical standards have been established, and they have been generally maintained.

The process of professional peer review has been highly developed, with hospital and medical licensing boards having the power to censure doctors or even to recommend the removal of their license to practice, in cases of negligence and misconduct.

Doctors generally maintain high standards of confidentiality and professional conduct. It is expected that intimate disclosures will be protected.

The key role of doctors as guardians of healthcare standards has been enacted into law in every state.

The downside to conventional medical care is that errors are inevitable in any human activity, and when medical errors or misconduct lead to injuries and suffering, doctors are liable to be sued. The high rates of malpractice litigation in the US have produced an atmosphere of defensive medicine. In many situations doctors may be inclined to act with caution or even fear – lest they be sued for acts of commission or omission. Defensive medicine leads to over-use diagnostic procedures (some of which carry serious risks), and to a tendency to intervene with invasive procedures lest the lack of intervention eventually provide grounds for a lawsuit claiming medical negligence. Some specialists have been sued so frequently, often for unavoidable problems such as childbirth injuries, that their insurance premiums have skyrocketed. Many obstetricians and gynecologists have chosen to leave their practices rather than have to pay hundreds of thousands of dollars annually for insurance premiums.

Sadly, the danger of malpractice litigation has grown to the point that many doctors practice in an atmosphere of distrust and fear. This has eroded the healing nature of the doctor-patient relationship.

Direct disadvantages of conventional medicine
There are two very practical matters and two philosophical issues that are highly problematic in medical care.

1. *Costs* of medical care in the US are excessive by the standards of every other developed nation in the world. Medications are one of the most expensive items.

These costs are becoming bones of contention between employers whose profit margins are squeezed by the costs of employee health programs and employees who are now being expected to pay increasing proportions of their own healthcare costs. Ironically, the higher costs are not purchasing better care. By all international assessments, the US ranks relatively low on the list of health ratings.

2. *Deaths caused by conventional medical care*, due to medical errors and side effects of medications properly prescribed, place medical care between the first and fourth leading cause of death in the US – depending on the source of the estimates.

3. *Death* is seen by many conventional medical practitioners as the end of existence, an evil to be fought at all costs.

While prolonging life is one of the primary goals of modern medicine, there comes a time in every life when this struggle is no longer appropriate.

Doctors are often trained (as I was) to believe that if a person under their care dies it may be the doctors' fault – because they either failed to make the correct diagnosis, did not prescribe the correct treatment, or prescribed a treatment that had disasterous effects. While this may be true in some instances, doctors have to consider this possibility in every instance, because in many cases they cannot know what the cause of death was, even after an autopsy.

4. *Life after death* is considered no more than wishful thinking and any discussion of this subject is often dismissed or relegated to the clergy.

While the average medical practitioner may not be familiar with these aspects of human experience, wholistic practitioners frequently address such spiritual matters, and some are specifically trained to do so.

> *Man's extremity is God's opportunity*
> *– William Blake*

CAM treatments

Complementary therapists often approach healthcare in ways that differ substantially from the views and methods of allopathic medicine.

1. *CAM theoretical constructs are more wholistic.* Most complementary therapies address the person who has the illness rather than the illness the person has. These approaches are based on the belief that a person functions as a unitary organism and cannot be understood from the examination of its individual parts. In fact, many of the CAM therapies include people's relationships with other people and with their environment as essential elements in the course of their assessments and treatments.

2. *Biological energies* are assumed to play an essential role in normal physiology and in pathological processes. Interventions may be made through acupuncture points and meridians, chakras, energy medicines, and biological energy interactions with the therapist.   Mental imagery can influence the body's energy patterns, as well as its neurohormonal and neuroimmunological systems.

3. *Diagnosis may relate to symptoms* but they are usually considered in the context of the entire person, and assessment may include analysis of the clients' relationships and environment. Treatments may be given to the whole person rather than focused on individual symptoms or on any one part of the body.

One of the most serious risks in complementary therapies perceived by Western medicine is that a medical problem that is potentially treatable through another modality – such as allopathic medicine – might be missed, and delay of conventional medical treatment could allow the illness to worsen.

The converse is also true, but almost totally ignored by Western medicine. For instance, acupuncture can halve the time for recovery after a stroke. Were the same standards of negligence to apply for failure to prescribe an effective CAM therapy, more people would enjoy the benefits of a variety of wholistic modalities.

4. *Diagnoses and treatments may vary between practitioners.* Just as each respant is unique, so is each therapist. The *person* of the practitioner may be as important as her *practices*. It is generally held that different approaches may be equally effective within systems of wholistic care, but this has yet to be substantiated in research. The question will probably always remain as to whether there aren't better treatments available than the one(s) prescribed.

5. *Treatments may produce side effects briefly*, as in emotional releases with deep massage, or symptoms that appear when a homeopathic remedy is started. These are usually transient and are viewed as *releases* of old, maladaptive patterns. People usually tolerate these responses much better than side effects of allopathic medications because practitioners let them know that they will be transient; that they are meaningful; that they are not harmful; and that they indicate progress.

6. *Psychological aspects of illness* are considered integral to many of the complementary approaches. Many people understand that their thoughts, memories, and emotions play important roles in the development of their health problems, and in the degree to which they are able to tolerate and deal with them. Similarly, many respants are able to accept that shifts in their attitudes, psychological conflicts, and relationships can bring about improvements in their condition.

7. *Exercise, nutrition and other aspects of lifestyle* are addressed by complementary therapists. This makes good sense and feels good to people who appreciate that they can contribute to the maintenance of their own health. People feel empowered when they can participate in their own treatments, and cures.

One danger, however, is that some people may begin to hope and believe that they can treat themselves without the help of conventional healthcare professionals. This is particularly true in the age of the Internet, since surfers can locate information on any condition and multitudes of treatments for it. In this context, a little knowledge may truly be a dangerous thing. I have seen many people misdiagnose themselves and their family members by applying limited knowledge, and even more who apply inappropriate remedies. There is a growing awareness of this problem, as witnessed by a Consumer Reports survey of 46,000 subscribers which found a higher rate of success when treatments were supervised by therapists than when they were self-prescribed.

8. *Respants are encouraged and empowered to explore and use self-healing approaches.* Many people are pleased to help themselves and not to be completely dependent upon a therapist. Others seek the expertise of a knowledgeable practitioner to advise them on approaches to self-care.

9. *Spiritual belief and practices* are important aspects of some of the complementary therapies.

One of the most common points of satisfaction is the fact that CAM therapists take more time to listen and to talk with clients. Respants also appreciate being addressed as people rather than as agglomerations of symptoms or walking containers of biochemicals. They feel that the psychological and spiritual aspects of their health problems are important, and they feel better understood when these are considered as integral aspects of their overall health.

> *All illness is curable, but not all patients.*
> – Keith Mason

10. *Chronic illnesses and conditions* such as backaches, arthritis, multiple sclerosis, and the like respond well to complementary therapies such as spiritual healing, homeopathy, and osteopathy. Sadly, because of our society's history of reliance on allopathic medicine, many people turn to CAM therapies late in the course of their illnesses, when it is actually less likely that they will have a strong effect. When

CAM treatments are given early on in the course of illness, most therapists feel that they have a better chance of helping.

11. *Particular illnesses may be more effectively and/or more safely treated by complementary therapies.* For instance, the newer anti-inflammatory and pain medications called NSAIDS, which are used in the treatment of osteoarthritis, may produce tens of thousands of cases of severe side effects annually – such as renal failure and gastrointestinal bleeding. On the other hand, glucosamine supplements have no serious side effects and they have comparable salutary effects to NSAIDS (Lopes). Chronic ear infections in children are often treated with antibiotics, with all of the potential risks mentioned above. Surgery for implantation of ear-tubes carries further risks. In comparison, significant numbers of cases of ear infection in children improve without treatment and with greater subsequent immunity to reinfection (van Buchen et al);[250] and with elimination of allergens from their diet (Dees/ Lefkowitz), with no serious risks involved.

For further discussion of problems where CAM may be of great benefit, see particular problems that respond well to CAM modalities. See Table II-8, *Complementary Therapies compared to Conventional Medicine,* for a summary of the differences between complementary therapies and allopathic medicine.

Two separate issues are relevant to any discussion of the benefits of complementary therapies.

Complementary therapies can be cost-effective. Studies of health promotion and disease prevention show clear cost benefits at various work sites. Most CAM therapies contribute substantially to health promotion and disease prevention. A study at a general practitioner's office in England showed that spiritual healing reduced expenses for 25 patients with chronic illnesses by $1,600 for the group over a period of six months (Dixon 1993). Disputing the cost-effectiveness of CAM therapies, A. White and E. Ernst noted a dearth of rigorous studies to support such claims.

Complementary therapies promote hope and positive attitudes towards illness and health management. Many of the CAM therapies include self-healing components. These empower respants with the feeling that they can contribute to their own healing.

CAM therapists stress caring rather than curing. This attitude focuses on the present, exploring all possible ways for enhancing quality of life *now*. Allopathic medicine, which focuses heavily on fighting disease, looks toward the future – to avoid death at all costs, even if this means seriously diminishing quality of life in the present.

CAM therapists offer hope by encouraging explorations of the spiritual dimensions of awareness. From this perspective, death can be seen as a transition to an afterlife rather than as the end of all existence.

Conventional practitioners caution against introducing false hopes of cure that can lead to severe disappointment, disillusionment, and despair. In ethical CAM practice, as in ethical allopathic practice, treatments are offered with the suggestion that they may help – not with promises of cures.

Another criticism of CAM interventions is that respants may feel guilty if they do everything that is prescribed but their disease continues to deteriorate. They may

Table II-8.

CAM Therapies	compared to	Conventional Medicine
Diagnosis		
Diagnosis may be unnecessary	Diagnosis required	
Diagnosis by intuitive perceptions that supplement history and observations	Diagnosis by history, physical examination, and laboratory examinations	
Syndromes – patterns of symptoms that involve body, emotions, mind, spirit	Symptoms – primarily physical; emotions, mind, spirit are considered secondary	
Diagnoses may vary between diagnosticians	Diagnoses should be consistent between diagnosticians	
Treatments		
Wholistic approach includes body, emotions, mind, relationships and spirit.	Discrete elements of therapies are introduced, focus is mostly on the body.	
Treatments may be specific or non-specific, may involve bioenergies, and may be focused by actions or by the mind of the therapist.	Treatments are discrete and specific within physical parameters. They are considered "objective," i.e. independent of the person giving them.	
Interventions to uncover underlying causes of problems, restore harmony	Treatments to repair malfunctioning or damaged organism	
Respant (responsible participant) takes active role in self-healing as possible	Therapist diagnoses, prescribes and/ or administers treatments	
Theory		
Symptoms and diseases are indications of disharmonies in body, emotions, mind, relationships and spirit.	Symptoms and diseases are evidence of malfunctions of the physical body.	
Spiritual aspects may be viewed as the most important elements of health.	Physical aspects are the most important; spiritual issues are relegated to clergy.	
Mind and body are unitary parts of one entity and constantly interact directly with one another.	Mind and body are separate; only words, symbols, and sensory exchanges are vehicles for their interactions.	
Healing action effective from any distance	Action is local, distance diminishes force	
All of time is present in the now, and treatment may be directed to "anywhere."	Time is linear, with past, present, and future; treatments are given in the present.	
Physical death is a transition to spiritual dimensions.	Physical death terminates existence.	
Death is a natural part of existence, and healing into death is a good healing.	Death is to be avoided and fought against at all costs.	
Explanations are "both/ and"	Explanations are in either/ or"	
Research		
Individual case reports and qualitative studies preferred, RCTs (with compromises in usual CAM practices)	RCTs are the gold standard; qualitative studies and observation based on individual cases are inferior.	

also come to feel that they are somehow to blame for creating or maintaining their illness. This is sometimes a problem with CAM bodymind fundamentalists, who insist that our mind-set or attitudes entirely determine what happens to us. I believe that this approach is unrealistic, in view of the multiplicity of factors that combine to determine one's state of health, including genetic endowment, exposure to infectious organisms, allergens, and toxins in the environment, and normal degenerative processes in the body. Many of these factors are clearly beyond any individual's control.

The opposite danger is of introducing *negative suggestions* that discourage hope, and this is far more common in allopathic medicine. Most doctors present statistics in a negative way, such as, "In a cancer of your type the life expectancy is about three years." This sets up the expectation that the patient won't survive beyond three years, which is similar to the casting of a hex. Some patients may take these suggestions on board and expect to die after a certain length of time and therefore program themselves to do so.[251]

Statistics are just averages of data from many individual cases. The CAM practitioner or the more wholistically oriented doctor might say, "While this is a serious illness, a certain number of people who have it live longer than others. No one but God knows how long any of us will live. I might get hit by a bus and you might live much longer than me. Let's see how we can help you be one of those people who lives longer."

Research: There has been little research to clarify which CAM approach is best for which problem.

In one survey (A. Long/ Huntley/ Ernst), single-modality providers were queried about the target problems that respond to their treatments. Modalities with 2 or more responses included: aromatherapy, Bach flowers, Bowen technique, chiropractic, homeopathy, hypnotherapy, magnet therapy, massage, nutrition, reflexology, Reiki, and yoga. The most common conditions reported to respond to particular therapies were the following (parentheses indicate lack of research support for claims):

Stress/ Anxiety – aromatherapy, Bach flowers, hypnotherapy, magnet therapy, massage, nutrition, reflexology, (Reiki), and yoga

Headache/ Migraine – aromatherapy, (Bowen technique), chiropractic, hypnotherapy, massage, nutrition, reflexology, (Reiki), and yoga

Back pain – (Bowen technique), chiropractic, magnet therapy, massage, reflexology, and yoga.

Contraindications were therapy-specific, as in avoiding massage in cases of skin disease.

While evidence comparing CAM and conventional therapy is limited, what is evident is that the safety of CAM approaches is on the whole is far greater than the safety of conventional treatments.

While much remains to be clarified on this subject, there are often clear advantages to the uses of CAM therapies (T. Chappell).

The best of both worlds can be found in *integrative care* practices, where conventional and complementary therapists work together. Attesting to the growth of this approach is the fact that about half of the medical schools in the US now offer courses in complementary therapies (Wetzel et al.; Pelletier 2000). There is now an American Board of Holistic Medicine, which was initiated by the American Holistic Medical Association, and an American Holistic Nurses' Association.[252].

People are spending more and more of their healthcare dollars on CAM therapies.

Out of 831 adults who used both CAM and conventional medical care in 1997, 79% believed that the two approaches combined were better than either one alone (Eisenberg, et al. 2001). Many cancer patients undergoing conventional treatments in the UK also seek CAM therapies. They choose healing, relaxation, visualization, diet, homeopathy, vitamins, herbalism and other therapies.

So how does one decide which therapy to use for which problem?
When there are obvious indications that a particular problem can be competently handled by allopathic medicine, such as a bacterial infection or a fracture, the initial choice is easier. However, there is no reason why treatments that help to deal with shock and pain, such as rescue remedy (a Bach flower remedy), arnica (homeopathic), or spiritual healing, should not be used at the same time. Similarly, my personal experience is that the pain of bruises, cuts, fractures and burns can be markedly lessened by applying these treatments, and that physical healing is more rapid – with no conflict in adding the healing to conventional treatments.

Complementary therapies may be helpful additions to allopathic treatments for almost any health problem. In some cases, however, there may be diverse or even conflicting recommendations from practitioners of these two approaches – and from different complementary therapists as well.

If your problems are more complex, particularly in the case of serious and chronic illnesses, complementary therapies may be the treatments of choice. One of the most thoughtful resources in exploring these clinical questions is the summary of Patrick and Christopher Pietroni from the (London) Marylebone Health Centre's experience in exploring integrative care. The physicians at this center explored how they could integrate conventional medical care with Chinese medicine, massage, counseling, relaxation, imagery, and spiritual awareness (in a clinic housed within a church). The summary of their work is broad, deep and very well presented.

Other excellent resources include the following:
Alternative Medicine (Burton Goldberg Group) gives succinct summaries of complementary therapies as modalities and also discusses various illnesses and therapies that may be helpful; and
Alternative Medicine: Expanding Medical Horizons (NIH – Workshop on Alternative Medicine) provides discussions of complementary therapies and extensive research references.

A spectrum of CAM therapies can be helpful in the treatment of psychological problems. Ruth Benor Sewell makes some specific recommendations for complementary therapies that may be most appropriate for people with different strengths in their characterological preferences, according to the Jungian polarities. She suggests that there may be similar characterological preferences for complementary therapies in treating various problems. For instance, people with strong intuition (and weak outer sense attachments) may prefer imagery, music and story telling to deal with pain, while people who have opposite preferences may benefit more from yoga, massage, and Autogenic Training.[253] (See Figure II-15.) While these suggestions are as yet unsupported by research, they would be easy to explore using the Myers-Briggs personality test.

In the more limited areas of using CAM in surgery, a variety of approaches were found to be helpful for related psychological and physical problems (Norred).

Figure II-15. Stress management approaches

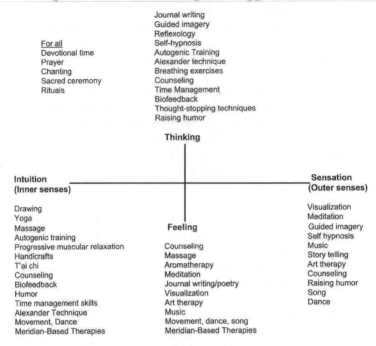

* Adapted for each primary functions, from Sharp 1987.

We still have so much to learn about integrative care. The challenges are great, but the benefits that are already apparent clearly indicate that the efforts will be worthwhile.

NATURAL HEALING ABILITIES AND
NORMAL RHYTHMS OF THE BODY

To do nothing is sometimes a good remedy.
— Hippocrates

*The art of medicine consists of amusing the patient
while nature cures the disease.*
— Voltaire

Having discussed an enormous spectrum of psychological approaches and CAM modalities for healing, it is worth emphasizing again the vast natural healing abilities that we all possess. Sometimes, doing nothing is the best medicine. Simply creating a healing environment in which a person can de-stress may provide sufficient rebalancing of enegies for natural healing to occur.

The urge to treat may be difficult for caregivers to resist, however. Two strong motivators often drive them to prescribe and intervene in invasive ways. The first is the obvious monetary motivation of earning their living. The second is their ego involvement, which produces expectations that they will provide cures and anxieties lest they should fail.

It is unclear where the body's memory of normalcy resides, but it is certain that within each one of us there are vast capacities for self-healing, when we honor and encourage our self-regulating mechanisms to resume their normal functions.

> *Our body is a machine for living. It is organized for that. It is its nature. Let life go on in it unhindered and let it defend itself, it will do more than if you paralyze it by encumbering it with remedies.*
> – Leo Tolstoy

Spiritual healers suggest that the biological energy body contains the templates for all of the body's functions. This could explain how organs and tissues know to grow to a certain size and shape but no farther; how cuts, bruises and burns are repaired by the body; and how fingertips can regenerate after they are amputated (even including the same fingerprint).

If the energy body is the template for the physical body, this could also help to explain how psychological factors and emotional traumas might alter the biological energy field, thus producing secondary subjective discomforts and even changes in the physical body (as in anger that seems to produce arthritis).[254]

Taking this several steps further, spiritual awareness and spiritual healing suggest that each of us is an expression of spiritual templates that manifest through the energy body, and are in turn expressed through the mental, emotional, and physical bodies.[255]

> *A person is neither a thing nor a process, but an opening or clearing through which the Absolute can manifest.*
> – Martin Heidegger

As a part of this discussion, we should also consider the factor of *time*.

First of all, it is important to take time to contemplate what is actually going on when disharmonies develop in body, emotions, mind, relationships, and spirit, rather than rushing in and trying to fix things according to the swift logic of clinical diagnosis. When we provide a healing atmosphere within which to heal, time can allow self-healing to occur.

Second, there are biological rhythms of several varieties that may facilitate or impede healing (Touitou/ Haus). The study of shifts in body rhythms over time has been termed *chronobiology*.

In women, the menstrual cycle may determine certain periods of sensitivity, receptivity, or resistance to therapeutic interventions.

Some believe that there are regular biorhythms – cycles of biological activity that correlate with a person's date of birth, as cycles with a fixed series of numbers of days in the life of the person. I have found no research evidence to support the influence of such regular biorhythms on health.

Astrological factors may also be relevant to medical problems and treatments within the discussion of time as an influence on healing.

Circadian rhythms are physiological shifts that occur, like the tides, in the 24-hour diurnal cycle. Production of adrenal steroids, melatonin and other hormones may rise and fall in regular patterns over the course of a day. Acupuncture is said to be more effective for certain problems at particular times of the cycle, related to greater activity at those times of the meridians associated with the affected body areas.

Ultradian rhythms are shifts in brain hemisphere dominance that occur in cycles of 90 to 120 minutes. These have not been studied in relationship to physical healing, but they could influence a person's receptivity or resistance to suggestion and other healing interventions.

Considering all of these factors, it is easy to conceive that each individual may have times of greater and lesser receptivity to healings of every sort. Repeated visits to complementary therapists, which are commonly spaced at weekly intervals, may provide more windows in time for greater therapeutic efficacy.

THE PERSONHOOD OF THE THERAPIST

The doctor's arrival is the first part of the cure.
                                        – Anonymous

I have been examining the issues addressed and the questions raised in *Healing Research* since I began my 13 years of adult education and throughout my entire professional career – spanning 35 years. I find that the person of the therapist is one of the most important ingredients in the level of satisfaction that people derive from their treatments, second only to the *chemistry* between therapist and client.

Qualities in the therapist that are important for good healing include openness, caring, compassion, ability to empathize, unconditional acceptance, integrity, and rich life experiences. When therapists have had treatments for their own problems, they are better able to appreciate the processes of healing in their respants.

No man's knowledge here can go beyond his experience.
                                        – John Locke

Another book, or at least an editorial, feels like it is percolating around this subject, so I will say no more here beyond emphasizing that therapy does not occur only in a therapist's office. All of life is a process of healing and every single thought and action has the potential to contribute to this healing journey.

The creative spirit creates with whatever materials are present. With food, with children, with building blocks, with speech, with thoughts, with pigment, with an umbrella, a wineglass or a torch. We are not craftsmen only during studio hours. Any more than man is wise only in his library. Or devout only in church. The material is not the sign of the creative feeling for life: of the warmth and sympathy and reverence which foster being; techniques are not the sign. The sign is the light that dwells within the act, whatever its nature or medium.
                                        – M. C. Richards

CHOOSING YOUR DOCTOR AND OTHER THERAPISTS

> *It's not enough for your doctor to stop playing God. You've got to get up off your knees.*
>
> – Marvin Belsky

Choosing a generalist or specialist and developing a treatment team to deal with chronic or difficult problems can be a challenge. Here are some factors that you may wish to consider:

- Establish a relationship with a primary care physician who gets to know you and who you know over a period of time, to develop mutual understanding and trust.
- Clarify your problems and learn as much as possible about them. If you are dissatisfied with the information or treatment you receive, the Internet offers a very broad range of sites with information about most problems. Be aware, however, that the quality of information and advice offered on the Net varies considerably from site to site.
- Prioritize your needs and wishes for the people who will treat you.
- Seek clarity of diagnosis for your problems, in words you understand. Don't hesitate to ask clarifying questions, and insist on clear, and comprehensible answers.
- Bring someone with you you trust when you go for a serious consultation. Your anxiety may interfere with your ability to absorb all you are told.
- If you want your caregivers to take charge of your problems and prescribe treatments without providing explanations, tell them so.
- If you want your caregivers to be your advisors, making decisions for treatment in consultation with you, be clear with them about this.
- Caregivers should:
  - Care for you as a person, not only focused on treating your symptoms and illnesses
  - Be open to your questions
  - Understand the contributions to your problems made by stress, and by psychological and relational issues
  - Have a spectrum of other caregivers available to refer you to for specialized interventions, and to provide him/her with consultations
  - Be open to your seeking second opinions
  - Be open to your exploring a variety of approaches for dealing with your problems

  Availability for urgent consultations
- Costs

Getting personal recommendations from satisfied respants is probably your best way of making an initial choice of caregiver. A wise and trusted caregiver can then be a resource for further consultations and interventions, as well as further referrals.

If you develop uncomfortable feelings about your therapist, seek a second opinion. Trust your intuition if the advice you are getting or the manner in which you are being treated feels wrong to you. Should you have more serious questions about the behavior or ethics of your caregiver, consult their professional associations regarding standards for practice in general, or to ask for information on the specific person you are concerned about.[256]

THE TRANSPERSONAL IN WHOLISTIC MEDICINE

No one can touch the full potential for healing by believing that one treatment is good for the body but in conflict with the soul, or vice versa... The fullest potential exists when the inner conse-cration and the outer action unify.

– Richard Moss

Transpersonal perspectives[257] can re-frame challenges within their worldviews, helping you to deal with them in more creative and satisfying ways. For instance, many transpersonal therapists are now including work on awareness of birth, pre-birth, and past life[258] experiences in their treatments. Though this may seem far-fetched, there is ample evidence to support the belief systems surrounding such work.

[W]e not only choose our responses, but perhaps more importantly, we choose the labels we give them. A rose by any other name is not a rose.
   The moment you step outside of your problem to observe it, you create a larger context for it. Observing or witnessing this becomes a key activity in therapy...

– Steven Wolinsky (p. 101)

The old/new methods of meditation are finding applications in modern psychotherapy, as the practice of wholistic medicine shades into and blends with transpersonal psychology.

In the past century there has been an increasing opening in Western society to awareness of an interdependence and interconnectedness between individuals as well as between humankind and all of creation. This awareness exists on many levels of consciousness, from linear deductions about limitations on natural re-sources and the consequent need for their better allocation and distribution, to the need to manage environmental pollution, to a growing sense of the need for global community, to awareness of interpersonal connections on other levels of reality (including karmic), to a more experiential appreciation of interconnections with the All.

The transpersonal includes insights from intuitions, meditation, altered states of consciousness, spirit guidance, and the like, which can point to a holographic organization of the cosmos.[259] "As above, so below," is a succinct statement of the concept that every single thing you do, think, feel, and *are* is an important part of the All. By clearing your inner self you enhance the state of the All, since you are part of it.

In terns of linear logic this appears at first to be superstitious nonsense. However, quantum physics[260] teaches that the observer and the observed are inseparable. Each of us is far more integrally connected with the universe than we generally believe in our materialistic Western culture.

Clinical science has always viewed the state of a system as a whole as merely the result of interaction of its parts. However, the quantum potential stood this view on its ear and indicated that the behavior of parts is actually organized by the whole.

– Michael Talbot (p. 41)

Along with transpersonal awareness of oneness with the All comes a reverence for nature, concern for our fellow creatures on this planet, and anxiety about the excesses of modern materialism – which places a higher premium on personal gains and emphasizes regional economic, political and sectarian interests over global concerns for all life.

Chief Seattle observed in 1854:

The shining water that moves in the streams and rivers is not just water but the blood of our ancestors. If we sell you land, you must remember that it is sacred, and you must teach your children that it is sacred and that each ghostly reflection in the clear water of the lakes tells of events and memories in the life of my people. The water's murmur is the voice of my father's father.

The rivers are our brothers, they quench our thirst. The rivers carry our canoes, and feed our children. If we sell you our land, you must remember, and teach your children, that the rivers are our brothers, and hours, and you must henceforth give the rivers the kindness you would give any brother.

When making important decisions, Native American elders would always consider the consequences their actions would have upon the seventh generation following their own. Contrast this with Western time frames for governmental concern in decision making!

The awareness of our oneness with nature has not escaped the observation of Western naturalists, poets, artists and mystics. Sadly, our society is allocating ever fewer resources to further explorations of how we can live in harmony with our environment, and how we can teach our children these vitally important lessons. Instead, competition and self-seeking approaches to life are often promoted in our schools. An ever growing emphasis is placed on promoting the global consumer society. Public schools are increasingly cutting or even eliminating their budgets for teaching the arts and humanities, from elementary school through university.

In any weather, at any hour of the day or night, I have been anxious to improve the nick of time, and notch it on my stick too; to stand on the meeting of two eternities, the past and the future, that is precisely the present moment, to toe that line.

– Henry David Thoreau

I recall a time not many years ago when I viewed discussions of spiritual awareness as "preachy" and found myself put off by what seemed more like evangelical scientisms than scientific observations. I have no intention to preach here – only to share what I and others have observed by letting our intuitive awareness complement our sensory awareness. If some of these observations are shown to be projections of our fantasies, I am willing to respect all evidence in this regard. The personal experience, however, of opening to greater awareness in transpersonal realms carries a feeling of inherent truth to it. This can only be appreciated through experiencing it.

There has recently been a tide of millennial predictions that we may be coming to the end of an age of materialism, and should be soon moving onward and upward into more spiritual ways of organizing our affairs. Whether these awarenesses and predictions are merely wishful thinking or contain elements of precognitive perceptions remains to be seen. But perhaps such a dream can be actualized if enough people lend themselves to the cause (Benor 1985).

I will discuss the subject of spirituality in much greater detail in Volume III. In the present volume we will continue with our explorations of energy medicine.

INTEGRATIVE CARE: HARMONIZING CAM
AND ALLOPATHIC THERAPIES

> *The problem is not that there are problems.*
> *The problem is expecting otherwise*
> *and thinking that having problems is a problem.*
> *– Theodore Rubin*

We have reviewed many ways in which biological energies can manifest in illness, and have discussed how they can be used through various CAM approaches to promote healing. Our understanding of these vastly expands our appreciation of energy medicine as a part of wholistic healing.

For a summary of the theoretical and practical differences between these approaches, see Table II-8.

One of the most important differences in these two approaches concerns the process of determining what is wrong in the first place. Allopathic medicine emphasizes precision in diagnosis, and this approach has facilitated huge advances in medical research and treatment. With clear diagnoses it is possible to identify specific physical and psychological malfunctions, and to clarify what causes them and how to treat them. Students of medicine, nursing, and the counseling arts are trained to identify various symptom clusters that manifest within particular processes of dysfunction and disease. They rely on patients' historical reports, focused questioning by the examiner, physical examination and laboratory studies. Objective criteria are emphasized, and multiple examiners are expected to arrive at similar if not identical diagnoses after considering given sets of data. (While this precision is the ideal, it is very rare to find it even closely approximated.)

CAM therapies are much broader in the range of data collected for patient assessments. Symptom clusters that are meaningful in CAM diagnosis may have no relevance to conventional medical practitioners. The color of a person's tongue, a tooth that is in need of dental care, and sensitivity to hot and cold may be relevant to acupuncture diagnosis for seemingly unrelated conditions. Similarly, discomfort with tight collars and lack of motivation to engage in activities may be highly relevant to the choice of a homeopathic remedy. CAM practitioners often focus on people's subjective experiences of their illnesses; their relationships with family, friends, colleagues, home and work environments, and society as a whole; their spiritual life, and other factors that may influence bioenergies.

Diagnoses may vary much more widely between individual CAM practitioners than between allopathic physicians. This is particularly true if therapists are working within different modalities, but diagnoses may also vary between practitioners of the same modality. It is as yet unclear to what extent this is or is not correlated with efficacy of treatment. The explanation commonly accepted by CAM therapists is that there are many roads to health and all of them can be effective in releasing patterns of illness and promoting patterns of health. The therapist is also a part of the treatment, which introduces another source of variability in treatment effects and outcomes.

Many conventional medical practitioners have minimal training in dealing with non-physical issues that affect health and illness. I was shocked to find that many medical schools do not include training in bedside manner and public relations. It is apparently assumed that basic common sense will always prevail, and that doctors and nurses must possess these skills innately. Not only is this far from the truth, but the experience of going through medical or nursing school can discourage and even deaden the inborn interpersonal sensitivities which caregivers-in-training bring in with them. In conventional medical training the emphasis is placed very heavily on physical diagnosis and interventions. Patients' eagerness to discuss the psychological and social aspects of their problems is often viewed as a hindrance in the caregivers' attempts to obtain a complete and accurate medical history, focused on physical issues. Doctors and nurses tend to cut short such discussions, which in any case may take more time than they feel they can devote to a given patient under the pressures of their job requirements.

Conventional caregivers, who focus on the physical causes of problems, naturally prescribe physical interventions. Medicines and surgical procedures are the primary tools they are trained to use. Patients are presumed to be ignorant of the true causes of their problems, and it is seen as the caregivers' job to cure them.

CAM practitioners usually spend much more time exploring the complex issues surrounding the problems that cause patients to seek their help. They tend to label the people they treat as *clients* rather than *patients*. CAM therapists see their roles as teachers who can help people to develop better lifestyle appreciation and habits. They seek non-physical roots of problems, and develop self-healing strategies and practices with which clients can address their own health issues.[261]

It is not surprising that in the US, more visits are paid annually to CAM practitioners than to physicians. Many find that simply telling their story to a respectful and caring listener is a healing interaction. Spiritual healers and other CAM therapists are often good listeners, and many will deliberately promote self-healing practices. Qigong, meridian based therapies, and psychoneuroimmunology are particularly helpful in this regard.

Another contrast in the focus of CAM and allopathic approaches is in *caring* vs. *curing*. In conventional medicine, practitioners are taught and encouraged to strive toward a cure as the ideal goal. Death thus becomes an enemy to be fought, as it represents ultimate, irretrievable failure. By comparison, for many CAM therapists, particularly spiritual healers, a good death is considered a good healing.

Compounding their other difficulties, doctors and nurses often work under unhealthy, dehumanizing conditions. They function under the combined pressures of long work hours; night call, night duty, and rotating shifts; very brief time allotments for each patient; economic and administrative requirements to see increasing numbers of patients; a besieged mentality generated by the ever-present danger of malpractice litigation; lack of peer support; and no training or experience in stress management techniques for their own needs. In fact, medical personnel are encouraged to ignore their feelings or to swallow them down. Throughout the challenging years of their training and practice, these stresses accumulate and take multiple tolls. Family life is stressed by job pressures, so there may be less than optimal support or nurturance at home. In the competitive atmosphere of modern professional training, asking for help is felt to be a weakness. It is no surprise that doctors have a very high rate of alcohol and drug abuse and even of suicide.

One of the major benefits offered by CAM therapies is stress management and healing techniques for the practitioner. I know many health caregivers who were first introduced to CAM methods through their own personal need for help. Some of the clearest introductions I've had to CAM therapies have been through enjoying their benefits for my own stresses and stress-related pains and other symptoms. I've been especially pleased with the results of spiritual healing and meridian and chakra based therapies.

There has been interest in working together on both sides of the divide. CAM therapists have offered to help doctors with patients who have difficult problems, and doctors have invited CAM therapists to work in their clinics and private offices. The results of such collaborations have been mixed. They seem to work best when they evolve gradually, from shared experiences of helping patients together. In that way, each side gets to understand how the other side works, and therefore has more realistic expectations when closer working relationships are forged. The richness of these therapeutic interactions is often highly stimulating and deeply satisfying to all participants. While a number of large clinics for integrative care have been started, some of these have not lasted for long. The greatest obstacle to success seems to be financial in nature. The high overhead expenses of maintaining large conventional medical facilities require that more patients be seen than most CAM therapists can comfortably manage without limiting their interventions to the point that their added benefit would be lost. More frequently successful are the working relationships in which doctors refer to CAM therapists in their own offices. However, the element that is often missing in these referral relationships is the close collaboration and mutual learning that occur when therapists with varied expertise and approaches work in closer collaborations organization.

When the CAM-allopathic marriage does work, both sides usually benefit and all involved learn a great deal from each other. As in any working relationship, the personalities and good will of the participants are major determinants in the success of the partnership. This marriage, like any other, needs the nurturing of time budgeted for discussions and clarifications of the working relationships. The people who benefit the most from integrative care are the respants, who enjoy the best of both CAM and allopathic therapies.

Acknowledging the engagement, if not yet the marriage of CAM with conventional medical care, The Federation of State Medical Boards (Euless, Texas) introduced "Model Guidelines for the Use of Complementary and Alternative Therapies in Medical Practice" in April 2002. They recommend that state medical boards should be given the options of adopting, modifying, or ignoring these guidelines:

> 1. The guidelines are grounded in an evidence-based approach. Conventional and alternative medicine are placed on an equal ground, and the limitations of both approaches are acknowledged.
> 2. Conventional and alternative therapies are addressed accurately and with parity. Patients can choose the therapies they want and physicians will not be disciplined based solely on their use or recommendation of CAM.
> 3. The guidelines are the vocabulary and evidence-based approach of the National Center for Complementary and Alternative Medicine (NCCAM). By adopting the definition of CAM used by NCCAM, the Federation established a link to the major NIH center responsible for evaluating alternative medicine in the United States.
>
> – Bonnie Horrigan and Bryna Block

This mixed marriage will require exhaustive pre- and post-nuptial contracts in order to make it a success. To help smooth the problems of diagnostic differences between the two systems, Alternative Link devised over 4,000 codes covering a wide range of CAM procedures and supplies, which are categorized as Alternative Billing Concept (ABC) codes. These codes have been given a trial run at a several medical centers with integrative programs. Their adoption on a nationwide scale will significantly advance the development of integrative care.

CHAPTER 3

The Human Energy Field

Big fields have little fields
Upon their backs to fight 'em;
And little fields have lesser fields
And so ad infinitum.
— Edward W. Russell

Heat and other measurable energies emanate from the human body. These may be what healers sense when they pass their hands around the body to assess its condition. It may also be that laying-on of hands healing works through these known, conventional energies.

Many people can sense these fields. You might just take a moment to explore this yourself. Hold your hands opposite each other, separated by about an inch. Slowly move them to about 18 inches apart, then back to their starting position. Repeat this about ten times. Pay attention to any sensations in your palms and fingers. (The endnote at the bottom of this paragraph describes what many people experience.) Now, rapidly make fists with your hands and then open them, about 20 times. Repeat your initial explorations. If you can find several people who are willing to explore this with you, repeat the process of moving your hand closer and farther away from one of theirs. Then reverse hands through all the possibilities of right opposite right, right opposite left, and left opposite left. Do this with each person in turn. [262]

Gifted, sensitive people may develop a detailed tactile vocabulary and learn to interpret these sensations as indications of specific energy blocks, illnesses, and psychological states.

Some of the fields that healers sense appear to involve energies that conventional science has difficulty in identifying and measuring. For instance, there are gifted sensitives who report that they can see an aura, or halo of color, around the body. A few very gifted sensitives can perceive the physical body itself as a complex energy field. In effect, they seem to have "X-ray eyes" with which they can observe the bioenergetic aspects of organs and biological processes as they occur in the living body. Some of these healers report that they can see the standard acupuncture meridians as well as many other meridians that are not mentioned in conventional acupuncture texts. They also see the chakras – as wheels of color from the front, and cones from the side.

Healers can diagnose people's physical, mental, emotional, and spiritual conditions by examining their auras and chakras. Healers may perform various manipulations on the auric fields that "cleanse," "unblock," and/or heal these abnormalities in the aura, thus producing secondary healings in the physical body, the mind, the emotions and the spirit.

Some healers claim that it is in these fields and in a *higher self* that the true essence of our being resides. Many healers believe that the fields are shaped by the non-material spirit and soul, and the physical body is shaped by a *higher self*, which is an energetic aspect of the person, in and through these fields.[263]

Let us start our discussion of the human energy fields with a review of reports on the auras that are sensed by healers. We will then consider studies exploring energies that may account for many aspects of auras.

AURAS

> *The real voyage of discovery consists not in seeing new landscapes,*
> *but having new eyes.*
>
> – Marcel Proust

Gifted clairvoyants[264] have reported that they see colored auras or halos around all objects.[265] They tell us that the auras of living things change according to their physical, mental, emotional and spiritual states, as well as in response to interactions with their surroundings. Various healers have reported differing observations of auras.

The late Dora Kunz, a gifted clairvoyant and healer, learned to make medical diagnoses by sitting with a physician named Shafika Karagulla and describing what she saw when Karagulla described her patients' medical conditions (Karagulla/ Kunz 1991). Kunz (1981) explained: "That's how I learned, for instance, that little red bricks in the aura mean that the person is on insulin."[266] Kunz could then diagnose people's illnesses from her readings of their auras. She identifies three concentric layers of the aura: the *vital* (*etheric* – relating to the physical body); the *astral* (emotional); and the *mental*.

Kunz, like other clairvoyant healers, also identifies health problems by observing the appearance of the *chakras*. The chakras are focal energy concentrations within the energy field. Seven major centers along the midline of the body appear as cones of swirling energy that interpenetrate the auras through all their layers. (See Table II-7.) Distortions in chakra color and shape correlate with illness in that region of the body. It is interesting that Kunz locates the second (splenic) chakra well to the left of the midline of the body, and the fourth (heart) chakra slightly to the left. Most other clairvoyants report that these chakras lie along the midline of the body.

Sensitives like Kunz have learned to systematically correlate these fields with specific conditions of the organism. They can diagnose states of health in any living organism at a glance.

Dolores Krieger (1979), Professor of Nursing at New York University, developed the Therapeutic Touch (TT) method of healing in collaboration with Dora Kunz. TT healers pass their hands around the body of healees, holding them several inches away from the skin, to obtain intuitive impressions about states of health and illness from tactile sensations of the aura. Areas in which there are physical problems may feel warmer, cooler, tingly, or different in some other distinctive way from normal areas of the body.

I can personally attest to the efficacy of this method for locating problem areas, though I am not sufficiently gifted or practiced in this method to be able to identify much more than the general location of a physical problem with my hands, and even this only works for me some of the time. I find it easiest to identify asymmetries in the right and left sides of the body that can provide clues as to the areas where problems reside. Chronic problems often produce a diminished intensity of sensations, while acute problems may feel hot, tingly or prickly. I am far more sensitive to picking up emotional components of dis-ease than physical ones, which is consonant with my specialization in psychiatry.

Barbara Brennan, an astrophysicist who now teaches aura reading and healing, observes at least seven concentric levels to the aura. Each is related to a distinct aspect of a person's being:

1. *etheric* – physical body;
2. *emotional* – emotions;
3. *mental* – thinking;
4. *astral* – I-thou emotions and desires;
5. *etheric template* – higher will;
6. *celestial* – higher feelings;
7. *ketheric* – higher concepts.

Each level envelops all of those below it. [267]

Brennan (1993) discusses additional energy levels within the aura. She calls these the *hara,* which relates to intentions; and the *core star,* which represents the divinity within us.

Brennan (1987; 1993) reports that the auras of people who are physically close to each other interact, which indicates bioenergetic exchanges between people.

The late Gordon Turner, a British healer, was gifted with the natural ability to see auras (and spirits). He described clear changes in the auras of healees during healings:

> [T]he process of spiritual healing can be traced through the auric field and, although there are variations in pattern according to the nature of the disorder and the personality of the person concerned, there does appear to be some similarity in the phenomena observed in all cases. When a healer places his hands upon a patient there is an immediate blending together of their auras. Within a few minutes all other colours that were previously observable become subordinated by a prevailing blue, which extends greatly beyond normal and seems to fill the room in which treatment is being carried out. Physical vision is

not impaired by this and it is still possible to see furniture in the room or the patient's features; but more than a moment's concentration on them causes the auric colour to become fainter and frequently to vanish altogether. It is still possible to see the colours that had denoted symptoms, but these float away from the body of the patient and become surrounded by a yellow coloured light which seems to be spinning. What follows is for all the world like the action of a "spiritual penicillin." The yellow light gradually overcomes the duller colour of the disease and it becomes flattened out and much less intense. Only about five minutes is required after the healing for the aura to return to normal and, if the cure has not been instantaneous, the disease colours return in lessened intensity according to the degree of benefit evoked by the healing, but still surrounded by the yellow light seen during the healing. When the healing is complete, the colours that signified the original disorder become flattened and very small, like minute scars. These may remain in the auric field for a varying length of time, from weeks to years, according to the gravity of the disorder.

Turner's description is consistent with the reports of Philippine healers who claim that they can tell by looking at the auras of prospective healees whether they have been treated previously by other healers.[268] In some instances they even claim to be able to identify *which* healer did the healing. They do not report which parts of the aura are used in this process.

Healers frequently direct their attention to the chakras, in addition to the parts of the body that are symptomatic. The chakras provide information about the condition of the body area adjacent to each chakra, and also give healing access to these local tissues and organs. These observations are in complete agreement with the Chinese descriptions of *chakras.*

Research:[269] I share greater details in this area of my particular interest.

Susan Marie Wright developed an energy field assessment (EFA) questionnaire, to identify particular qualities observed during assessments of the biofield. Her study explored the reliability of the EFA in assessing the location and intensity of pains, as well as in identifying generalized fatigue and depression.

The 52 people studied suffered from chronic lower back or cervical pain, fibrositis/ fibromyalgia, osteoarthritis, and other musculoskeletal pains, excluding cancer and rheumatoid arthritis. The duration of pain symptoms ranged from 2 to 480 months (mean 83.4 months).

The following results were reported:

Significant correlations were found between the sensed field abnormalities and subjects' reports of pains in the neck, upper back, and lower back.

There were not enough subjects with pains at other locations for the study to achieve a level of statistical significance.

Wright notes that subjective experiences of pain vary widely between people, despite the presence of apparently similar objective pathology. She suggests that in future studies it might be helpful to include assessments of *organic pathology*, as this might correlate more highly with energy field disturbances than do subjective experiences of pain. Further suggestions include replications with larger samples and inclusion of a control group of subjects who are pain-free.[270]

Table ii-9. Subjects' and Experimenters' reported locations of pain		
Site	Subjects	Experimenters
Head	4	4
Right shoulder	10	8
Left shoulder	7	7
Chest	4	2
Right elbow	1	0
Left elbow	2	1
Abdomen	1	2
Right hand	2	3
Left hand	3	5
Pelvis	2	0
Neck	25	28
Upper back	21	34
Right arm	3	4
Left arm	2	2
Low back	36	43
Right leg	9	5
Left leg	9	10
Right knee	6	7
Left knee	4	9
Right ankle	4	0
Left ankle	2	0

Two experiments (Schwartz et al 1995) were performed to establish whether ordinary people who were blindfolded could detect the hand of an experimenter that was held several inches above one of their hands. (Subjects had made no claims of healing abilities.)

The first of these experiments included 20 subjects, the majority of whom were not previously familiar with the experimenter.

In each trial, the blindfolded subjects used either their left or right hand to sense the presence of the experimenter's hand, and the experimenter used either his left or right hand to test the subjects' abilities. Experimenters sat opposite the subjects, holding their palms together with their hands placed in their lap. This was intended to maintain an equal temperature in both of their hands. During the trial, experimenters held their left or right hand palm down, 3 - 4 inches above the subject's right or left hand. When an experimenter had her or his hand in place, they would say "ready." Subjects then reported which of their hands they felt was covered by the experimenter's hand. Experimenters withdrew their hand after the subject's choice was stated. Subjects then rated their confidence in their guess on a scale of 0 to 10.

At the end of the series of 24 trials, subjects completed a questionnaire about the sensations they believed were associated with correct guesses, and they made an estimate of their total percentage of correct guesses.

Results: Mean correct guesses by subjects were significantly above chance, while estimates of performance were 12 percent lower (not significant). Subjects' mean confidence ratings were significantly higher for correct guesses than for incorrect ones. This suggests that they were partially aware of whether their guesses were correct.

The second experiment included 41 subjects, most of whom were familiar with the experimenter who tested them. The same procedures were followed as in Experiment 1.

Results: Subjects' guesses were 69.8 percent correct, which is significantly above chance. Again, estimated performance was 12 percent lower than actual performance.

Combined results of both experiments: Results were highly significant, and could have occurred by chance only five times in 100,000 trials.. Both groups also had higher confidence ratings regarding correct guesses compared to incorrect ones. Subjective sensations that were reported when subjects felt more confident of their guesses included temperature (usually warmth), tingling, and pressure.

Out of the 61 subjects, 47 were able to identify the correct side (left or right) at significantly better than chance levels, with an overall correct rate of 66 percent.[271]

This study clearly demonstrates that ordinary people can sense when another person's hand is near their own. This supports claims by healers that they are able to sense an energy field around the body.

This study does not prove that biological energies exist outside of the known and currently accepted electromagnetic spectrum. As noted by the authors, effects of heat, electrostatic energy, or electromagnetic resistance could have produced the results in this study. No conclusions can be drawn relevant to healing, other than that healers might experience sensations in their hands and healees might experience sensations in their bodies due to effects of known physical energies.

> *As a hands-on therapist, what you touch is not merely the skin – you contact a continuous interconnected webwork that extends throughout the body.*
>
> – James Oschman, 2000 (p. 47)

In contrast with the last two studies, the next one is of interest primarily due to its publication in a prestigious American medical journal, and its demonstration of the readiness of conventional medical journals to present what they perceive to be negative results of healing studies.[272]

In 1966 Linda Rosa's nine-year-old daughter Emily did a study of TT healers' abilities to sense bioenergy fields, for a fourth grade science fair project. Fifteen TT healers were tested over several months at their offices or homes (Rosa et al 1998).

In the experiment, healers were asked to lay their hands on a table, palms up and 25-30 centimeters apart. The experimenter sat opposite the subjects, screened from sight by a tall barrier. The healers inserted their arms through holes at its base, and as a further precaution a towel was placed over their arms so that they could not see the experimenter through the armholes. Each healer was tested 10 times, and was allowed to prepare mentally for as long as they wanted before each set of trials. The experimenter positioned her right hand 8-10 cm. above one of the healer's hands (chosen by coin toss) and then alerted the healer, who was to identify which of the healer's hand the experimenter was covering.

For significant results, healers had to identify the targeted hand correctly 8 out of 10 times. In the first series only one healer scored 8, but on a retest the same healer scored only 6.

Healers' explanations for their failures included the following:

1. A tactile "afterimage" made it difficult for healers to distinguish the actual hand from the "memory" perception. However, the initial trials in each series did not produce scores greater than chance either.
2. Healers' left hands are usually more sensitive receivers of biological energies than their right hands, which are usually more potent projectors of such energies. Out of 72 trials with healers' right hands, 45 (62 percent) demonstrated incorrect responses. Out of 80 incorrect responses, 35 (44 percent) were with the left hand. These differences are not statistically significant.
3. In a practice trial prior to the experimental test series, healers performed better if they were given feedback as to which hand was being tested. Rosa et al. feel that feedback should not be necessary, but concede that allowing it would eliminate this objection.
4. The healers felt the experimenter should be more active, by intentionally project-ing her energy field. Rosa et al. feel this should not be necessary, as no such de-mand is placed upon patients whose energy fields are being sensed by TT healers.
5. Some healers reported that their hands felt so hot after several trials that they either had difficulty or were unable to sense the experimenter's field. Rosa et al. observe that this contradicts statements by TT healers who claim that they can deliberately manipulate patients' energy fields during the course of a typical 20-30-minute TT session. This objection is also contradicted by the fact that only 7 out of 15 first trials produced correct responses.

In 1997 a second series was completed in a single day and recorded on videotape by a TV broadcasting crew. In this experiment healers were permitted to sense the experimenter's field, and each selected which hand the experimenter would use for the test. Healers correctly identified which of their hands was being tested in 53 out of 131 trials (41 percent). The range of correct responses was 1-7.

Healers made the following objections at the end of the study:

1. One healer said the towel over his hands was distracting.

2. One healer said her hands were too dry.

3. "Several" healers complained that the televising of the proceedings interfered with their concentration and increased stresses.[273] Rosa et al. believe that the presence of a TV crew should not distract or stress healers more than the usual hospital settings in which many TT healers practice.

The result of 123 correct responses out of 280 trials (44 percent) in the two series obviously does not support claims by healers that they are able to sense energy fields. No significant correlation was found in this study between healers' performance and their levels of experience.

Rosa et al. conclude that TT healers have no ability whatsoever to sense the biological energy field because the 21 TT healers studied did not succeed in identifying which of their hands was being tested. They state, "To our knowledge, no other objective, quantitative study involving more than a few TT practitioners has been published, and no well-designed study demonstrates any health benefit from TT."

George D. Lundlberg, M.D., then editor of the journal (*JAMA*) adds the following comment on this study in the issue in which it appears:

> The American public is fascinated by alternative (complementary, unconventional, integrative, traditional, Eastern) medicine. Some of these practices have a valid scientific basis; some of them are proven hogwash; many of them have never been adequately tested scientifically. "Therapeutic Touch" falls into the latter classification, but nonetheless is the basis for a booming international business as treatment for many medical conditions. This simple, statistically valid study tests the theoretical basis for "Therapeutic Touch": the "human energy field." This study found that such a field does not exist. I believe that practitioners should disclose these results to patients, third-party payers should question whether they should pay for this procedure, and patients should save their money and refuse to pay for this procedure until or unless additional honest experimentation demonstrates an actual effect.

I wrote to Lundberg, informing him that a doctoral dissertation examining the sensing of auras by healers had showed positive effects. Phil B. Fontanarosa, MD, the senior editor of *JAMA* replied that my letter "did not receive a high enough priority rating for publication in *JAMA*" and indicated no interest in this dissertation.

It is surprising that a study done by a 9-10 year old girl could be published in a prestigious medical journal. Editorial standards of such publications usually require that all research the publish must be performed by a medical practitioner or qualified scientist.

Three of the co-authors of this article are self-identified skeptics and the last two are members of an organization called Committee for the Study of the Paranormal. This organization is known to be dedicated to discounting all evidence for parapsychological phenomena. The methods it uses do not always meet the highest scientific standards, and many observers find them to be deliberately misleading. Several examples of such methods are also evident in the study by Rosa et al.

An example of misdirection in this study can be found in the statements by Rosa et al. about the extensive published healing research. "Of the 74 quantitative studies, 23 were clearly unsupportive."[274] The authors make no mention of the remaining 51 studies, which one would guess from their analysis must be supportive, and do not provide a list of which studies they are discussing. I know of several such studies, and Rosa et al. cite some of these in footnotes nos. 76-86 of their article, inclusive. *No discussion of the positive findings is presented, and I find no reference in the text to footnotes 76-86.* The authors' statement, "To our knowledge, no other objective, quantitative study *involving more than a few TT practitioners* [my italics] has been published." is again misleading. Most studies of healing involve only one or a few healers. This cannot be taken as a valid as criticism of the general research methods in this field, which have in fact produced significant results in many cases. The conclusion of the sentence, "and no well-designed study demonstrates any health benefit from TT" is clearly untrue.

Due to these omissions and falsehoods, at first reading the article looks quite convincing in its damnation of published TT research. It would appear that these omissions function to support the authors' and editor's skepticism, and one must wonder whether they were deliberate.

Rosa et al. and the JAMA editor assume that there is no validity to healers' claims that they are able to sense energy fields or to influence them. They therefore dismiss any complaints by healers regarding factors in the test situation which might influence their ability to sense such a field.

Healers' objections that the stress of performing in front of TV cameras could have a negative influence appear to me a valid criticism of the second part of this study. While the ambiance of a hospital ward might seem stressful (particularly to outsiders), it is composed of elements that are familiar to nurses and are therefore not as distracting as the unfamiliar presence of a TV crew.

There is evidence that one can influence one's own energy field and the process of healing by controlling one's mental state and intent. In one study, several nurses were able to produce significant results with TT when it was given with the intent to heal, as opposed to simply going through the motions of the therapy while doing arithmetic in their heads (Keller 1983; Quinn 1989). It has also been observed that skin resistance in the hands can be altered by changes in mental state. This would produce a concomitant change in the electromagnetic field around the hand. Kirlian photography has demonstrated that when people have positive feelings for each other their energy fields merge, and conversely, when they feel negatively towards each other their energy fields retract.

I can add anecdotal evidence from workshops I give on developing one's healing gifts. One person can project energy from a hand or foot and another person can identify when the first one discontinues this projection of energy. I support healers' suggestions that it is possible for experimenters to withdraw or to not project their energy fields, thus making it difficult for a healer to identify the energy field.

A further objection that can be raised in connection with this study is that part of the experience of sensing energy fields is dynamic. When I sense someone's field I move my hand towards and away from their body, as well as across their body.

This provides far stronger sensory perceptions than simply holding my hand still near the body.

I would also suggest that the presence of a skeptic during a study of parapsychological phenomena or healing practices could dampen or inhibit the effects under study. While this must appear to skeptics as an unfair proposal, this is in fact the nature of parapsychological effects. They are very much influenced by the mental states of participants and observers. Skeptics are likely to obtain negative effects, believers positive ones. This has been amply supported by studies of *sheep* and *goats* in psi research.[275] In the testing of energy fields, two studies of sensitives' abilities to see auras produced negative results (Ellison; Gissurarson/ Gissurarson).

The sweeping dismissal of TT as a valid therapeutic method by the authors of the Rosa et al. article and by the editor of the journal, based upon the evidence of limited research carried out by a 9-10 year old girl, is patently ridiculous. This study simply explored the ability of healers to sense the energy field of one experimenter under specific test conditions. In no way did it test healing abilities.[276]

Sadly, the popular media trumpeted the negative results of this study far and wide, and many people who had no access to the details of the study believed their dismissive conclusions.

Discussion of energy field sensing

Various energies that are well recognized in conventional science could account for some of the observed bioenergy phenomena. Schwartz et al. (1995) note that direct current (DC) skin electrical potentials can normally be measured on the hands. It's possible that the amount of sweat on the skin could modulate these DC potentials, and this could also alter the amount and quality of the heat radiated from the skin. Blood flow in the skin and muscles of the hands conduct cardiac electrical and sound patterns as well as generating heat, which is radiated as infrared pulses. The muscles in the limbs produce electromyographic (EMG) pulses. Movements of the limbs generate electrostatic fields. All of these energies combine to form a complex, dynamic energy pattern around the hands and other parts of the body.

Chien et al. (1991) also identified emanations of heat energy, which they measured as infrared signals in therapeutic touch healings.

Conversely, the hands contain nerve endings which can detect pressure, temperature, and the stretch of tendons and ligaments. These receptors could, theoretically, also respond to other energies. Electrostatic fields might produce subtle stretches or pressures which these receptors might be able to register. Minute breezes could also be detected through temperature, pressure, and/or stretch receptors. Perceptions of electrical or magnetic signals have not been empirically established as yet.[277]

Other energy field interactions

Gary E. Schwartz and colleagues (Russek/ Schwartz) note that the various measurable energies of two people may interact when they are physically close together. For instance, electrical cardiac energy interactions measured by an electrocardiogram (ECG) occur and they may vary with the degree of openness that the participants feel toward interpersonal communication. This team also found that the ECG patterns of two people sitting near each other are reflected in each other's electroencephalogram (EEG) patterns.

Valerie Hunt (1977) reported on aura changes during rolfing. Rolfing is a form of vigorous, deep massage that is used to loosen up tense areas of muscles and joints. Rolfing produces intense releases of emotions that are often associated with physical tensions. It is theorized that emotions are stored in the body either through conditioning or via an actual imprinting of memories in the body per se.[278] In Hunt's study, electronic readings of changes in muscle tension were recorded. Rosalind Bruyere, a gifted clairvoyant, simultaneously described the auric changes she observed in therapists and patients. Clear correlations emerged between the changes noted by Bruyere and those measured by bio-electronic sensors. Bruyere found particular visible changes in chakras that developed progressively through the series of rolfing sessions.[279]

Other scientists question the validity of visual aura perceptions.

Arthur Ellison was a Professor of Electrical and Electronic Engineering at London City University and a parapsychologist. He performed an experiment in which a sensitive who claimed to be able to observe auras reported the colors of the aura that he saw between the fingers of Ellison's hands, which were held close to but not touching each other. Next, he placed a cardboard box with a small window in it as a screen between himself and the sensitive. Only the space between his hands was visible to the sensitive, and his hands were screened. When he told the sensitive that his hands were next to the window, the sensitive confirmed that he could see the aura. When he told the sensitive that he had removed his hands, the sensitive reported that he saw no aura. Ellison then had the sensitive continue to report when he saw the aura and when he did not, and meanwhile Ellison led him to believe that at certain times he was holding his hands up and at other times not. In fact, he held his hands flat on the box below the window for the whole period of the experiment, or even removed them and placed them in his lap. The sensitive nevertheless continued to report that he saw an aura at the window at times when Ellison *indicated* that his hands were there. Ellison concludes that the aura "... was produced by what is sometimes called 'unconscious dramatization' and bore no relationship to 'reality' by way of the position of the fingers." He speculates that auric matter reportedly seen by sensitives may be a reflection of visual fatigue, after-images, and/or projections from the mind of the perceiver. Generalizing from this single case study, he suggests that such projections may be the mind's way of transforming unconsciously imaged material into the conscious mind. His conclusion is that the aura is a projection of the imagination of the alleged sensitive.

In a similar study, Loftur Gissurarson and Asgeir Gunnarsson challenged several people who reported that they could see auras to identify which one of four barriers a man was standing behind. They presumed that the auras would project beyond the edges of the barriers. Only chance scores were achieved.

I was surprised to find that no one had studied whether several sensitives would report they perceived the same colors in the aura if they all observed a patient at the same time. I set up a pilot experiment (Benor 1992) on making assessments based on auras with the help of Dr. Jean Galbraith,[280] an English general practitioner. Eight sensitives simultaneously observed a series of people with known diagnoses. The sensitives drew and interpreted their perceptions of the subjects' auras. The overlaps between the drawings and interpretations of the sensitives were small compared to the differences between them. Yet when the patients who had been observed heard the diverse interpretations they resonated with seven out of the eight.

In a second pilot project with four healers who are more gifted and more experienced, we again found diverse observations of the auras and broadly differing interpretations of what they perceived. In addition, we found concurrences among the healers in observations regarding energy field abnormalities that bore no relationship to clinical diagnoses. The *interpretations* of the latter field abnormalities differed from one healer to another.

How can we understand the varying reports about auras?

My conclusion is that aura readings, as with other psi perceptions, are filtered through the unconscious mind and the perceptual apparatus of the sensitive. Psychic perceptions arrive in the deeper awareness of the mind, and only partially filter into conscious awareness. The data are thus colored by the individual during the processes of perception, translation into visual imagery, and cognitive/verbal interpretation.

Barbara Brennan[281] suggests that the difference between reports may be due to healers' resonation with different layers of the aura. The innermost aura layer, which is associated with the physical body, will appear different from the next aura layer, which relates to the emotional body; and similarly for the mental and spiritual layers. Many healers may not be aware that they are perceiving a particular sub-section of the aura. I believe that Brennan's assessment is probably correct for some instances of such discrepancies.

However, some sensitives intuitively or clairsentiently perceive the condition of a person's health without seeing their aura. The information may come to them as audible words, smells, tastes, body sensations in their own bodies which mirror those of the person they are observing, or direct, intuitive *knowing.*[282] This suggests to me that my original interpretation of the data may be more valid. It may also be that each of these explanations is partially valid.

Evidence from other areas of study may shed some light on the phenomenon of aura perceptions.

There are reports that a sense organ (eye, ear, etc.) can sometimes convey information obtained by unusual stimulation, of a kind that is not ordinarily perceived by that particular sense (Romains). This is technically termed *synesthesia.* An example of this fascinati8ng capability is that many people (about one woman in twenty, and fewer men) can *hear* color. That is to say, various sounds produce mental sensations of color.

Research on dermal optics, which is the sensing of color through the skin, may provide further information about aura vision. It may be that auras are manifestations of such synesthesias, with skin sensations or clairsentient perceptions that are translated by the brain into tactile or visual imagery. Several clairsentients have told me that they perceive auras even with remote viewing of healees or when looking at photographs and videotapes of subjects. One sensitive reported that when she looked at a picture of a woman who was drinking water from a

Japanese temple, she saw a white light around the water, indicating that it had healing properties.

Yvonne Duplessis (1985) found that the skill of perceiving the colors of pieces of paper through sensations in the hands could be learned. The distance of the hand above the paper beyond which a color could no longer be perceived varied consistently in each subject for each color. The height threshold for the same color also varied according to whether the illumination of the target colors was by natural light or artificial lighting. This research appears to parallel in a general way the studies of body aura perception with the hands. It may also provide a caution to investigators to note whether studies are done in natural or artificial light.

Carlos Alvarado and Nancy Zingrone explored the visual imagery styles of people who experience synesthesias (crossed-sensory perceptions, such as perceiving certain sounds in response to seeing certain colors). Those who perceive synesthesias have very vivid visualization abilities. While this enables them to produce internal imagery that appears very real to them, investigators may still find it difficult to clarify and assess what actually occurs in the process of synesthesias.

I tested a musician who reported that he "heard" colors, by playing various tones on a tape recorder and having him select paint color chips that approximated the colors he perceived. He found the task exhausting, and required many repetitions of the tone and careful sorting of the paint colors. He often ended up dissatisfied that he could not find precisely the right match. He believed that he was absolutely consistent in his perceptions, so I re-tested him two months later. His color selections were 90 percent consistent, but several tones produced distinctly different colors the second time.

Tactile perception of the energy field is much more commonly experienced and reported by healers and ordinary people than are synesthesias.

Synesthesias demonstrate that the mind may interpret sensory inputs from one sensory modality as subjective perceptions that are experienced in another modality. This supports the speculation that bioenergy aura perceptions could be translated into various sensory perceptions.

Overall, clairsentience appears to me the more likely explanation for auras.

The process of diagnosis within the frameworks of other complementary therapies may overlap with the clairsentient perceptions reported by healers. Robert Duggan, a gifted acupuncture practitioner, reports:

> When I first learned to read the pulse as used in relation to the practice of acupuncture, I though I was observing what occurred on the wrist of the other person. Later, I realized that what I observed was what occurred in my fingertips as I experienced my fingertips in the presence of the other. Another practitioner placing finger on wrist would experience a very different phenomenon.

Other experienced acupuncturists report that they can sense and reliably identify the locations of acupuncture points with their fingers and can tell when the meridians have a proper flow of Qi or are blocked (e.g. Upledger). This tactile sensitivity supports the claims of healers that it is possible to sense the human energy field through one's hands.

Further support for the existence of energy fields comes from the phenomenon of *phantom limb* sensations following amputation. People frequently report that they continue to experience pain and other sensations where an amputated limb used to be, even though it no longer exists physically. It can be a most annoying experience to feel a physical itch they cannot scratch! Conventional medicine interprets this as an effect of persistent brain or mental images that produce fantasy sensations of the limb. It is further speculated that the nerve ends from the amputated limb may still send messages to the brain, which interprets these as though they were coming from the now non-existent limb. Healers suggest that phantom limb perceptions may be energy field phenomena. Healers may be able to sense the presence of an energy limb after the physical limb has been removed. Spiritual healing given to the energy limb may reduce or eliminate the phantom limb sensations.

Phantom limb phenomena parallel the phantom leaf effects of Kirlian photography, described later in this chapter.

How can we explain the intensity of skeptics' criticisms of healing (and other psi phenomena)?

The willingness of a major medical journal to publish a study done by a 10-year-old girl; the exaggerated criticism of spiritual healing levied by the editor of that journal; and the degree of publicity surrounding this study are remarkable. all These (and similar critical reactions to reports of healings and healing research suggest that there is considerable resistance to accepting evidence supporting the validity of intuitive assessments and spiritual healing, and a great readiness to accept evidence, however flimsy, that suggests these are not valid phenomena. It is apparent that intuitive awareness and spiritual healing push the boundaries of Western scientific paradigms, and it is a natural reaction to resist change.[283]

Discussion of aura phenomena

We still have much to clarify about the perception of auras. The visible aura described by sensitives does not appear to be a wholly consistently or objectively observable phenomenon – both within and between individual aura perceivers. Gifted sensitives report they see the aura all of the time, but many others see the aura only some of the time. The differences in aura perceptions between sensitives is striking.

There are some who propose that the visible aura is nothing more than a visual after-image (Fraser-Harris). They note that it is normal to see colors if you close your eyes after staring at an object. The colors perceived in this case will be primary complements to the real-world colors that they reflect. You may test this yourself by staring at something with a single strong color, in bright light, for about a minute. Then close your eyes. Your brain will now perceive the after-image of the object in its complementary color (e.g. if the object is red, you will see green with your eyes closed).[284] Given the fact that the eyes flit around constantly as we gaze at objects, Fraser-Harris hypothesizes that some alleged aura phenomena are blurred after-images from the edges of the objects being gazed at.

This theory might account for a small portion of reported aura phenomena, specifically those connected with the aura that is seen immediately adjacent to the body. However it cannot account for the portions of the aura described as the chakras, or the portions extending many inches and even several feet away from the body, nor for interactions of auras when people are physically close to each other. It also cannot account for sensitives' correlations of the aura with physical, mental and emotional processes, which they perceive in colors that not only differ from the primary color complements of the object observed, but change constantly as well.

Some have suggested that auras might be instances of bioluminescence, or the emission of visible light from living organisms (like the lights of fireflies). Carlos Alvarado surveyed reports of such luminous phenomena around the body and found that they are qualitatively distinctly different from the auras described by sensitives.

Western science tends to rely more on electronic sensors and to denigrate human sensors as being too full of "noise" to provide reliable readings. In my opinion, the human biocomputer is the most sensitive of all sensors. Symptomatic exploration with aura readers may offer us the most valuable information available, with the caveat that we must be cautious in accepting any single human "reading."

This last caution would apply equally to Ellison's study of a single subject's report of aura perception, from which he deduces that auras as described by healers do not exist

Charles Tart (1972b) and others suggest there may be psychological constructs of psi perceptions or of projected mental imagery, thoughts or feelings that manifest in the conscious mind as auras. I have found support for this view in reports of a number of healers who perceive auras. For instance, the late Olga Worrall was one of the better-studied healers in America, and she claimed that she could perceive auras with her eyes closed. She speculated that the visual information was detected by her *third eye*, a spot between the eyebrows alleged by many mystics to be the sense organ for clairvoyance. Other healers have told me that they perceive auras with their *third eye* or some other "inner perception."

Harry Oldfield, an English healer, and Valerie Hunt, an American scientist, have developed methods of videotaping the aura. Sensitives who have seen these videotapes report that they closely resemble the auras they perceive visually. Hunt's methods involve processing the tape after the recordings are made. Oldfield and Hunt have not revealed their methods as of the date of this publication, and this unfortunately leaves their work open to question.[285]

Why some people perceive auras and others do not is unclear. One hint comes from the work of James Peterson, who studied descriptions by children of "the colors they saw around things." He found that many children had such perceptions, although they might differ in range and quality from one child to another. He adds (1975):

> In my experience, clairvoyant children have been very reluctant to talk
> about their unusual vision, usually because their reports have been re-
> buffed, condemned or ridiculed. Even a kind parent is likely to say the

experiences aren't "real." And a concerned and sensitive teacher might well call the perceptions "imaginary." More stern adults may scold the clairvoyant child for lying. The sum of it all is apt to be confusion, self-doubt, even self hate. (One seven-year-old, Stacy, told me she hated herself because her visions distracted and disturbed her so much.) And it's not only adults who can disturb the clairvoyant child. Peers are quite likely to make fun of the one who "sees things," often less gently than adults.

Imagine the strain on the child who is scolded by her parents, disciplined by a teacher, and ridiculed by friends – all because she sees things that others don't. To cope with the stress and rejection, she may convince herself that what she sees isn't really there at all. Or she may simply learn to keep quiet about what she sees.

Peterson reports that children were often very relieved that they could discuss their perceptions with him. An adult who Peterson interviewed also confirmed that she would have been much happier if, as a child, she been able to find someone who understood her clairvoyant perceptions. Peterson speculates that children may actually lose these psi abilities, partly through their attempts to conform to expected social norms, and partly due to physiological maturation. He concludes with a plea for sensitivity to the needs of such children, who require and deserve understanding on the part of the adults in their lives.

> *When I was the age of these children I could draw like Raphael; it took me many years to learn how to draw like these children.*
> – Pablo Picasso

A decrease in aura sensing ability with maturation may be similar to observations of a peak age for photographic memory in children. This peak occurs around age ten, with gradual waning of memory abilities thereafter (Feldman). Further studies should clarify whether social rather than developmental factors contribute to or cause these changes.

While we don't yet have research to demonstrate the functions of the aura, Barbara Brennan and other healer report that the innermost layer of the visible aura is a template and matrix for the anchoring of body matter. Changes in the aura that indicate disease processes may become apparent as unusual aura colors several months prior to the appearance of the physical problems. Brennan and John Pierrakos "... observed that an energy field matrix in the shape of a leaf is projected by the plant prior to the growth of a leaf and then the leaf grows into that already existing form" (Brennan 1987).

John Pierrakos is a New York doctor who sees auras and specializes in bioenergetics. He claims that the aura represents *both* a life-field that is a sort of template for the physical body, and also a product of life processes within the body – indicating a dual nature for the aura. This explanation seems the most convincing to me.

In effect, the aura may be a part of the energy aspect of physical, material life processes. This would correlate with Albert Einstein's theory of relativity. Quantum physics has amply confirmed that matter and energy are interconvertible. Newtonian medicine has been slow to accept that the human body can be addressed as a form of biological energy.

> *What is Matter? Never mind.*
> *What is Mind? No matter.*
>   *– Punch*

On the basis of conventional science, it would be hard to differentiate between healers' claims that they can influence the *etheric body* which in turn influences the physical body, and the alternative that healers influence the physical body *directly* and the etheric body reflects these changes. Clairsentients, however, are unanimous in observing that it is the etheric body which changes first, preceding the resulting physical changes in some cases by many weeks or months. Changes indicating illness that are observed in the aura do not have to manifest in the physical body. They can be altered and cleared by self-healing and healer-healing.

Several sensitives have reported that they can predict the impending death of a person by the presence of a black aura or by the total absence of an aura. Such observations have been made not only in patients who are ill, but also when a sensitive has noticed such auras around a group of people boarding a plane that subsequently crashed. This raises many fascinating questions regarding the phenomenon of death, precognition, and predestination of events (all of which lies beyond the scope of our present discussion). It supports the hypothesis of the aura as a construct of the mind that brings psi perceptions into conscious awareness.

Some sensitives suggest that relationships exist between portions of the aura and the astral body of the *out-of-body experience* (OBE),[286] and also with non-physical or spiritual aspects of man's being. It may be possible to test these observations. For instance, one could explore further how different sensitives agree and disagree in their readings of *spiritual* aspects of the aura; what different sensitives perceive when a person is dying and their spirit separates from the body; whether such observations correlate with other assessments of spirituality, meditative practices, and more.

What seems clear is that a biological energy field exists around the body that is visible to some people, probably more though clairsentient perception than through visual perception. Others can sense such fields with their hands. This ability is much more common than the ability to perceive auras visually.

Let us now turn to a discussion of the energy fields on and around the body that are measurable with various instruments and technical devices.

KIRLIAN PHOTOGRAPHY

> *If you conduct a study and the data doesn't agree with your theory,*
> *the scientist throws away the theory.*
> *The quack, on the other hand, throws away the data.*
>   *– David Bresler*

The late Russian scientist Semyon Davidovich Kirlian and his wife Valentina developed an electrophotographic technique in the 1940s for recording auras around animals, plants, and inanimate objects. No light or lenses are used in this process. Objects photographed are placed directly against the film in a darkroom and a pulsed electric current of high voltage and low amperage is passed through both the object and the film.

For diagnostic purposes, Kirlian photographs are usually made of the palm, fingertips, foot or toes. The shape, density and color of the Kirlian aura have been found to correlate with states of health and disease in plants, animals and humans. This is a new field for research that may help us greatly to understand the energy nature of life. In Eastern Europe numerous practitioners utilize this diagnostic technique (which they have termed *bioelectrography*). Sadly, Western medical science has not invested in this promising mode of diagnosis, and most Western researchers have had to finance their work out of pocket.

Relevance of Kirlian photography to healing
1. Various states of physical and emotional health and disease in plants, animals and humans can be identified using this method. Kirlian photographs in color add dimensions to the readings, but they also add to the variability of the process and considerably increase costs. Generally speaking, illness, tiredness, or physical and emotional imbalances may be reflected in a narrow, thin, broken and irregular aura. The field is broken into *streamers* (See Figure II-16, below.) A healthy state usually correlates with a broad, robust, dense and unbroken aura (See Figure II-17, on the next page.)

Figure II-16. Fingertip with irregular, ragged Kirlian aura, typical of illness prior to healing.

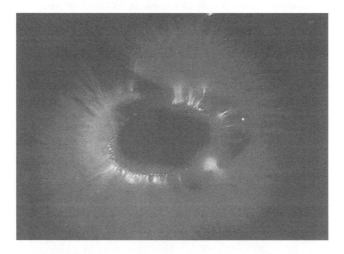

These criteria are applicable for many conditions, but with cancer the corona may be dense and unvarying, in contrast to normal auras, which show cyclical variations with time (Mallikarjun).

A careful study correlating Kirlian auras with illness was performed by Dr. Ramesh Singh Chouhan and P. Rajaram, Professor of Obstetrics and Gynecology, in Pondicherry, India. Using black and white Kirlian fingertip images, they studied fifty normal peri- and post-menopausal women to obtain a normative baseline for such images. They then studied the Kirlian photographs of 100 women aged 45 - 60 years, whose only illness was cancer of the cervix. In all cases biopsies and/or vaginal cytology were also examined. No anti-cancer therapies were started prior to the initial Kirlian photography. The study focused on "increase in intensity and character of the emission pattern."

> The film was processed on an automatic processor and the electrogram was then analysed densitometrically for the intensity of the emission... Palmar sweating/ hyperhidrosis was seen only in 6% of the subjects. 60% showed dryness of the skin to touch. Analysis of electrograms revealed that there is a definite increase in the intensity of emission in cancerous and precancerous stage as against normal. The coronal midzone increase is linear to the advancement of disease. The streamer density was plotted on a graph after densitometric measurement. Though slight fluctuation was seen in the intensity of individual images they all fit into a pattern which could be distinct to each stage of the disease... Correlation with histopathologic and clinical staging was 100%...

In cases where follow-up evaluations were made, staging of disease progress by Kirlian photography correlated closely with clinical and laboratory results for staging of the disease. An unpublished extension of this series to include 1,000 cases confirmed the results (Chouhan).

Figure II-17. Fingertips with regular, robust Kirlian aura, typically seen in healthy people and following healing.

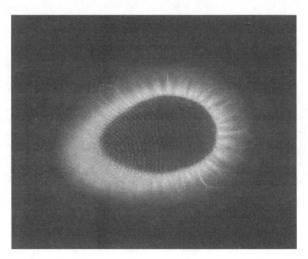

2. Valerie Hunt et al. found correlations of Kirlian photography with results of structural integration treatments (rolfing, or deep body massage). Those treated showed a significant finding: greater numbers of white bubbles in their Kirlian auras after rolfing.[287]

3. Healers' and healees' Kirlian auras may change reciprocally from before to after a healing treatment. Typically, healers' auras are robust prior to healing and less so afterwards; and conversely for healees' auras. If a healee's aura is ragged prior to healing, it may be more full after the treatment is received. Autogenic training, a system of self-healing, is also said to alter Kirlian images (Roman/ Inyushin; Steel).

Hans G. Engel is a Los Angeles physician who is also a healer. With the collaboration of Thelma Moss at the University of California, Los Angeles, he obtained Kirlian photographs for each person he healed, and for himself, prior to and following each treatment session over an 18-month period (Engel/ Cole). An assistant selected a representative 120 paired samples from thousands of pictures taken before and after every phase of treatment, representing every type of response to giving and receiving healing. The pairs of *befores* and *afters* were randomly arranged on pages of an album.

> After these 120 pairs were mounted, each pair to a page, the set was given to three judges in turn. These three were individuals working in the laboratory but not involved in the energy healing experiment. They were asked to evaluate the corona discharge on the pictures according to three standards: darkness (i.e., intensity), length of emanations, and gaps in the pattern, to a total of 360 evaluations.
>
> There was a strong tendency of all judges to score the therapist's corona discharge as more intense before than after treatment; however, they did not find that patients showed a significant increase in the corona discharge after therapy... neither of these results was found to be statistically significant. Concordance between the judges' evaluation was subjected to blind, independent rating; statistics reveal significant correlation in their collective interpretations.

4. Kirlian and others claim that they can identify illness in plants or animals through their Kirlian images even prior to the appearances of outward signs of disease that are visible or detectable by other measurements. Rosemary Steel studied the clinical correlations of Kirlian hand images, finding links with specific physical and emotional problems. This suggests that there may be a holographic representation of the whole person in the hands.[288]

5. A correlation is reported between some aspects of Kirlian photography, and acupuncture points and acupuncture treatments. Particularly bright flares appear at acupuncture points and their intensities are altered with acupuncture treatments. Steel finds that her interpretations of Kirlian hand images correlate well with hand maps of acupuncture and kinesiology.

6. Dumitrescu has an electrophotographic technique that he calls *Electronography*. He has demonstrated flares emanating from parts of the body that correspond with acupuncture points.

7. Plants and food products that have been grown organically (without pesticides) and are fresh typically demonstrate much brighter and broader Kirlian auras than those grown with chemical fertilizers and pesticides. Food products treated with preservatives and especially those that are irradiated show particularly dull and narrow auras.

8. Water that is given healing and water from holy springs demonstrates a very bright Kirlian aura.

9. In rare Kirlian photographs of leaves that have had portions cut away, the Kirlian aura of the missing segment may still appear. This has been labeled *the phantom leaf effect*. This effect has been difficult to replicate but it has been reported in a sufficient number of laboratories to confirm its existence. The parallels between phantom leaf Kirlian photographs and phantom limb effects are consistent with a theory of energy fields that exist within and around living organisms.

10. Interactional effects have been found in Kirlian auras of pairs of people who are photographed simultaneously on the same film. In exposures of their fingertips (held adjacent but not touching) their Kirlian auras will coalesce if they have positive feelings for each other. Conversely, if they have negative feelings for each other the auras withdraw from each other.

Problems with replication of research results
The interpretation of these Kirlian photographic halos is still a controversial subject.

As with many other aspects of energy medicine, Kirlian phenomena have not been consistently replicable by all investigators, or under all circumstances by the same investigators. This has unfortunately contributed to the rejection of a potentially useful tool for medical diagnosis.

Numerous technical factors may influence the appearance of Kirlian images. These include voltage; electrical pulse width and rate; frequency of signal pulse; moisture (e.g. sweat) and dirt on objects photographed; atmospheric gases; pressure of object on film; exposure time; film type; flatness of film; angle of objects relative to the film; barometric pressure; atmospheric temperature (Poock); grounding of subjects – which may be influenced by leather vs. rubber-soled shoes, or the type of chair the subject sits in (Steel) – as well as parameters of film development such as temperature, freshness and agitation of processing solutions. In the phantom leaf Because these parameters have not been standardized or consistent among investigators, it has been difficult to obtain consistent results in different laboratories.

In addition, psychological/ emotional factors in the subject and in the other persons present in the laboratory may influence the photographs. It appears possible that the operator of the equipment or other observers may influence the Kirlian photographs, and that believers may obtain positive results while disbelievers do not.

Yvonne Duplessis (1985) found that in color sensitivity tests of dermal optics, perceptions shifted according to whether the subject was tested in daylight or artificial light. Sensitives have told me that the size and nature of the room in which Kirlian photographs are made and in which other energy medicine phenomena are observed may influence the results. Jacob Liberman makes a strong case for deleterious bioenergetic effects of ordinary fluorescent light bulbs, which is the most common type of lighting in scientific laboratories. We must take such cautions seriously when investigating phenomena that differ substantially from conventional subjects of study in Western science. These factors may contribute to some of the variability that is repeatedly found in replications of subtle energy studies.

Some researchers believe that the operator of the Kirlian equipment may contribute an energetic component to the Kirlian photographs, thus adding yet another confounding factor to the list of variables that can influence these pictures.

Other researchers contest the validity of all of the above-mentioned positive findings, citing conflicting theories and confusion in experimental parameters.

Implications of Kirlian photography

It is unclear as yet what Kirlian pictures actually represent. The majority of scientists studying Kirlian photography believe that the image reflects the biological energy state of the subject. If wse assume this to be a valid theory, then interactional effects between Kirlian auras of several persons suggest that there are field interactions among living things when they are in close proximity with each other. This suggests a possible basis for how spiritual healing may work. Sadly, other than the limited experiments cited above, no controlled studies have been published to support this view.

Some skeptics think that Kirlian images represent only the photographic effects of electric currents or magnetic fields that flow through and/or around the object being photographed. They do not believe the pictures correlate with any unconventional fields or emanations from the subjects, or that they reflect their internal states. They suggest that variations in photographs of the same subject *simply reflect successive technical variabilities* in the system. Fluctuations in skin moisture has been particularly implicated as a variable that could produce these effects, but many other factors could also produce variability in the Kirlian photographs.

Others see skin moisture as an intermediary condition influenced by neurohormonal states (as when one "gets into a sweat" with anxiety or other emotions), which could provide a recognized indicator for limited internal mind-body conditions.

Where spiritual healers' Kirlian auras are less robust after giving treatment, and healees' auras are more robust after receiving healing, it is suggested by Kirlian researchers that an energy transfer must have occurred from healers to healees. One avenue for studying the bioenergy transfer hypothesis suggests itself for investigation. One would expect to see more robust Kirlian auras after healings in those healers who claim to channel external energies (particularly those who report they feel energized by the process) than in those healers who report that they are projecting their own bioenergies. It would also be of interest to see simultaneous Kirlian photographs on the same plates or motion pictures of healer-healee Kirlian images to detect any direct interactions that might confirm energy transfers between healers and healees. A difficulty with this suggestion is that such procedures would be likely to interfere with the healing treatment by distracting the healer from focusing on the healing.

> *A scientist wished to study the neglected natural phenomenon of the cat's purr. He implanted electrodes in the cat's brain and throat and connected them to sophisticated electronic devices. His efforts were in vain. The cat refused to purr.*
>
> – Anonymous

It is imperative that investigators fully describe parameters such as instruments, photographic film, developing techniques and other relevant factors if the confusion reigning in this area at present is to be sorted out. In addition to the known factors mentioned above, I would suggest paying attention to the many factors that could potentially influence healing research (listed in Chapter IV-3), and especially to geomagnetic activity, time of day, and lunar phases (per Chapter II-4).

Although it is clear that extraneous factors do alter Kirlian photographs, there appears to be much more to Kirlian effects than mere artifact. There is a growing body of anecdotal literature evidencing relationships between Kirlian images and states of health and disease in animals and plants.

The Kirlians, Oldfield/ Coghill and Hunt developed instruments for direct, live aura observations. These should be able to provide even more detailed information on this subject. Russians investigators report that in motion pictures of Kirlian auras there are discharges, flares, and pulsatory, dynamic phenomena.

There are also similarities between Kirlian photography and aura perceptions in the ability to identify acupuncture points.

The phantom leaf effects seem to support contentions by sensitives that an energy body surrounds the physical body of all living things. The interactions between Kirlian auras of people who are photographed simultaneously also support this claim. These observations imply that the Kirlian image represents an interaction of electric current with leaves and the people and their biological fields.

The reports of sensitives and Kirlian photographers are similar in *predicting* the development of physical illness, according to changes observed in the auras. This suggests that: 1. the Kirlian aura and the aura perceived by healers may be similar or identical in origins; and 2. the aura may be an organizing energy field, so that a disharmony in the field is secondarily reflected in the physical body.

Interactional effects between Kirlian auras of several persons also suggest that there may be energy field interactions amongst living things that are in proximity with each other. The same is true for interactional effects between the operator of the Kirlian instrument and the subjects being photographed. The energy field interaction hypothesis of how spiritual healing works may find support here.

Sensitives suggest that the energies concentrated at acupuncture points are exchanged between the body and the energy fields around it, as well as with energies flowing within the body. The reports of more intense Kirlian aura activity at acupuncture points supports these claims.

Though the validity of many of the observations from Kirlian photography is still considered by many to be questionable, they are consistent with observations from other energy medicine observations and studies reviewed in this book. The presence of an energy field surrounding living things has been reported repeatedly by sensitives who see auras, and by healers who feel them. No studies have been reported to verify that the Kirlian aura is similar to or identical with aspects of the aura that sensitives perceive. An observation of Jack Schwarz (who sees auras) that only a small portion of one of the aura bodies that lies close to the physical body is represented in Kirlian photography is the only relevant comment I have seen.

Other diagnostic methods have been developed using photography. For instance, Alain Masson has developed a "biotonic instrument" that produces aura photographs using an electric generator and chemicals (phyllosilicates) present in beeswax. The results are dependent on the operator of the instrument.

Possible applications for Kirlian photography
Kirlian photography appears to hold the promise of providing a system for screening and diagnosing energy states of health and disease.

Much as the *A.M.I. instrument* of Hiroshi Motoyama assists in evaluating activity in acupuncture meridians, and the *Mind Mirror* of Maxwell Cade helps to clarify mental states via electroencephalograms, *Kirlian devices* could provide a method for assessing the effects of healing. It could also provide a feedback device for students who are learning to heal.

Now that we have surveyed a range of evidence for a biological field that can be perceived by sensitives and healers, and fields in Kirlian photography that appear to overlap with these, let us examine reports from other studies of biological energies.

LABORATORY MEASUREMENTS
OF BIOLOGICAL ENERGY FIELDS

> *The universe in which we find ourselves and from which we can not be separated is a place of Law and Order. It is not an accident, nor chaos. It is organized and maintained by an Electro-Dynamic Field capable of determining the position and movement of all charged particles.*
>
> *For nearly half a century the logical consequences of this theory have been subjected to rigorously controlled experimental conditions and met with no contradictions.*
>
> – Harold Saxton Burr (1972)

Recognized energies
Conventional science recognizes four energies or forces:

1. *The strong nuclear force* binds neutrons and protons in the atomic nucleus. It is relatively strong but acts only over short distances.
2. *The weak nuclear force* also contributes to nuclear structure and to radioactive decay. Both (1) and (2) have little effect outside the nucleus.

3. *The electromagnetic (EM) force* pervades all of our cosmos, from atomic structures, to chemical molecular interactions and electrical power. It is also active in stars, including our own sun.

4. *Gravity* is weaker than the others over short distances and is active in proportion to the mass of an object. On the planetary, solar, and cosmic scales it is the dominant force. Although its effects are measurable, its nature is least understood amongst the four forces. We can measure its effects with great precision, but as yet we have no clear theories to explain *how* it works.

In our everyday world it is the electromagnetic (EM) force that we have harnessed to fill our energy needs, and with which we are most familiar.

Studies of healers and psychics are inconclusive, reporting correlations of healing effects with EM fields in some cases but not in others (Balanovski/ Taylor; Taylor/ Balanovski). Theoretically, the fields might explain some aspects of local psi effects, but they cannot explain psi effects that do not appear to diminish over enormous distances, and that transcend time. We will consider these studies in detail below.

It may be that some form(s) of energy exist that we have not yet identified, and which may have EM components or aspects (Rein 1992). Albert Einstein speculated:

> It is possible that there exist human emanations which are still unknown to us. Do you remember how electrical currents and "unseen waves" were laughed at? The knowledge about man is still in its infancy.

Mind may interact with energy and matter in ways we have yet to understand. The following sections explore such possibilities.

Electromagnetic fields and the body
Let us start by reviewing research on the energies that are recognized by conventional science, looking first at studies of EM fields that are present in and around the body.

Electrochemical reactions in nerve cells create electrical impulses that are used for communication amongst nerve cells, and between nerve cells and the various organs and tissues of the body.   The electroencephalogram (EEG) is used to identify the summed fluctuations in EM activities of countless brain cells. EEG brainwaves are recorded with electrodes placed on the scalp.

When muscles contract they create EM impulses that can be measured on the surface of the body by an electromyogram (EMG).

The electrocardiogram (ECG or EKG) is used to record the contractions of the heart muscle, which produces the most powerful EM activity found in the body.

These EM activities have been thoroughly studied over the course of many decades. There are other EM fields within and around the body whose presence and functions have not been studied as thoroughly and are therefore not as well understood. They have also been ignored by mainstream science for reasons that are not entirely clear or obvious.

Findings with much broader implications have resulted from careful measurements of biological EM fields. Harold Saxton Burr taught at the Yale University Department of Medicine for over four decades. He developed reliable methods for measuring differences in electrical potentials between points on the bodies of animals and plants. Using this method he established that every living system has a complex direct current (DC) EM field that can be measured with electrodes on its surface. Organisms studied included slime molds, plant seeds, trees, amphibian eggs, amphibians, rodents, humans, and many other organisms. These EM fields vary over time, and are highly correlated in regular patterns with growth, development, physiological processes (e.g. ovulation), disease (e.g. malignancies), wound healing and emotional conditions. Patterns of variation were noted with external factors, such as correlations with atmospheric and earth potentials as well as with lunar cycles and sunspots.

Labeling this phenomenon the "L-field" (*Life-field*), Burr speculated that it provides a template for the maintenance of relative structural and biochemical constancy. Molecules and cells are replaced through the normal turnover of chemical materials throughout the life of the organism. It appears that the organism requires a mechanism to assure that appropriate replacements will be made in an orderly fashion, to provide for continuity of physical integrity and to maintain the health of the organism. Burr's L-fields may provide the necessary templates for this process. Similarly, he speculated that the L-fields may also function as organizers for growth and development of the organism. For instance, Burr found that frog eggs demonstrate an electrical polarity that predicts which side of the egg will develop into a head and which will become a tail.

Leonard Ravitz, an American physician, took Burr's research a step further. He reviewed numerous measurements of electrodynamic states in humans in a wide variety of conditions, and found that field perturbations accompanied many physical symptoms. They also correlated with schizophrenia and depression.

He confirmed that periodic field shifts correlated with lunar and solar flare cycles, and extended the connection several steps further. He noted periodic shifts in human potentials and those of plants and other animals which all occurred in the same time intervals. Furthermore, behavioral and physiological changes in people over time could be predicted on the basis of anticipated periodicities in environmental field shifts. Human behavior correlated most closely with quantitative shifts in field intensity, while somatic changes correlated more with polarity vector readings.

> *I sing the body electric.*
> – Walt Whitman

Ravitz argues that the polarities measured relate to global organismic fields of living organisms, and are not directly dependent on nerve transmissions or other somatic elements such as ionic shifts in the body as a whole. [289]

In other studies, Robert Becker and Andrew A. Marino extensively investigated the effects of EM fields on the mammalian body. They believe that the fields observed by Burr and his followers cannot be adequately explained as the products of underlying physiological mechanisms such as cellular metabolism. [290] Becker and Marino see no adequate explanation that would account for how metabolic activity could be converted into the observed electrical potentials.

Becker and colleagues review a large number of experiments (some their own and some by other colleagues), and build a convincing argument for their hypothesis of an organizing function for DC fields within the body. In one experiment, they built a model of a salamander, including a wire analog of the salamander's central nervous system. They then were able to measure a similar electrical pattern surrounding the model as was found around a live salamander, suggesting that the salamander's nervous system could produce the DC field that is measured around the live salamander. This and other evidence suggested that the DC fields (which are probably associated with the nervous system more than with the body in general) are products of overall physiological processes in the nervous system.

Becker and colleagues postulate several functions that may be served by the DC current system in the body. First, they think that it may help to integrate the entire activity of the brain, whose functions are too complex, in their opinions, to be accounted for by the digital neuronal model alone.

Second, DC fields may integrate processes of organ growth. This hypothesis is supported by research on the *planarian* flatworm, a rather winsome creature measuring less than a centimeter in length, with large spots on its head resembling eyes. (When viewed under the microscope, it appears to be looking back at the person viewing it!) When cut transversely into pieces, it regenerates an entire worm from any piece, preserving the same electrical polarity of head and tail in the regenerated worms as was present in the original.

The electrical orientation of the worm is also maintained by the pieces. That is to say, the head of the worm is positively charged and so are the ends of the pieces that were oriented towards the original head. But if an externally generated current is applied to the pieces in reverse to the original polarity, a tail will usually develop where the head should be and vice versa. This is the clearest demonstration I have seen of an organizing property for DC fields.

Becker and Marino found further evidence for the organizing properties of DC currents that are applied from outside the body. In their own experiments, small DC currents markedly enhanced healing of human fractures that had previously refused to knit (as sometimes occurs for unknown reasons). With externally applied fields they also produced complete regeneration of limbs of frogs (including the joints) and partial regeneration of limbs of rats. This had been considered impossible prior to their work

An empirical observation reinforces the evidence presented above. If the fingertip is sheared off in an accident at a point distal to the first joint, and the end of the finger is left unsutured to heal on its own, often an entire fingertip will regenerate, complete with a fingernail and a fingerprint identical with the original. This occurs more often in children under the age of ten. It is hypothesized by Becker that an organizing field must exist to account for this.

A completely different line of research is suggested by the observation that biophotons are emitted by living organisms. These minute quanta of energy may be triggers for some aspects of bioregulation. (See further discussion on light emitted from the body below.)

With the helpful clinical EM treatments that are now being developed, further studies are proceeding on biological EM fields within and around the body. These are discussed in chapter II-2. To recapitulate briefly, pulsed EM fields (PEMFs) can help with healing in cases of chronic failure of mending in fractures, in osteoarthritis, pain, depression, and many other syndromes.

The precise mechanisms by which EM fields influence living organisms has yet to be established, and several hypotheses are being pursued.[291] A likely locus for EM effects is the cell membranes. Minute EM forces might alter the transporting mechanisms that shuttle material across these membranes by modifying chemical receptors.

Naturally occurring EM fields, such as those in nerve cells, might also be modulated by external EM fields with information that promotes healing. Similarly, specific EM frequencies may trigger particular cellular biological processes that facilitate physical healing. EM fields might also facilitate bio-energy flows to promote healing.

Energy fields near the body
The late Canon Andrew Glazewski, a British theologian, scientist and healer, proposed a theory based on more than forty years of investigations in healing. He observed that each person emits a unique pattern of infrared (IR) radiation, due to wave interferences that are peculiar to the individual. He also noted that EM and sound patterns must surround the body, as they are products of physiological functions. Such radiations, he postulated, must carry information relating to the body of origin, and they may thus form a basis for a spiritual healer to analyze and diagnose. The crests and waves of the interference patterns could account for the various sensations (such as heat, tingling and vibrations) described by healers when they are giving touch and near-the-body healing. He theorized that some day it may be possible to analyze this biofield with suitable instrumentation, but that scientific equipment of this kind will never surpass the human hand in sensitivity or the mind in its ability to interpret such sensation. He also makes an unsupported observation that the field around the body rotates once in twenty-four hours.[292]

J. Bigu points out that a very complex set of known energies and fields may emanate from the body to produce the visual aura reported by sensitives. These energies may include: electrical, magnetic, radio frequency and microwave, infrared, ultra-violet, X-ray, gamma ray, beta ray, neutrino, chemical, mechano-acoustical scattering, diffraction and refraction auras. The perceived aura may represent a sensory or psi perception of these fields individually or in combination(s), perhaps in the form of interference patterns. These are variations in energy waves produced by adding and subtracting the energy strengths of wave pulses as they combine with each other.

Jan Szymanski, of Warsaw, Poland identified a stationary electromagnetic field (EF) as well as a quasi-stationary or slow-changing field around the body. This can be detected from a distance of several centimeters from the body and it appears to correlate with aspects of normal and pathologic physiology. His instrument is a "high sensitivity static-electricity meter" with a probe that is held five centimeters above the surface of the skin. Measurements "at 40 skin measuring points" were performed on 9 *bioenergotherapists* (Eastern European term for healers) and 20 "common persons" inside a Faraday cage, which excludes extraneous EF. Szymanski found that:

> 1. [P]ersons with various ailments show relatively high potential difference, from -3V [volts] to +3V at various points of their body but positive potentials generally prevail;
> 2. Healthy persons with a good general feeling show more often negative potentials and there are not high potential differences between various points of their bodies (-1V to +1V only)...
> 3. All the bioenergotherapists, 7 men and 2 women, showed with almost no exception negative potentials only (-1.1 V to -0.2V); the only positive potentials, if any, could be observed exclusively around their heads and were very low (less than +O.5V)... ; and
> 4. [A]ttention has been given to the quasistationery EF of the therapists' hands. It was found that only negative potential could be detected...   mean value -0.5V to -0.6V[C]ommon persons have shown...   the mean value...   0.0V to -0.1V.

Szymanski found that EF potentials of the hands may change slowly or rapidly. In common people, 10% fluctuations may be noted over a period of two hours. In two bioenergotherapists, after performing single brief treatments of patients, EF potentials of their palms dropped 200 - 300%, to about -1.5V. During treatments, the bioenergotherapists' hands also radiated EFs of high intensity to a distance of about 3 centimeters.

He speculates that healers may be able to diagnose problems by detecting alterations in the fields around patients' bodies, and to treat them by influencing the patients' EFs with their own.

John Zimmerman, at the University of Colorado School of Medicine, reports that he can identify a magnetic field around the entire body by using a modified EEG. Zimmerman (1990) documented that EM pulsations emanate from TT healers' hands at frequencies shifting from 0.3 to 30 Cps.. The most common frequency is in the range of 7 to 8 cycles per second, which is also one of the more common brain rhythm frequencies.

These findings were confirmed in Japan through studies of various healers and martial arts experts. Seto and colleagues found that extremely strong biomagnetic fields could be measured near the hands of experts in a wide range of healing and martial arts, such as meditation, Qigong and yoga. Fields measured up to 0.0010 gauss, or approximately 1,000 times more intense than the cardiac field, which is the strongest field in the body, and 1,000,000 times stronger than the brain's electromagnetic fields.

Chinese researchers report that infrasound (sound waves that are below audible levels) is regularly emitted from the hands of qigong healers. Mechanical emitters of infrasonic sound can reproduce many of the beneficial effects of qigong healing.[293]

Significant decreases in gamma radiation counts have been measured around the bodies of people receiving Polarity Therapy.

SQUID (superconducting quantum interference device) technology can detect EM fields around the body. The SQUID is particularly sensitive to the EM currents that are created by ions (charged molecular particles) in the blood as they stream through blood vessels. Alterations in these currents can be mapped from the changes in blood flow through the brain during particular mental activities. This process has led to entirely new ways of studying activity in the brain. Newer technology will make it possible to identify whether certain parts of the brain are activated during healing. J. Zimmerman (1990) reported that biomagnetic pulses from the hands of a Therapeutic Touch healer could be measured with a SQUID magnetometer. Pulses between 0.3 cps. (cycles per second) and 30 cps. were found, with the greatest activity between 7 - 8 cps. Non-healers were found to produce no such pulses.

A. Seto et al. confirm that the hands of qigong healers (as well as those of people who practice yoga, meditation, and martial arts) emanate EM pulsations between 8 - 10 cps, with an intensity about 1,000 times greater than that of ordinary human biofields. This is within the range of alpha brainwaves, and within the frequency that is found to be most beneficial in enhancing physical healing of wounds: 2 - 50 cps.

While there is as yet no study demonstrating direct effects of EM pulsations from healers' hands upon healees' EM pulsations, J. Oschman (1997) suggests that the entrainment of bioelectrical EM pulsations is theoretically quite feasible. Physicists have noted that EM pulsations of similar frequencies in different EM devices have a tendency to become coupled to each other. This could occur in living organisms as well. Early research with EEGs (summarized below) appears to confirm this speculation.

W. R. Adey and S. M Bawin present some interesting investigations of EM effects on living systems. It is speculated that biological organisms may be exquisitely sensitive to EM fields, and that they may be able to distinguish meaningful signals from the cacophony of EM "noise" that is constantly present in the environment. There is further speculation that arrays of cells, or even arrays of molecules which are polarized within cells, could act as EM sensors for detecting meaningful signals. These would be similar to the arrays of antennas that are used in radio telescopes to detect faint signals from heavenly bodies that may be billions of light years away. By summing up differences between several sensors, more information is derived from the signals. The simplest example of this is in depth perception which is achieved by having two eyes view the same object from slightly different angles.

> Bodywork and other repetitive practices such as yoga, Qigong, tai chi, meditation, therapeutic touch, etc. may gradually lead to more structural coherence (crystallinity) in the tissues, facilitating both the detection and radiation of energy fields (Oschman & Oschman 1997). Arrays of water molecules associated with the macromolecules are probably involved as well.
>
> The process has been described as the formation of "coherence domains" in liquid crystal arrays (Sermonti 1995). The mechanism involves that stabilization of the positional and orientational order of

millions of rod-shaped molecules, as in cell membranes, connective tissues, DNA, muscle, the cytoskeleton, the myelin sheath of nerves, and sensory cells (Oschman 1997). Stabilization spreads from molecule to molecule, throughout the system. Del Guidice (1993) describes the process as one in which individual molecules "lose their individual identity, cannot be separated, move together as if performing a choral ballet, and are kept in phase by an electromagnetic field which arises from the same ballet."

— James Oschman (2000, p. 221-222)

Elmer Green and colleagues (1991) at the Meninger Institute followed up on an unusual observation from meditation literature, recorded in 1882 (Barker). It was recommended that Tibetan student monks sit on a marble bench isolated from the ground by glass, and stare at their image mirrored in a copper wall, with the north pole of a bar magnet suspended by a string over their heads. Green et al. constructed a room with copper walls and replicated this arrangement, attaching sensitive instruments to the walls to measure any EM effecs.

Studying 10 meditators in 45-minute sessions they found no body-potential surges reaching as high as 4V [volts]. In contrast, healers who meditated in the copper-walled room produced surges of 4 to 221V lasting from one half to twelve seconds. During non-contact healing sessions the same healers demonstrated body-potential surges between 4 and 190V. Most of the surges had a negative polarity.

These surge values are 1,000 times greater than EM changes observed with emotional responses, 100,000 times greater than EKG voltages, and 1,000,000 times greater than EEG voltages.

Others are also studying EM biofields.

The Institute of Heartmath in California has developed a meditation and biofeedback system for teaching people to develop coherent patterns of heartbeats. During healings, healers' and healees' heart rhythms become entrained.

Linda Russek and Gary Schwartz found that EEGs in frontal regions of subjects' brains became entrained to the ECG rhythm of the experimenter. Experimenter and subject sat facing each other, with their eyes closed, without touching. The effect was more pronounced in those subjects who felt that they had been raised by loving parents than in subjects who felt that their parents had not been loving.

In these studies we see early evidence of EM interactive effects between healers and healees. These suggest there may be an EM aspect in bioenergy fields and that fields of healers and healees may interact during healing. It is unclear whether a single EM healing energy is being measured along segments of its full spectrum, or whether there are several different healing energy fields.

EFFECTS OF ENVIRONMENTAL EM FIELDS

Geomagnetic effects on biological systems are well recognized but as yet they are little understood. The molten core of the earth contains a high percentage of iron.

This produces EM fields around the earth, including the magnetic polarity that is reflected in compass needles. The sun also radiates EM fields that fluctuate with solar activity. When solar flares erupt, these fields can be so strong that radio and TV communications are disrupted.

Living organisms are influenced by EM fields in ways that have yet to be clarified and explained. For instance, there are certain naturally occurring EM frequencies around the earth, and it is speculated that they are relevant to biological systems. One is the Schumann resonant frequency of 7-8 cycles per second, a regular EM pulsation produced by standing waves that bounce back and forth between the surface of the earth and the ionosphere. Biological systems on earth appear to have adapted to these constant EM pulsations. In one study, when people were shielded from environmental EM radiations, their biological rhythms of sleeping and waking and the regular fluctuations of various hormone levels were disrupted.

Gross magnetic fields and chronic environmental EM pollution may have negative effects on health.

M. F. Barnothy reviews the literature on the effects of magnetic fields on living things to 1964, and Vinokurava reviews related Russian research. In the laboratory, gross magnetic fields produce headaches, fatigue and other symptoms of malaise. These were disturbances of sufficient severity to warrant concern and recommendations for removal of the subjects from exposure to such fields. Vinokurava also reviews research on naturally occurring fields, such as that of the sun. Specific brain centers (hypothalamus) and types of brain cells (glia) were noted to respond to magnetic influence.

Deliberate exposure to EM fields at the frequency of EEG theta waves altered short-term memory.

Robert Becker and colleagues review a variety of evidence strongly suggesting that there are serious health risks associated with environmental EM pollution from power lines, transformers and other such equipment. Environmental medicine has also clarified that combinations of EM fields from household appliances and electrical wiring in the walls can be irritating or harmful. These may include phones (especially cell phones used without earphones), electric blankets, and various computer and entertainment equipment. It is a wonder that the public is not more aware of and concerned about these issues. Personnel exposed to the enormously powerful magnetic fields that surround modern devices for imaging the inside of the body also would appear to be candidates for related health problems, although early research does not as yet support this conjecture.

Several researchers found a relationship between depression and overhead power lines.

Svetlana Vinokurava found that strong fields produced negative symptoms, including headaches, fatigue, loss of appetite and insomnia. Physical changes included edema, decreased pain sensitivity, heart pains and itching. Other studies showed that magnetic fields increased the ability of white blood cells to eliminate foreign bodies; decreased non-specific immunity to bacteria and viruses and increased cell mutations.

Anecdotal reports suggest that in its simplest expression, EM radiation from fluorescent lights may cause fatigue and headaches. People with multiple allergy syndromes often complain that they do not tolerate fluorescent lighting. In more complex exposures, EM radiation appears to contribute to more serious symptoms, including arthritis, allergies, and susceptibility to infections.

Evidence is now emerging that long-term EM pollution may contribute to a variety of illnesses, such as heart disease and depression; various allergies, including to EM radiations themselves; chronic fatigue syndrome; psychological effects, and more. Much of this evidence is as yet partial and in need of further confirmation, as some studies have shown no negative effects.

Of particular concern is evidence that children and adults who are exposed to environmental EM fields may be prone to developing cancer. This is further supported by laboratory studies showing that cancer cell growth in the laboratory is enhanced with exposure to EM fields.

Cyril Smith, a Senior Lecturer in the Department of Electronic and Electrical Engineering at Salford University in England, in collaboration with Ray Choy and Jean Monro, two doctors specializing in allergic disorders, explored the reactions of people who are hypersensitive to EM radiation. One person was so sensitive that she would convulse whenever she was within 200 meters of overhead power lines.

This team reports that a simple laboratory oscillator tuned to relevant frequencies can bring out allergic symptoms, and that other frequencies neutralize them. They found that the particular frequency was far more of a factor than signal strength. Patients identified frequencies producing symptoms identical to those they developed with exposure to specific chemical allergens, such as foods, medications, gasoline fumes and perfume. Although experimental blinds are mentioned, they are not described – which leaves these reports open to questions about experimenter effects that could have contributed to the findings.

While a great deal of skepticism has been expressed about the dangers of environmental EM radiation, simple tests of EM influence on non-human subjects have also produced negative effects. These have demonstrated significant detrimental effects on purified water, alkaline phosphatase (a liver enzyme), and fruit fly larvae. Samples protected by a Faraday cage and placed inside an incubator were significantly shielded from measurable EM effects, as compared to samples placed on a shelf adjacent to the incubator.

Various devices have been developed that allegedly can protect a person from negative environmental EM effects. Shealy et al. (1998) demonstrated in a controlled study that the Clarus Q-link could indeed offer significant protection against environmental EM disturbance of the EEG.

Replications and extension of studies on EM effects are sorely needed, as there is the clear possibility that some results may represent placebo effects.

SPIRITUAL HEALING AND ELECTROMAGNETISM

Spiritual healing appears to have some similarities or actual points of overlap with EM effects.

Studies by Robert Miller showed that both healers and strong magnets could alter water in such a way that its surface tension was decreased, and this water enhanced plant growth. In separate studies, Justa Smith and Hoyt Edge demonstrated that both a healer and an extremely strong magnetic field could enhance the activity of the enzyme trypsin.[294] Much further work remains to be done in order to clarify the relationship between electromagnetism and healing.[295]

John Zimmerman studied the magnetic fields around the bodies of healees. Regardless of where on the healee's body Therapeutic Touch healing was being applied, he observed alterations in the entire body field. Some of these signals appeared to parallel brain wave frequencies. This seems similar to the work of Motoyama on acupuncture meridians and chakras.

Benford et al. found that Polarity Therapy decreased the amount of gamma radiation emitted by healees' bodies.

Unusual EM phenomena have been noted around people who have psi experiences. Boguslaw Lipinski studied the teenage children who reported that they saw the Virgin Mary appear frequently in a church in Medjugorje, in the former Yugoslavia. Healings are also said to have occurred when people prayed there before and after these apparitions. Lipinski was following up on reports by Professor Henri Joyeaux, of the Cancer Institute at the University of Montpellier in France, which claimed that the alpha waves in the EEGs of these children increased in amplitude at the beginning of an apparition. Lipinski hypothesized that an increase in concentration of ambient ions (electrically charged air molecules) might be responsible for the altered EEG patterns. Using a portable electroscope (ion detector) he did in fact record exceedingly high readings of up to 100,000 ions per cubic centimeter.

Lipinski then shielded the instrument with a metal sleeve to prevent registration of ions from the air, and the instrument still continued to show high readings. Ordinarily this could only be caused by such a high level of radioactivity that physical damage and even fatalities would be expected among the participants. Lipinski hypothesizes that an *unknown type of energy* must be responsible for the observed effects. Oddly, the highest reading occurred *prior* to the arrival of the visionaries. He cannot explain why other researchers have obtained only brief positive electrostatic recordings at the site, or none at all. He postulates that as the operator of the instrument, he may have contributed to the effect.

Lipinski also discovered an unusual effect on a tape that was used to record a conversation at the home of the children. Upon replaying the tape after returning home, he noted a low frequency sound (15 - 20 cycles per second) that had not been noticed at the time of recording. He presumes that it was caused by a magnetic pulsating field of unknown source.

Others have used Geiger counters to record reduced background readings during healing sessions.

Lu Yan Fang, Ph.D., of the National Electro Acoustics Laboratory in China, recorded infrasonic sound emitted from the hands of qigong masters during external qi healings. She was able to produce healing effects with synthetic infrasonic sound at similar frequencies, and reported benefits for pain, circulatory disturbances and depression. On the basis of these explorations, the infrasonic QGM is now being studied in America.

Fritz Grunewald, a German engineer, studied a medium named Johannsen around 1920 (Stelter). He reported the following:

> ... Johannsen could do simple feats of psychokinesis such as depressing one side of an evenly balanced scale. Grunewald found that each time, just before the scale descended, the magnetic field strength in the medium's hands – which he held out toward the object to be moved – grew markedly weaker, only to increase after the psychokinetic act. It looked as if something which had produced the strong magnetism in Johannsen's body – perhaps the turbulent cold plasma postulated by Sergeyev – displaced itself outward and released psychokinetic effects.
>
> A few times Grunewald, by means of iron filings strewn on glass plates, was able to obtain pictures of the magnetic field within Johannsen's hands. In this way, he found several magnetic centers in the hand's magnetic field which Grunewald believed were evoked by electrical eddies in the medium's hands – another startling similarity to Sergeyev's theories of turbulent cold plasma. But strangely, the magnetic centers seemed at times to lie outside the medium's hand. We must recall the hypothesis that the biofield can move outside the body.

Photons and ultrasound may be produced in dividing cells, perhaps during shifts between liquid and crystal states of the involved molecules. Such mechanisms may underlie mitogenetic radiation in plants, Gurwitch, below.

I have heard anecdotal reports of other researchers working along similar lines, but I have not seen publications of their results.

UNCONVENTIONAL FIELDS AND RADIATIONS

Scientists have identified a variety of unusual fields and radiations that can be found on and around humans and other living things. While the existence of these fields has not been accepted by conventional science, the evidence suggests that there may be fertile ground for further study in these reports.

Measurements of conventional EM fields around the body in relation to their effects on healing have not produced consistent results. Glen Rein suggests that self-healing and healer-healing may be mediated by unconventional EM fields that are postulated to exist when two opposing EM fields neutralize each other's conventionally measured EM effects. Drawing on the writings of David Bohm, he suggests that such fields may act through higher dimensional energies, or that they may be described as repositories of information rather than as fields.

The existence of such energies has been investigated by a number of scientists, in addition to Rein: "They have been called non-Hertzian energy... scalar energy, longitudinal waves, motional fields, time-reversed waves, radiant energy, gravitational waves... free energy and cosmic energy to name a few. It is presently unknown whether these energies are identical or distinct from non-Hertzian energy... " (Rein 1992). These energies cannot be measured using conventional EM devices.

The body may respond to the influences of such fields through its positive and negative ions; through the liquid crystals in cell membranes, bones and other tissues; through bioenergetic patternings in body fluids; and/or through subatomic biopotentials in the atomic nuclei.

One device that is theorized to produce non-Hertzian fields is a specially designed Möbius strip that traps EM fields. Such Möbius strip devices are commercially available in certain wristwatches, and they are alleged to generate non-Hertzian fields as well as EM fields between 7 to 8 cps. Rein showed that this kind of device could influence the growth rates of nerve cells and immune cells in tissue culture.

Because there is as yet no instrument for measuring non-Hertzian fields, it has been impossible to test directly Rein's hypothesis that these may be the mediators for the effects of healing. Rein took a step towards clarifying this issue himself when he introduced a device that was alleged to produce non-Hertzian fields. He used this device to study the hands of a healer who was producing measurable conventional magnetic field patterns:

> ... prior to addition of the device, the magnetic pattern was repetitive containing numerous sharp, small positive peaks. Upon addition of the device, the magnetic field pattern was substantially altered. The new pattern was qualitatively similar in shape but gradually increased in overall magnitude. These results suggest that non-Hertzian quantum fields enhanced the magnetic field emitted from Laskow's hand during holoenergetic healing.

These observations echo reports by healers who say that healing involves interactions between energy fields that surround the bodies of both healers and healees.

Dubrov (reviewed in Krippner 1980) speculates that all living things may emit gravitational waves, which could possibly be produced by the rhythmic movements of cellular molecules. Others have speculated that there may be a relationship between psi and gravity, as both appear to reach everywhere.

Various unusual energies are said to be produced by a range of unorthodox electronic gadgets, some of which are based on the inventions of Nikola Tesla and Antoine Priore. These instruments supposedly produce combinations of EM and gravitational waves which are claimed to travel faster than the speed of light, cause levitation of objects, and produce rapid cures of illnesses. If verified, these reports may explain some of the effects of healing. The role of the observer is said to be a crucial aspect of these phenomena, and therefore healing may reciprocally help to explain some of their unusual aspects.

In Eastern Europe and America there are Psychotronic Associations that study these devices. The USPA publishes a journal of their reports.

Physicists are now postulating (M. King) that enormous energy resources are available from empty space, which in turn would indicate a source for healing energy. Edward Russell (1971) hypothesizes that the thoughts (*T-fields*) of one person can telepathically affect the biofields (*L-fields*) of another person, and that this may explain a host of psi and healing phenomena.

Burr further speculates that *L-fields* act as guiding principles in the evolution of living things, or bridges between the spiritual and the material worlds. There may be overlaps in this regard with Sheldrake's theory of *morphogenetic fields*.

Otto Rahn reviews numerous experiments on what he has labeled *mitogenetic radiation*. This effect was first discovered by A. G. Gurwitsch of the USSR in 1923. Its name originates from the biological system in which it was noted – the growing tip of an onion root. When one onion root was pointed toward the tip of another (See Figure II-18), the second root demonstrated increased cell division (mitoses) in the segment towards which the first root was pointed.

Figure II-18. Onion roots used to test mitogenetic radiation

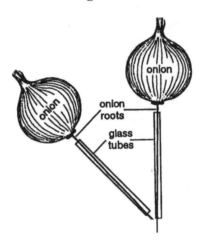

Gurwitsch and associates found numerous organisms and tissues that emitted this kind of radiation, including bacteria; yeast; eggs of annelid worms; chickens (during the first two days of incubation); blood; intact contracting muscle; neoplasms; and more. Non-radiating organisms and tissues included adult animal tissues (except brain); blood, muscle; blood of cancer patients and of starving rats, and more. The common denominators for active emitters seem to be that they are either undergoing glycolysis (sugar metabolism) or proteolytic processes (breaking down of proteins).

Intermittent, pulsed mitogenetic radiation was found to be more powerful than steady radiation. The effects of mitogenetic radiation are generally positive and growth – enhancing, especially in bacteria and yeasts, and cultures of these organisms eventually came to be used as indicators instead of onion roots. Gurwitsch also cites a study in which wounds in tadpoles healed more rapidly when this form of radiation was applied. From these and other experiments he concluded that the mitogenetic rays are actually UV light.

Rahn also observed evidence for radiations that had negative effects. For instance, he found that radiations from menstrual blood could alter the cell forms of microorganisms in the laboratory or even kill them. This effect was stronger in summer than in winter. He also reviews several reports about particular women whose presence affected bacterial cultures negatively during their menses. He noted that in other instances laboratory workers of both sexes had negative effects on a particular strain of yeast. Rahn determined that this effect was related to emanations from their fingers, which could kill a particular yeast strain at a distance of a few millimeters within a period of five minutes. With other yeasts the effect was less severe.

A variety of researchers have reported similar positive results with rnitogenetic radiation, but several attempts at replications were negative. These studies therefore were abandoned. It is not clear whether the entire series took into account all of the factors mentioned by Gurwitsch and others. For instance, it may be that certain experimenters are able to obtain positive results while others are not, as in the *sheep/goat* effect[296] and some aspects of radionics. It may also be that seasonal effects and geobiological or other influences contribute to these variations.

With the observation that pulsed UV light may transmit bioenergetic information, it is fascinating to survey other pilot studies considering similar phenomena.

In Eastern European countries there has been a strong interest in the fields surrounding the body. V. M. Inyushin is a respected Russian scientist who researched biological fields that he and others believe consist of "bioplasm." He quotes Victor Adamenko (1972) in explanation of this theory:

> ... until recent times, three states of matter were known, solid, liquid, and gaseous, differing principally in the degree of packing of the molecules. Then the "fourth state of matter" was discovered, called plasma, in which the particles are ionised and charged, with free electrons mixed with them; we may have hot plasma such as occurs in stars, and cold plasma, which according to the doctrines of bioplasm, can be found in living organisms. Because the particles are charged, they can affect the electrical fields used in Kirlian photography, and so become visible on the photographic film.

Inyushin reports that bioplasma emits ultraviolet (UV) light, which he has been able to detect using photo-cells, and to record on special photographic film using cryogenic (ultra-cold) techniques to eliminate hot objects as extraneous sources of UV light.

He also found that sensitive photomultipliers were able to pick up UV emanations near the eyes of animals and humans. Variations were noted in the intensity of these emanations, related to emotions and diurnal cycles. Yet these radiations seem to consist of more than just UV light. Inyushin reports that he was able to obtain exposures on "special emulsions particularly sensitive to 'hard' components of radiation" even when metallic screens were interposed between the emulsions and the subjects' eyes so that no UV radiation could reach the film. This was successful even with exposures as brief as one-thousandth of a second.

Inyushin also reports on experiments in which healthy chicken tissues were placed in two containers next to each other, with quartz windows in the adjacent faces of the containers. When tissues in one of the containers were infected with a toxic virus, with every precaution taken not to contaminate the second one, the tissues in the second container nevertheless demonstrated identical changes, and died just as those in the first container did. Regular glass blocked this effect. This suggests that UV light may be involved in "transmitting" disease, because UV light penetrates quartz but not regular glass.

This type of experiment has been repeated a number of times using frog hearts separated by quartz glass, with similar transmission of the effects when one of the hearts was physically damaged. The second heart developed identical damage, even though it was protected from physical damage. Of tangential interest is the fact that this experiment worked with spring and summer frogs but not with winter frogs. At times pulsations of UV light were observed coming from the infected or poisoned heart tissues, suggesting an association of these emanations with certain stages of biological processes, infection or toxicity.

Larissa Vilenskaya refers to further observations by Inyushin. He found that two onion roots will produce an ultraviolet interference pattern when pointed in the same direction. This indicates that each root is emitting UV light. Such observations led him to experiment with weak, pulsed (rapidly flashing) laser light. He found that this could stimulate seeds to germinate faster.

Viktor Adamenko confirms yet another aspect of the pulsed emissions of UV light in mitogenetic radiation. He reviews evidence that pulsating light appears to have salutary effects in arthritis and asthma; that pulsed stimulation of acupuncture points is more effective than steady stimulation; and that pulsed illumination of plant seeds enhances the growth of plants grown from these seeds.

Chinese researchers also report that brief pulses of light were found to emanate from a psi subject during clairvoyant perception experiments.

Russian researchers report on UV emanations from healers' bodies, especially their hands and eyes. This suggests that UV light might be the source of healing energy that we are seeking. However, *UV light does not penetrate beyond the most superficial layers of the body's surface.* A. P. Dubrov (1982) hypothesizes that UV light may cause alterations in biological systems via interactions with the biological field of the organism.

Inyushin postulates that there are emissions from the tissues that act as carriers of information, possibly analogous to telepathy at a molecular level (Krippner 1975):

> A structure in the bioplasmic field is produced which acquires temporary stability, conveying mitogenic information from the living organism. This structure endures for up to five minutes, long enough to make an impression on the film emulsion. Telepathy, or biological communication, can be looked upon as a product of resonances in the bioplasmic bodies of two organisms.

He further states (Inyushin 1972):

> We envisage microbioplasmons or excitons carrying a 3-D hologram, conveying with it information relevant to the bioplasmic field of the entire organism.

The Russians have emphasized the information-carrying properties of these apparent energies. Kaznacheyev details studies of luminescence of blood. He postulates that "... blood in the human organism might be not only a carrier of nutrient substances, but also a carrier of information that might be 'written' on it in the form of a hologram that is given to tissues and organs through ultra-weak radiation in the ultraviolet or/and other ranges of the electromagnetic spectrum" (Vilenskaya 1985). UV radiation could imprint patterns in blood elements at the surface of the skin, and this would explain how UV light emanating from a healer could be a vehicle for healing in humans. It would be difficult to see how this could apply to animals, however, as their fur would block UV patterning of blood in skin capillaries.[297]

Gennady Sergeyev reports on measurements of biological radiations in a healee prior to, during, and following a healing given by Nina Kulagina. He noted changes in the frequency of emissions from the healee.

The Russian researchers do not propose how the UV emanations might originate, although they seem to imply that they are the result of ordinary metabolic processes.

Yvonne Duplessis studied the phenomenon of dermal optics, which is another aspect of information sensing. She found that people could learn to identify colors through sensations that they experienced when holding their hands on – or even several inches above – colored papers. Most remarkable of all, she found that *they could still do this when the colored papers were covered with metal plates.* Various colors were regularly detected at different specific heights above the papers, even with the metal plates intervening. The height at which individual colors were perceived differed systematically according to whether daylight or artificial light illuminated the laboratory. Duplessis' work suggests that there are energies involved in color perception that we cannot as yet identify, and that the skin may pick up information from the environment in ways that we do not understand.

Dietrich Luedtke mentions that laser light can pick up and transmit information from a liquid through which it passes. The informational component of the laser beam is not blocked by solid substances, even though the light component is blocked.

In the mid-nineteenth century, German industrialist Karl Von Reichenbach investigated energies associated with magnets. He found that sensitive people could feel sensations of cold or "pulling" when a magnet was passed near their body. Some also saw luminous emanations in the dark from the poles of strong magnets and from crystals. (Some healers today report similar perceptions with magnets.) Reichenbach called this magnetic force *od* or *odyle*. Searching for other sources of odic energy, he found that much of the material world could, under suitable circumstances, produce it.

W. Edward Mann summarizes Reichenbach's findings on the properties and potentials of *odyle*:

1. Odyle is a universal property of all matter in variable and unequal distribution in space and time.
2. It interpenetrates and fills the structure of the universe. It cannot be eliminated or isolated from anything in nature.

3. It quickly penetrates and courses through everything.

4. It flows in concentrated form with heat, friction, sound, electricity, light, the moon, solar and stellar rays, chemical action, and organic vital activity of plants and animals, especially man.

5. It possesses polarity. There is both negative odyle, which gives a sensation of coolness and is pleasant; and positive odyle, which gives a sensation of warmth and discomfort.

6. It can be conducted, with metals, glass, resin, silk and water being perfect conductors.

7. It is radiated to a distance and these rays penetrate through clothes, bed-clothes, boards and walls.

8. Substances can be charged with odyle, or odyle may be transferred from one body to another. This is affected by contact and requires a certain amount of time.

9. It is luminous, either as a luminous glow or as a flame, showing blue at the negative and yellow-red at the positive[and] can be made to flow in any direction.

10. The aura around the body is produced by odyle, because living things contain odyle which produces a luminosity. Over 24 hours there is a periodic increase and decrease of odylic power in living things.

These observations were confirmed and extended by other researchers. The most famous of these was Wilhelm Reich, a physician and psychoanalyst who trained with Sigmund Freud. Reich was impressed that in sex as in many other functions of living organisms there is a basic, four-beat rhythm consisting of mechanical tension; bioelectric charge; bioelectric discharge; and relaxation. This is most dramatically seen in orgasm but it is also evident in rhythmic pulsations of the heart, lungs, intestines, and other body systems. Reich postulated that there is a basic energy that he called *orgone* behind this pulsation.

Reich reported finding *bions* (basic units of orgone) in many different preparations. Bions were microscopic vesicles (sacks) that appeared to be organized at times into cells like protozoa, yet were distinctly different in their behaviors and properties. Reich found that cancer cells were immobilized when placed near bions. Investigators reported that their eyes were irritated with prolonged observation of bions, which suggested that bions radiated an irritant energy which Reich labeled *orgone radiation.* Certain bions could also produce discoloration, pain and inflammation of the skin when held on a glass slide in a person's palm. They also fogged photographic film. They induced the ability to see auras in people who previously had not possessed this ability. Organic insulating substances such as paper, cotton and cellulose absorbed orgone energy and could then discharge an electroscope. Such experiments led Reich to believe that the electroscope measures orgone and that static electricity is not electricity at all, but orgone.

Reich constructed a box with metal walls on the inside and organic material (such as wood) on the outside. He anticipated that orgone radiating from bion cultures within such a box would be kept within the box by the metal inner layer, while the outer layer would prevent external orgone radiation from entering. When bion cultures were placed in the box, bluish moving vapors and yellow points and lines were produced. These visual phenomena persisted in the box even after it was ventilated, dismantled and thoroughly washed. This result led to the use of such boxes as orgone accumulators. Alternate layering of metal and organic materials in the walls of the boxes was found to increase their effectiveness as accumulators of orgone energy.

Further experimentation with orgone boxes showed that a thermometer placed above an accumulator would register 0.2 to 1.8 degrees Centigrade higher than room temperature, which suggested that orgone might be a physical energy.

Orgone also was found to have biological effects. Protozoa grew more slowly inside an accumulator, but faster when placed above one. Mice with malignant tumors who spent half an hour daily in an accumulator survived markedly longer than untreated mice. Reich also used various orgone-storing and transmitting devices to treat a variety of human illnesses.

Reich believed that orgone energy flows relatively slowly through the body, and that in some people there are blocks to the flow due to chronic tensions. When unacceptable emotion is elicited by life's circumstances, the neurotic person will unconsciously block the full, conscious, unpleasantness of the feeling, diverting it into tensions in particular parts of the body. These are comparable to body armoring, designed by the unconscious to protect the conscious mind (the *ego*) from external and internal dangers.[298]

Reich's ultimate goal was to help patients achieve an unblocked flow of energy from head to pelvis. Followers of Reich continue to focus on relaxing the physical armoring at particularly tense points. They find that this can change the patient's emotional defensive patterns. One study supports this theory. A sensitive who sees auras observed patients treated by Rolfing, which is a variant of Reich's methods. She reported clear changes in the patients, closely correlated with changes noted simultaneously in EM monitoring devices.

Reich's experiments – with apparatus that seems to demonstrate the existence of a biological energy – have been repeated by numbers of other experimenters. They have independently reported similar findings of apparent energies that can be blocked in the body, radiated by living organisms, transmitted by wood and silk, etc.

Two controlled studies on orgone treatments were published in German. Clinical controlled studies have yet to be published in the US due to the harassment of the FDA, so at present experimenter effects cannot be ruled out in most of the available research. Nevertheless, anecdotal reports continue to suggest that there may be considerable value in orgone therapy. For instance, Myron Brenner, a psychiatrist in Baltimore, reports that orgone treatments were helpful in treating chronic infections that had not responded to conventional treatments. Other therapists continue to use and study the approaches of Reich.

Mann briefly reviews the sad and unfortunate response of the American medicolegal establishment to Reich's work. He was hounded to jail in the early 1950's for espousing views and recommending treatments that ran counter to accepted beliefs and practices, and his books were publicly burned. He died after two years in jail. The existence of this sort of threat partially explains why these and other such unconventional energy-related phenomena have not been better studied.[299]

Further types of energies, which have been observed using unconventional methods, are suggested by other experiments.

In England, L. E. Eeman explored bioenergy transmissions within single individuals and between various people, using copper wires as conductors. With single individuals, copper gauze mats were placed under a subject's head and buttocks (at the base of the spine). A wire from each mat was held in either of the subject's hands. With the head (H) mat wire held in the left hand (L) and the spine mat wire (S) in the right hand (R) subjects reported feeling relaxed within a few minutes. Eeman called this configuration a relaxation circuit. (See Figure II-19.) If the wires were held in the opposite hands (H-R and S-L) the person soon felt tense, restless and uncomfortable. Eeman called this a tension circuit.

Figure II-19. One subject in a relaxation circuit, showing copper gauze mats and wire connections.

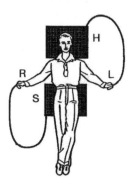

Eeman assumed that these effects are due to polarities of unknown energies in the respective parts of the body. He arbitrarily designated them as positive and negative, presuming that opposite *charges* attract and like charges repel. (See Figure II-20) He later discovered that left-handed subjects have a reversed polarity relative to right-handed people.

Figure II-20. Classical diagram of human polarities

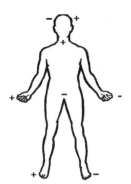

Eeman found that when people used the relaxation circuit (or any other methods for muscle relaxation), their muscle tensions were markedly reduced. However, they remained ready to contract their muscles with the least thought of doing so. He demonstrated this to them by having them close their eyes, saying he would lift their legs for them. He started by lifting both legs, pulling up on their trouser cuffs. He then gently released one cuff but continued to pull on the other. Both legs continued to rise in 90 percent of people he tested! In another variation of this exercise, he held the cuffs with both legs up in the air for a few moments and gently released them. People continued to hold their legs up in the air, assuming he was supporting them. They were astonished to find they had been holding their own legs up – totally unaware of the tensions they were maintaining in their muscles. They had been absolutely certain they were completely relaxed and having their legs raised passively. People must therefore hold the conscious intent to relax and release all tensions from their muscles in order to achieve full relaxation.

In another experiment, Eeman connected several subjects in one circuit. He found that if positives were connected to negatives, an even more marked sense of relaxation was produced, and conversely for like-charged connections. Subjects regularly fell asleep for a few minutes in relaxation circuits, and awoke invigorated, with a feeling of having rested well. Numerous subjects can be connected in series using similar mats and wires. (Fig. II-21.)

Figure II-21. Two subjects in series

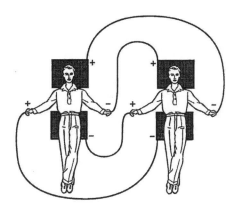

Eeman identified several different types of individual according to their characteristic functions as "valves" in his energy circuits: emitters, conductors, resisters and relayers. Further, he found that many illnesses were relieved by spending some time in a relaxation circuit. Conversely, normal subjects could sense the symptoms of ill people within the same circuit. A drunk in the circuit produced a mild sense of intoxication in sober participants. Only a few attempts at controls for suggestion were reported in Eeman's experiments, and the controls did not diminish the reported effects.

Eeman hypothesizes that people radiate a carrier wave that transmits information from one person to another. Conversely, the bodies of others can resonate with the originator of a state or sensation, and through this resonation they will acquire information about its source.

Eeman also discovered that if he placed a medicine such as aspirin in a liquid solution and connected it into relaxation circuits, subjects responded within two minutes as though they had taken the medicines. Fevers could be lowered this way using aspirin.

Studies were done of various medications under blinded conditions, where subjects had no knowledge of the substances that were in the circuits. Consistent effects of the medications were observed in the subjects.

Aubrey Westlake suggested that the energies Eeman was investigating might be transmitted by materials other than copper wires. Eeman checked this hypothesis and found that silk was also effective as a conductor.

Leslie Patten and Terry Patten review many further experiments by Eeman and others. In one of these, an acute illness appeared to be ameliorated through the influence of another person in a circuit who had recuperated from that illness. This suggests that antibodies may have an energy field component. Placing left-handed people in circuits with right-handed people introduced tension, which was dissipated if lefties' heads and feet were placed next to the feet and heads, respectively, of the righties' heads and feet. The Pattens' review contains many other interesting observations on these apparent energetic phenomena.

Julian Isaacs and Terry Patten report on a double-blind controlled study of bio-circuits' effects on EEGs, EMGs and GSRs. The EEGs and EMGs demonstrated significant relaxation responses. Subjective reports differentiated between real and placebo circuit effects on relaxation and other sensations.

Some of Eeman's approaches and findings appear to be echoed in the healing methods of *Polarity Therapy,* where healers intuitively sense body polarities and rebalance those that are disharmonious.

Recent research by William Tiller (2003a; b), Professor Emeritus in Physics at Stanford University shows that intent to alter water can be imprinted on an electrical device. The devices were imprinted in one laboratory, then mailed to another laboratory hundreds of miles away, with identical control devices. Each was marked with a code so that the second lab researchers were blind to which was the imprinted device. Intents imprinted in these devices to either increase or decrease the acidity of water were able to significantly alter the water acidity in the predicted directions. This suggests that intent may include a force or energy that can influence matter. As Tiller notes, this is very similar in action to a healing intent that brings about physical changes in biological systems. Even more fascinating is the imprinting of intent to alter water in a laboratory in England - prior to the arrival of the IIED in the mail (Tiller 2003c).

LESSONS FROM BIOLOGICAL ENERGY FIELD STUDIES

There is convincing evidence from the numerous research and anecdotal reports reviewed in this volume and in Volume I of *Healing Research* that biological energy fields are found around all living things.[300] There would appear to be many levels of fields, including those that are found in cells, organs, and the entire living organism.

The reports reviewed suggest that these fields interact with environmental energies and with inputs from several types of more local external fields, which I will describe briefly here.

Electromagnetic fields: Minute inputs of external EM energy facilitate physical self-healing of some physical disorders, such as fractures. Chronic exposures to mild fields and shorter exposures to stronger fields appear to be deleterious.

The work of Burr, Ravitz and others correlating L-fields with physiological and geobiological processes suggests that all living things resonate with each other and with geological and cosmic fields. Their hypotheses on the *organizing* nature of DC fields, though logical, are still speculative. These fields may be produced as a result of biological processes involved in metabolic and/or neuronal activity, as postulated by Glazewski.

The studies cited by Burr in which predictions are made of behavioral and physiological changes in living organisms, which can be anticipated through periodicities in external field shifts, support the hypothesis that external fields may influence biological systems. This is especially true where such periodicities are noted across numerous species. Alternative hypotheses are also possible. Seasonal changes in the length of day, atmospheric ionic concentrations, or other, unknown factors may account for some of these cross-species periodicities. That is, factors such as changes in the length of the day may trigger physiological adjustments that secondarily influence the fields produced by the organism.

The evidence from experiments with flatworms seems to prove conclusively that fields can organize body processes. Becker's work with salamander limb regeneration adds weight to these arguments, as does the example of the perfect regeneration of severed fingertips.

An alternative explanation for the fingertip regeneration, however, is that there are organizing fields generated from within the body that maintain its integrity. These may be summations of minute atomic and/or molecular fields from protein molecules or from clusters of individual cells, which may be expressed via processes that are just starting to be clarified under *chaos (complexity) theory*.[301] Organizing fields could also be generated by the nerve cells, as suggested by Becker and his co-authors. Chaos theory explains how simple, repetitive summations of mathematical equations can produce regular patterns that are commonly found in nature, for example in the shapes of plants. It is possible that similar summations of biological EM fields might organize various aspects of body structure and functions.

That external fields may reorganize body processes is suggested by the healing of fractures and by the successful treatment of cancer with DC currents. This, in turn, suggests a possibility that such EM healing effects may operate through body/organ energy fields. Some self-healing and spiritual healing effects might also be mediated by EM effects within the body, which are initiated by neuro-hormonal mechanisms triggered by suggestion or by spiritual healing.

Becker's work with mechanical models suggests that the nervous system is a source of DC fields. It may also be that the nervous system acts as an antenna or channel for external fields. Gary Schwartz and colleagues (1996) confirmed that the human body can act "as a strong antenna and/or receiver for electrostatic body-motion" at a distance of 5 to 25 cm. from an electronic sensor. Schwartz and colleagues also note that with hypnoanalgesia, a suggestion can be given that a person's sense of touch will be anesthetized as though a glove were covering one hand. Not only does the suggestion reduce pain perception, but it also reduces electromagnetic field gradients over the entire hand. This is particularly interesting, because the analgesia does not follow the patterns of the nerves in the hand. That is, several nerves running to the hand begin producing a weaker EM field, starting at the wrist. This shows that the mind can influence EM aspects of bioenergy.

Some people appear hyper-allergic to EM fields, become severely symptomatic when exposed to certain EM frequencies. Conversely, alleviation of allergic reactions have been reported through exposure to particular EM frequencies.

The enhancement of bone knitting and chronic wound healing with DC field inputs is marvelous in and of itself. This phenomenon makes it clear that there are latent regenerative potentials in the body. Sadly, this discovery has also illustrated the initial reluctance of the medical establishment to explore unconventional findings.

In summary, at this stage of our study of bioelectromagnetics, we can say that there appears to be an organizational level within the body at which EM fields can at least transmit information about body growth and physical healing. The EM fields may act as templates for growth and physiological functions. It is conceivable that this EM level could act as an antenna or resonating field for healing that is directed from outside the organism. It may also mediate mind/body or spiritual self-healing.

Spiritual Healing and EM effects: If the fields around living things have organizing properties, then healing may act via these fields. In touch healing or near-the-body healing, the agent or channel of healing may be EM, UV, infrasound or other emanations from healers' bodies. Alternatively, healing could act via resonations, transdimensional coupling, or other sorts of interactions between the fields of healers and those of healees. Such field interactions might explain sensations experienced by healers and healees (warmth, tingling, vibrations, etc.).

EM effects might also be produced indirectly via telepathic influence on the healees, who then activate their own self-healing powers through their bodies' EM fields.

Eeman's observations of polarities in the body overlap with the work of Burr, Ravitz and Becker. Eeman's experiments with interconnections of polar points on the body using various wires or silk as conductors seem to be worth following up. The existence of a type of energy other than the EM spectrum is suggested – particularly if effects of medications and resonations with the illness of someone in the biocircuits can be sensed by others linked in the biocircuits.

Reich's orgone energy may be similar to Eeman's energies, in that it can be transmitted via wires. Reich's observations on the induction or enhancement of aura perception via exposure to orgone radiations are most interesting. Perhaps exposure to such energy sensitizes one to experiencing its effects.

Ultraviolet light and biophotons: The report by Rahn demonstrating that mito-genetic radiations enhanced wound healing in a salamander appears at first glance to point to UV light as a likely agent for healing effects. Kaznacheyev proposes that blood may transmit information to tissues and organs via the UV light that it emits. This provides yet another alternative means (in addition to interactions with organizing fields) through which UV light from external sources might affect internal organs, despite the fact that the original light cannot penetrate deeper than the skin. In addition, UV light may act upon total-body fields, which then influence physical processes. The observation that water demonstrates changes in its UV range after healing treatments are applied supports this possibility. It may be that water in the blood or body tissues is patterned by UV light or by subtle energies.

The reports by Rahn and Adamenko (1982) regarding the efficacy of pulsed light may indicate another fertile area for exploration in the relationship between field effects and healing. Perhaps more successful healers have oscillations in their fields that enhance their effectiveness. The vibrations of healers' hands and the sensations of vibration and tingling that are experienced during healing by healers and healees alike may be related to such field oscillations.

Eeman's observations on the transmission of the effects of medicines and im-munity via wires connecting people in his healing circuits seem revolutionary. They may point to an efficacy of medications that does not function via chemical effects but rather through field or healing energy interactions with the fields and energies of the body. This is supported by Smith and Best's reports on electro-magnetic patterning of allergies, and by subtle energy observations from the modalities of homeopathy, other complementary therapies, radionics, Kirlian photography and recent research with crystals and lasers.

Distant healings: We cannot explain distant healings as the result of EM effects because the strength of EM fields decreases with distance from their source. Therefore the strength of EM signals could not be sufficient to influence healees across many miles, though healing effects have been confirmed at such distances in randomized controlled trials.[302]

One might hypothesize that healers influence healees' EM fields directly via PK. This possibility is supported by studies demonstrating significant psi effects reg-istered on EM equipment, such as random number generators showing psi effects over great distances. This is not meant to explain distant healing per se, since psi effects over great distances have yet to be explained too. It does suggest, how-ever, a possible way in which EM fields may be involved in distant healings.

Distant healing effects may also be explained eventually as *tunneling* through other dimensions, or through as yet unidentified processes. There is considerable speculation on the role of consciousness as an organizing and healing agent for physical as well as for psychological health problems.[303]

The sensations felt by healees during distant healings are hard to explain on the basis of field interactions.[304] It is possible that these sensations are independent of healer-healee field interactions, and the field hypothesis still holds. One would have to postulate an unknown energy source in this case, because healing seems to work regardless of distance. Alternatively, the sensations may be produced by processes that are triggered by self-healing within the healees' bodies, regardless of whether it is initiated through touch or distant healing.

In summary: A substantial body of evidence suggests the existence of bioenergies that are not recognized within conventional science. Western science assumes that there are no energies beyond the basic four discussed earlier. However, in quantum physics there is a growing acknowledgement of the role of consciousness in selecting processes that determine which of several quantum pathways are followed. The precise mechanisms by which consciousness could interact with matter and energy have not yet been clarified.

The East Europeans' theories on bioplasma and UV rays seem at variance with Western scientific thinking. They appear far ahead of the West in developing practical applications for such effects, such as Kirlian photography for diagnosis of biological processes in health and disease. For many years they have been more open than the West to studying healing phenomena and to utilizing healers in clinical settings. In part this may still be due to the economic straits in the East that make healing and other complementary therapies attractive.

My own best guess is that there are biological energies that are as yet unidentified by conventional science. These energies might overlap in some respects with EM energy. Alternatively, they might produce EM energy secondarily during phase shifts of whatever brings about or accompanies healing, possibly through various dimensions of reality beyond our familiar three dimension – much as heat may be produced when liquids change to solids, or as a byproduct of electrical transformers.

It seems certain that healing energy interacts with the mind and emotions of all participants in experiments on healing effects. These bioenergies may link with the mind or be an aspect of mind. The general acknowledgement of such a mind/energy or mind-energy link could conceivably advance the search for a unified field theory in quantum physics. Consciousness may eventually become a variable in the equations of a future elaboration of quantum physics.

Living organisms are probably the most sensitive sensors for these energies, though people may require practice to perceive them consciously and to identify them reliably. Our extreme sensitivity leaves us open to distractions and distortions from extraneous "noise," such as geomagnetic forces. Rather than rejecting biological sensors on this basis, I see room to refine their focus and their ability to screen helpful signals. For instance, we might schedule our measurements to take into account geomagnetic fields, sunspots and other influences that alter biological systems, so that we can increase the reliability of human sensors. Multiple sensors can be used to seek common denominators of perceptions, which would likewise help to sift out some of the "noise."

The above-mentioned reports and speculations on fields and energies are clearly only an early beginning in our exploratory explanations for the mechanisms of self-healing and spiritual healing. Clairsentients and mystics have been talking about visible and palpable *energy bodies* around the physical body for several millennia. Our western materialistic conditioning makes it hard for us to accept such reports from a gifted few, when the rest of us "normal" folk cannot validate them for ourselves. How much moreso with observations of mystics about astral bodies and other levels of existence. Readings on instruments that indicate various quantifiable physical forces and energies seem much more believable. However, even with so-called objective measurements we have not arrived at definitions and explanations of our world that are beyond question. We often forget that we must add our own interpretations to these instrument readings in order for them to have any meaning. Furthermore, mechanistic science starts with axioms of belief just as energy medicine does. Both provide models that are useful, each in their own domains, but they all will inevitably be altered with further study.

See Table II-10 for a comparison of the world of quantum physics and the world of Newtonian physics, and Table II-8 for a comparison of CAM therapies with conventional medicine, or – in the light of our discussion in this chapter – we might say this is a comparison of energy medicine with Newtonian medicine.

Table II-10. Various ways to define the world	
Quantum physics $E = mc^2$ Newtonian physics	
Particles and energies are interconvertible.	Matter and energies (mechanical, electromagnetic, gravity) are distinct.
Action can occur from any distance.	Action is local, and effects diminish with distance.
Holographic world	Linear/ spatial world
Observer may determine reality.	Mind is separate from the physical world, a product of the brain.
Time is reversible.	Time is a linear stream.

Hopefully, other researchers will confirm and extend these pioneering works that have enhanced our comprehension of mankind's energetic relationship with the universe. We may then see the development of instruments that measure biological fields reliably, or we may learn to refine the biological instrument itself. Then we can develop frameworks that more satisfactorily explain spiritual healing.

Western scientific paradigms will have to change to accommodate these findings, and quantum physics appears to be moving already in this direction. Particularly in its observational theories we find hints that mind may interact with matter, and thus we may find within quantum theory a reciprocal basis for understanding healing.[305]

We should not delay the use of *biological energy medicine* or *vibrational medicine* techniques till definitive theories are developed and validated. There is already sufficient empirical evidence that these techniques are effective.

Our life is frittered away by detail... Simplify, simplify.
– Henry David Thoreau

Let us proceed to the next chapter, which examines natural fields that may interact with biological fields.

CHAPTER 4

Geobiological Effects

Men often stumble over the truth
but most of them pick themselves up
and hurry off as if nothing had happened.
         – Winston Churchill

In the preceding chapter we examined a variety of fields and forces that exist in and around the body. Some are within the electromagnetic (EM) spectrum that is recognized by conventional science. Other energy phenomena seem to contradict the basic laws of conventional science, and provide strong hints that the accepted energy spectrum must be expanded to include several new types of fields and energies.

In this chapter we shall examine fields in the natural environment that may interact with biological energy fields. Some of these can be measured by electromagnetic devices, while others are only perceptible to particularly sensitive people.

We shall start with various geobiological[306] effects that have been observed by dowsers and supported by scientific research. Then we shall consider evidence for astrological influences that may interact with biological systems.

RADIESTHESIA (DOWSING) AND RADIONICS

At one of his trials, Jurion was testifying about patients he had cured by dowsing remedies when, suddenly and savagely, the judge turned on him to shout sarcastically: "This tribunal is not objecting to your curing people but to your treating them."
         – Christopher Bird

The Chinese have studied the effects of *feng shui* from at least the ninth century AD. Experts in this field can sense earth energies and advise people about the selection of sites for houses and graves, or about positive and negative vibrations at a certain location that may bring good or bad luck.[307] According to this system, certain architectural structures and configurations within a home are health-promoting and others may have deleterious effects on inhabitants' health. Strategically placing mirrors, plants, and other objects can correct bad energy configurations. Various parts of a home and areas within each room relate to different aspects of one's life.[308]

Sacred geometry is the study of how aesthetically and spiritually pleasing shapes of rooms and buildings can influence the way we feel within those spaces. Thomas Moore terms this "*Genius loci*, the spirit of a place." It has been recognized for ages that certain proportions of length, width and height are inherently aesthetically pleasing. Mystical properties have been attributed to particular measurements, some of which appear repeatedly in nature, as in the chambers of a snail shell and the structure of plant leaves.

I have not made a study of sacred geometry, as I have not found research to validate the reported effects on health. Sacred geometry was also applied by ancient cultures to the study of the planet Earth.

Beyond aesthetics of ambience, there are intuitive perceptions of positive and negative subtle energies that are inherent in any location. You have probably experienced a sense of positive energies when visiting particular places in nature, or perhaps some houses of worship. Conversely you may have sensed negative energies in other places in nature or in particular buildings that appear to induce a sense of gloom, tension or foreboding. People who are sensitive to subtle energies have many explanations for these perceptions. The simplest is that the presence or lack of healing energies can produce such sensations. These energies may occur naturally in particular locations or they may be the result of prayers or healing activities that are conducted there. Electromagnetic and chemical pollution may produce negative feelings in a given place.[309] In addition, our intuitive and bio-energy awarenesses can connect with the vibrations of a place, giving us an inner knowing of its positive or negative nature.

One way of detecting earth energies is through dowsing. *Dowsing,* or *geomancy,* has been used in Western culture for centuries. The earliest published report, *De re Metallica* by Georgius Agricola, dates from 1556.

Dowsers are gifted people who are able to locate water, oil and other minerals in the earth with the aid of various simple instruments. While dowsing may appear odd to many readers of this book, dowsers' abilities have been used to great advantage in numbers of situations. Dowsers have helped in the U S Army Corps of Engineers and the military to clear minefields and to locate enemy installations underground, and by various civilian utility companies to locate buried pipes and power lines.

Various devices are used by dowsers. Some use forked sticks or Y-shaped, flexible plastic rods, which they hold, flexed in front of them in a state of tension, while walking back and forth over the land they are exploring. The dowser holds the image of the desired material in his mind, and when he passes over it, the forked branch will bend sharply downward or upward. Others use L-shaped wires held parallel in each hand, with handles encased in a loose metal or plastic sleeve so that they are free to swivel. When passing over the sought material the wires will diverge or converge from their initial parallel positions. Some dowsers use a pendulum, which they typically hold over the ground or over a map of the territory while the dowser is thinking about a specific question relating to the material in the ground.

Dowsers may use their intuitive powers to answer any yes/no questions, including those relating to health and illness. Various types of pendulum motion give the dowser answers. For instance, a swing away from the body and back may indicate a "yes" and a swing parallel to the body a "no"; or a clockwise turn may indicate "yes" and counterclockwise, "no." The pendulum may also be swung above a radial chart to indicate the degree to which a certain factor is present, such as the rate of flow of an underground stream, the degree of severity of an illness, or the required strength of a medication. Dowsers report that they themselves are not consciously manipulating the devices, although many acknowledge that their unconscious minds are probably providing the impetus through their muscles. The more sensitive dowsers rely on sensations such as heat in their hands, pains in various parts of their bodies, smells, etc. as indicators, and do not use any mechanical device.

Map dowsing

Many dowsers claim that they can dowse for items within a territory by using a map. The map seems to function as a *witness,* which in dowsers' terminology is an object that connects the dowser psychically with whatever she wants to focus upon. In some instances dowsers claim greater accuracy when they are facing in a particular compass direction – either for map or field dowsing.

Others may use *radionics* devices (sometimes affectionately called *black boxes*) for diagnosis and treatment. These have a range of dials and compartments for specimens from the patient. In an earlier model of the box, a rubber diaphragm was rubbed with a finger until a particular sensation was felt, which indicated that the device was tuned to the vibration of the item that was being sought mentally by the dowser. More modern devices have electrical dials for assessing health problems of patients, described below.

The distance of dowsers from the object of their dowsing is no obstacle to success in locating it or in projecting healing. Many dowsers find that they are equally effective in dowsing a map of the territory as they are in the field, and this is equally true with radionics devices, which may be located many miles from the *target* person.

Dowsing for diagnosis and treatment

Dowsers may ask their pendulum or other device to identify illnesses in people, animals and plants. They arrive at the answers through a series of Yes/No queries or through swinging the pendulum over radially distributed lists of problems, percentages of deficits, doses of medication and the like. When the patient is not present, dousers usually prefer to use a *witness,* which can be any object closely associated with the healee, in order to link with her. The witness may, for example, be a lock of hair, a drop of spittle, urine or blood on a piece of blotting paper, a photograph, or an object belonging to the healee. Lacking these, the healee's name written on a piece of paper may suffice.

Devices with electronic dials plus visual and/or tonal outputs have accompanied dowsing into the modern age. The devices may utilize sealed vials of toxic and medicinal materials in place of the dowser's mental image as a focus for tuning. A person with chronic tiredness, for example, will be told to hold an electrode attached to such a dowsing device. As the dowser puts each of a series of vials of toxins in the diagnostic chamber, he places an electronic probe on an acupuncture point. The dial will give a reading indicating whether the healee's body contains the given chemical at deficient, normal or toxic levels. Similarly, tests can be made for allergens or vitamin deficiencies, and for predicting the efficacy of therapeutic agents.

With all of these devices, the operator appears to be an essential link with the instrument, though many dowsers who use them tend to project the responsibility for the results entirely onto the devices. This is patently impossible with the rubber diaphragm radionics device, as the boxes have no intrinsic circuitry that can do more than provide mental focus and/or feedback to the operator. Some radionics practitioners propose that these devices, in and of themselves, hold and/or project healing energies (of an as yet undetermined nature), once they are tuned by the practitioner.

One unique contribution of dowsing to the field of energy medicine is the ability to identify illnesses that are caused by underground streams or other sources of negative earth energies, called *geopathic zones*. These are said to stress people who spend time over them, for example when sleeping or working regularly above a geopathic zone. Moving one's bed or workstation away from these zones has been reported to cure a variety of problems, such as insomnia, arthritis, chronic fatigue syndrome and more. Alternatively, spikes or pipes can be driven into the ground at particular points along the negative energy line to neutralize its effects, or to transform its emanations to positive energy.

Radionics practitioners claim that they can tune their devices to send healing vibrations to correct a wide variety of problems that are causing illness or harm to plants, animals and humans. Radionics treatments consist of tuning the dials on the device to vibrational frequencies that are corrective for chemical deficiencies, allergies, infections and toxicities. Radionics specialists have also reported successes in treating infections, possession by errant or malevolent spirits,[310] and infestations of insect pests in crops. The recipient of radionics treatments is a passive subject to the ministrations of the radionics operator.

Radionics devices have also been developed to produce homeopathic remedies. They utilize vibrational patterns printed on cards to transfer therapeutic vibrations to the carrier solution or to the sugar pills that are used for homeopathic treatments.

Sensitive medical dowsers may gradually develop powers of clairsentience so that eventually they rely on their instruments less or not at all. Then they can simply ask their questions mentally, and the answers come to them intuitively. Some also develop healing abilities that operate independently of their devices.

Some skeptics have suggested that dowsers may simply be well-versed in geology and/or keen observers of various cues that they can translate into intuitive impressions (as in pattern recognition based on accumulated unconscious knowledge), which are projected onto their devices through unconscious minor movements of their hands. Others have hypothesized that dowsers may be extrasensitive to various EM or other known radiations.

Your reasoning is excellent - it's only your basic assumptions that are wrong.

– Ashleigh Brilliant

Let us examine the research evidence, starting with field dowsing and extending into medical dowsing.

Research

Field dowsing is the term commonly applied to the locating of materials and objects in the greater world using intuitive means.

The classical use of dowsing is to locate underground streams for wells. Under sponsorship of the German government, physicist Hans-Dieter Betz studied dowsers in Sri Lanka over a 10-year period. In 691 drillings they achieved a success rate of 96 percent, compared to the 30-50 percent success rates anticipated when drillings in this area are based on geological recommendations. Even more impressive was the fact that the dowsers predicted the depth at which water would be found and the amounts of flow, within a 20-30 percent margin of error, *prior to drilling.*

A. M. Comunetti discovered that Hoffman-La Roche, a major drug company in Basle, relied on two sensitive employees to dowse for underground sources of water for their chemical plants around the world. Comunetti tested these dowsers in the corridors of the multi-story Basle factory for their abilities to identify a source of water that was several floors below. Even with blindfolds or blinkers (which prevented them from seeing the walls or the floor of the corridors) they were reliably able to identify the location of the source of water. As Comunetti had each of the dowsers approach the area of the water source from both directions, it became apparent that one dowser was sensitive to the borders of the water zone, and the other to the body of the zone.

Continuing his investigations, Comunetti set up a series of parallel pipes along the floor of a warehouse. The pipes were places so that a stream of water could be directed through each of them individually, in parallel. The pipes were made of glass, 5 cm in diameter and 2 meters long. One was clear and the others were filled with sand. This enabled the experimenter to vary the amount of flow, up to 10 liters/ minute. The dowsers walked along a platform that was 8.8 meters long, and raised 2.1 meters above the water source. One dowser could identify when water was flowing in the sandy pipes but not in the clear one. The other could not sense a flow of water, even when he knew the water was turned on. When a layer of sand 10 - 15 cm thick was placed on top of the pipes, both dowsers felt the flows much more clearly.[311] Comunetti tested the dowsers with blindfolds, both when walking and riding on a cable-trolley that was remote-controlled. The dowsers knew the location of the pipes but not when the water was turned on and off – that was determined by the toss of a coin for each trial. Intervals between trials were 2 to 4 minutes. The dowsers were successful in 4 out of 8 series of between 10 and 11 trials each, which is a highly significant result.

Comunetti initially intended to vary the position of the water pipes. In exploratory trials he found that there was a linger effect at the initial location that lasted for 5 - 15 minutes. That is to say, the dowsers would identify the previous location of the water pipes during the first 5 to 15 minutes after the pipes had been moved.[312]

J. B. Rhine, a methodical parapsychology investigator, challenged two dowsers to identify whether water was flowing in two hidden underground pipes over which they walked carrying dowsing rods. The dowsers scored significantly lower than chance in one series of trials and somewhat above chance in another series. There was a decline in success rate as the experiment progressed.

Remi Cadoret asked dowsers to locate a penny that was hidden under one of 25 tiles. The dowsers produced results that were statistically marginally significant in a series of trials. In another experiment dowsers used a map corresponding to a grid in Cadoret's back yard to locate a buried penny. Again, marginally significant results were obtained.

Karlis Osis, at the Parapsychology Laboratory of Duke University, tested a dowser who worked for a gas company. Osis placed 18-inch long segments of pipes randomly in ten trenches he had dug in the ground, and covered them with boards. In tests where Osis was blind to the location of the pipes, the results were marginally significant; for the entire series, the results were highly significant. Osis also tested the dowser for the ability to locate money hidden under one of 25 tiles. Results were marginally significant.

D. H. Pope reported on results of experiments by a lecturer in biology at Harrogate Training College in England. A dowser was challenged to locate a coin under pieces of cardboard. Despite the fact that only 63 trials were run, the results were highly significant. Unfortunately, sensory cues were not entirely ruled out. Stage magicians have demonstrated that such cues can very often reveal hidden objects to a person who is seeking them. When people know the location of a hidden object, they very often provide non-verbal indications, such as glancing at the location or tensing up as the magician moves closer to it.

L. A. Dale et al. found only random results in a study of 27 dowsers who tried to locate natural sources of water and to estimate depth and rate of flow.

Benson Herbert,[313] an English parapsychologist, pointed out that the pendulum used by dowsers does not move of its own accord but rather due to minute motions of the dowsers' hands or via their breath. Herbert clearly demonstrated this by holding the string of the dowsers' pendulums in a fixed clamp and/or under a glass bell. In such cases the dowsers were unable to make the pendulum sway. Benson tested a dowser by asking him to identify under which of two paper wrappings a coin and a rock were placed. Only random results were produced. Herbert was doubtful that any psi effects are involved in dowsing.

N. B. Eastwood found that if dowsers' hands and forearms were covered with aluminum foil their ability to dowse with forked twigs was blocked, but their dowsing ability with pendulums and rods was unchanged. Foil over the chin and jaw blocked only the pendulum, and foil over the upper face and upper abdomen blocked only the rods.

Dowsing of EM fields has been studied to explore whether dowsers might obtain information on EM wavelengths.

Zaboj V. Harvalik was a professor of physics retired from the University of Arkansas and a former adviser to American Army Advanced Concepts Materials

Agency. He describes a series of tests with a German master dowser, Wilhelm de Boer. The dowser walked perpendicular to the current flow of 5 milli-amperes (thousandth of an ampere), which was gradually reduced in successive tests to 2.5 micro-amperes (millionth of an ampere), and de Boer was still able to identify the signal by dowsing it. Rest periods of 5 to 10 minutes were needed between every 10 to 12 runs. He was successful 100% of the time when his left side faced the negative electrode, and unsuccessful 100% of the time when his left side faced the positive electrode.

In another experiment, Harvalik blindfolded de Boer, who walked in circles past one of two generators.[314] Without the dowser's awareness, the generators were switched on and off at random. Forty runs were made with the generators on. The position and orientation of the generator coils was varied so that as he passed the generators, he sometimes crossed the magnetic lines and sometimes did not. The dowser reliably identified when he crossed the radiation beam. A copper mesh screen interrupting the beam prevented him from receiving a signal. If the copper screen was used as a mirror to deflect the beam into his path, he did note a signal.

No blinds are described by Harvalik, nor are the numbers of trials or successes given. It is implied that the dowser was entirely accurate. The only discrepancy noted was on an indoor trial where the beam was pointed vertically towards the ceiling and the dowser reported a weak signal. This was explained as a possible detection of reflected signals.

Harvalik proceeded to test de Boer with partial screening of the dowser's body by copper wire mesh. Placed before his solar plexus, this screening totally interrupted the dowser's ability to identify the signal, and partially obstructed his ability when his head was shielded. Harvalik postulates that the presence of two parts of the body where dowsing sensors are apparently located may enable dowsers to discriminate gradients of magnetic fields. The sensing of EM fields from two points on the body might provide indications of the materials and objects for which they are dowsing, as the EM fields (or other bioenergy vibrations) of objects in the environment may have different "tonal qualities" when perceived through two separate sensors. This has parallels with auditory perceptions. It is possible to set up an interference pattern within the brain by inputting different sound frequencies into each ear. Having two sensors for dowsed vibrations may set up interference patterns that provide identifying clues to the dowser on the nature of items that are being perceived.

Having two sensors could also provide perceptions that are similar to the depth perception that is possible when two eyes view an object from different angles. This may explain dowsers' reputed abilities to identify the depth at which minerals are located, just as stereoscopic vision enables depth perception.

Harvalik repeated the blocking experiments with fourteen dowsers, using a low-power, high-frequency EM field and pieces of aluminum sheet placed over the kidneys and brain. In 694 trials they were able to guess correctly whether the field was on or off 661 times. This is one of the most convincing studies, as it was conducted with a double-blind design and the field was switched on and off on a random schedule. It is unclear, however, whether the dowsers were aware of the experimental hypotheses about the locations of sensitive body zones, so one still has to view with caution the blocking aspect of this study.

Harvalik concludes from a long series of studies that sensitive dowsers can respond to changes in very weak magnetic fields,[315] and exceptional dowsers can detect changes 100 times weaker. This is consistent with my own observations of the varying abilities of medical dowsers.

Sol Tromp, a Dutch geology professor and director of the Bioclimatological Centre of Leiden, tested dowsers' sensitivity to EM fields with a tangent galvanometer and a coil of wire. Elaborate precautions were taken to limit extraneous cues: using noiseless switches on the electrical equipment, blindfolds, and cotton earplugs, and keeping the experimenter who was recording responses blind to whether the current was on or off. Using U-shaped rods, dowsers were able to detect alterations in the strength of the EM field at very low gradients.[316] They could identify shifts and changes in the field, but not field strength per se. In the first 20 trials sensitive dowsers had an 80% rate of accuracy, but after this they complained of fatigue and their success rate subsequently declined.

Tromp noted that some dowsers were able to detect EM fields with the aid of pendulums when they had failed with the U-shaped rods. Pendulum dowsers were also able to identify differences in field strength.

Yves Rocard, a physics professor at the École Normale in Paris, also confirmed that dowsers could identify alterations in a DC EM field using rods (of a different configuration from those used by Tromp). He found that at the level of the chest their sensitivity was highest[317] when the dowsers were walking at normal speed (1 to 2 meters/ second). Gradients above a certain level (not specified) were not detected and were presumed to produce *saturation* or fatigue of the sensors. Magnets attached to the forearms of the dowsers also blocked their perceptions of fields. Responses were poorer with pendulums. Hansen, my source for the review of this French study, makes no mention of blinds.

R. A. Foulkes, testing only one dowser, failed to replicate Rocard's work.

P. Kiszkowski and H. Szydlowski found that it was impossible to reproduce Rocard's results when they replicated his experiments. They then explored dowsers' sensitivity to AC EM fields over a range of voltages,[318] using aluminum electrodes 10 cm in diameter. They found that different dowsers were able to detect EM fields over different parts of their bodies. The dowsers did not know when the current was switched on. When electrodes 12 cm in diameter were held near the hand of a dowser, the pendulum often swung in a particular direction, which was frequently parallel to the direction of the electric fields. Positive results were noted over a wide range of field strengths.[319] Factors that were found to influence the results included the duration of the sessions and the time of day. After 2 hours of experimentation they could not obtain reproducible results.

H. L. König and colleagues also explored dowsers' responses to EM fields. The dowsers were required to identify one of the following:

1. Where an EM field was located within a given area;
2. When a field from a known source was switched on or off; or
3. Which of several EM devices was switched on.

The last two produced clearer results, as only yes/ no responses were required. Following the format used by Fadini,[320] spools of half a meter in diameter with 24 windings of wire were mounted on wooden supports about 1.5 meters high. No shielding was used over the leads, so stray currents[321] were detectable at distances from half a meter to one meter around the coils. Subjects who felt that they could tell the difference between on and off conditions were challenged to identify which one of a row of 8 coils was switched on. In the initial trials the subjects were blind to which coil was on but the experimenter was not. The dowsing rods moved for most subjects when they were still 1 - 2 meters or more away from the coils.[322] The series of 8 coils is preferable because the repetitive testing procedure with only one coil is fatiguing to the dowsers. In this series situation a frequency of 30 cps. was used, and the current (which determined intensity) was varied. Under single-blind conditions the correct coil was identified in 23 out of 46 trials, which is highly significant.

People who trained to develop their sensitivity to EM fields spontaneously developed an ability to dowse for water. However, the experimenters could not identify EM fields around the water sources identified by dowsers.

Duane Chadwick and Larry Jensen, two electrical engineers at Utah State University, asked ungifted subjects to mark places along a prescribed path where their dowsing rods indicated a reaction. Chadwick and Jensen then measured EM variations along the path. Various dowsers' marks clustered significantly around particular locations and these were more likely to be areas with a particular gradient of intensity.[323] Statistics for correlation between clustered and other measured locations are not presented in their report.

W. H. Jack, an instructor in parapsychology at Franklin Pierce College in New Hampshire, asked twelve ungifted subjects to use dowsing rods to detect whether a weak current[324] was or was not flowing through an electrical wire. His subjects achieved significant results, but proper blinds were not included in the study.

Colin Godman and Lindsay St. Claire report on attempts to demonstrate the effectiveness of dowsing by using it to map underground caves and locating men who were hidden in them. Results were partially successful but no quantification of the data was built into the study design.

J. L. Whitton and S. A. Cook tested 27 people, two of whom claimed dowsing abilities, using weak EM fields produced by alternating current. They tested another 11 people (none of whom claimed dowsing ability) using a direct current coil. Using L-rods, only chance results were obtained.

E. Balanovski and J. G. Taylor found dowsers insensitive to magnetic fields of 100 gauss, and to high-frequency, low-power electromagnetic fields.

Electrodermal responses during dowsing
Dowsers often complain of severe physiological reactions, such as dizziness, nausea, and pains, when exposed to negative earth energies. Changes in the voltage gradient of a person's skin correlate with stress (which provides the physiological basis for lie detector tests). Recordings of *electrodermal activity* (EDA) during dowsing have thus provided measures of dowsing-related stress responses.

Tromp connected the wrists of dowsers to an instrument that records skin electrical potential. Insulated grips were provided for the loop-shaped rods. Alterations in EDA were noted immediately after a nearby magnetic field was turned on. Similar readings were obtained with dowsers walking through "dowsing zones." Tromp presents evidence to counter the possibility that the altered galvanometer measurements were due to emotional reactions or induction potentials. For example, similar measurements were recorded with dowsers walking through "dowsing zones" without rods. Less sensitive people demonstrated similar, though slower and less marked EDA when walking through such zones. Tromp found that sensitive dowsers had a baseline skin resistance that was much lower than that of other people. Sketchy mention is also made of EDA that was recorded when dowsers moved rods over the heads and feet of subjects.

Kenneth Roberts, a historical novelist, reports a st udy by American electrical engineers of the EDA of Henry Gross, a famous dowser. They noted changes in his EDA during several trials at map dowsing, and a 100-millivolt change when he walked over underground water. A subsequent series of map dowsing trials did not produce significant results. In another series of tests, skin potential changes of 100 to 200 millivolts were noted in a Canadian dowser, Desrosiers, when he walked over a known water vein. Desrosiers worked without instruments, dowsing through sensations of pain in the soles of his feet and in the small of his back. Non-dowsers showed only 10 - 30 millivolt changes when walking over the same territory.

Berthold E. Schwarz noted some inconclusive changes in the EEG of Henry Gross during dowsing performed in the laboratory, as well as irregular respiration, decreased skin resistance, increased pulse rate and blood pressure.

Underground dowsable energy lines (*ley lines*) and geopathic stress

Dowsers can detect lines of energy within the earth that are unrelated to EM energies and undetectable except through the person of the dowser. Many call these *ley lines,* though some prefer the term *dowsable earth lines.* The Chinese refer to these as *dragon paths* or *dragon currents.* Mapping ley lines is a hobby for some, has produced fascinating historical information. Many ancient roads and modern tracks of wild animals follow ley lines. Ancient holy places were often built at points of confluence of several ley lines. In Germany and Austria a regular grid of energy lines running 3 to 4 meters apart has been identified. This is called the *Curry net.*[325]

There may be harmful earth radiations above ley or *Curry lines* that are alleged to contribute to or even cause disease. The danger points, called *geopathic zones,* are above intersections of two or more lines or of ley lines with underground water streams.

Ilse Pope discusses geopathic stress in German and Austrian patients with various disorders:

> In 1929 a German scientist named Freiherr von Pohl was curious about anecdotal reports connecting ley lines with illness. He convinced Dr. Blumenthal of the Berlin Centre for Cancer Research to review the 54 cancer deaths in Vilsbiburg, a village in Southern Germany with a population of 3,300. This is an unusually high number over the brief period when records were kept of cancer deaths. Freiherr von Pohl drew onto the map of Vilsbiburg all the subterranean water veins which had a strength of above 9 on the Pohl Scale... This

scale, which went up to 16, Freiherr von Pohl had worked out over his many years of research into the phenomenon of earth radiation. After three days his plan was compared to the records of the district hospital and it was found... that every single cancer death had occurred exactly above the lines which Freiherr von Pohl had drawn as being above the strength of 9 and therefore cancer producing... When Freiherr von Pohl was called back to Vilsbiburg 18 months later because another ten people had died of cancer, the beds of these ten people again were exactly on the lines he had drawn on the map.

These results were so impressive that they were published in the *Journal of the Centre for Cancer Research.* While no blinds are mentioned, the last 10 cases occurred in predicted zones.

Dr. Rambeau, the President of the Chamber of Medicine in Marburg, heard of Freiherr von Pohl's work. Using a geoscope, "an instrument used by the Geological Institute to locate geological fault lines," he mapped the geological fault lines in the villages around Marburg. He found that "the beds of all his severely ill patients were above these geological fault lines." He could not locate a house that was not over a geopathic zone in which a person had lived for a long time just prior to the development of cancer, and felt that cases of cancer did not occur on neutral ground. No controls or blinds are mentioned.

In Stettin, Dr. Hager studied the 5,348 cancer deaths that occurred between 1910 and 1931. All were associated with dowsed subterranean water lines. *Only 1,575 premises were associated with one cancer death each. All the rest involved multiple deaths.* All premises with more than 5 cancer deaths (199 people in 28 houses) were located on crossings of water veins. Five premises were associated with more than 10 cancer deaths each.[326]

Kaethe Bachler, an Austrian teacher, compiled an excellent review of dowsing. She studied the influence of geopathic lines on children with learning disabilities. She reports that moving the beds or school desks of such children (when these were located over water or *Curry crossings)* often resulted in improved school performance. She also found correlations between cancer and such geopathic zones. No controls or blinds are mentioned.

O. Bergsmann, a Viennese consultant in medicine, explored the effects of geopathic stress on 24 laboratory parameters. These included electrodermal response; heart rate; systolic blood pressure; orthostatic changes in blood pressure (changes when people rise from recumbent positions); time required to warm fingertips that were cooled in a standard manner; tendon reflex time; muscle electrical potentials; blood sedimentation rate; circulating immune system proteins; and levels of calcium, potassium, zinc, serotonin, tyrosine, and tryptophan in the blood. Three dowsers identified areas of geopathic stress and neutral areas in eight hospital rooms around Austria. The stress areas involved crossings of water lines or crossings of water and earth energy lines. Bergmann studied the 24 parameters in 985 people. Each subject was given the battery of tests three times: after sitting for 15 minutes in a neutral area, after 15 minutes in a stress area, and after another 15 minutes in a neutral area. Subjects did not know which were the stress areas.

Results showed significant changes in 12 parameters. The serotonin level is the only test identified specifically by the reviewer of this German report. Serotonin levels change with mood and sleep, and changes in this variable may be related to sleep disturbances and depressions reported by people suffering from geopathic stress.

Herbert Douglas investigated 34 cases of arthritis. He dowsed underground veins of water that crossed precisely under the affected part of each arthritic's body. In 18 out of the 34 cases he was able to convince the patients to move their beds. In each case there was partial or complete improvement within one day to three months following the relocation. No controls or blinds were instituted in this study, so effects of suggestion cannot be ruled out.

Vlastimil Zert of Czechoslovakia reports that tree tumors are also found more frequently over geopathic zones, and other studies have shown various further anomalies occurring over geopathic zones.

In one very interesting summary of dowsing research, Herbert L. König et al. mention that infrared radiation from human bodies is altered when they stand above geopathic zones.[327]

Petschke performed extensive experiments on laboratory blood test results in relation to geopathic zones. In 62 series he observed differences in results when tests were run over a neutral zone, in a dowsing zone, and at a crossing of dowsing zones – all carried out in the same area, only a few meters apart. He found that the blood sedimentation rates[328] were either accelerated or retarded over dowsing zones and over crossings, relative to the rates over neutral zones.

E. Hartmann repeated these tests in the homes of a series of people who had died of cancer. He had several erythrocyte (red blood cell) sedimentation tubes that were placed 6 cm apart in a rack, with some of the tubes over the point in the bed where the cancerous organ would have been positioned and others outside of this zone. The sedimentation rates in the tubes over the geopathic zones deviated markedly from those that were not over these zones. Germination of seeds of vegetable such as cucumbers and corn was suppressed over these zones. No blinds or controls are mentioned.

Changes in the weather were also noted to alter the sedimentation rates in the above-mentioned studies.

E. F. Scheller studied ionizing radiation anomalies that he found at particular locations which he felt were injurious to health. Wherever there was an elevated level of radiation he found that blood samples developed fibers, granules, globules, and vesicles. The *Scheller test* for darkfield microscopic examination of red blood cells was developed in the belief that this could identify people at risk for the development of cancer because of geopathic stress.

Hartmann found that "reaction times" (unspecified) were 1 to 10 percent slower over geopathic zones. Hartmann observed 3 groups of 4 mice. The first cage was kept over a geopathic zone, the second over a neutral zone half a meter away, and the third in a Faraday cage (which blocks EM radiation) 2 meters away. Over a 6-month period there were 124 mice born in the neutral zone, 118 in the Faraday cage and 56 in the geopathic zone. No blinds are mentioned.

Hartmann injected rats subcutaneously with Yoshida tumors. He studied 12 series involving 3 rats in each of 3 cages, following each series over a period of 3 to

4 weeks. In the initial 4 series one cage was placed over a geopathic zone, one over a neutral zone and the last in a Faraday cage. The cages were 1 to 1.3 meters apart. Just after their inoculation the rats in the Faraday cage were given two exposures of 15 minutes each to high-frequency radiation.[329]

In the last 8 series a fourth cage with 3 mice was placed in a second neutral zone about 30 cm from one of the control cages, as a check on whether small distances unrelated to geopathic zones could produce observable differences in tumor growth. In the last 8 series the rats in the Faraday cage received no EM exposure after their inoculation.

Tumor growth was estimated by palpation followed by molding in plastiline and weighing. In the first series the rats over the geopathic zone had the most rapid growth of cancer, those over the neutral zone had slower growth, and those in the Faraday cage the slowest growth. In the second series the rats in the Faraday cage had the fastest growth, followed by those over the geopathic zone, and those over the neutral zones had the slowest growth.

Magnetic field intensity was measured over the various geopathic points. A probe that was passed over the geopathic zone in one direction registered a decrease in magnetic field intensity of about 80 percent compared to other places in the room. No blinds are mentioned in this study.

Hartmann found magnetic anomalies over a geopathic zone, using a dual compass. J. Wüst measured magnetic anomalies over such points with a variety of instruments, and reports that the EM resistance in the ground was substantially increased at such points. S. W. Tromp found that ground conductivity over geopathic zones was increased but also noted resistance peaks in some of these areas. G. Lehman found significantly lower gradients in electrostatic fields over geopathic zones. Lehman also noted increased conductivity in the air over dowsed water veins. F. Bürklin found that lightning strikes were more frequent at low-voltage power transmission poles that were located at geopathic zones. A grounding wire provided protection for these poles.

Brüche found that measurements of radioactivity over water veins could be elevated or decreased periodically, and that this seemed related to weather conditions. Endrös identified infrared and microwave emissions over underground water veins. Stängle developed a scintillation counter using sodium iodide, which he mounted on wheels and used for measurements of radioactivity over geopathic zones. He studied the sites identified by von Pohl (where people living over geopathic zones had died of cancer) and found radiation intensities close to twice as high as over adjacent areas. The scintillation curves in these areas were similar to curves obtained over underground water veins. Hartmann found that gamma radiation varied at heights of 12 to 25 cm above ground over geopathic zones (usually producing 10 to 30 percent higher radiation counts). He noted periodic rises and falls at intervals of 15 minutes and 3 hours. Again there were variations correlated with the weather. Lead shielding of the instrument probe decreased the counts over geopathic zones, but not to the same degree as it did over normal areas. Shielding with paraffin-graphite blocks of about 10-cm thickness increased the counts.

J. Wüst showed that very high frequency (VHF) radio transmitters performed differently over geopathic zones. Hartmann found VHF anomalies around sick beds, unrelated to geopathic zones. Physician D. Aschoff studied VHF field intensities in the rooms of 125 people with chronic health problems that had been unresponsive to conventional treatments. Of 85 who moved from areas of high VHF intensity to areas of low intensity, 28 reported immediate improvements.

Hartmann developed a VHF transmitter and receiver with which he measured the DC resistance between the hands of subjects. He found that the time course of body resistance varies when subjects are over geopathic points, as compared to when they are over neutral points. These findings are also related to weather conditions.

Various devices have been developed for neutralizing negative earth energies. Hartmann claimed excellent results with *bioresonators* that he developed for this purpose. H. L. König studied the elastic, double brass coil that is at the core of this instrument. He found that its natural mechanical resonance is around 10 Cps., which means that is biologically active. Therefore it could easily be activated by vibrations in the floor. However, König is skeptical that this could neutralize other EM fields and thus eliminate geopathic stress.

Discussion

Dowsers have had difficulty convincing scientists that their perceptions are anything more than lucky guesses. As with other forms of psi and intuitive perception, they are irregular in their successes.

The research in dowsing is not well publicized and most scientists are unaware that any has been done at all. The studies summarized here strongly suggest that dowsing produces significant results. Although suggestion cannot be ruled out in many of the studies, due to lack of controls and blinds, there are sufficient studies with rigorous design to confirm there dowsing is effective and to encourage further research.

Why dowsers scored significantly lower than chance in the series by Rhine is unclear. Perhaps this poor result was related to the attitudes and interactions of the dowsers and experimenters. Declines in success are typical of many psychological and psi experiments. This may be due to factors of fatigue and boredom with experimental tasks, as well as with the dowsers' perception of a lack of true need for the application of their psi abilities in many laboratory conditions.

It is unfortunate that Pohl's and König's reports on medical dowsing do not review the German literature critically, and that Bachler shows little appreciation for scientific methods in her reports. Dr. Blumenthal's investigations appear to be the most rigorous, especially his last ten cases, in which predictions were made ahead of time identifying locations where cancers later developed. The opposite seems the case with the work of Rambeau, Hager, Bachler, Douglas and Zert. These investigators presumably knew at the time they were dowsing that a cancer death had occurred or that a learning-disabled child lived in a particular house, and dowsed there for that reason. When dowsers are seeking correlations with dowsed phenomena and they know the expected outcome, their unconscious minds might bias the results in the direction they anticipate. A more scientific procedure would be to give a dowser a randomized list of addresses to dowse, including equal numbers of houses where residents have health problems and others which are problem free. However, even in this case experimental results may reflect only the clairsentience of the dowser. That is to say, the dowser might psychically (and unconsciously) detect the fact that a person with cancer had been in particular rooms, and the dowsing results could then be influenced by this awareness. Further evaluations, as in the last ten cases of Dr. Blumenthal, would be even more convincing. With this model, however, precognition on the part of the dowsers could still influence the results.

The fact that *multiple* cancer deaths occurred in particular homes is strongly suggestive of a geopathic effect. Other factors, such as EM radiation or other known environmental stressors, would still have to be ruled out in these cases.

The studies of electrodermal responses of dowsers help to confirm their subjective claims and add support to the theory that they may be responding to unconventional energies.

Surprisingly enough, these are the only scientific studies of dowsing that I could locate. It seems incredible to me that so few serious investigations have been made of a potentially valuable method of searching out natural resources, identifying harmful influences on physical health and mental conditions, and providing healing therapy.

More on medical dowsing
Medical radiesthesia is an area that has been even more meagerly explored than field dowsing. Here again, a plethora of anecdotal evidence is available, attesting to dowsers' successes in:

1. Identifying areas of geopathic stress where underground energies appear to emanate a negative influence;
2. Locating and diagnosing plant, animal and human diseases;
3. Selecting medications and determining dosages that are appropriate for treating the diagnosed problems;
4. Suggesting innumerable biological and horticultural applications, the range of which is limited only by the dowsers' innovativeness in asking "either/or" or "yes/no" questions. For instance, a common use of dowsing in agriculture is to match soil components with seed, and to recommend appropriate mineral and fertilizer additives.

The first of these applications has been discussed above. The other three differ little from any other sort of clairsentience, and seem to represent the dowsers' use of the pendulum or wand to make their psi impressions consciously perceptible. I know of no formal research in these areas to clarify whether dowsing has any intrinsic advantage over clairsentience without dowsing instruments, but a wealth of anecdotal reports on the efficacy of radiesthesia and radionics suggest that this is a fertile area for further study.

The Chinese have a rich tradition of folklore that describes states of health and disease, harmony and disharmony, as related to *dragon lines* and other earth forces.

Christopher Bird, who had a wide-ranging interest in parapsychology, prepared a very attractive, well-illustrated book on dowsing. He mentions a number of items that are relevant to spiritual healing (unfortunately these are not reviewed with scientific rigor, but they are nevertheless interesting and suggest rich possibilities for further research):

1. Abbe Alexis Bouly was a well-known dowser in France. He was able to identify specific types of bacteria in a laboratory using a pendulum. As with dousing results achieved using a radio receiver, orientation of the dowser to different compass points could influence the readings.
2. Father Jean Jurion, inspired by Bouly, successfully extended the investigation of dowsing to the diagnosis of medical problems that were puzzling to doctors.

Aubrey Westlake, a British physician, investigated dowsing and radionics over the course of many years. He postulates several levels of sensitivity at which a dowser may function:

1. The physical level, at which the operator appears to function like a radio receiver tuned to presumed vibrations of various substances.
2. The level of divination, in which the dowser utilizes sensory and psi faculties. Here the dowser appears to have a wider range of perception, and is not restricted to utilizing sensory and psi faculties. At this level, dowsers are not restricted by their orientation within the earth's magnetic field or other such factors. (Westlake considers this to be another physical level of dowsing.)
3. The level of consciousness, where the sensitive "... appeared to be on a mental level of full consciousness and became independent of the limitations of both time and space, in the sense that it was possible to recover the past, and neither witnesses[330] nor actual remedies were required and orientation was unnecessary."
4. Westlake also identifies "... still higher levels, of clairvoyance and clairaudience, but not in the ordinary psychic sense, as the vision and the speech were inward and not outward. It is the inner vision and the still, small voice that is apprehended in full consciousness and not the apparition or the trumpet of the seance room under trance conditions."[331]

Westlake notes that in (2) and (3) a technique of question and answer is often very helpful. Yes/no dichotomies are put to the pendulum, which provides answers. This can be an extremely helpful aid in clarifying medical diagnosis and treatment, yet Westlake feels that this should not be used as a *mechanical* approach to treatment. In his practice he does not focus on diagnosis, except in very broad terms:

> One deals with a sick person, a person who is out of balance, out of harmony physically, mentally, emotionally, spiritually - the object of therapy is to restore that person to a harmonious functioning as a whole.

Westlake observes that the *witness*

> ... is subjected to forces tending to restore the patient's health pattern by the removal of blockages, restoration of flows and a rise of con-

sciousness. This is mystery enough, but the main mystery is the nature of the relationship of the blood spot to the patient, as for all practical purposes the blood spot and the actual patient can be regarded as identical.

This is consistent with LeShan's theories on the mythic level of reality, in which a part of an object and the entire object may be identical in some essential, functional way.[332]

There are anecdotal reports of broad disparities in results when several dowsers simultaneously or serially gave readings on the same subjects (for both diagnosis and treatment). Dowsers explain these objections away by claiming that each individual dowser picks up on different aspects of the subject's problems, filtering them through the various aspects of their various devices and prescribing accordingly. They assert that there are many ways to shift an organism from disharmony towards greater wholeness.

Westlake found that radiesthetic readings often indicated an improved condition when the patient was close to death or even dead already. He believes this indicates that the radiesthetic readings relate to the condition of the *auric* body rather than the *physical* body. Under normal conditions the physical and etheric bodies coincide closely enough that a reading on one reflects the condition of the other. At the time of death, when the energy body is separating from the physical body, the reading reflects the condition of the auric rather than the physical. Death may be a release from suffering for many people, in which case the etheric, spirit part of the person that the dowser is reading might register as being improved.

In a similar manner radionics treatments may affect the auric body rather than the physical, and the auric body could then secondarily influence the physical. Dowsing for the condition of the aura could provide a warning of illness prior to its appearance in the physical body. Radionic treatments may also facilitate separation of the auric from the physical when death is near, thus theoretically hastening death. This can be seen as a form of healing, especially when the healee is suffering, weary and ready to die.

RADIONICS

Treating healees at a distance using a radionics device is a clear example of absent healing. Radionics practitioners claim a greater precision than healers, who do not project vibrations specific to the identified problems. They also claim that their devices may be effective in storing and projecting healing energies, and that they can tune a device and leave it to project specific healing vibrations as long as necessary. All of these claims require further investigation and substantiation.

Langston Day and George de la Warr report their extensive observations on the users of radionics devices that were developed in England a few decades ago. In connecting with a healee, Day and de la Warr wrote, "For at least one second he [*the operator*] must hold in his mind a single thought – as a result of which his solar plexus emits a wave-form which resonates with the blood specimen."

Relevant to healing, Day and de la Warr observe the following:

1. There appears to be a resonation between an object and any part of the object, including a picture of it. This enables the operators to make contact with patients via specimens of blood, urine, etc. that they place in the radionics device.

2. If a subject is rapidly rotating during the operation of the device this blurs the results. Linear directional motion of the subject did not seem to have adverse effects.

3. A magnet placed near the specimen, and rotated to a specific orientation relative to the specimen and to the earth's magnetic field, would markedly enhance the sensitivity of the device.

4. De la Warr developed a photographic diagnostic device based on these principles. It could produce pictures of the target object using a *witness*. In addition, with proper setting of the dials, it could produce photographs of the future potential or the past of that object. For instance, from a seed the device could produce a picture of the flower of that species. From a blood specimen of a pregnant woman he obtained pictures of the fetus in stages of development that were both earlier and later than its age at the time of the picture. The more displaced the images were in time, however, the hazier they appeared. The specific person who inserted the film in the camera was as critical to the success of its operation as was the operator of the dials.[333] Only a few operators were able to obtain photographs of this sort.

5. Plants removed from their original place of germination grew best if their original orientation to Earth's magnetic field were maintained at their new location.

6. De la Warr's instruments, when suitably tuned, produced distant healings of a gradual (not instantaneous) nature.

7. Though these devices seemed effective in curing bacterial infections, they failed to kill bacteria in laboratory cultures. De la Warr attributed this to a selective intelligence inherent in the cosmic forces that are involved in these processes, which would work for the greatest good.

8. These devices could be used to clear plants of insect pests. If an aerial photograph of a field were used as a *witness*, with a section of the field marked off with a pen and the operator's intention focused upon it, the insect pests from the area indicated in the photograph could be eliminated. Many experiments were done that verified this use of radionics.

9. Spring water and water consecrated by a cleric produced markedly different registrations on these devices than did untreated tap water.

Day and de la Warr speculate on the mechanisms involved in these processes. They feel that there is a resonance between the parts and the whole of an organism, and also between the whole of an organism and other members of its species. The influences of magnetic fields seem to be involved, but there may be other "fundamental rays" involved that have yet to be identified. Day and de la Warr also comment on emanations that seemed to originate in the operator's solar plexus. This was deduced from the fact that a sheet of perspex (heatproof glass) placed in front of the solar plexus partially cut off the emanations.

Much of their book is devoted to stories of the difficult times that Day and de la Warr had in trying to get the scientific community to pay attention to their experiments. The general skepticism has even led to outright refusal to consider their experiments as anything more than trickery. This resulted in part from the fact that proper controls were not instituted in the experiments.

Despite these problems, Day and de la Warr's observations seem to warrant further investigation. For instance, Cleve Backster reports results that are similar. Backster placed wires from a polygraph into a human semen sample. The donor, who was sitting about forty feet away, was then asked to sniff amyl nitrite, which is very noxious. Two seconds later his sperm showed a response. Control specimens from other donors did not respond.[334]

Lyall Watson similarly reports that when one sample of tissues from a donor is damaged with concentrated nitric acid, a second sample at a distant location often can be shown to react as well, using electronic monitoring. Watson speculates that this is a cellular response, which originally evolved as a species-specific means of communication, possibly for defensive purposes. In single-cell organisms it would be the primary means of inter-individual communication. In plants and animals it is overshadowed by other inter-organism mechanisms, but is still present as a residual ability.[335]

Edward Russell presents an excellent review of radiesthesia and radionics. The following are some items of note:

1. Experiments demonstrated that a screen of cardboard covered with tin foil is impervious to human energy fields. (No mention is made of blinds or other controls for suggestion.)
2. Ruth Beymer Drown was able to produce photographs of the internal organs of patients using radionics devices. An anesthetized patient could not be successfully photographed in this way.
3. T. Galen Hieronymous obtained a patent in America for a device with which he could grow healthy green plants in the dark (as compared to control specimens, which were pale and seemed to lack chlorophyll). Energy was conducted to the plants via wires.

Anthony Scofield is a lecturer in animal physiology at the University of London. He has investigated the influence of geopathic lines both in his own dowsing and in the practice of a wide range of other dowsers. He feels that the so-called geopathic zones may in many cases be created either by the ill person or by the dowser who is seeking them. Ley lines are presumed to be vertical "walls" of energy that stand above geopathic zones, yet when Scofield examined rooms in a building that were below rooms in which geopathic lines had been dowsed, he was not able to identify similar lines that theoretically should have been present beneath those rooms where such lines were dowsed. He notes further that he has found some lines (called "black lines") that make him feel ill when he dowses them.

Scofield has also created energy lines by visualizing them, and other dowsers have subsequently been able to identify them by dowsing. Scofield's observations are anecdotal and suggest a variety of experiments that would be easy to perform.

Scofield notes that *Curry lines* have been identified in Germany and Austria by dowsers in those countries, but not in Britain by British dowsers. When a German dowser visited England she was able to demonstrate Curry lines and local dowsers could identify them as well. However, after she left the local dowsers could no longer identify them.

Sig Lonegren, another dowser, also observes that the results of dowsing depend on the question that the dowser holds in his mind during the procedure. He points out that historically, *ley lines* correspond with the energy lines that have been identified between ancient sacred sites, and that these may be qualitatively different from other energy lines.

The Chinese identified *dragon lines* that seem similar, if not identical, to ley lines in their effects on health and illness. The Chinese have extensive systems, called *feng shui,* for concentrating or accumulating positive earth energies as well as for neutralizing negative ones.

THEORIES OF RADIESTHESIA AND RADIONICS

If we assume that dowsing is essentially successful clairsentience, this raises some interesting points.

Numerous attempts have been made to increase subjects' abilities to demonstrate psi powers reliably. Feedback has been highly successful in bringing many psychophysiological mechanisms under the control of the conscious mind. Using this method, practitioners have been able to alter their heart rate, blood pressure, skin temperature and more. All of these physiological processes were previously thought to be controlled exclusively by the autonomic (unconsciously regulated) nervous system. Extending the experience of biofeedback into research in extrasensory perception, it was hoped that if proper feedback were given for successful psi perceptions, then subjects would be able to learn to perform better with their psi abilities. Neither the receptive nor the expressive aspects of psi have responded more than minimally to feedback in the average person. If we assume dowsing to be a clairsentient skill, it would appear that this is the psi area in which feedback has come the closest to being successful for large numbers of people.

There seems to be a contradiction here between laboratory evidence of biofeedback as a method to enhance psi effects and the feedback observed with dowsers' devices in their practices. Why the former should be unsuccessful while the latter appears highly functional is as yet unclear. This may support the hypothesis of the importance of *need* as a vital factor in the expression of psi and healing.In other words, people may be more successful in producing psi and healing effects when they feel there is a true need for the use of their abilities – rather than demonstrating them to meet the needs of a laboratory researcher. Another possibility is that people who self-select to become dowsers are highly intuitive.

The same seems to apply in spiritual healing. People have been highly successful in learning to develop their healing gifts, in a wide range of courses that teach how to heal.

Dowsers' subjectively report that they tune in to vibrations of the thing that they are seeking. When it comes to treating disease by radionics, which is in fact a mode of healing, dowsers claim that they can return to normal the vibrations that have gotten "out of tune"; reimpose a healthy vibration; or identify missing elements that are needed to reharmonize total body vibrations. It seems reasonable to propose that radiesthetic devices are aids to clairsentience and that radionics is actually a form of spiritual healing, which the practitioners of radionics attribute to the devices they use. The reports on dowsing add to evidence from other research covered in this book, supporting the growing awareness of bioenergy forms of medicine.

The evidence from published reports of dowsing strongly suggest that this topic seriously warrants further study. Such study must take into account the intrinsic differences between dowsing and conventional science. For instance, we ought to give careful consideration to dowsers' explanations and theories of dowsing. For instance, it seems to be a general property of psi that it is expressed more readily in response to true, serious needs, rather than according to the demands of laboratory situations. The need factor may explain why there is a higher percentage of significant results in studies of spiritual healing than in studies of other psi effects.

There are also numerous reports from psychics and healers that skepticism and negativity in observers can inhibit the expression of their psi gifts. Non-believers will of course see this as an excuse for the inability to produce psi under scrutiny, and will interpret this as proof that psi consists of nothing more than wishful thinking, selective reports of random successful guesses, self-delusion motivated by ego or desire for fame and fortune, or deliberate fraud.

While I don't agree with the skeptics' interpretations of the evidence or of dowsers' motivations, I do agree that there is reason to ask for more research. Until more and better controlled studies are run, dowsers have only a limited scientific basis on which to lay their claims. More work is needed of the caliber of Harvalik's, Hager's, Von Pohl's and Tromp's explorations.

Research of medical dowsing would be very easy to set up with rigorous controls. This task awaits only the people to do it.

William Tiller (1971) is a professor in the Department of Materials Science and Engineering at Stanford University. He studied at Oxford University on a Guggenheim Fellowship, during the course of which he extensively investigated radiesthesia and radionics. He defines radiesthesia as

> ... sensitivity to radiations covering the whole field of radiations from any source, either living or inert. As such, this would appear to include clairsentience and telepathy. Radionics is the use of instruments to augment the sensitivity to radiations.

Tiller observes that the pendulum, the divining rod and radionics devices all serve to reduce the signal/noise ratio. They are of help to the average individual who is not blessed with the gifts of concentration that are apparently inherent in gifted healers, who can enter meditational states very rapidly and easily. He feels that psi abilities are not required for dowsing so much as a well-disciplined mind and sensitive emotional structure, although psi abilities may develop with prolonged practice of dowsing, to the point where the devices are no longer required. Tiller proposes:

... A basic idea in radionics is that each individual organism or material radiates and absorbs energy via a unique wave field which exhibits certain geometrical, frequency and radiation-type characteristics. This is an extended force field that exists around all forms of matter whether animate or inanimate... The fundamental carrier wave is thought to be polarized with a rotating polarization vector.

... The information concerning the glands, body systems, etc., ripples the carrier wave and seems to be associated with a specific phase modulation of the polarization vector of the wave and also with frequency modulation of the wave for a specific gland. Regions of space associated with a given phase angle of the wave constitute a three dimensional network of points extending throughout all space. To be in resonance with any one of these points is to be in resonance with the particular gland of the entity. The capability of scanning the waveform of the gland exists for the detection of any abnormalities.

Tiller then explains spiritual healing as follows:

Likewise, if energy having the normal or healthy waveform of the gland is pumped into any one of these specific network points, the gland will be driven in the normal or healthy mode. This produces a tendency for its structure to reorganize itself in closer alignment with the normal structure; i.e., healing of the gland occurs. Cells born in the presence of this polarizing field tend to grow in a healthier configuration, which weakens the original field of the abnormal or diseased structure and strengthens the field of normal or healthy structures. Continued treatment eventually molds the healthy organ structure and the condition is healed.

Tiller integrates Eastern cosmologies into his explanations of how dowsing works.[336] His recent work, exploring how intention can be imprinted on electronic devices, also supports the reports of Scofield regarding imprinting of ley lines through mental focus.

Larry Dossey suggests that our everyday expectations may mislead us to believe that some kind of energy must intervene in order for perceptions or physical changes in the world to occur. Nevertheless, awareness and action at a distance may occur without energetic exchanges, according to the theories of modern physics, psi research and reports of mystics through the ages.

Discussion

Field dowsing appears to have a basis in an energy form that can be blocked by various types of metal shields, and possibly by other materials as well, just as EM energies can be blocked. It may be that the human body is far more sensitive to EM radiation than has previously been appreciated by conventional science, as evidenced by Harvalik's and Tromp's experiments. The parapsychological studies of remote psi perception[337] suggest a close parallel with dowsing, which would seem to be a kind of instrument-assisted clairsentience.

Critics have objected that movements of the various mechanical devices that are used in dowsing (pendulums and rods) are not automatic but rather controlled by the dowsers themselves. Critics imply that the dowsers are deluding themselves and/or others, or even defrauding others, in representing these devices as instruments that are effective in and of themselves. There is validity to these criticisms insofar as the instruments are concerned, but this mechanistic Occam's razor cuts at a point too close to the device. Since clairsentience may manifest itself via unconscious processes within the dowsers' minds, a different hypothesis may therefore be proposed. If the dowsers themselves are the instruments that identify whatever they are seeking, their devices can be seen as feedback devices that identify what their unconscious minds are perceiving, rather than the devices themselves locating things directly in the outside world through inherent properties of the devices. In other words, the dowsers are the receivers for the information, and the instruments are like dials that provide readings from the dowsers' unconscious.

Other factors may help to explain why various devices work well for dowsers in facilitating their psychic impressions.

Numerous healers report that it is more comfortable to work in a group, or to "turn the healing over to a higher power" rather than to focus on doing the healing themselves. By taking less responsibility for making the healing happen, they become less ego-involved in offering healing. This allows them to be more totally immersed in the healing state, not worrying about how they are doing with the healing – which would become a distraction from being fully engaged in the healing process.

Similarly, in meditation practices it is a common joke that when you are thinking about how well you are meditating you have lost your focus on the meditation itself.

Applied Kinesiology is very similar to dowsing. It relies on changes in muscle strength to access unconscious, intuitive, and psychic impressions.

It would thus appear that dowsing is well within the spectrum of approaches that help people to access their intuitive and psychic awarenesses.

There is so far only limited and not very convincing evidence that map dowsing of distant locations is effective. If solid evidence is produced for map dowsing, this would suggest that a type of energy other than EM may be involved in field dowsing because of the diminution of strength of EM signals with distance. It would also indicate that clairsentience rather than sensitivity to energies emanating from dowsed items is the mechanism for dowsing.

The significant studies of Harvalik, Hager, Osis Von Pohl, and Tromp provide strong evidence of a dowsing effect. However, it is unfortunate that relatively little rigorous research has been done to establish the validity of dowsing and to explore the range of its efficacy. Numerous anecdotes attest that dowsers have successfully located natural water sources, forgotten water mains, buried electrical lines or gas pipes, oil and other minerals, missing people, archaeological remains, and land mines, and have determined the missing minerals that contribute to poor soil conditions. Dowsers have also identified the quantities of underground resources that will be found, such as the rates of flow of well and spring waters.

Research questions

Why are there differences between varying perceptions when several dowsers explore the same geographical or medical territory? How can we explain the disparate findings of British and German dowsers regarding Curry lines? The skeptic will say that it is the different projections of the imaginations of the dowsers that produce these discrepancies. In fact, there is probably a component of this sort in most dowsing, but I suspect that there are two further explanations. First, clairsentient perceptions are often colored by the perceiver, as are all data that filter through to consciousness from the unconscious mind.[338] Second, some of the geopathic zones and medical diagnoses may be projections of the minds of the dowsers, as when Scofield seemed able to visualize a dowsable line into existence, which other dowsers could then identify. Much research will be needed to clarify which hypothesis is more relevant, and to what degree.

Dowsing as a wholistic therapy

If we accept that wholistic healing is the harmonizing of energies within healees, then this should also be the goal of radionics treatments. Within this framework of healing we may more easily accept that there is indeed a range of prescriptions that might each achieve positive therapeutic ends, although the results might differ. This is similar to the variations seen with many of the CAM modalities, where assessments and responses to treatments by different caregivers applying the same modality may differ.

Although these explanations are consistent with energy medicine theories, they leave me most uneasy. The chances seem quite high that we may fall prey to Type I research errors, and allow ourselves to be convinced of "facts" that are in fact not true.

In considering the specificity of radionics from within its own conceptual framework, I have a further uneasiness. The very specificity of the modality, which is alleged to be beneficial, may also be a dangerous pitfall. If the dowsers ask the wrong questions or fail to ask the right questions, they may obtain limited or erroneous information and may therefore make poor or misleading recommendations or interventions. My pilot studies of aura perceptions, in which several sensitives observed the same patients with known medical diagnoses, seem to indicate that intuitive diagnosticians may perceive only *part* of the picture. It remains to be clarified whether dowsers and radionics practitioners can guard against this danger by asking the question, "Is there anything more I should ask or know?"

Healers who direct their unconscious minds or higher selves to identify health problems and to prescribe and/or administer the necessary vibratory treatments may be less prone to such errors. These healers' energies may also be directed toward a wider spectrum of problems. On the other hand, it may be that the broader spectrum approach is not as potent for some specific problems. It may also be that different energy medicine practitioners convey different forms or qualities of subtle energy intervention, and that each tunes in to the particular aspects of their healees' problems that they are best suited to address, and provide the interventions that their healees are most ready to receive.[339]

The current state of radionics and dowsing practices leaves so many questions unanswered that they can only be seen as more of an art than a science. In seeking medical advice from dowsers on any serious medical problem, there are two basic rules of thumb: 1. Select a dowser with a good track record, preferably based on trustworthy personal recommendations from satisfied healees. This is the usual way of selecting a healer. 2. In any case, you must not rely only on your intuition to determine whether the healers you consult seem to match your expectations and needs. You must also use common sense to assess whether they present themselves professionally, ethically, and sensibly. When in doubt, as with medical consultations, a second opinion may provide a measure of protection against misinterpretations due to the idiosyncrasies of individual dowsers. However, although it might seem logical and prudent to consult a number of experienced dowsers separately and to follow the consensus of opinions, this can sometimes be confusing.

Conversely, if we are too cautious, we may lose the benefits of intuitive diagnoses and treatments that are particular to specific dowsers.

In the end, we are left to make our personal decisions (employing logic along with intuition) as to what will cure our ills, whether we turn to conventional or to complementary medical practitioners. We might learn from dowsers to ask our own unconscious minds' advice more clearly, perhaps with the aid of their devices. At times I have personally found a pendulum or bent wire rod helpful in letting my unconscious express an opinion. The process of learning to communicate with my unconscious has been, in and of itself, a form of healing.

Dowsers have not been able to demonstrate their abilities consistently in the laboratory. Skeptics suggest that reports of successful dowsing are old wives' tales, with occasional lucky "hits" or selective reporting of chance accurate predictions, while inaccurate ones are ignored. Dowsers I have spoken with say that the powers of their trade are not to be used frivolously and that their work is accurate when used for legitimate, real-life needs. It is less successful when used in parlor games or laboratories.

Dowsable energy lines in Gaia, our planet

It has been suggested that ley lines on the earth are analogous to acupuncture meridians on the body. Further observations suggest that our planet may be a huge, living organism in its own right. Fascinating observations have been gathered to support this view.

James Lovelock pointed out homeostatic interactions between life on earth and its geological evolution. Over many eons, algae, bacteria and plants have altered the balance of gasses in the atmosphere and have stabilized the planetary temperature. Lovelock proposes that the earth's flora and fauna have transformed the planet into an extension of life at an interactional level. He named this ecosystem Gaia, after the Greek earth goddess.

> You... interact individually in a spiritual manner through a sense of wonder about the natural world and from feeling a part of it. In some ways this interaction is not unlike the tight coupling between the state of mind and the body...
>
> – Lovelock (p. 211)

Every living creature has homeostatic mechanisms that maintain its internal environment within the acceptable boundaries of temperature, hydration, nutrition, etc. that are necessary for life. If temperatures rise, for instance, the organism sweats, seeks the shade, breathes faster, or pants. Lovelock proposes that aspects of the planet earth suggest that it too has homeostatic mechanisms that maintain various conditions within particular ranges. For example, the oxygen and nitrogen contents in the air remain at fixed values, despite man's gross alterations of the environment, both in decimating or eliminating large numbers of life forms and in polluting on a massive scale. Temperatures also remain within particular limits over many centuries. The amount of water frozen in the polar caps may ebb and flow, but these shifts also remain within particular limits.[340]

John Barrow and Frank Tipler have gone so far as to hypothesize that this ecological stability must imply an inherent guiding intelligence in the cosmos. They speculate that this transcends mankind's influence by so great a factor that it overshadows all of human endeavor, making us no more than a tiny speck in the vastness of the universe. Others hold that man is analogous to an organ of the planet, acting much as nerve and brain cells. Some view man as a cancer, growing unchecked, fouling and destroying the earth-body that nurtures mankind.

> *By avarice and selfishness, and a groveling habit, from which none of us is free, of regarding the soil as property... the landscape is deformed.*
> – Henry David Thoreau

Those who live close to nature and are intuitive describe an awareness of sentience in trees, water, wind and earth. They believe it is a logical extension to suggest that healing may be effective at planetary levels, either through species-specific, collective fields, through the ecosystem as a unit, or piecemeal through successive transformation of small units at a time.

Though our focus has been on the scientific aspects of radiesthesia and radionics, these practices touch upon the spiritual as well.[341] I will close with the observations of Rev. J. C. C. Murray:

[R]adiesthesia reveals most clearly the fact that there is no hard and fast frontier between matter and spirit. The artificial divisions created by centuries of materialism taken as a matter of course until very recently, have been abolished. In their place, we begin dimly to see a continuum of vibration, of radiation, extending unbroken from the heart of so-called "dead" matter, right up through the octaves of the rays of flesh and blood and the etheric processes of the mind, to a region beyond the human spectrum in which powers from another dimension begin to be apparent. It is therefore more than possible that just here the long battles between science and religion will find their truce at last and that the radiations found and plotted out by man's intellect will coalesce with and intermingle with those discerned by the spirit. We shall discover something of the unity of creation, a unity which must be reflected in His works. We seem to be presented once again with that strange pattern of the ascending spiral which leads without a break from the heart of the stone to the heart of immortality.

COSMOBIOLOGY AND ASTROLOGY[342]

At present we can only suspect a general relationship of some kind between the whole of the human species and the whole of the electro-magnetic phenomenon that includes the sun, other stars and the galaxies.
— Robert Becker

Astrology interested us, for it tied men to the system. Instead of an isolated beggar, the farthest star felt him and he felt the star. However rash and however falsified by pretenders and traders in it, the hint was true and divine, the soul's avowal of its large relations and that climate, century, remote natures as well as near, are part of its biography...
— Ralph Waldo Emerson

Claims have been made over thousands of years that the sun, moon and planets influence our lives. Western science has considered all this to be mere superstition, but in the last few decades research has confirmed that the positions of the moon and the planets, as well as solar flare activity, are correlated with biological fields and with the behaviors of plants, animals, and man.

After H. J. Eysenck and D. K. B. Nias, I distinguish here between the following disciplines:

1. Cosmobiology – seeking correlations between the positions of heavenly bodies related to limited, discretely observable phenomena such as birth, surgical bleeding, personality characteristics, and death by murder or suicide; and
2. Astrology – seeking correlations between the positions of heavenly bodies, astrological signs, and aspects of people's lives such as compatibilities in their relationships with others, propitious and unpropitious days for various activities, and predictions of the future.

The evidence for cosmobiological influences on living systems is impressive. The research evidence supporting most of the claims regarding astrology as a science is not substantial, although there are some overlaps with cosmobiology.

An excellent place to begin our scientific review of astrology is the work of Michel Gauquelin (1969). With the help of his wife Françoise, Gauquelin has done more than any other person to establish the validity of particular correlations between planetary positions at time of birth and people's success in their professions.

His first study examined 576 members in the French Academy of Medicine. These were men who had achieved outstanding success in medical research. Gauquelin found that their birth times correlated beyond chance with the rising of

Mars and Saturn, or with the passing of these planets through the mid-heaven. As a control group he checked the same correlations for people whose names were randomly chosen from the electoral register, who had been born during the same time period as the doctors. The astrological correlations for the control group were only at chance values.

Gauquelin repeated the study with a second group of 508 French doctors who were involved in significant research, and found similarly significant correlations.

To rule out the possibility of an anomaly peculiar to his initial test populations, Gauquelin (1969) charted the positions of the sun, moon and planets at the time of birth for 25,000 prominent people in five European countries. He found that success in one's chosen career was significantly correlated with positions of the moon and of several planets at the time of birth.

Separating out 3,647 successful people involved in the sciences and 5,100 in the arts, Gauquelin found that Saturn was ascendant significantly more frequently than chance at the time of birth of the scientists, or had just passed the mid-heaven. The artists were significantly less likely to have been born with these correlations. Mars and Jupiter were correlated significantly more frequently with the births of military leaders.

Such correlations were found only for the births of people who had distinguished themselves in their careers, and not for ordinary people. Clarifying this point further, Gauquelin checked the birth dates of soldiers whose careers had been truncated by crippling injuries or death, but who had received military decorations for bravery. These soldiers also showed significant correlations between their birth times and the positions of Mars and Jupiter. This suggested that the crucial factor in determining success or failure was not a matter of destiny but rather of the innate characteristics of the individual.

Gauquelin also tested this theory with successful figures in sports. Those who had a firm determination to succeed showed similar significant correlations, whereas those who lacked ambition and vigor showed no such correlations.

This was a turning point in his conceptualizations about the relationships between heavenly bodies and human experiences. It became clear that *it was not the choice of career which was related to time of birth, but the personal characteristics correlated with certain times of birth that made for success in particular careers.*

Gauquelin et al. (1979) then classified famous people according to personality characteristics evident in their biographies, including 1,409 actors, 2,089 sportsmen, and 3,647 scientists in his subject group. Distinguishing factors included introversion and extroversion, tough-mindedness, and emotional instability. Sybil Eysenck rated each of the subjects according to these personality criteria, while remaining blind to their birth times. Irrespective of profession, the personality variables correlated significantly with the relevant planets' presence in the critical zones in the sky at the time of birth. The traits that correlated with particular planets included the following (Eysenck/ Nias):

> *Mars* – active, aggressive, quarrelsome, dynamic, fearless, daring, willful;
> *Jupiter* – ambitious, authoritarian, assertive, debonair, independent, bantering, vain;

Saturn – formal, reserved, conscientious, cold, precise, melancholy, timid, industrious; and

Moon – amiable, sociable, good-hearted, generous, imaginative, easily influenced, poetic, tolerant.

Once it was established that there were indeed relationships between time of birth and personality, the obvious question presented itself: How could the planets and the moon influence personality?

To begin teasing out answers to this question, Gauquelin studied the relationships between times of birth of successful people and of their parents. He found highly significant correlations between planetary and lunar positions at the time of birth of children and of both of their parents. Correlations are twice as strong for each parent with their child when both parents have birth times under similar heavenly bodies as their child. Correlations apply for Mars, Venus, Jupiter, Saturn and the moon, but not with the sun or other planets. *These correlations hold for natural births but not for births induced by chemicals or by or caesarian section, nor for births assisted with forceps.* Rather than concluding that the heavenly bodies influence a person's career, Gauquelin suggests an alternative hypothesis: People are born at the time which is appropriate for their dispositions.

What sort of signals could pass between people and planets? Gravity is a force that knows no limits, while electromagnetic forces diminish rapidly with distance. Gauquelin checked the correlations of births on days when planetary geomagnetic fields were disturbed. Such disturbances may occur in relation to sunspots or without known cause. He found that children were more likely to have planetary correlations with birth times corresponding to their parents' correlations with planetary birth times on days when earth's magnetic fields were disturbed. There is no hypothesis as yet to explain this association.

Being the meticulous scientist that he is, Gauquelin replicated the study on children and parents twice, examining groups of more than 15,000 couples with their children. All of the previous findings were confirmed.

Gauquelin (1980) did not find correlations between births under heavenly bodies and mental illness.

It would thus appear that either cosmic influences may result in a particular time of birth for each individual, or that births are initiated to coincide with propitious conjunctions of heavenly bodies. Eysenck and Nias suggest that it is the baby who chooses the time to initiate the birth process. They note, however, that this is a very complicated proposition because labor commences 5-15 hours prior to birth. Labor averages 9 hours in first births and 5 hours in subsequent births, and is 25% shorter when it occurs at night rather than during the day. Eysenck and Nias do not even consider the multitudes of factors influencing conception, which add further complexity to their hypothesis.

Gauquelin's studies do not question or refute the claims of astrologers that heavenly bodies continue to influence people's destinies. However, there is no research evidence as yet to support these claims.

This research was very carefully reviewed and confirmed by H. J. Eysenck, Professor of Psychiatry at the London University Institute of Psychiatry, in collaboration with his colleague at the same institute, D.K.B. Nias. Eysenck and

Nias carefully consider the responses of skeptics to Gauquelin's research. They find that criticisms by such groups as the Belgian Committee for the Scientific Investigation of Alleged Paranormal Phenomena (Committee Para) and the American Committee for the Scientific Investigation of Claims of the Paranormal (CSICOP) have serious biases, of the kind that is not consistent with forthright scientific inquiry. These skeptics claim that it is impossible to assess time of birth with sufficient accuracy to permit this sort of analysis. What they consistently ignore is the fact that control groups do not show these effects, while groups of people whose births conform to the stated criteria repeatedly demonstrate the effects to a significant degree. The Gauquelins emphasized this point again and again, using samples from several countries, and repeatedly demonstrate that people who excel in their professions show these effects while other people do not.[343] Eysenck and Nias go so far as to state:

> We have looked carefully at the arguments concerning statistical evaluation and experimental design, and we have inspected with great interest the debates between the Gauquelins and their critics on various points. We have come to the definite conclusion that the critics have often behaved in an irrational and scientifically unusual manner, violating principles they themselves have laid down, failing to adhere to their own rules, failing to consult the Gauquelins on details of tests to be carried out, or failing to inform them on vital points of the results. We have not found any similar misdemeanor on the part of the Gauquelins, who seem to have behaved throughout in a calm, rational and scientifically acceptable manner, meeting criticism by appropriate re-analysis of the data, by the collection of new data, however laborious the process might have been, and by rational argument. We do not feel that the "scientific" community emerges with any great credit from these encounters. (p. 202)

Solar effects

Relationships between heavenly bodies and other biological systems have also been observed (Gauquelin 1970). Gauquelin found negative health effects associated with solar flare activity, including heart attacks, deaths from tuberculosis, eclampsia (hypertension in pregnancy) and epidemics.

He reviews research of other scientists demonstrating the following findings:

1. An inorganic chemical reaction may be influenced by sunspot activity. Giorgio Piccardi, Director of the Institute of Inorganic Chemistry at the University of Florence, is credited with clarifying the mysterious variability in a process for removing *scale,* a calcareous deposit, from industrial boilers.

> ... Household saucepans are an example of this... and, in industry, boilers follow the same rule. These calcareous deposits would impair their function if a procedure had not long existed for descaling them. The procedure is simple: at regular intervals *physically treated* water is put into the boiler. This special water, called "activated water," re-

moves the carbonate of limestone when it is heated; instead of forming a hard and thick crust, like ordinary water, it removes the crusts already formed in a kind of scum. The procedure is very simple, but at the present time the way it works is completely incomprehensible to scientists...

... a glass phial containing a drop of mercury and low-pressure neon, is gently moved about in the water. As the buoy is moved, the mercury slides on the glass; the double layer of electricity between the mercury and the glass splits and produces a reddish glow through the neon. The water which comes in contact with the buoy thereby becomes "activated"... (Gauquelin 1970, p. 211-212)

Many scientists were skeptical that the process described above could affect the water, especially as there were no observable chemical changes detectable in the activated water. Furthermore, activated water was not reliably effective, and results might vary with the time of day, or the date. When Piccardi found that the variability in the effectiveness of the activated water was reduced by placing a metal screen over his laboratory test tubes, he was encouraged to seek an outside influence for this phenomenon. In a decade of exploration he gathered convincing evidence that this variability correlated with minor sunspot activity, which caused short-term changes; major sunspot activity, which caused eleven-year cycles of changes; and months in the year (March and September) when the earth's course through space intersects galactic lines of EM force at a particular angle, which caused lesser changes.

2. Human serum albumin changes its chemical properties in correlation with a number of solar factors. Maki Takata, a Japanese doctor, developed a test in which serum albumin flocculates (clumps) when a particular chemical reagent is added to it. The degree of flocculation correlates with women's ovarian hormonal cycles, and this test was therefore useful in gynecological evaluations. In men the degree of flocculation remains constant. In 1938, after many had been successfully using the flocculation test for several years, doctors began to report extreme, unpredictable and unexplained variability in their results with this test. Takata confirmed that this was true even in testing men.

Takata methodically examined the new responses of serum albumin in his test, discovering that identical, simultaneous rises and falls in reactivity were noted in serum from patients in distant parts of Japan and in other countries as well. In 1951, after thirteen years' work, he found conclusive proof that the variations were related to the sun. Flocculation indices rose markedly just prior to sunrise, and when the test was performed in a high-flying airplane. They fell during a solar eclipse or when the test was performed in a deep mine shaft. It was also found that the sudden variability in 1938 correlated with a periodic increase in solar flare activity. The particular aspect of solar radiation responsible for these changes is not known. Laboratory exposure of people to X-rays, gamma rays or neutrons produced effects similar to but not as marked as those of the sun.

3. German scientists G. Caroli and J. Pichotka demonstrated that both inorganic (*Piccardi type*) and organic variabilities (such as the Takata test) occurred during the same time periods.

4. Russian scientist N. Schulze found that sunspot activity correlates with reductions in numbers of white blood cells in healthy people.

Gauquelin's observations on correlations of inorganic and organic reactions with sunspot activity present a mystery as well as a caution. Students of subtle energies may themselves be subject to variability related to sunspots. This may help to explain why healing works on some occasions and not on others.

A variety of subtle energy observations appear similar to those reviewed by Gauquelin.

Burr and Ravitz report extensive correlations between geophysical conditions and changes in the biological fields of plants and animals. A. J. Becker found that sunspot activity correlated modestly with aggravated assaults and with cases of murder and non-negligent manslaughter. Victor Yagodinsky reports solar and magnetic effects on virus and bacteria.

The underlying mechanisms linking these reactions with the sun have yet to be elucidated. Viktor Adamenko reports on a study by Velkover demonstrating that certain characteristics of bacteria could reliably be used to predict solar flares one week before they occur. Adamenko proposes several possibilities to explain this effect:

1. The bacteria may respond directly to solar EM or corpuscular emanations;
2. They may respond to changes in the earth's magnetic field; or
3. They may react to some unknown emanation that has specific biological effects.

From the accumulated evidence, it is evident that solar influences upon biological systems exist. These are subtle but distinct and measurable. Further work is clearly warranted to clarify the extent and nature of these effects, which may well be relevant to bioenergy therapies.

Lunar influences
Lunar influences on various aspects of life are legendary, though many consider such reports to be no more than myth and fable. Yet various studies suggest that there may well be correlations between phases of the moon and earthly events.

In the most thorough analysis of these possible effects, Dean Radin and Jannine Rebman review reports on lunar correlates with human behaviors. These include *anecdotal reports* of: problem at or near the full moon, including increased postoperative bleeding; psychiatric disturbances, and alcoholism. Research shows significant correlations with homicides, psychiatric hospital admissions, and various other crises. Other studies show *inconsistent correlations* with madness and homicides, and other findings that could be simply coincidental, as in calls to fire and police stations. A meta-analysis in 1985 concluded that there was insufficient evidence to support correlations of lunar phase with lunacy (Rotton/ Kelly), but later published a reconsidered opinion suggesting that an effect was present but was very small, on the order of 25.7% vs. the 25% expected by chance. A review of 20 studies on lunar phases and suicide was also unconvincing (S. Martin et al).

Radin and Rebman then summarize their study in Clark County, Nevada on the correlations of lunar phase with 37 variables, including weather (sunlight, maximum, minimum and range of daily temperatures, precipitation, wind speed, humidity, and barometric pressure); geophysics (daily planetary geomagnetic indices, sunspot number, and radio flux); abnormal behavior (911 telephone emergency service crisis calls, suicides, admission to a county mental health department for observation and for treatment); crime (homicides); death rates (total, motor vehicle, and other accidents); financial behavior (average of residuals of 250 de-trended mutual funds); and "Pick 3" state lottery payouts (6 individual states and their average).

They point out that there are actually five ways to measure lunar cycles,[344] which may account for some of the variability and conflict in research reports.

Radin and Rebman present a series of analyses of data collected throughout the entire year of 1993.

1. Linear correlations were calculated for the moon phase with each variable. Then averages were calculated for periods of 1-15 days before and after the full moon, and a correlation was calculated on a 29-step sine curve of the lunar phase vs. the 29-element average variable array.
2. Correlations of maximum and minimum values with the time of the full moon were calculated, with particular focus on maximum deviations found relative to the full moon.
3. The mean values of data were calculated for each item 14 days prior to the full moon and compared to the means for 14 days following the full moon.

Significant positive correlations were noted between lunar phases and psychotic behavior; total deaths; death rate for motor vehicle accidents for men; and stock prices. Correlations were also found with the geophysical variables of daily planetary magnetic indices; sunspot numbers; and solar radio wave fluctuations. The average of 6 states' lottery payout percentages showed a significant negative correlation.

Of particular interest are findings that result when correlations with maximum and minimum values are calculated. Very high correlations were noted with the full moon for minimum temperature; maximum temperature; precipitation; barometric pressure; and crisis calls; strange behaviors; homicide overall; male homicide *increases*; female *decreases*; male deaths; female deaths; and female motor vehicle accidents.

Abrupt changes were also found in the rates of suicides (rising with the waxing moon, dropping sharply at the full moon); total deaths (dropping 7-9 days before and 2-6 days after the full moon); and crisis calls (rising sharply on the day of the full moon).

Complex spectral analyses of the data confirmed that the results are unlikely to represent chance anomalous findings.

Discussing the results, Radin and Rebman note that two types of theories explaining lunar effects include the variable of tidal effects influencing biological systems and lunar/weather interactions.[345] Critics suggest that the tidal fluctuations involve such small gravitational changes that effects on humans are unlikely, although effects on fish and on small mammals have been demonstrated. Other critics observe that just because there are correlations between lunar phase and behavior does not necessarily mean that these are related in a causal manner. A simpler correlation might be with stormy weather, which is related to moon phase, and can have a negative influence on mood – both for psychological reasons and because of changes in ions in the air.

It is also apparent that the magnitude of these changes is quite small in terms of actual numbers and percentages, despite their statistical significance. Thus the increase in psychiatric admissions from one day prior to the full moon to one day afterward was only a tenth of a person, and the increase in deaths from one week prior to the day of the full moon was only one person. Crisis calls increased by only 1.5%.

There are many other reports of phenomena on Earth which correlate with positions of heavenly bodies. Here are a few of these:

1. At or near the time of the full moon there are more homicides; aggravated assaults, as well as a wide variety of other crimes; psychiatric admissions and emergency room admissions. A slight but not significant increase in suicides was noted at the time of the full moon and the new moon.

One difficulty in these studies is to determine at which point a meaningful causal relationship might have existed between moods, mental states, behaviors, and consequences of these behaviors. For example, a crime or emotional breakdown might have occurred hours after a particular conjunction of heavenly bodies.

2. Lunar influence seems to be demonstrated in a classical study on oysters. When Frank Brown transported a dozen oysters from the seashore in Connecticut a thousand miles away from their native ocean beds and placed them in a laboratory in Illinois that was shielded from outside light, the oysters had some unknown means of identifying when the local tides would be high. After an adjustment period of about 10 days they opened their shells during these hours, even though no clues from outside light or ocean water could reach them.

3. Brown found that a rat which remained in a cage under unchanging light and temperature was half as active when the moon was above the horizon as it was when the moon was below the horizon.

4. Brown measured the activity of four hamsters for two years, recording their use of an activity wheel. Lights were turned on and off at regular intervals in the lab. The hamsters learned to anticipate the timing of the changes in lighting, decreasing their activity just prior to the lights coming on, and increasing it just before they went off. They also demonstrated significantly greater activity for four days following the full moon and for several days following the new moon.

M Klinowska studied a male hamster for a year and could not demonstrate correlations of activity with lunar phases. The difficulty with these studies is that they included small numbers of animals.

Arnold Lieber proposes that biological effects of lunar influences may be due to altered permeability of cell membranes and blood vessels. He does not present adequate evidence to support his hypothesis.

Variations in plant growth in several studies also have suggested lunar effects.

N. Kollerstrom found that potatoes grew 25 percent better if planted when the moon was in earth signs of the zodiac than when it was in water signs.

F. Brown and Chow found that the amount of water absorbed by bean seeds (controlled for temperature) was greater during the full moon. Jan Joy Panser, a biologist, found that water intake and germination of seeds correlated with moon phases.

Harold S. Burr, Professor Emeritus of Anatomy at Yale, and Leonard Ravitz, a Neurologist at Duke University, measured direct current EM fields on a wide variety of animals and plants. They found that there were periodic variations in these measurements that were consistent across the entire range of measured species, and that correlated with atmospheric and geomagnetic potentials, lunar cycles, and sunspots. These scientists were able to reproduce their findings many times, but their experiments still await replication by others.[346]

Vlail Kaznacheyev noted that frog hearts studied in the laboratory responded differently in different seasons to various experimental procedures.

Geomagnetic energies appear to be possible sources for many of these observed effects. For instance, the research on biological resonations with the Schumann standing waves was mentioned in Chapter 3.

All of these plant and animal studies await replication before any firm conclusions can be drawn. However, they appear to suggest that biological systems – including human beings – are sensitive to and influenced by geomagnetic and other geobiological energies.

Psi and geobiological effects

George B. Schaut and Michael Persinger, at Laurentian University in Canada, found that telepathic transmissions were more likely to succeed on days when there was low Earth geomagnetic activity, relative to attempted transmissions on the preceding or following days. This effect was not observed with precognitive reports. Several confirmations of these observations have been published. They suggest that extremely low frequency (ELF) bands may be implicated as carriers for telepathy.

Stanley Krippner retrospectively reviewed results of his dream telepathy experiments. He found statistically significant differences in successful telepathic transmissions, correlated with phases of the moon. The second quarter, around the time of the full moon, was the most favorable.

A Russian psychiatrist, Dr. Soomere, reported findings exactly opposite to those of Krippner. There were significantly fewer cases of spontaneous telepathy in his series during the full moon.

In another experiment, Krippner found results similar to Soomere's, thus contradicting his own initial findings. There were fewer successes with a test of clairvoyance during the full moon.

An unidentified editor of the journal *Spiritual Frontiers* reports on a number of healing studies related to geobiological effects:

1. Dr. Setzer performed a double-blind study on the effects of water left in church sanctuaries on the growth of radish plants, compared to the growth of radishes

given tap water. Those that got the church water grew more, overall, but at an erratic rate that was related to moon phases. A high degree of correlation was noted but no numbers or statistics are presented. Water "taken from church close to the second and fourth lunar quarters (when the gravitational pull of the moon is increasing) always produced spectacular plant growth[W]ater... close to the first and third quarters produced growth less than or no better than the [control] plants... "

2. Edward Brame, an industrial scientist, found that water kept in churches during services showed an alteration in its infrared spectrophotometric pattern on Sundays near the full and new moon, and no effect at the half moon.

Discussion

Evidence is accumulating that the positions of heavenly bodies and solar flares may be correlated with physiological processes of living organisms, as well as with various biochemical and industrial processes. The nature and import of these correlations are still a matter for conjecture. In some instances we may hypothesize causality (e.g. ionic radiation from solar flares, or tidal gravitational effects of the moon), though in others (e.g. positions of planets) the links between heavenly and earthly events may be tied to non-linear levels of causalities.[347]

Influences of the moon and of solar flares on health appear to be negative. This may have to do with gravitational effects, especially in the case of the moon. *How* these forces influence living organisms is as yet entirely unknown. The sun may emanate a field and/or rays that affect biological systems either directly or secondarily – after interacting with the Earth's atmosphere or fields (perhaps by shifting atmospheric ionic balances). Gravity, EM fields, cosmic rays, or other unidentified energies or fields may be involved.

Although we view lunar effects as being caused by the moon, they are usually maximal when the moon and sun are aligned in gravitational opposition to the earth, so a solar contribution may be relevant to lunar geobiological effects.

It is worth noting that "activated" water, which cannot be distinguished chemically from normal water, has a different interaction with calcareous deposits compared to the effects of normal water. This suggests that the effective alteration in activated water may be the result of an energy field alteration. Spectrophotometric analysis of activated water might reveal changes similar to those identified in healer-treated water.[348]

The manifestation of bacterial sensitivity to sunspot activity a week prior to the appearance of the sunspots suggests that there may be forms of energy emitted by the sun that are detectable by living organisms but as yet unidentified by modern science. Interference in psi perceptions by geomagnetic activity likewise suggests that there may be an unidentified energy that is common to both, or that telepathy is somehow related to electromagnetism (despite the fact that it does not diminish with distance between participants). Alternatively, the effects upon psi may be secondary to effects upon the brains or other physical features of the participants.

Kaznacheyev's observations on seasonal variability in frogs' hearts may relate to geobiological influences, or to hormonal differences due to seasonal variations in frogs. These might be related to temperature or life cycle fluctuations and unrelated to direct influences of heavenly bodies.

Of relevance to spiritual healing research is the caveat that healing responses may fluctuate with geobiological conditions. This would mandate that appropriate controls be instituted in all experiments. The simplest method would be to pair experimental and control trials as closely as possible in time. At the least, such influences should be retrospectively sought and factored out of the data. This may potentially be another factor that could explain some of the seemingly irregular expressions of healing and psi effects.

Ecopsychology

In a more immediate sense, we are closely related to the planet Earth. Theodore Roszak coined the term *ecopsychology* to indicate this relationship. He focuses on our innate need to commune with nature both physically and psychologically.

This review of bioenergies suggests that our relationships to Gaia are even more intimate than we may have supposed, due to our energetic relationships with the cosmos. We are an integral energetic part of the ecobioenergetic system of our planet. I discuss this subject further, as well as our spiritual relationship with Gaia, in the next two volumes of *Healing Research*.

> *Just as light and gravity extend forever into the cosmos, connecting galaxies and stars and planets across the universe, so our consciousness extends everywhere and everywhen.*
>
> – D. B.

CHAPTER 5

Self-healing approaches and exercises:
Bringing in light to deal with shadow

... and the day came when the risk to remain tight in a bud was more painful than the risk it took to blossom.
– Anais Nin

INTRODUCTION

Self-healing can offer enormous benefits for physical and psychological problems. You can explore many avenues for dealing with your symptoms and issues through the many paths to self-healing described below.

As detailed in earlier chapters, your body, emotions, mind, relationships (with other people and with your environment) and spirit all work together to create the state of health you are experiencing. Some of the self-healing methods described below are designed to address specific levels; others invite engagement on all of these levels. A shift on any one level can facilitate shifts on all of the others. When you relax physically, you will have an easier time relaxing mentally and emotionally. When you meditate, you also relax, focus and discipline your mind, learn to choose when and how much to engage your awareness with your emotions, and may open to spiritual awareness and healing. Being open to changing on all levels and using healing practices to help access your resources on each level can markedly facilitate your self-healing.

Western society generally addresses the body as a physical thing to be treated mechanically and biochemically. Wholistic medicine views the body as an intimate part of your entire being, a participant in your emotional, mental, relational and spiritual life. An aspect of your inner self may speak to you through your body – for instance, when tensions are building up in your mind or relationships and you start to get headaches, backaches or stomach cramps. Listening to your bodymind when it speaks to you in such ways can help you de-stress.

If you address your symptoms, dis-ease or disease as challenges that invite you to learn more about yourself, you may come away enriched through these self-healing exercises – rewarded by resolution of your symptoms, but also rewarded even when your symptoms are not always eliminated. You can learn how to deal with them in new ways, and can learn to listen to what your inner self is inviting you to become aware of.

BACKGROUND

Our need for rigidity and structure stems directly from our unwillingness to face the pain of our childhood experience. Mythology tells us that the wound is both necessary and inevitable – necessary to initiate the growth of the child into an adult, and inevitable to our individualism.
Michael Greenwood and Peter Nunn (1994, p. 145)

It all starts when you allow a child to program your lifetime computer. As we observed in Chapter II-1, a child's best way for handling disappointment and pain may be to stuff away the hurt and angry feelings deep inside, beyond the reach of conscious awareness. It can be an enormous relief when you no longer feel the pain.

Denial, ignoring pain, and repressing it in your unconscious mind may be helpful as well when you experience traumas as an adult. You may function better by denying the seriousness of a problem – as when you respond to a physical crisis, to the first shock of being told you or someone in your family has a serious illness, or when someone who was close to you is unexpectedly unable to be there for you. Without some measure of denial, you may feel overwhelmed and may find it difficult to carry on with your life. By going into a denial mode, you conserve your energies for managing the crisis and the challenges that it presents.

While denying or stuffing away your problems relieves your distress, it may also create a series of problems at the same time. When you stuff your unpleasant feelings, it leaves you dragging around a bucket of old garbage. When you are older and no longer helpless to deal with stress and distress, your inner computer will still be programmed as it was in childhood: when something new comes along to upset you, your habit will be to stuff it away. You may eventually reach a point at which your bucket is so full that it sloshes over whenever something further is dumped inside.

This is why people erupt in excess anger over minor issues, as when someone "makes you angry." No one can make you angry other than yourself, as we noted in the discussion on defense mechanisms in Chapter II-1. Rather than responding to a provocation with anger, you could respond by avoiding that person, by asking him what is upsetting him, or by asking yourself what you might have done to contribute to his anger.[349]

Another childhood program is to run away from unpleasant experiences. Again, this is helpful in when we are young, when we don't have the understanding or the power to sort out, control or change unpleasant situations. Running away from issues and distancing ourselves from threatening situations reduces anxieties and fears. However, this easily becomes a habit that serves us poorly as adults. Running away from our *shadow* – that part of ourselves which we are not comfortable looking at or feeling – simply perpetuates our problems.

Most of us have these childhood programs, and we tend to notice our bucket when it ends up overflowing. This is a wake-up call to deal with the bucket in more constructive ways.

This chapter offers you many options for dealing with whatever may upset you.

REASONING YOUR WAY THROUGH STRESS

Personality factors in stress

> ... the dream of a country where every man will respect the dignity and worth of the human personality.
> That is the dream...
>
> – Martin Luther King, Jr.

Each of us has our distinct and unique personality – characteristics that are composed of hereditary traits, shaped by our life experiences. Understanding these factors and taking them into consideration can help you understand yourself and those who are near and dear to you, but whose personalities may clash with yours in significant ways. Understanding your differences can help you adapt to them.

Alexander Thomas and colleagues identified a series of traits that were evident when you were a month old, and will persist as predispositions with minimal changes throughout your life. These include:

1. *activity levels* – high or low in general, being more awake in the morning or in the evening;
2. *rhythmicities* in eating, sleeping and other activities – preferences for regular periodicity or for irregular schedules;
3. *adaptability* – flexible and going with the flow, or unbending and easily rattled by changes;
4. *approach/ withdrawal* – extroverted and reaching out spontaneously, or quiet, introverted and passive;
5. *threshold for response* – sensitive and quick to respond, or unbothered and slow to respond to noise, intrusive touch and other environmental stimuli;
6. *intensity* – preferring soft, gentle and quiet exchanges, or rough and tumble interactions;
7. *moods* – even, with a narrow range, or punctuated with wide-ranging ups and downs;
8. *distractibility* – shifting gears easily or with difficulty from one awareness or activity to another;
9. *persistence* – remaining focused on tasks with greater or lesser intensity.[350]

Understanding these factors may help you adjust your life to achieve greater harmony in many ways.

First, write down a list of ways in which these factors apply to you. These are not to be viewed as *either/ or* items, because we all have some measure of each polarity. So give yourself a number from 1 to 10 (10 being the strongest you can imagine anyone being in regard to that factor). On item #1, you may have high activity levels during one part of the day, lower levels at other times.

Next, go through the list, asking yourself where any of these factors contribute to stresses in your life. For instance, adaptability (#3) is a common rub. You may be festering over the ways that things are or are not unfolding for you; or feeling you are too easy-going and flexible to the point that you let others push you aside sometimes when it's not in your best interests to give in so easily. Your threshold for responses (#5) may be leading you to over-react to minor stresses or slights from people you care about; or people may complain to you that you seem insensitive to things that are bothering them.

In general, when your numbers are towards the polarities of 1 or 10, you are more likely to find yourself uncomfortable with life's challenges or in conflict with others whose numbers on these factors differ from yours. When you are in the middle range, you may find it easier to compromise over issues related to these factors.

Having done this self-assessment, look over the list and see whether there are items you might want to examine, perhaps to work towards changing them or perhaps towards accepting that this is the way you are and making your peace with them.

Then, make a list on a separate piece of paper for someone you are close to and with whom you are feeling stressed. Better yet, see if you can get them to fill out their own responses to the list and discuss it with you. Hold your list and theirs next to each other and see where there are major differences. Often, these polarities can give spice and pleasure to your relationships. A person of great intensity, who is lively and outgoing may bond well with someone who is quiet and a good listener. A person who is a homebody may be the homemaker who gets along well with the mover and shaker who goes out to conquer the world, and returns to enjoy the warmth of their nest.

When there are major differences between people, however, there may be differences between them in their personalities that are so great or so grating that they become uncomfortable. Common differences I've helped couples sort out include:

- One who likes soft music and another who jives to Latin beats and jungle drums;
- One being wide awake late at night and raring to go, and the other who is falling asleep after 9:00 o'clock;
- One who likes to sit in the sun in a beach chair, partnered with someone who is bored just sitting still and wants to go shopping or sightseeing;
- One very focused and persistent (who liked doing puzzles with 1,000 pieces) and another who flitted from listening to a tune to doing a smattering of housework and then might want to go out for a walk;
- One who is easy-going about routines and schedules, and could have lunch any time between 11 and 3:00, or dinner as late as 9:30, and a partner who got irritable if lunch was delayed much after 12:30 or dinner past 7:00.

You may easily imagine how these differences could be challenging! Simply identifying the factors that are causing friction can clear the way for negotiations and compromises that reduce stresses. When solutions aren't obvious, friends, family or professional counselors can often suggest ways to work around these differences, or to make peace with the disparities in each one's nature and respect each other's individuality.

The same types of sifting and sorting of differences can be helpful within the framework of the Jungian polarities, represented in Figure II-2.

Vicious circles – and how to deal with them

> You suppose you are the trouble
> But you are the cure
> You suppose that you are the lock on the door
> But you are the key that opens it
> It's too bad that you want to be someone else
> You don't see your own face, your own beauty
> Yet, no face is more beautiful than yours.
> — Jelaluddin Rumi

When we are stressed we get up tight. If this happens frequently or constantly, our tense muscles will ultimately start to complain by hurting. Backaches and headaches are common results of stress, but other muscles can also spasm and ache. Once we feel the pain, the vicious circles set in:

PAIN → ANXIETY → MUSCLE TENSION → SPASM → PAIN IN-CREASES → MORE PAIN → MORE ANXIETY → and so on.

These vicious circles can be truly vicious. A traumatic experience can leave you with truly troublesome residues of tension. You may have vague anxieties or very vivid nightmares that replay the original trauma. This is a post-traumatic stress disorder (PTSD). It can include a host of physical symptoms, such as headaches, stomach aches or muscle pains associated with an original physical trauma, panic attacks, sweating, sleep onset delays, frequent waking at night and waking very early in the morning, with multiple fears and phobias all day long. In a PTSD, your fleeing response is working overtime, with alarms going off at the slightest hint of perceived danger. It doesn't matter that you can see logically that there is no reason to be afraid. Your automatic alarms have been set to such a sensitivity that they are triggered by the slightest hint of possible danger, and you cannot find the shut-off button.

In some cases it feels helpful to have a highly sensitive alarm system, because it promises to keep you very safe. The problem is that it tends to go off so often that it is exhausting, and it often goes off without anything resembling a real danger being present. Your vicious circles are then activated and strengthened, ultimately perpetuating and even worsening your problems rather than helping or resolving them.

There are many self-healing approaches for dealing with your stress and distress – at each point in the vicious circles.

CASE: "Josie" was molested by an uncle when she was eight years old. Her mother refused to believe her when she reported her uncle's inappropriately touching her in the bathtub and when he tucked her into bed at night. She didn't even bother to talk with her father, who was a workaholic and rarely at home.

Her mother's betrayal of her trust and failure to provide for her safety – even more than the sexual abuse – frightened Josie so much that she became hyper-vigilant whenever she was around men. Her unconscious mind, seeking to provide extra protection, led her to eat and put on excess weight so that she wouldn't be attractive to predatory men.

Even though she was intelligent and had a pleasant personality, she was by na-ture on the shy side. Though she went out on a few dates in high school, she would always end her relationships before they became too intimate. This pattern continued till she came for therapy when she was 33 years old. At this time, she felt awkward in all social situations, which she avoided as much as possible.

Josie's alarm system worked overtime to protect her from further sexual moles-tation. While it succeeded in its goals of keeping her safe from harm, it was so over-protective that it kept her from having normal relationships with people who could have been safe, warm and nurturing. She felt lonely much of the time and was often depressed – sometimes to the point of having difficulty dragging herself out of the bed in the morning, and occasionally even to the point of wondering whether there was any point in living.

Josie's vicious circle was:

> anxiety when getting close to people, especially men → distancing from close relationships → low self confidence → gradually increasing anxiety and awkwardness in social situations → further distancing from close rela-tionships → etc.

Many of the self-healing techniques can help to turn down the sensitivity settings on your alarm system, allowing you to respond appropriately to dangers with ap-propriate concern and action, without getting yourself into unnecessary fear and panic because of traumas in your past.

CASE: Josie used WHEE, a self-healing technique to tone down the alarm reac-tion that was ringing because of her childhood trauma. She found she was able to relax enough with men to go out on dates, but still held back from any intimacy.

When there are more serious problems, such as Josie's, a psychotherapist or counselor may be helpful.

Case: A cognitive behavioral therapist was able to help Josie work through her remaining issues, adding several relaxation techniques to her self-healing reper-toire for dealing with anxieties and fears.

The fact that this was a male therapist was also helpful to Josie to learn to relate to and trust a man. Her self-healing techniques were invaluable in reducing her anxieties – within the therapy sessions and when they arose in her interactions with men in her everyday life. She learned to identify when her alarms were going off, to pause and assess whether the situation truly warranted an alarm reaction, and when it didn't (which was nearly always the case), to calm herself down so she could respond out of place of concern rather than one of panic.

Over a period of six months Josie was able to turn a corner in her life, leaving most of her old patterns behind and setting out on a path in her life that felt firm and secure.

Old habits of anxiety occasionally were still awakened, triggered by issues related to her early trauma that she had not cleared. For instance, she discovered that climbing steps or being on an escalator when someone was close behind her made her nervous. This was because her abusing uncle had followed her up the stairs to the bedroom.

Josie had the confidence of success in confronting so many other issues that she was able to deal with these residual issues rapidly, knowing that she could reduce their negative impact immediately and then eliminate them entirely, using her self-healing techniques.

Building on successes – developing sweetening spirals

Out of clutter, find Simplicity.
From discord, find Harmony.
In the middle of difficulty lies opportunity.
                                         – Albert Einstein

Healing exercises can help in developing sweetening spirals:

With healing we may FEEL BETTER → BE LESS TENSE → HAVE LESS PAIN → FEEL BETTER → and so on...

A variety of self-healing approaches are introduced below. Please use common sense when following any of these suggestions. If your body is injured or particular muscles or joints are in pain, be gentle with them. Just as you would build yourself up to a strenuous physical workout with gentler initial exercises, the same applies with the healing exercises. If you feel uncertain or if an exercise does not appeal to you, you should not do it without consulting a therapist.

It should be clear that in considering self-healing exercises you are not being told that you are to blame for making yourself symptomatic or sick. As discussed earlier, who you are today is the product of your genetic endowments, influenced by your nutrition; physical and emotional stresses; environmental toxins in the air, water and food you take into your body; infectious organisms; allergens; and degenerative processes. Even though you may not be able to arrest or reverse all of the factors contributing to a problem, you may be able to significantly alleviate much of your discomfort and pain by working on any or all of those factors which are within your ability to change.

You have vast potentials for self-healing that you can activate through various exercises and practices. In some cases, your self-healing may activate sweetening spirals that far exceed the expectations and explanations of conventional medicine. People have started using self-healing approaches for symptoms of pain and stress, and then find that their underlying illness may improve dramatically. I have known people who had their arthritis, irritable bowel syndromes, chronic fatigue, fibromyalgia and even cancers improve significantly, and in some cases even disappear.

Regardless of how much you influence the physical aspects of your illness, your problems may prove to be amazing invitations to deep inner awarenesses, maturation and growth in insights and wisdom, and invitations to enhancements and deepening of relationships. Many people with serious illness have actually come to be thankful for the lessons they have had in the process of dealing with their problems.

> *A time of deep despair can create personal growth that we have otherwise been unable to achieve. The struggles of daily life may not be enough to break through those emotional blocks that keep us from reaching our potential. For some people, the change comes in response to a debilitating or life-threatening condition caused by an accident or illness. It may result from the process of grieving the loss of a loved one and eventually healing from the trauma of separation. I often hear or read about life-renewing spiritual development that was brought about by physical or emotional struggle. These events were horrible to live through, but many are aware that they would not have made the changes without the wakeup call.*
> – Deena Zalkind Spear (p. 47)

Most people find that they resonate with particular approaches and not with others. The more you practice these, the more quickly and profoundly they may help you.

Facing and owning your issues

> *We avoid the things that we're afraid of because we think there will be dire consequences if we confront them. But the truly dire consequences in our lives come from avoiding things that we need to learn about or discover.*
> – Shakti Gawain

If you run away from your shadow it will follow you relentlessly. This is as true of your psychological shadow as it is of the shadow you cast on the ground in the light of day.

Case: "Val" was very sensitive to the slightest hints of criticism. She would become defensive if her boyfriend looked upset when she arrived late for her dinner date; when her boss asked her if she had finished typing his letter; or if anyone seemed to be looking at her critically.

Val blamed all of these people for "making her nervous and upset." From her point of view, she was fine until these other people did things that disturbed and upset her. She had no awareness of her own behaviors that sometimes contributed to the ways people responded to her.

It was only after she began wondering why she kept losing friends and couldn't stay in a relationship that Val woke up to the fact that she herself was the root of many of her problems. One day, her older sister Cindy – whom she loved dearly and greatly respected – pointed out that Val was blaming her for making Val angry, when Cindy had had no intention of doing this and had been unaware that she was bothering Val by simply asking how Val's day had gone.

As obvious as this appeared in hindsight, it was a major revelation for Val.

No one makes anyone else upset or angry. Being upset is usually a sign of feelings that are stirred but not clarified or not fully expressed. Being angry is a choice. Instead of being angry, one might ask, "Why is my boss so demanding today?" "What could be upsetting him?" or "What have I done that upset him?"

Case: Val sat down with Cindy and helped her examine how she frequently got upset with other people. Val started to wonder out loud what it was about the situations that made her react as she did. Several interesting facts emerged.

Val came to realize that she was a very territorial person, protective of her personal space. She felt intruded upon when people came within her comfort zone without her invitation or permission, particularly when they spoke in loud voices. Many of the people who annoyed her tended to walk right up in her face to speak with her and had loud or strident voices.

Val was embarrassed to ask people to back off, even though she was extremely uncomfortable with their behaviors. She was by nature a private person and lacked confidence in asserting her needs.

Once you are ready to ask, "Why am I upset?" the doors open to understanding your feelings and reactions. You can then make the changes that will free you from your upsets.

Case: Val learned to pay attention to her needs for space and her stressing over loud voices and other noise. When possible, she made her sensitivities known to those she felt were intrusive. When not, she used self-calming techniques, such as common-sense methods of distancing from the proximity stressors and diminishing noise levels she was exposed to. When these practical measures were not sufficient, she used variations of WHEE and other relaxation and self-calming techniques.

Blaming may be stimulated by some of the shadow junk we carry around in our buckets. These are unacceptable feelings that we experience but have been told are improper, bad or against the teachings of our family, society or religion. Because we feel embarrassed, ashamed or guilty for having such feelings, we do our best to deny, ignore and bury them.

If we see behaviors in others that evoke these feelings, we may dump some of the self-critical load from our (mostly unconscious) guilt and shame buckets on those whom we catch in unacceptable behaviors. Our unconscious mind then feels better, because we have punished others for that which is buried inside, and unacceptable to ourselves.

Healing communications

"I-messages" and "You-messages"
It may be difficult to be on the opposite side of the fence when blaming is causing problems. When someone points a finger at you, the natural reaction is to feel attacked, setting off a multi-person vicious circle:

> Person 1 blaming → Person 2 feeling attacked → Person 2 becomes hurt, angry and attacks back → Person 2 (often not even aware they had been blaming and were perceived as attacking) becomes hurt, angry and attacks back → etc.

Have you ever noticed that there are people who seem able to enter a room that is tense with negative feelings and disagreements, and these unusual people simply don't get flustered? They are able to speak with hot-headed, angry and hurt people and help to calm them down. How do they do that?

Some of the secrets for dealing with stressful situations are detailed beautifully in a book by James Gordon, called *Parent Effectiveness Training (PET)*. One of his helpful suggestions: When you find yourself in a tense or conflicted situation, Gordon points out that it is wise to ask, "Whose problem is this?" You can save yourself a lot of stress, if your answer is "It's not my problem." Simply let the owner of the problem deal with it, and don't stress yourself over it.

My own response is to picture to myself that there is a good, strong fence between me and others who are agitated or upset. I stay respectfully on my side of the fence, and do my best to point out to them what part of the situation I believe is on my side of the fence and what part I feel may belong to them.

Notice that I really am staying on my side of the fence, even when I'm speculating on what part of the tense situation might belong to them. I express this as *my feelings of what may belong to them.* So, in the first place, I am stating that these are my own observation, and then I allow that there are parts of this which *may* belong to them – in both instances staying on my side of the fence by not suggesting that I know what is on their side of the fence.

Case: "Ted Fox" was still sputtering and complaining as he walked down the hall with me for a psychiatric evaluation of his four year old daughter, "Kelly." Due to an error in scheduling, he had had to wait with this severely oppositional and defiant girl, who could not sit still for more than half a minute, and was constantly getting in arguments and fights at home and in her pre-school. I apologized in the name of the clinic over the scheduling problems. He responded in a loud voice with complaints about how our clinic is run, and how insensitive secretaries are in general to the needs of the public.

I continued with an acknowledgment of his justifiable anger. "I can understand your being upset over the confusion in the appointment."

He continued, with considerable anger, "You haven't a clue how frustrating it was to have to wait for two for this appointment, to take the day off from work, and then to be told we couldn't' be seen – I'm just not ready to put up with that kind of crap."

Despite his upset, we managed to navigate through the formalities of a thorough history, the details of Kelly's difficult behaviors, and the frustrations Mr. Fox and his wife were having in their struggles to deal with her. It was difficult managing this interview, as Kelly was constantly moving from one toy to another and having trouble abiding by my rule that she had to put away the one she was playing with before taking out another. (Her father was very ineffectual at setting limits on her behaviors.) When I suggested that counseling might help in addition to the medications Mr. Kelly was anticipating I would prescribe, he exploded in anger again, shouting at me, "So now you're blaming me and my wife for making our daughter behave this way!"

Taking a deep breath, I responded, "I see that Kelly is quite a handful. She's also very clever, and I think she may have figured out ways to get around you and her mother."

"You're saying we don't know how to handle a four year old girl!" he growled.

I responded, in as calm and firm a voice as I could manage, "I'm saying I hear how frustrating it must be having a daughter who is constantly getting in trouble and arguing all the time. I've treated many children like Kelly, and I've helped many parents like you and Mrs. Fox to sort out ways to help their children behave better."

He responded a little less angrily, "You're trying to tell me you know how to raise my kid better than me and my wife do. You haven't lived though her hour-long tantrums like we have."

"No," I said, "I haven't had that very frustrating experience. I can feel just how challenging that must be. What I'm saying, though, is that I've seen enough children with problems like Kelly's that I can sometimes save the parents I see considerable time in figuring out the best ways to help their child settle down when she's getting upset."

Notice that I am staying on my side of the fence, even when I'm speculating on what part of the challenging situation might belong to Mr. Fox and his wife. I express this as my feelings and understanding of what may belong to him. So, in the first place, I am stating that these are my own observation, and then I allow that there are parts of this which may belong to him – in both instances staying on my side of the fence by not suggesting that I know what is on his side of the fence.

I avoid using the word "you" in a blaming way. Whenever I say "you" it is likely that a person who is upset will feel I am pointing a blaming finger at him. I do my best to keep to my side of the fence, using "I-messages" to explain how I understand the situation.

This invites the other person to state how he understands and feels about the situation. If he points fingers and blames me, I don't respond defensively and don't attack even when I feel I am being attacked. This is not to say that I just lie down and let myself be verbally beaten or unfairly blamed. If I sense this is happening, I may say, "I feel hurt that I'm being accused of --- when I don't see what I have done to earn this blame." (Notice that I remain firmly on my side of the fence with "I-statements" and don't say, " -- that you're accusing me of --)

This invites the other person to say what I may have said or done that upset them – from their side of the fence. Even if they state their complaints and accusations in "you-statements," I don't bite the blame-bait and respond with a counter-blame or attack. I stay firmly on my side of the fence and continue to state my own opinions and feelings.

By staying firmly on my side of the fence, and clearly owning my feelings and opinions, I avoid provoking others and keep from adding fuel to the fire.

This is the principle of non-aggressive defense. While it may appear to open you to further attack, it leaves you (hopefully more calmly than if you engage in aggressive responses) observing and commenting on your side of the fence, and not adding fuel to the fires.

> *Communication is to a relationship what breathing is to living.*
> – Virginia Satir

Experiential exercise: Conjugations
How we say things to each other can soothe or provoke. It can be fun and helpful to practice "conjugating" various statements in order to sensitize ourselves to the "how" of our communications.

Here are several examples:

> I'm a teeny bit overweight.
> You're kind of chubby.
> He's a fat slob.

> I tend to say what I have to say very directly.
> You're rather blunt at times.
> She's a sarcastic ass.

> I can be distracted sometimes when I'm driving.
> You're a bit careless changing lanes.
> He's a frustrated LeMans racing driver.

> I'm upset.
> You're angry.
> She's a flaming fury.

> I slipped up.
> You made a mistake.
> He screwed up

Such exercises are not just for humorous entertainment. They can help us to choose the most healing approaches when we're expressing angry thoughts and feelings, cutting others the slack that we allow for ourselves.

Active listening

> Between
> What I think
> What I want to say
> What I believe I say
> What I say
> What you want to hear
> What you believe you hear
> What you hear
> What you want to understand
> What you believe you understand
> What you understand
> There are 10 possibilities we might have difficulties to communicate.
> But let's do it anyway.
>
> – Anonymous

Many misunderstandings occur because we misperceive or misunderstand each other's words, feelings and intentions. A way to assure that we are truly understanding each other is to practice *active listening*. To do this, you simply repeat what you have heard, putting it into your own words, before you respond to what the other person is saying. If you have heard it accurately, the person you are speaking with will simply listen as you respond. If you have not understood it correctly, the person will explain it further until you have caught their full meaning.

While this might appear to you to be a tedious process, it is actually one that usually leads to a good feeling between people who use it. They feel heard and understood, and know that there is good intention in the communication process.

Active listening is best appreciated through trying it out and practicing it.

Cognitive behavioral therapy (CBT)

> *When you lose, don't lose the lesson.*
> – HH The Dalai Lama

CBT addresses problems through logical analysis and reason. If you have an unrealistic fear, you can assess the degree of likelihood that there is actual danger in what you fear and then reason your way around it, and develop ways of dealing with it.

While this usually requires a therapist, you may be able to help yourself. You can sit down and assess your situation, then figure out a variety of ways to let go of some the stress and distress you are experiencing. A trusted family member or friend can be helpful with CBT.

CASE: "Carol" had a fear of dogs ever since she had been bitten by a Rottweiler when she went into a neighbor's yard to retrieve a ball when she was 5 years old.

At 32, her fears were an embarrassment to her, as she would cringe and draw to the side of the street, and if possible cross to the opposite side of the street if a dog was being walked towards her. Her children were also starting to fear dogs, following her behaviors.

Carol realized that in the 27 years since she had been bitten, she had rarely seen another dog on the street who really looked likely to bite her. She was eager to let go of the alarm system she was carrying that rang whenever a dog came near – due to her old childhood trauma.

She reasoned that she could probably force herself to stand still while smaller dogs were walked by her on a leash, as a start in overcoming her fears. So the next time a small dog came along, she waited by the curb, at a gap between two cars, so that her escape route would be assured should she need one. To her enormous relief, the dog completely ignored her. This gave her the courage to repeat her challenges to the anxieties her unconscious mind was raising whenever a dog approached. Gradually, she worked her way up to allowing larger and larger dogs to pass her while she remained ready to flee if she should feel she was really in danger.

In this way Carol was able to overcome most of her troublesome fear of dogs. She had no wish to be friendly with dogs or to own one. She was happy to be able to walk down a street with her family and not be embarrassed – although she did still keep a wary eye out when larger dogs were near her.[351]

A cost/ benefit analysis (CBA)

> *The price of anything is the amount of life you pay for it.*
> – Henry David Thoreau

Focused and organized sorting and sifting of issues and alternatives can bring order to what feels like hopeless chaos and confusion. This can be done as a cost/ benefit analysis of your situation, which can help you decide on where to invest your energies, when to put issues on a back burner, and when to relinquish struggles to a higher power.[352]

For instance, listing how your symptoms help you and how they hinder you can be a good start at dealing with a stressful situation. Actually putting this down on paper in black and white can often give you a new perspective on your issues.

CASE: "Zack," a housing contractor, had had recurrent severe headaches for over 20 years. They started in his late teens when he was cramming for exams. Initially he handled these tension headaches with over-the-counter painkillers. Gradually, he found he was needing higher and higher doses, and started suffering constipation, which is a side effect of the medication. He was reluctant to use the stronger pain medication his doctor had prescribed, because his father had a drinking problem and his brother was struggling with multiple drug dependencies.

He sought advice from friends. Some were disappointingly lacking in sympathy for his situation, and he regretted even mentioning his problem. Others – often those who had suffered headaches or other pains themselves – empathized with his struggles to overcome the pains in order to work and carry on with his life. One mentioned that she had found relaxation techniques enormously helpful in making her headaches less severe and less often. Another pointed out that psychological stress often worsened his backaches, which alerted Zack to start thinking about the stresses in his own life. A third related how she had had to make a difficult decision about whether to stay in her high stress job as assistant manager in a fast food restaurant, when she found her headaches ruining her marital relationship and seriously detracting from her enjoyment of life in general.

Putting it all together, Zack spent the better part of a weekend examining the stresses in his life and what he could do about them. To his surprise, his wife was tremendously helpful in discussing his analysis, adding many observations and suggestions for dealing with his headaches. Previously, he had generally been reluctant to burden her with his pains, which he had seen as something he simply had to bear, making the best of life despite their debilitating drain on his energies.

Zack realized that his job was enormously stressful, with many problems every day due to late deliveries of building materials, delayed schedules of one part of the construction that put off other parts which depended on the earlier work being completed, and site owners constantly pressuring for prompt completion of the contract. Then there were personnel issues, with one worker who was lazy and needed constant supervision, another who was sarcastic and annoying to work with, and a secretary whose mother was ill and needed someone to accompany her on hospital visits. Finances were tight and bills for his three growing children's clothing and his own home repairs were also stressing him. His wife, Trudy, had been staying home to mother the children, and had not been able to find work in the six months that their youngest child had started kindergarten.

Zack made several lists. The first had two columns: one for problems he could influence and the other for those which were beyond his control. He found that just making this list was a small relief, because it identified some problems that he had been stressing over when there was absolutely nothing he could do to change them. These included the high level of impatience of one of the site owners and his wife's unemployment. Both seemed likely to be resolved within a reasonable time.

The second list was for the time that would ideally be budgeted to handle each of his problems, and whether he wanted to invest that time. Notable with this list was that it helped him truly appreciate the past excellence and loyalty of his secretary and resolve to support her during her mother's illness in every way he could; to plan to replace his lazy worker as soon as possible; and to promise himself he would regularly discuss his problems with his wife.

His third list proved more difficult. This list arose from his strong impression that two of the friends who had spoken with him had made when they mentioned they sometimes found their pains offered unexpected benefits. One friend's headaches seemed clearly to be a message that her job stresses were more than she could handle. His other friend found it was helpful that he had a bad back when his wife wanted to visit her mother, who lived a two-hour drive away

Zack realized his headaches were like red lights on his truck panel – warning him when his emotional radiator pressure was too high, that he needed to check the lubricants in his relationships, and that in some situations. His emotional fuel reserves were running low. He resolved to carry a little notebook with him and to write down what stressors preceded each headache.

At the end of the week, he sat down again with Trudy after the children were in bed to review his scribbled notes on possible contributors to his headaches. He was struck by the fact that they seemed to come on very frequently, but not in-variably, after someone made him angry.

Trudy reminded Zack about how she had gotten a lot of stomach cramps when she was around her former employer, who was constantly criticizing her secretarial work and never let her know when she was doing a good job. His sarcastic manner in particular had left her constantly worried and feeling she was no good. Her worst cramps came when she sorely wanted to tell her boss off but held back out of fear of losing her job. In discussing this with Zack, she came to a deeper understanding of how she had been swallowing down her feelings of frustration and anger, which ended up in stomachaches.

Listening to Trudy, Zack realized that his worst headaches came when he was biting his tongue, holding back his frustrations and angers. During the week, he noted that there were times that he was just as angry but said or did something to discharge the anger and then did not get headaches. He resolved to carry a stress ball in his truck and to take every opportunity to release tensions when he was driving between work sites. Trudy encouraged him to close the windows of the truck and yell out a few choice words that he was probably better off not saying directly to the people who were frustrating him.

Trudy also pointed out that his headaches might alert him to problems that he could address through practical responses – such as he had done already by replacing his lazy worker.

In essence, CBT generally offers common sense solutions to problems. There is absolutely no reason why you shouldn't do some of this yourself, as self-healing. The difficulty may be in standing outside your situation in order to see and understand what the problems are. It may be difficult to realize how you could be contributing to a problem or how you could change the situation when you are in the midst of a conflict or simply stuck in problematic ways of seeing and hearing yourself and others.

A trusted family member or friend may be enormously helpful (as was Trudy with Zack), by providing a new view on issues that may have you stuck in ruts of habit – both in thinking about your problems in certain ways and in responding to your problems out of old habit programs. A therapist can also add many dimensions to this work – through her knowledge of psychological defenses, therapeutic ways of addressing issues, and clinical experience of having helped many people with similar issues and problems.

Other forms of therapy could be effective in addressing anxieties and fears, depending on your preferences.

See also: Breathing; Conditioning; Imagery/ Visualization; Muscle relaxation

Personal space, ambience and sacred space

> *I fill the rooms with the vibration of love so that all who enter, myself*
> *included, will feel this love and be nourished by it.*
> – Louise Hay

Stress can sometimes be subtle, perhaps even outside of our conscious awareness. The vibrations of the space we live in and work in can be healing or stressful. Most of us have had the experience of coming into a room and noticing that it had positive vibrations which made us feel warm and welcomed, or negative vibrations which made us fee we'd rather not stay there. This is a bioenergetic reality, not just our imagination.

Positive vibrations are built up when there is peace, harmony, acceptance, love and healing in a space. Negative vibrations accumulate when there is frustration, impatience, anger and hatred.

We can enhance our abilities to deal with stress by choosing environments with positive vibrations, avoiding those with negative vibrations (to the extent possible), and seeking ways to bring healing vibrations into negative spaces.

The first attention should be to your personal space. This starts with everything that is outside your skin. Finding the soaps and creams that make your skin feel comfortable, taking the time to bathe or shower and to nurture your skin prepares you to meet your environment with a clean slate, so to speak.

Choosing clothes which you find comfortable, including fibers, textures and colors that suit you can make an enormous difference in how you feel about yourself. Clearing clutter and making your home and work space tidy and appealing creates positive spaces in which you can feel an inner calm in resonation with the outer calm. There are specialists in environmental energies who can help you enhance the bioenergies of your space, particularly when you feel strong negative vibrations there. For negative bioenergies you might seek a *Feng Shui* consultant; for negative earth energies a dowser; and for electromagnetic pollution an expert in environmental medicine.[353]

Meditating, praying and inviting healing into a space can markedly improve the bioenergies. This is something you can readily do yourself. Regular practice will improve your abilities to do this and will build an increasingly positive ambience in your personal spaces.

Interpersonal space

> *Distance can be deceptive*
> *Sometimes when I'm close to you,*
> *I find you're very far from me.*
> – Ashleigh Brilliant

Your bioenergies extend into the space around you. They project the energies you are emanating – be they peacefulness and healing or negativity and irritation. Others will be able to sense your energies, just as you sense theirs.

Depending on your sensitivities, you may be uncomfortable when others, particularly strangers or people you don't trust, enter the space within which your energies may interact with theirs. Most people have a comfort zone that extends 1-5 feet in front of them, somewhat less wide to their sides, and again wider at the back. Some may find their interpersonal comfort zone to be wider yet. Knowing this, you may prevent stress by keeping a reasonable distance between you and others.

Turning worry into concern

> *A young boy had a phobia about monsters under his bed which kept him from going to sleep at night. Numerous conventional counselors and therapists were unsuccessful in helping him overcome his fears. Pulling at straws, his parents took him to a rabbi who had a reputation for solving unsolvable problems.*
> *The rabbi's advice: Cut the legs off the bed.*
> *The problem disappeared when they followed his advice.*
> – Anonymous

A problem can feel overwhelming in its enormity.

CASES: Gloria, a mother of six young children was widowed when her husband was killed at a bus stop by a hit and run driver. Joshua, a high school teacher in the prime of his life and career, was diagnosed with a malignancy that has spread beyond surgical cure. Twelve year-old Delia, removed to a foster home following a rape by a family member, had to be moved yet again because another foster child in the same home touched her inappropriately.

The best of caregivers may feel seriously challenged when asked to help to deal with such problems. Self-healing may seem utterly inadequate to deal with issues of this magnitude – yet they can be enormously helpful and in many cases can actually help a person deal effectively with their challenges.

Taking stock
The first commonsense approach is taking stock. Listing problems and resources puts perspective to a problem, shape-shifts a monster-sized issue out of the worry and panic category, partializes it into manageable chunks, and moves it into a series of *to do now* and *to do later* boxes.

Take stock and make lists of all resources – current and potential. There are often relatives as well as friends and colleagues at work, at church or in schools who are available and willing to lend a hand if asked.

Do an internal check on whether you're holding back from asking for help. Many times we hesitate to request assistance when others are more than willing to offer it. Ask a trusted family member or friend whether they feel you are as open as you can be with asking for help. You may be surprised to learn that they find you less open to receiving help than you realize. (More on asking, below.)

If finances permit, hired help such as extra childcare or home care may be invaluable.

List all problems and issues needing your attention and decide which require immediate attention and which can wait for a period of time – entering calendar dates next to those allocated for future resolution. Mark in red any delayed issues that have critical consequences if ignored for too long, such as bills, medication refills, mailing out employment résumés, registrations for school or other critical and time-sensitive jobs.

Start each day by reviewing the list, to see if there are any critical issues to attend to immediately.

Turning troublesome worry into appropriate concern
Lists are not just for managing outer-world problems and resources. They can also help deal with stress and anxiety. They can help you turn worry and panic into appropriate levels of concern and action plans.

Your stressing over your problems can be an enormous drain of energies. You may find yourself stressing and anxious about your worrying; blaming yourself for creating or perpetuating the problems; or fretting that you aren't dealing better with the situation. I call this *meta-anxiety*.[354] This is a layer of worry you can definitely release with self-healing.

You may add to your list those exercises and approaches from this chapter that are most likely to help you deal with problem items on your list. You may create a column for helpful resources such as these on the problems page, or on a separate sheet. (Lists such as these, by the way, are good to keep in a journal where you log your progress and put your experiences and feelings into written words.)[355]

If you still find yourself stressed from worrying over practical problems – after you have made your lists and sorted out what you can do about pressing issues – you may wish to re-assess how you are allocating and using your inner resources. Ask yourself if worrying is helping you solve your problems and deal with them. Worrying will usually waste inner resources rather than being productive. (See *cognitive behavioral approaches*, above, for suggestions in how to reason your way through issues like these.)

Once you've attended to the urgent items list for the day, set it aside. You've done what you can do for that day and can now use your energies constructively for enjoying life. Yes, it is possible to enjoy life even though there are problems to deal with.

> *I was asking myself why I was having these obstacles in my life... then I suddenly became aware that these obstacles were my life, and I began to enjoy them.*
> – John Kanary

Partializing
A few more words are in order about partializing problems. If you have a huge stack of bricks and think of building a house out of them, the task may at first appear utterly daunting. But if you take one brick and set it firmly in place, and

follow it with another and another, pretty soon you will have a wall, a room and then a complete house.

Brainstorming
Good old common sense can often sort out even knotty, chronic problems. (*See cognitive behavioral therapy, above.*)

Thinking outside the box can often reveal solutions to problems we feel stuck with. Set aside ten minutes to open yourself to any possible solutions to your problems – however weird, wacky or unlikely to be successful. Write down each and every one that comes to mind. Don't censor or criticize them in any way, just jot them down as they appear to you.

When you've run through whatever surfaces in your mind, look over the list and see if any brilliant solutions lie among the items you've brainstormed. While an initial idea may be impractical or unfeasible, it may contain the seed that will grow into the precise flower or fruit you need for dealing with problems that have gnawed at you for ages.

Don't forget that your intuition, your higher self, your spirit guides and guardian angels, any and all spiritual beings, and God are all available to provide support and inspiration. You can connect with these by asking for their help; in dreams; through meditation; and prayers; (*See Dreams; Meditation; Protection; Spiritual approaches for self-healing*)

Ask for help in sorting through problems and issues
We might not be able to see the light, however, if we've dug deep habitual defensive trenches for ourselves. If you cannot see the light at the end of the trench, then seeking the advice of family and friends, or consulting a therapist will often uncover overlooked inner and outer resources to deal with problems.

Discuss your problems with people whom you trust and respect. Show them your brainstorming lists. They may be able to suggest a variation to one or more of the ideas which you might have overlooked or rejected.

I have been repeatedly surprised and amazed at how consultations can help when I feel stuck – both in my own life and in my position as a therapist. Having regular consultations and supervision with a colleague is almost always refreshing and enlightening.

Ask for help in dealing with problems and issues
You may want or need to call in other experts to help with installing plumbing, electricity, doors and windows. You may not have the resources to put it all together immediately. With patience and persistence, however, you will be able in time to complete the job.

The same is true of dealing with your physical and psychological problems. If you look at the problems facing you initially, they may seem like an impossible pile of bricks and boards to sort out. They might even look more like a house hit by an earthquake – needing considerable dismantling and clearing away of old psychological rubble – before you even start the rebuilding. Take it a stick and a brick and a problem and a challenge at a time. Before long, your life will be much clearer of old emotional debris, and your new self will be a more comfortable abode.

You can reduce the intensity of your worries and even change them into manageable concerns by using the stress reduction techniques that follow.

THE BODY

Touch

> *Too often we under estimate the power of a touch, a smile, a kind word, a listening ear, an honest compliment, or the smallest act of caring, all of which have the potential to turn a life around.*
>
> – Leo Buscaglia

Physical touch can be wonderful for nurturing and de-stressing. In infants, touch is so important that without it a child will not thrive and may even die. We may experience lack of touch as "skin hunger," a craving to be given this vital form of nurturing and healing.

The caring touch of family members is probably the most nurturing.

Massage can be wonderful for de-stressing.[356]

Touching can be done through the heart as well as through the skin. We acknowledge this in common phrases, such as "He touched me deeply." "A touching moment." and "Her loving presence was touching."

Muscle relaxation exercises

> *Man is so made that he can only find relaxation from one kind of labor by taking up another.*
>
> – Anatole France

As with any exercise program, you will probably find that starting with a few minutes of an exercise and building up to longer times is easiest. However, if an exercise feels particularly good and is working effectively, you may choose to practice it several times in a day or for longer periods.

Use common sense in doing these exercises. Do not tighten any muscles during if they are injured, strained or in pain. Painful or tight muscles will often relax if you practice relaxing other muscles, particularly your hands and arms – which respond quickly because they are used to taking orders.

Single muscle group relaxation

Using your dominant hand, clench your fist and bring it up tightly towards your shoulder. Hold the tension for about half a minute, connecting with your hand and arm muscles through their tightness. Take a deep breath and *slowly* begin to release the tension in these muscles. Pay attention to how they let go of their tightness. *Slowly* let your arm relax so that your hand, which is also relaxing, gradually lowers itself until it comes to rest on your lap or at your side. Tell the muscles to continue releasing their tension while your hand and arm remain still.

Don't force your fingers to open. Let them stay curled in a relaxed position. When you feel they are about as relaxed as they can get, take another deep breath and blow out any further tension that might remain, in preparation for moving your hand. Notice any differences you can feel between your two hands.

Now do the same with your other hand. Your hands respond readily to such exercises because they are used to taking orders to grasp and release, to gesture and serve you in so many ways.

Have the muscles in the rest of your body been listening in as you tell your hands and arms to relax? As we relax any part of the body, the remaining muscles tend to relax as well.

Progressive muscular relaxation:
If you have the time, you might give yourself the pleasure of a deliberate, total-body relaxation, starting with your toes and extending upward, one muscle group at a time, through your calves, thighs, buttocks, lower back, belly, chest and upper back, hands, arms, shoulders and neck, and face.

Check back over your body after a total-body relaxation job. Look for any straggling, unrelaxed muscles. Invite them to join the rest of the crowd that are unwinding.

Benefits of muscle relaxation
Muscle relaxation is good as a general tonic, lowering body tensions. It slows or even stops vicious circles involving physical tension. Muscle relaxation is an excellent way to let go of a day's worries, or to ease yourself to sleep.

Muscle relaxation can help with specific pains. Headaches are notoriously associated with stress – as witnessed by our calling them *tension* headaches. The same is true of neck aches, where we often identify a source of stress as a *pain in the neck*, or back pains when you *get your back up* over something, or are stressed by a situation that leads you to *bellyache* about it.[357]

Tension headaches are often felt around the temples. Here is a simple exercise that will show you why. Place your fingertips lightly on your temples while you clench and relax your teeth. Notice how the muscles on your temples tense when your jaw is tight. These are your masseter muscles, amongst the most powerful muscles in your body. They connect at one end to your jaw (you can feel them tense at the angle of your jaw too when you clench your teeth) and at the other end on your skull at your temples. If you are unconsciously clenching your jaw – *literally*, in accompaniment to your *figuratively* biting your tongue – you are putting tension into these muscles. It is very common to clench the jaw unconsciously when there are words of complaint, hurt or anger on the tip of one's tongue – which we feel we cannot safely express. If these masseter muscles get overworked, they can go into spasm and will complain by hurting – letting you know they have been too tense for too long.

Muscle relaxation can therefore be of enormous help in reducing such muscle tensions, thereby stopping tension headaches and other pains due to muscles that are complaining of excess tension. Neck and back muscles, which are constantly in use – keeping your body and head upright – may also complain through pains and will be grateful for relaxation exercises.[358]

See also: Imagery/Visualization; Massage; Meditation

Massage

> *The hands of those I meet are dumbly eloquent to me. There are those whose hands have sunbeams in them so that their grasp warms my heart.*
> – Helen Keller

At workshops that I lead, simple foot, hand, back and face massages are among the most appreciated of relaxation and healing techniques. While it is lovely to have someone else massage you, there is no reason you can't enjoy simple hand or face massages that you administer to yourself.

While it is easier and better to demonstrate this than to write about it, a few simple guidelines can be helpful.

In a foot, hand or fact massage, explore to find the pressure that feels best to you. Stay flexible, even after you find a pressure you like, because on different occasions you may prefer to work with greater or less firmness. Let your own body be your guide, searching first for places that feel normal or just a little tight and working on these before you address stressed or painful muscles. If there is pain, be very gentle and again let your body guide you as to whether to persist or suffice with a light massage.

Don't put pressure on bones, as they are unhappy with kneading.

Joints may enjoy being stretched – again letting them guide you regarding the intensity of pressure you use on them.

Breathing slowly and deeply as you massage, and imaging that you are kneading in and/ or breathing in healing energies to facilitate the massage can enhance the results.

Remember that your body participates in memories. As your muscles are massaged, they may release stored up images of past physical and emotional stresses, along with the feelings that were experienced around these events. This is not a bad sign, although the experience may be as pleasant as having a tooth pulled or a boil lanced. If you go with the flow of the release, perhaps using some of the other techniques in this section to help you deal with the released feelings (such as breathing out stress and negative feelings), you will come to a place of relief. Your unconscious mind will thank you for relieving it of the burden of carrying these old hurts and keeping them outside your conscious awareness.

Exercise and wholistic fitness

> *Physical fitness is not only one of the most important keys to a healthy body, it is the basis of dynamic and creative intellectual activity.*
> – John F. Kennedy

Muscles (including your heart), ligaments, bones and joints are made for movement. These body parts are happiest when given regular exercise that keeps them toned and fit. If you haven't been exercising for any length of time, it is important to work your way gradually into a program of fitness, where you will be giving your body a workout that keeps it in good shape.

We often think of exercise in terms of jogging, going to a gym, or participating in sports activities. These are concentrated doses of exercise. Longer periods of gentle exercise can be just as beneficial, and sometimes more enjoyable. A long walk, dancing, or yoga practice can be a meditation, a social event, and can bring you healings on many levels.

People often complain that they have no time to exercise. Small doses of exercise may still be scheduled into your day, as in climbing stairs instead of taking elevators, and parking your car a few blocks from work so that you get your circulation moving after sitting for periods of time during your commute and on your job. While such brief periods of exertion will not give your heart its best possible workout, they will keep your locomoting muscles in shape.

Exercising puts you in touch with your body and its functions. When your body knows you are attending to its needs and caring for it, it is more likely to participate in and facilitate your wholistic self-healing programs. You also get in touch with your body through practicing the muscle control required for exercising. It is certainly more pleasant to get in touch with your body through health and fitness than through illness, when your body is complaining about disharmony in your life!

Exercising your physical body is also good for your bioenergy body. This is the energy field that surrounds and interpenetrates your physical body and connects you on all levels of your being – physical, emotional, mental, relational (with other people and with your environment), with your spiritual self and with the All.[359] Bioenergy flows through and around your body in a variety of ways. You have acupuncture meridians running from your toes to your head; chakras along the midline of your body; and a bioenergy field surrounding your entire body. Each of these contributes in its own way to your wellbeing on all levels.[360]

When you exercise, you also enhance your awareness of your body. This can make it possible for your unconscious mind to speak with you, especially at times when you get distracted in the outer activities of life, becoming a *human doing* instead of a *human being*, and lose touch with your inner self. At times such as these, your unconscious mind may speak to you through your body, calling your attention to dis-ease in your life through tensions, pains or other symptoms of disharmony in your body.[361] After you have responded to the messages your deeper self wants you to hear, you may thank and reward your body by making it a point to meet its needs for exercise and fitness.

Exercise can become a meditation. As such, it can bring us into *peak* or spiritual experiences.[362] Yoga, T'ai chi and Qigong are movement meditations.[363]

Your body also stores memories, particularly the traumatic ones. In some cases it can act as the "bucket" where you hide away feelings from your conscious awareness. These stored traumas have been described as *energy cysts*. With various types of healing, energy cysts can be released.

CASE: I was running to answer the phone when I slipped on a piece of paper, bashing my left knee on the floor. In the following two weeks, although I had no pain from moving my leg, the tendon below my kneecap was exquisitely tender to touch. When I saw it was not improving, I contacted a gifted medical intuitive, Wendy Hurwitz, for her advice and help. She asked me, "What happened when you were 7 years old? I couldn't recall anything happening to my knee at that age. "No," she responded, "What happened in your LIFE at that age?" My brother had been born then, necessitating the usual sibling adjustments to a new baby. Half an hour after releasing some of my long-buried feelings about this event, the pain diminished by about 70%, and cleared entirely by the next day.

Emotions stored away in the body may be released during exercise, massage, meditation, psychotherapy, bioenergy therapy and spiritual practices. If you just go with the flow, do your best to not get too upset or panic, and seek the support of a knowledgeable therapist, the release is likely to be a healing experience.

The greatest difficulty with emotional releases come when people get into meta-anxiety,[364] becoming fearful or panicking over the uncomfortable feelings associated with emotional releases. Many of the techniques in this chapter can help you deal with emotional releases and the associated meta-anxiety.

FEELING YOUR WAY THROUGH STRESS

Emotions: experiencing and expressing them constructively

> *But whatever the threat, if it is faced and dealt with, if we express our feelings and go for the truth there will be a reward beyond all imagining.*
> – John MacEnulty (2002)

Emotions have lives of their own. They play as strong and major a part in our lives as our thinking but in western society they aren't given the acknowledgment they deserve. Most of our school years are spent in honing our thinking and ignoring our feelings. Most of our educational funding supports this bias.

Emotions can help in many ways to enhance our appreciation of our relationships to ourselves, to each other and to the wider world. Conversely, emotions may initiate and perpetuate stress-related illnesses through buried, unacknowledged feelings, which can start or may worsen vicious circles.

You can do a lot of self-healing through emotional awareness.

Acknowledging feelings is an essential first step. Hints that emotions may be stirring in your unconscious mind include: being out of sorts; not feeling like your usual self: being edgy and short tempered with others, being moody, depressed and even tearful for no apparent reasons; withdrawing because you don't feel like socializing in your usual manners; or feeling that the rest of the world is not resonating with you. If you find yourself responding to life like this, then you ought to stop and ask, "What is it that I'm feeling?"

If you catch yourself feeling out of sorts like this, the chances are your feelings have been stirred but you haven't attended to their messages and haven't given them their acknowledgment, expression and release.

Here again, your childhood protective programs may be working against you – encouraging you to run away from awareness of feelings they sense as unpleasant and therefore potentially dangerous; leading you to deny the feelings even exist. Your automated, child-programs will help you go on ignoring them by burying them in the buckets and caves it carves deep in your unconscious mind with the help of your psychological defenses.

At the same time, some part of your unconscious mind is protesting, saying that perhaps you are really stronger and safer now, and could handle these buried feelings. It is this part of you that opens little windows of awareness into the dark corners of your shadow, inviting you to uncover the buried emotions that are festering and ready to be released – as the old emotional pus they have become.

Relationships stir awareness of buried feelings and cherished but problematic beliefs. Often, it is only through our relationships with significant others that we come to realize we have these defensive programs. Without someone who is close to us, whom we care about and who cares about us, it is very difficult to become aware of our automated defenses. It may be challenging and at times even unpleasant to have our belief systems and behaviors confronted and questioned. Married couples often tell of horrendous arguments over the silliest things, such as whether glasses and cups should be stored with their open ends up or down; the toilet paper should be set with the paper unrolling at the top or at the bottom of the roll; or which drawer in the dresser should hold his or her underwear.

Case: I recall as though it were yesterday my two days of running arguments, a month after I was first married, over whether to put the paring knives point up or point down in the dish drainer. It seems utterly incredible that two intelligent people would spend two days making themselves and each other miserable over such an apparently trivial issue.

It wasn't actually the knife that was the main issue, of course. It was a whole raft of questions about which would prevail and be honored: my personal preferences and opinions or my wife's; her family traditions or mine; her right as the primary cook to dictate what happens in the kitchen or my right as the primary dishwasher to make this important decision; and meta-level questions about how we state our opinions and feelings; how we settle differences of opinions; and how we listen to each other.

We both came away from these arguments frustrated and bitter, convinced that the other was unreasonable, opinionated and rigid. It was an enormous relief to speak with a fellow medical student – who could speak from the wise vantage point of having been married six months longer than us – who laughed and reassured us that this was just part of the honeymoon adjustments that most couples experience.

Close relationships bring out some of the best lessons about ourselves; they confront us with choices which we never suspected might exist, forcing us to decide whether we wish to keep our childhood programs for handling feelings and our accumulated beliefs and habits, or to re-evaluate and alter them – to be more in tune with adult awareness and values.

Close relationships also challenge you to rise above yourself, to reach out from your heart; to learn and ever deepen your acceptance, love and forgiveness for others – and, as well, for yourself.[365]

> *The unique personality which is the real life in me, I can not gain unless I search for the real life, the spiritual quality, in others. I am myself spiritually dead unless I reach out to the fine quality dormant in others. For it is only with the god enthroned in the innermost shrine of the other, that the god hidden in me, will consent to appear.*
>
> – Felix Adler

Relating through your heart

> *The heart is like a garden. It can grow compassion or fear, resentment or love. What seeds will you plant there?*
>
> – Gautama Buddha

Daniel Goleman has written an excellent discussion of *emotional intelligence.* He explains that we all have emotional awareness that is as important as our thinking intelligence. In fact, attending to what your emotions are telling you can provide you with a radar that is far more sensitive than many of your other ways of interacting with the world around you.

We may be stressed over not understanding why we feel a certain way or over not knowing what to do about problems. These are questions posed by the head. They may have ten answers or no answers – in either case leaving us without a clear basis for responding to challenges. We may ask questions like:

Why am I angry at people who haven't done anything to hurt me?

Why am I unhappy about my job?

Why don't I trust my partner?

Why can't I let go of my grief over losing my (father, mother, partner, job, or other important piece of my life) – when it's been years since the tragedy and everyone else has adjusted to the situation and returned to a normal life?

Our cost-benefit analysis and logical reasoning may not be adequate to answering these questions in satisfying ways.

In cases like these, it is often the feelings we have about the situation and about issues that it is raising which are the problem. It is not the logical reasons surrounding the problem that are causing our unhappiness. What disturbs us and makes us comfortable are the feelings that are raised by the attitude of someone we are dealing with. We may not have adequate reasons to explain our distrust of a person who is close to us, but our feelings may alert us to something that feels wrong about the way they are relating to us – something in their tone of voice, their touch or the way they don't quite listen to us may be triggering inner alarm bells. There may be no *logical* reasons apparent for the ways that we feel about relationships or how our lives are unfolding – but there may be *feeling* reasons (rather than logical explanations) behind our frustrations, stressing and unexplained emotions.

Learning to identify and trust your feelings may be doorways into much deeper understandings of yourself. How you feel when you are young may set your emotional thermostat and determine your ways of relating to others for the rest of your life.

Taking this several steps further, we may learn to relate to others from our hearts as well as from our heads. Responses from the head tend to come from sets of expectations and rules, imposing structure on our perceptions, our interpretations of situations and our responses. Responses from the heart come from a healing, spiritual place – where every experience may be an invitation to become more heart centered, responding with compassion, love and healing rather than with logical and reasoned responses.

> *Each difficult moment has the potential to open my eyes and open my heart.*
> – Myla Kabat-Zinn

Journaling

> *In order to be as honest as possible with myself, I wrote everything down very carefully, following the old Greek maxim: 'Give away all that thou hast, then shalt thou receive.'*
> – Carl Jung (1961, p. 187)

Writing down your experiences, particularly your feelings, can be an enormous help in sorting them out, resolving internal conflicts and releasing negative emotions. Finding the concepts and words that express what you are experiencing helps to clarify what you are feeling and may take much of the sting out of a hurtful incident. The physical act of putting words on paper adds to the process of releasing the distressing emotions. Seeing the words on paper may help to view an experience in new ways and to find new approaches to understanding and dealing with it.

When you are upset and alone, you may be surprised at how much better you feel after journaling. If you are in therapy, your journal can also serve an auxiliary memory – bringing up details for discussion that you might otherwise have forgotten.

Revisiting your journal periodically can add depth to your understanding of your dis-ease and disease processes.

I have enjoyed watching the TV detective, Columbo, who meticulously questions and writes down his observations of minute details about the people he is investigating. I often recommend to careseekers that they mimic Columbo, reviewing their journals to see whether they can identify patterns that may explain their symptoms and underlying issues.

By using their journals as a detective's notebook, many people have identified items such as

- Food sensitivities that cause or worsen symptoms

- Days of the week when symptoms are regularly worse

- Particular people or events that resonate with buried issues

- Recurrent themes in dreams that point to underlying conflicts

Such items may not stand out enough in your daily routine for you to notice them. For instance, if you find that your symptoms are more severe on particular days, you can then identify stressors at work or in your home life on those particular days that make you up tight and worsen your problems

Another use of journals is to acknowledge your progress. On a day-to-day self-assessment, you may not notice the tiny increments, the hard-won little changes in your lifetime accumulations of unconscious self-limiting habits – as you work on yourself with various self-healing approaches. It is rather like seeing a child whom you haven't seen for a period of time and noticing how they've grown – when they themselves may not have noticed this, due to the slow and gradual changes that are not noticed from one day to the next. When you revisit your journal after several weeks, months or years, you will readily see your growth in understanding, emotional awareness and improved relationships.

Gestalt Therapy

> *... He would sit on the stone day after day wondering whether he was the one sitting on the stone; or was he the stone that felt it was being sat upon? This problem raised by the speculation was never solved. But he had no doubt that he was in some secret relationship with the stone. Also that the dialogue thus begun was in terms of a greater, more permanent and irreducible reality as represented by the stone...*
> — Laurens van der Post (1976, p. 74)

Physical symptoms often speak for the unconscious mind, which may otherwise have difficulty being heard. In gestalt therapy you dramatize the symptoms and problems, giving voice to whatever part of the body is complaining through the symptoms. By expressing the dis-ease that is attached to the problem, you can often release a considerable portion of the tension surround the problem – thereby decreasing the intensity of the vicious circle.

Case: "Vanessa" had severe headaches that were becoming a major burden in her life. They occurred two or three times a week and could come on at any time of day. They made it difficult to concentrate at work and were adding stress to her relationships with her husband and children. She had had to take several days' sick leave. Pain medications were becoming less and less effective and she was unwilling to take stronger medications containing codeine because of her con-

cerns over the possibility of addiction. Extensive medical workups were all nega-
tive, and Vanessa came reluctantly for psychotherapy at the suggestion of her
family physician.
  I invited her to describe her headaches. "They're not all in my mind," she an-
nounced, "even if they are in my head. I'm not just making up these pains. They
are very real and very painful."

When a doctor says, "There is no physical cause for this pain." it is a common
misperception to think she is saying, "You must be making this up." It would be
unusual for a doctor to say this, even though caregivers may sometimes think this
way, out of frustration and a feeling of failure – not being trained to understand
the mind-body connection.

Case (continued): I shared the picture of the balance of energies and issues (Fig-
ure II-4) and explained how stress and anxieties could contribute to whatever
physical problems were behind the headaches. Vanessa was able to accept this
explanation, so we proceeded to explore how to understand and deal with her
headaches.
  She had been working for years as the managing secretary in a busy coroner's
office, where she was under constant pressures to deal with urgent accident in-
vestigations and promptly get out the reports. At home, her duties as wife and
mother to three children (8, 11 and 13 years-old) were no more demanding than
they had been in the five years prior to the onset of her headaches. She was proud
of being a very competent and reliable office manager and homemaker. Nothing
stood out in her mind that could be causing the headaches.
  Even though Vanessa thought my suggestion to sit in another chair and speak
for her headache was pretty weird, she complied. She was surprised to hear her-
self saying, after a few clarifying exchanges between herself and the headaches,
that her pains were suggesting she needed to take more time to care for own
needs. They were helping her to take some time off from work, were getting her
husband to help more with the children and chores around the house, and al-
lowed her to beg off going out to some of her husband's business parties which
she found boring and annoying – because he was always talking with colleagues
and leaving her to her own devices.
  These revelations opened Vanessa's eyes to issues her unconscious mind had
been festering over – behind the doors of the closets where she stashed away
many of her feelings about issues she felt helpless to deal with or to change. Once
aware of them, she was able to consider more constructive and less painful ways
of dealing with them. Within two months, she had asked for additional secretarial
assistance in the office, had gotten her husband's support to insist that the chil-
dren help more with chores in the home, and had negotiated with him to spend
more quality time with her. Her headaches were much less frequent, and when-
ever she did start to feel one coming on, she would take it as a red flag that was
alerting her to attend to something stressful in her life.

Playing the role of a symptom or part of your body invites awarenesses about
underlying feelings and opens new insights. It also invites your to devise new

ways to deal with your problems. The spontaneity of the interchanges between yourself and "whoever" is sitting in the chair opposite you will often spur you to creative and constructive solutions to your issues.

Gestalt therapy is a very potent form of self-healing. Initially, when you are first learning this approach, it may be helpful or even necessary to have the guidance of a therapist to introduce you to using this approach.

Case: I (Dan Benor) still vividly recall a dream I shared in a gestalt therapy workshop 25 years ago.

I parked and locked my old, beat up convertible car on a street in Israel, where I was living at the time. After walking half a block away, I thought to myself that it wasn't wise to have left my camera in the car. I turned, just in time to see a teenager who slit the convertible roof of the car and made off with my camera. I gave chase and soon cornered him at the top of a stairway by a locked door. I reached for a stick to hit him, but then realized I didn't want to hurt him – but just to have my camera back.

The workshop leader had me speak for the old car. I was surprised to hear myself saying, "This beat-up old wreck is all he deserves." The intensity of feelings in my exchanges with the car on the empty seat took me to a great depth of emotional awareness very rapidly.

As you get used to gestalt therapy for exploring and activating your inner resources, you may be able to apply this technique on your own.

There are countless other approaches through feelings into healing, mostly focused on identifying and acknowledging feelings, releasing buried feelings, allowing yourself to experience feelings rather than running away from them, and learning to express them in appropriate ways.[366]

We are healed of a suffering only by experiencing it to the full.
– Marcel Proust

UNCONSCIOUS ROOTS OF STRESS

Conditioning

Surprisingly, behaviorism comes the closest to spiritual language, for it attributes pain to the conditioning that people receive.
– Brant Cortright (p. 33)

Repetitive patterns of emotional responses and of behaviors usually suggest that you have an unconscious habit of reacting to a given stimulus or situation. When you identify that you have problems with repetitive patterns, conditioning may explain them and could be helpful in resolving them.

Carol's fear of dogs (described under Cognitive Behavioral Therapy, above) was a habit of this sort. Without realizing it, Carol used her common sense to alter her conditioned response of fear whenever she saw a dog. By forcing herself to allow small dogs to come near her, she overcame her habit of running away from them. While her running away had reduced her anxiety, it was an awkward and embarrassing response to have. By forcing herself to not run away, she overcame the childhood programming from when the dog had bitten her. As a child, it was helpful to avoid this danger by keeping well away from all dogs – because she was not able to differentiate between neutral and potentially dangerous dogs. As an adult, she could be much more discerning and selective about which dogs she might choose to keep away from.

Systematic desensitization
Here is a systematic way of desensitizing yourself to things that make you anxious or uncomfortable in other ways.

Practice a relaxation technique until you feel comfortable and competent using it. In addition to muscle relaxation, there are breathing, meditation, imagery, WHEE and other exercises that could help you unwind. Choose whichever works best for you. You should practice your chosen technique until you are able to relax within 1 to 3 minutes from a mild to modest starting state of stress to a state of being comfortable and not stressed. Do not proceed with this exercise until you have achieved this level of competence with one or more technique.

When you know you have one or more ways to reduce stress, make a list of all the things that make you uncomfortable. Keep separate lists for items that fit within different categories. For instance, if you're anxious about speaking in public, list all the situations in which you feel uncomfortable when you have to speak. Rate each one of the items from "0" (doesn't bother you at all) to "10" (the worst you could possibly feel about this item). Re-write the list, listing these from worst feelings at the bottom of the list to least at the top. If you have access to a computer this task can be easier, and periodic updates can be readily inserted as you make progress.

For example, you might have twenty items on your list (more or less is also fine) about speaking in public. The least intense might be having to ask your spouse to help you do something in public (vs. it doesn't bother you at all in the privacy of your home); intermediate items might be asking directions of a stranger at a train station and asking a clerk at a department store where to find the toilet; and your top item might be having to give a public talk in front of an room full of people. (You might have separate, though related lists of such categories as fears of being criticized by different people; self-doubts about succeeding in various endeavors; or other such issues.)

The gentlest way is to start with just one of the milder items at or near the top of your list. First situate yourself comfortably, where you won't be disturbed for about half an hour. Use your relaxation technique to unwind until you feel very relaxed. Then, picture to yourself that you are in the situation where you feel mildly anxious, such as asking your spouse in public to help you. When you feel the anxiety associated with this situation rising to a modest degree (e.g. up to a 5-6 out of 10), release your focus on this image and return to practicing your relaxation technique until you are again as relaxed as when you started this exercise.

Repeat the process, picturing yourself asking your spouse to help you and relaxing until you find that you can hold the image of asking without feeling anxious. Well done! You are on your way to eliminating this whole list of problems.

If you feel you have the time and energies to work on another item from your list, go ahead. If not, then make a date with yourself to do so later.

Once you have eliminated the anxiety from your image of several of these items, check out how you feel when you actually do these things in real life. If, for instance, you no longer feel anxious when you are out in public and ask your spouse to help you, you now have feedback that this is actually working.

When you are confident with this technique, you can then skip several items, working on those that raise your anxiety levels to higher numbers, closer to the maximum of 10. You can then proceed to relax your way through the entire list.

In self-healing, you will ease your way through various exercises and techniques. If you can arrange to have the help of a counselor or therapist who is familiar and competent with such techniques, you may be able to proceed more rapidly.[367]

Benefits of self-healing using conditioning
Conditioning can help best with anxieties, fears and phobias; and is often helpful with troublesome habits and a negative self-image.

See also: Cognitive Behavioral Therapy; Imagery/ Visualization; Neurolinguistic Programming; WHEE

Dream analysis

> *The future belongs to those who believe in the beauty of their dreams.*
> – Eleanor Roosevelt

Dreams are invitations from your unconscious mind to pay attention to inner awarenesses that are important to your life. They include interplays of:

- Partly digested or undigested bits of day residues – experiences that made an impact but were not fully processed to resolve strong emotions or conflicts (internal or interpersonal). These are impressions that your unconscious mind identifies as important – when it goes to file them away in your mental databanks.

- Associations from your past experiences, stored in the mental and visceral records of all of the experiences and feelings you ever had. It is as though the day residues are settling into their place in the vast filing system of your unconscious mind, stirring the various records that lie in likely places where they are getting tucked away. Some of these memories are readily available to your conscious mind, should you be invited to search through your filing systems. Others lie in the *shadow* portions of your awareness – those aspects of yourself that you would rather not explore.[368] A few of the memories that are unsettled in this filing process become parts of the dream.

- Your operating systems for how to run your life, including your beliefs, disbeliefs, *shoulds* and *shouldn'ts* that were programmed into your automatic pilot by your child in response to teachings and experiences with your family, religious teachings, school teachers, media and other avenues for acculturation. These are the backdrops you have developed which set the stage for the performance of your life; and, in miniature, for the staging of your dreams.

- Your wishes, hopes and plans for the future, as well as your anxieties, fears and doubts about how the future might unfold.

- Psychic elements, such as telepathic and clairsentient awarenesses, past and future life experiences,

- Spiritual elements may enter your dreams – such as creative, intuitive perceptions, visits from spirits who want to communicate, angelic and other mystical communications, and a sense of your connection with the All.

When you wish to connect with this wonderfully intuitive part of yourself, you can write down your dreams every morning. It is best to do this immediately upon awakening. If you delay by going to the bathroom or even by letting thoughts about the coming day cross your mind, you are likely to lose much if not all of the information your unconscious is inviting you to explore.

You can enhance your recall significantly by reminding yourself as you go to sleep that you want to remember your dreams. Having a pen and paper or a small tape recorder by the bedside. Scribbling a few words during the night immediately after a particularly juicy dream can cue your memory in the morning. Even if it is just a single image or feeling, this can often open the doors of your memory to reconstruct the entire dream.

Dreams are like the tail of a tiger that your unconscious mind waves in front of you. They carry information from your shadow, and your unconscious mind is unsure whether you really want to remember these. You must grab that tail firmly and hold onto it if you wish to retain and benefit from these rich materials.

Every single element in your dreams represents something about you, yet it may be difficult for you to perceive some of the deeper layers of your dreams.

I do not recommend books that purport to give you the answers to your dreams. No one can do this but you, yourself.

Having someone to help you interpret the dreams can add many dimensions to your dream analysis. While a trusted friend may help, a trained therapist is even better. You should not expect them to give you the answers to any questions you may have about the dreams, but rather to help you ask your own questions more clearly and to sharpen the focus on the answers that your own unconscious will provide.

CASE I had pondered many of the elements of the dream described above from a gestalt therapy workshop – in which my camera was stolen from the old car. I had seen within the dream several clear statements about how unsafe I felt in living in Israel – prior to sharing it with the workshop leader. I was utterly surprised, however, by his invitation for me to speak for the old, beat up car, and to sense why I was driving what turned out to be an unsafe car in my dream, and to hear myself saying for the car, "This is all he deserves."

I would never on my own have come to this deeper question, which proved to be enormously enlightening regarding my feelings of not deserving greater measures of success or security.

You are the director, choreographer and producer of the dramas in your dreams, with all of their potentials for healing. The more you can own your dreams, the deeper will be your understandings of the lessons your unconscious is offering you. This may not always be easy, however. While many dreams have a single principal message that is fairly obvious, your understanding of a dream will often have layers upon layers of meanings that you can peel your way to with diligent sleuthing.

The assistance of a respectful, trusted friend or therapist can be an enormous help in noticing elements and layers of your dreams that you may overlook, and in deepening your understanding of them.

CASE: "Steven," a sculptor who was struggling in therapy with issues of low self-esteem and self-doubting, dreamed that he was in a studio, struggling to work into a lump of clay the image of beauty which he held in his mind's eye. Again and again he crushed the forms he created, utterly dissatisfied and frustrated with his work. Pausing to calm himself, he glanced over to the next table, where his wife (who in real life had no particular creative gifts) was putting the finishing touches on a glowing, perfect rendition of the very image that he had been striving so dismally and unsuccessfully to produce. He was jealous of her work, and returned to his own efforts to produce this image – with no greater success than before.

Steven felt that in this dream his wife was able to achieve what he had failed to produce, which paralleled her greater abilities to actualize herself and achieve success and satisfaction in real life. I suggested that in his dream he could have choreographed himself as the successful sculptor, because he had given the perfect sculpture to his wife. It took him three therapy sessions to acknowledge that he had given away his creation to his wife in the dream, and that it had not been his wife who created the sculpture.

It is the very nature of dreams that they both invite you to explore and understand your deeper self and that they disguise and hide elements and layers of your unconscious, buried in the past – due to the child programs that seek to protect you by forgetting and ignoring frightening and painful experiences. Dreams are invitations for you to reach into those old buckets and closets and caves where hurts are hidden, to do an internal house-cleaning, now that you are no longer in the original painful or dangerous situations.

Dreams can open into spiritual awarenesses. Everyone has a measure of intuitive, psychic abilities,[369] but most of us have so much mental chatter and emotional noise in our minds that we drown out the more subtle psi awareness that is in the background. We are also socially conditioned to discount these awarenesses as fantasies, so we become uncomfortable with them through being unfamiliar with them. When we are asleep and our mind is quieter, our psi impressions are often incorporated into our dreams. As with any other dream element, there may be considerable distortions in the translation of a telepathic or clairsentient perception into dream images and dramas.

Case: "Rosemary" dreamed that she was in her office, typing an urgent, angry letter from her boss to a hospital, complaining about his treatment there. Her boss came in just as she finished the letter and was angry that she had made two errors in the typing. He went on and on, letting out his anger at her and at the hospital. He started to turn red with anger, then blue and fainted.

  Early the next morning, Rosemary had a call from her mother that her father had had chest pains and fainted and was rushed to the hospital during the night. Her parents had to wait a long time before a doctor saw them, and there was confusion because the doctor had picked up the wrong chart. Her father was admitted for observation and tests, even though his pains had cleared up and he felt ready to return home.

Rosemary seemed to have picked up psychic information about her father's problems. Her unconscious mind brought them to her attention but displaced them, choreographing her boss as the person with the problems rather than her father. The unconscious mind will often do this with psi impressions that are upsetting. It reduces our anxieties by casting into the leading dream roles people who are not as close to us and therefore less likely to upset us in having serious problems in our dreams.

  Psychic awareness in dreams is often related to family and close friends, but apparently random psi perceptions may occur between strangers who have no known relationship. Here is a typical example of this type of spontaneous psi communication:

  ... in... 1910... I related to my husband that I had had a horrible dream the previous night. He looked at me inquiringly, and I said, "I dreamed of a man and a woman with a team on a wagon. One horse was a big bay. They drove onto a bridge which had sides like an inverted 'V.' When they got to the middle of it, the bridge went down. The bay horse reared and tried to go backwards. I saw the man. He had a piece of board right through his chest. We discussed the entire incident for what it was, as we thought, a very bad dream. As a matter of fact, I explained to my husband that I knew neither the man nor his wife and did not recognize the road.
  The next day my husband went to town. When he came home, he looked at me with a strange look and said, "Your dream came true... Mr. And Mrs. _____ came into town to the mill to get grain ground. They left about four o'clock to go home. The _____ bridge collapsed with them. Both were killed. There was a piece of wood driven through his chest. The one horse was a big bay. There was an eyewitness to the tragedy.
  This occurred at least twelve hours or more after my dream. I did not know the people or the locality where it occurred.

                                                              – Louisa Rhine (p. 117-118)

It is therefore impossible to know in most cases from the dream content alone whether it is simply playing a nightmare on the screen of our awareness or alerting us to an occurrence in the outer world.

With practice, one may learn to identify a feeling tone to intuitive and spiritual dreams. This is very difficult to describe in words. My own perception is that spiritual components in a dream often are associated with feelings of inner certainty and knowing of the truth/ rightness of those elements. When touched with the love of the Infinite Source, the sense of being totally and unconditionally accepted can be so strong that is feels close to overwhelming, and is clearly unforgettable.

Dreams are metaphors for our lives. When we seek understanding for these openings into our higher selves, particularly when we ask, wish and pray for such insights and guidance, our dreams can become wonderful windows and doorways into deeper spiritual experiences.

To some extent, our lives are lived out/ orchestrated/ choreographed through our expectations, beliefs, disbeliefs, wishes and anxieties – in the same ways that our dreams are. Working on our dreams can help us recognize and respond appropriately to spiritual experiences in our lives. We can address experiences in our lives - particularly recurrent or challenging ones, as elements in a dream can be addressed. By analyzing why a certain block is present to your progress, you may discover aspects of yourself that are inviting that variety of experience into your life – just as you may discover such elements in your unconscious mind as you analyze your dreams.

Applied Kinesiology (AK) – muscle testing

> *Intellect must be balanced by intuition and caring, so that information will be used appropriately, for the good of all and for the future generations.*
>
> – Kenneth Cohen (2003, p. 79)

AK originally was developed as a therapist-generated treatment, focused on acupuncture meridians. Meridians influence local muscles. If a particular muscle is weak, it indicates that its meridian is weak. Treating this meridian can then correct problems in the body organs that are associated with that meridian.

Aspects of AK are now used also for self-healing.

AK is particularly helpful for accessing your intuitive wisdom, using your body as an indicator for yes/ no answers to your questions.

The Bi-Digital O-Ring Test (BDORT) – Hold the tips of your left thumb and little finger together, forming an "O" or ring. Hook your right thumb through this ring, just where the left thumb and finger are touching and see how firmly you have to pull in order to break the grip of these fingers. Now, ask yourself, "What does my *yes* feel like?" and repeat the process, noting any change in the strength of your grip. Repeat the process, checking the strength of your grip while you are asking yourself, "What does my *no* feel like?" Most people will find there is a distinct difference in the strength of their grip with a *yes* and a *no*.[370]

Index finger kinesiology – While sitting, rest your left hand on your leg, near your knee. Raise your index finger. Use your right index finger to press down on your raised left index finger, to check the strength of your left finger. Now, repeat this while you think of a question that can be answered with a *yes* or a *no*. For instance, you might ask, "Is chocolate good for me?" (You may substitute any other food you have cravings for.) See if you notice any change in the strength of your left index finger. Weakness generally indicates a *no*, strength signifies *yes*.

Thumbnail kinesiology – Gently rub your first finger back and forth across the nail of your thumb, while asking "What is my *yes*?" and "What is my *no*?" Note any differences in what you feel with your finger. Extend this to practice with other questions. You might say out loud, "Today is ___" (stating the correct day) and explore the feeling of your finger running across your thumbnail. Then say, "Today is ___" (stating the wrong day) and again check your sensation.[371]

Your arm as your indicator – Extend your arm out to your side, parallel with the floor. Have a friend test the strength of your arm muscles by pressing down on your wrist to establish your baseline strength to resist his pushing down. (She should press firmly, but not so hard as to "break" your position.) Think silently to yourself of a situation that makes you feel sad. (Don't tell your friend what you are doing, so there will be no question that your arm is being pressed down either more or less firmly according to her expectations.) Note whether your muscle strength is different when she pushes down a second time, as you are focused on sadness. Then rest your arm a moment and have her press down on your wrist again while you're thinking of something that makes you happy. Note the strength of your arm. See the endnote for the most common responses to this sort of testing.[372] (Many therapists use arm kinesiology as their way of helping you to answer diagnostic and therapeutic questions.)

Imagery instead of muscle AK – Bring up a blank screen in your mind's eye. Ask your unconscious mind to insert an image on the screen that stands for *yes*. After receiving your *yes* image, blank the screen again. Then ask for a *no* image.

Having established your *yes* and *no* responses concerning neutral issues, you can proceed to ask yourself questions about your physical or psychological well-being. Simpler questions might concern whether various foods or medicines are likely to be helpful or harmful. We often find that the foods we particularly crave are the ones that AK will indicate are bad for us. Chocolate, coffee and white sugar are frequent culprits.[373] You may also explore more complicated questions, such as whether to engage in certain experiences or not, or whether psychological factors could be contributing to a stress state or illness. Any question at all can be posed, as long as it is simplified to allow a *yes* or *no* reply or series of replies.

Record your questions before or as you ask them. Your unconscious mind and higher self are extremely literal and will respond to the exact words you used in framing your questions. If you feel the answers you are getting are too illogical or feel wrong, ask your question in different ways.

Case: "Frank," a middle-aged participant in one of my workshops, became agitated and tearful when he started using the kinesiology. We asked him what was upsetting him. He replied, "I have cancer, and I asked, 'Will I die?' and the answer was yes. I asked several times and the answer was still yes."

Several of the other participants in the group started to laugh. Though I was startled by this laughter, I then realized that the answer to Frank's question could only be yes – for anyone who asked that question!

What Frank really wanted to ask was, "Will I die soon from this cancer?"

So be very precise and specific in asking your questions!

I repeat here the cautions mentioned in Chapter 2:

One must be extremely careful in interpreting the results of kinesiology. As with any diagnostic procedure (intuitive or physical), there will always be a percentage of false positive and false negative findings.

Several ways to reduce the risk of error include:

1. Use common sense and logical reasoning to analyze information that arises intuitively. Don't act rashly on the basis of intuitive impressions that contradict reason, and reject intuitive urges that go counter to ethics and moral principles.

2. Examine your introspective, emotional and intuitive responses to the information provided through kinesiology. The information you bring up may be similar to dream imagery, which can be distorted. (See Dreams.) That is, the *yes* you receive may be a yes to part of a question rather than to the whole question. When in doubt, consult friends and professional therapists.

3. Record the precise words you use in asking the questions, so they can be re-evaluated in the light of later analysis. This then allows you to tweak the questions for greater clarity and confidence in the answers.

4. When there are questions about results obtained with AK, use multiple readings and supplement them with readings by others, preferably by clinicians who are experienced and expert in the use of these methods.

The help of a knowledgeable clinician can be invaluable. Clinicians trained in kinesiology know the ways in which innate characteristics and learned patterns of beliefs and behaviors tend to cluster and manifest – both physically and psychologically. Clinicians may identify psychological issues that we ourselves are blind to – particularly around traumatic experiences that we have buried in our unconscious mind, and relating to habit patterns that we are blind to. Good psychotherapists will know ways to help unravel the complex structures of defenses built up over a lifetime of human interactions, and bioenergy therapists may recognize blocks or overactivities in various meridians that would not be apparent or even suspected by anyone who is unfamiliar with these patterns.

Where there is any doubt or question you must proceed with the greatest caution when using these techniques. Your unconscious expectations, hopes, wishes and fears may all influence your self-explorations – leading you to ask questions in ways that provide answers more comfortable to your wishes and expectations, or conversely, to avoid asking questions that might produce painful or uncomfortable answers. The same may apply for therapists, whose own unresolved issues may make them blind, insensitive or uncomfortable with particular problems their clients may have.

See also: Divination

HEAD WORKING WITH HEART

> *If you want to be truly understood, you need to say everything three times, in three different ways. Once for each ear... and once for the heart. The right ear represents the ability to apprehend the nature of the Whole, the wholeness of the circumstance, the forest. The left ear represents the ability to select a sequential path. And the heart represents a balance between the two.*
>
> – Paula Underwood Spencer (p. 16)

Transactional Analysis

Eric Berne developed a simplified language for psychoanalytic understandings of how people tick. He observed that everyone (regardless of our age) has three basic *ego states* (See Figure II-22):

- An inner *Parent* that tells us what we should and shouldn't do. This is the part that was programmed by our own parents, school teachers, religious teachers and authorities our broader society. This Parent can speak with a supportive voice or a critical tone.

- An inner *Adult* that computes the logical likelihood of our succeeding in getting what we want in life (like Mr. Spock in *Star Treck*) , taking into account our inner and outer awarenesses

- An inner *Child* that wants to be able to express its feelings and have what it wants when it wants it. Our inner child may express itself in a simple, *natural*, unfettered way; it may *adapt* its expressions of feelings in order to be accepted/ not be rejected; or it may *rebel* in order to get its own way in the face of opposition or criticism.

Figure II-22. Ego states

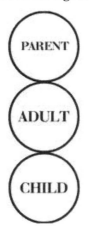

This is an extremely helpful map for self-healing. If you find yourself in conflict with other people, and you listen to *how they are speaking* and to *how you are speaking*, you may very quickly identify why there is friction between you.

Case: "Louise" asked her teenage daughter, "When are you going to clean up your room?" Louise's conscious intent was simply be to know when the floor would be clear so that she could vacuum it. Tammy responded angrily, "Why are you always nagging and criticizing me?" Louise was surprised to hear her so upset, when she was asking a simple question and looking for a factual answer.

When we re-enacted the encounter in a family counseling session, it became clear that while Louise's words were coming from her Adult ego state, her tone of voice had a distinct edge of Critical Parent in it (because she had actually asked Tammy this question more than just once before). Tammy was responding to her mother's Critical Parent tone rather than to her factual, Adult message.

It is extremely common to find that you and others respond more to the feeling tone of a message than to its content. So if you get an unexpected response, you might ask yourself, "What feeling tones are being expressed here?" This may rapidly help you understand where you are coming from when you get into conflicts, especially when these seem illogical relative to the content of your verbal exchanges.

The second helpful aspect to this map is that it immediately suggests alternatives to the conflictual exchanges. You could change your tone of voice and feeling focus to Supportive Parent. This might get a better response: "I know this isn't your favorite of all things to do on a Saturday morning, but I need to vacuum and I'd really appreciate your help in getting the house cleaned." Or you might shift to Adult (with a neutral tone), "When you've cleaned your room, we can go out shopping for your school clothes;" or to speak you're your own Child ego state, "I hate to have to do the cleaning as much as you do, but if we get it done quickly and without fuss we can both have the rest of the day to enjoy ourselves."

Anger management

> *Anger is a choice.*
> Daniel J. Benor (2003)

Here is a place where you can apply many of the approaches we've considered.

Anger and other ways we respond to upsets are choices that we make. To some extent these choices are unconscious and may be difficult to control once they are activated, particularly in a given situation when we feel provoked. However, our habitual ways of responding to provocations are subject to assessment, analysis and changes – if we choose to confront our habitual responses.

Anger is such a difficult feeling to deal with that a detailed discussion about handling this reaction to stress is presented here.

Anger is a natural response to being endangered or hurt. Challenges that commonly elicit anger include:

Being attacked verbally or physically

Being threatened verbally or physically

Intrusion upon or disrespect of our boundaries
- Physical
- Social

Not receiving
- Something in the outer world that was promised or expected (material or benefits)
- Behaviors or attitudes that are expected (respectfulness, courtesies, attention)

Acute anger is usually a visceral, emotional reaction. Our stress hormones kick in, and we may flush as blood is diverted from our internal organs to our muscles. Adrenalin makes our heart beat faster and our breathing deeper and faster. We prepare to respond to the challenge.

Many of our anger responses will be based on unconscious habits of reacting to similar stimuli in the past. If we have observed or have been treated with aggression by others when they were angry (particularly our parents and other family members), we are more likely to respond with aggression ourselves. If we have been successful when we reacted with aggression, we are likely to respond again with aggression. If we fared better by withdrawing from previous stimuli to anger, we are more prone to withdraw again in the future – from the scene of the challenge or simply into ourselves, either withholding or actually burying our response in our unconscious mind.

The mind: issues of choice and control

> *Between stimulus and response, there is a space. In that space lies our freedom and power to choose our response. In our response lies our growth and freedom.*
>
> – Victor Frankl

Most of the issues around anger relate to aspects of not being in control, feeling out of control, or feeling a loss of control.

Acute anger is a natural response when we are in situations of actual physical danger. Anger can be helpful because it activates the stress hormones that facilitate fight or flight. If a man with a gun enters the room I am in, I may respond more quickly and forcefully with the help of these hormones, which increase my alertness and enhance my muscle strength. I may be able to duck or run away more quickly, which could save my life.

Chronic anger may be unhelpful, however, when fight or flight responses are not necessary or appropriate. If I am sitting behind the wheel of my car in rush hour traffic, late for my appointment and unable to see what is causing the traffic delay, my stress hormones may build up and I may have no way to discharge them immediately, and no way to focus my energies in ways that could resolve the outward causes of my frustration. When I finally speed up towards my destination, if a car cuts in front of me and endangers my life, I may be frightened and angry, again without any way of addressing the person who stirred these feelings. When my cell phone doesn't connect with the office, the elevator is out of order when I arrive, already late for my meeting. I get pushed aside in the stairwell by a workman carrying a chair downstairs. The secretary who could smooth matters is away from her desk. My boss may bawl me out for being late, my IN box may be overflowing, and my wife may interrupt me urgently – just as I feel I am moving towards getting matters in hand - to ask what to do about a leak under the bathroom sink.

Unexpressed anger from numerous frustrations, large and small, can build up tensions and lead to expressions of anger. Often, we stuff these angry feelings away because we have been taught that expressing anger is wrong or because we feel there is no good or safe way to express them. Getting angry with a supervisor could endanger your employment; getting angry with a stranger could provoke them to violence. We may sometimes release feelings in verbal aggression towards those who offend us, perhaps screaming at the car that cuts in front of us, growling at someone who interrupts us, or pushing back against someone who jostles us rudely. While these responses may provide some release for the raging temper, they may also aggravate confrontations and conflicts into more angry interchanges, making matters worse rather than better. Angers that are expressed openly may thus escalate rather than get discharged and reduced. We therefore learn to suppress anger.

We often end up stuffing our angers away somewhere inside ourselves. Most of us carry around buckets full of stashed angry feelings (along with other negative, unexpressed emotions). When something else comes along to anger us, we may then respond with an excess of anger. This explains a lot of road rage, office rage, marital discord, and social conflicts. When our buckets are full to overflowing, any little stimulus to anger can give us the opportunity to dump other, stored up angers from our buckets along with the angers that are provoked in the current situation.

Furthermore, holding in anger is not good for our health. Chronic stresses and tensions can lead to physical dysfunctions. The neurohormonal, cardiovascular, pulmonary and genitourinary systems are particularly prone to such disorders, but they can occur in any organ system in the body. In Chapter II-2, I explored a long list of body language terms that reflect this awareness, such as "I got my guts in an uproar," "I was really pissed off," "I took that insult to heart," and many more.

Anger expression management

Letting your feelings out in acceptable manners is one of the healthier ways to deal with anger.

Sports activities provide helpful physical outlets for pent up tensions. When I was under emotional stress in the Air Force during the Viet Nam war, I played racquetball or squash six or seven days a week, even in the heat of Texas summers that often reached over 100 degrees. I consciously pictured to myself that I was venting my angers at various individuals and situations that challenged my belief and ethical systems, making it impossible for me to offer medical or psychiatric care as I felt they ought to be practiced.

Another release for anger can be through voicing your feelings. Giving my boss a piece of my mind, in no uncertain terms, at the top of my voice, can be a great release – in the safety and privacy of my car, with the windows rolled up, on my way home.

Letting it out directly towards the other person can be helpful, when this is done with respect. The risks of provoking anger in return can be considerably reduced by diplomatic phrasing. What has helped me is the picture a fence between myself and the person with whom I'm angry. If I stay on my side of the fence, stating that I am angry and why I am angry, I am less likely to provoke anger in response. In other words, I use "I" statements, stating what has angered me and explaining why.

I might say to my boss, in private, "I am really frustrated and upset over being bawled out by you for being late. I understand that you're angry you couldn't get very far with the meeting until I got here, but I feel it's unfair of you to call me on the carpet in front of customers without giving me a chance to explain. I was held up in a traffic jam on the expressway, my cell phone didn't connect, and the elevator wasn't working when I arrived. I left home early, but not early enough to accommodate all of these delays. I'm particularly upset because this isn't the first time I've experienced responses like this from you."

I avoid reaching over the fence in any way, refraining from using blaming or attacking *You-statements*. I don't say, "You have some nerve, blaming me for being late without bothering to ask what happened to make me late! I left home early and it wasn't my fault that there was a jam-up on the expressway and that my cell phone and the elevator weren't working. I'm really fed up because you always jump on me without asking what the problems were."

When I've stated my feelings, from my side of the fence, even if I've done this with considerable emotion and emphatic expressions, I'm inviting the other party to listen to my side. They are more likely to begin to see matters in a new light. In contrast, if I direct my comments at the person on the other side of the fence, the other party is likely to feel attacked and to respond defensively – often with further anger.

At other times, particularly under situations of bullying, the use of firmness and even an angry response in return may be appropriate. Bullies enjoy being one-up over those they feel they can cower. Showing them that they can't get away with it will usually discourage them from continuing with their harassments. This still works better for me as firmness from my side of the fence.

On energetic levels, anger sets up negative vibrations, within and around those who are experiencing and expressing the anger. You may have had the experience of entering a room where people have been upset or angry, picking up negative vibrations without anyone having said an angry word in your presence.

Many bioenergy practitioners surround themselves with protective biological energy shields. Such shields block negative energies and diminish or totally prevent the unpleasant and harmful effects of negative vibrations.[374]

All of the above may sound rather idealistic. The easiest, and unfortunately the most common response, is to strike back if we feel we have been attacked, and/or to pass along any unpleasantness we have received.

Case: In The Inspector General, a film starring Danny Kaye, one of my favorite actors, a scene of anger unfolds in a police station. The Chief of Police is bawled out roundly by his wife, who storms out of his office, slamming the door. With smoke coming out of his ears, he blusters over to the Desk Sergeant and excoriates him for no obvious reason. The Sergeant reams out the Corporal of the guard, who is just passing by on his way out of the door. Stomping down the steps of the police station, the Corporal brushes against a beggar who is passing by (Danny Kaye). He furiously shoves the beggar into the gutter, shouting at him for getting in his way. The beggar, having no idea why he is the object of this abuse, turns around and kicks at a passing dog.

Holding in angers is another common response. As children, we are usually told in school to not respond to aggression with our own aggression. The better alternative, we are told, is to tell the teacher or other person in authority.

Without learning to explore and deal with feelings, we are often left with these buckets full of resentments and angers sloshing around inside, waiting for an opportunity to be unloaded.

Cost/Benefit Analysis for anger
Advantages in releasing angers: Venting angers may be beneficial in a variety of ways. Holding in anger is unhealthy, leading to accumulation of angers that can spill out with excessive responses when we are again provoked to anger. Angers held over long periods of time may contribute to ill health. Letting out anger, particularly in unprovocative ways, can provide a safe release that does not escalate into further angers.

Disadvantages of releasing angers: There are several dangers in expressing anger as a way of dealing with loss of control. In the heat of anger, it may be difficult to stay on your side of the fence. You may provoke more anger and may end up the worse off for it. When you deal with anger from strangers, there is no background of mutual experiences of problem-solving, and there may be no good will to overlook slights or seek common grounds or mutual understanding. Staying on your side of the fence may not lead to the desired effect of having your situation heard and understood. Your best efforts may still be perceived as attacks, and may provoke further anger.

Venting angers at convenient targets provides immediate release for angers. However, like a stone cast into a pond that spreads circles of waves, sooner or later waves come bouncing back towards the point of anger that is splashed out.

The shadow and projections of blame
We also carry around buckets of unacceptable feelings that we experience but have been told are improper, bad or against the teachings of our family, our school, our society at large (through general social interactions and the media) or religion. Because we feel embarrassed, ashamed or guilty for having such feelings, we do our best to deny, ignore and bury them.

If we see behaviors in others that evoke these feelings, we may dump some of the self-critical load from our (mostly unconscious) guilt and shame buckets on those whom we catch in unacceptable behaviors. Our unconscious mind then feels better, because we have upheld the teachings we have internalized, but also because we punish others for that which is buried inside and unacceptable to ourselves.

> *It all started when he hit me back!*
>   – Anonymous

Responsibility and blame

It's all too easy to suggest, "It all started when he hit me back!" rather than to examine what we might have done, how our actions might have been perceived or experienced as a negative blow – that precipitated what we then experienced as an attack on ourselves.

In school we are not encouraged to analyze why we were attacked, and only rarely are we taught methods and processes for looking inward or for self-examination and analysis, and so we have no education in doing other than stuffing angers away inside.

When our anger is stimulated, the first reactions are often blaming ones. When someone does something as simple as to step on my toe, I may respond in pain and anger – not noticing circumstances that may have explained or mitigated the blame in the actions that led to my pain. If I happen to be carrying buckets full of anger from other threats, attacks, or disrespectful intrusions on my autonomy, I may be all the more ready to take this opportunity to vent some of my stored up anger.

If my pain is not too severe, or my stored up angers not at levels that tempt me to dump them, I may pause long enough before responding – to take into consideration possible mitigating circumstances.

I am bemused by the synchronicity of the arrival of the following anonymous internet "passalong," precisely at the time I was writing about this. I have slightly modified this to better illustrate my points.

PRAYER OF UNDERSTANDING, ACCEPTANCE, FORGIVENESS

Heavenly Father, Help us remember that the jerk who cut us off in traffic last night is a single mother who worked nine hours that day and was rushing home to cook dinner, help with homework, do the laundry and spend a few precious moments with her children.

Help us to remember that the pierced, tattooed, disinterested young cashier who can't get your order right when you most need someone competent to help you is a worried student, balancing his apprehension over final exams with his fear of not getting his student loans for next semester and worrying about whether he can pay both his rent and his tuition bill this month.

Remind us, Lord, that the scary looking bum, begging for money in the same spot every day (who really ought to get a job!) is a slave to addictions that we can only imagine in our worst nightmares because he was put on pain medication after being blindsided by a truck.

Help us to remember that the old couple walking annoyingly slowly through the store aisles and blocking our shopping progress are savoring this moment, knowing that, based on the biopsy report she got back last week, this will probably be the last year that they go shopping together.

Heavenly Father, remind us each day that, of all the gifts you give us, the greatest gift is love. It is not enough to share that love with those we hold dear. Open our hearts not just to those who are close to us but to all humanity.

Let us be slow to judge and quick to forgive.

Bless us with patience, empathy and love.

AMEN!

Most of us are able to see and appreciate circumstances that explain behaviors which stimulate us to respond with anger. When we empathize with those who have offended us, we can often understand, accept and forgive their behaviors. Our initial angry feelings dissipate, and may even be replaced with compassion and forgiveness for the person who wronged us and forgiveness for ourselves for responding too quickly or for over-reacting.

At other times, we feel that circumstances did not adequately explain, mitigate or excuse behaviors that made us feel bad, and we may continue to nurture our resentments.

Anger at self is a common cause for internal stress. We may have meta-emotions in response to anger (or other emotions). These are reactions to our own reactions such as, "Damn! I promised myself I wouldn't shout at my kid when he spilled his food, and I just did it again!" or "How could I have been so stupid as to blast that silly old woman who just had to stick her nose into my business at the office meeting when I asked for an explanation of my benefits?" Those who hone this skill and practice it often can even develop meta-meta-emotions, such as, "Here I go again, picking at myself again! I'm so terrible at catching myself when I do these things!"

Now, anger can be constructive or it can be destructive – depending on how you respond and what you take away from it. If someone bawls you out, you can take it as an attack on your personhood and stuff a rancid load of "I'm no good" or "He's a real so-and-so!" into your bucket.

Along with meta-emotions, we have meta-decisions about handling our emotions. You might resolve, "I'm sure going to stay away from Henry in the future when he's angry!" or "I'm no match for Henry. I'd better keep my lip buttoned at the office." or "You just wait, Henry, till I catch you making your next mistake!" or "I've had it! I'm quitting this job." It is really easy to get ourselves in a stew with such internal angers, which then raise our bucket's contents to simmering or boiling temperatures.

Alternatively, we could examine our behaviors that elicited the anger and change them so that we are less likely to provoke such reactions again; or we might ask ourselves, "What's the matter with Henry today, anyway?" – and perhaps replace anger with understanding and compassion, as in the passalong examples above. You might choose a healing approach to your angers, such as: "I wonder what I might have done to stir Henry's anger?" or "I need to catch Henry when we're both in a better mood and sort out our differences and how we can discuss them without dumping on each other in the future."

To summarize your options for when you feel angry: You always have choices. Anger challenges can be invitations to empty old junk you're carrying around in your buckets. This can give you the immediate feeling of unloading a burden – but the relief is usually only temporary. Anger usually begets anger in return (often paid with interest), so you end up in the long run with even more anger stuffed in your buckets.

If you choose a path of healing rather than a path of aggression, then anger challenges can be invitations to examine your feelings, your relationships, your meta-reactions, and how you would like to handle all of these. A healthy CBT approach is to ask yourself, "What choices do I have?" whenever you are confronted with a difficult situation. At the very least, this will help you "count to ten" before responding. With practice, it will help you make choices that are healing.

Moving deeper, you can come to a place of healing where you experience provocations as invitations to ask yourself, "Why does my bucket overflows with this particular type of issue, or this type of person?"

Practicing alternatives to anger responses, towards yourself and others – at times when you are not angry – can prepare you to respond in constructive ways when you are getting heated. (See "Conjugations," above.)

What has helped me enormously is practicing "reframing" – which I learned best from Jamshed Morenas, one of my most creative family therapy supervisors, when I was struggling in front of a one-way mirror, having outstanding instruction in dealing with families in conflict. I remember very clearly my first introduction to reframing. I was hopelessly mired, unable to shift a mother, father, and three teenage children out of their patterns of constantly criticizing each other, defending themselves and arguing incessantly. Jamshed called me out of the session for a discussion. I felt totally helpless to stop them from fighting each other long enough to even explore alternatives to being constantly angry and embattled.

Jamshed pointed out that the children were just being children and the parents were being parents. Working to stop them was an unproductive therapeutic frame of mind. This would only induct me into their system of arguing. A more constructive intervention might be to re-frame their arguments as expressions of caring for each other.

Although skeptical, I returned to the therapy room and observed, "This is a family of porcupines. You can't get close to each other without getting poked." They readily agreed with me, and we looked at ways that each one was good at poking at the others. Then I added, "But that's the way porcupines show that they care for each other – by needling each other." This had a stunningly positive effect. All of the members of this family of porcupines were quickly able to acknowledge that they did really care for each other. With a little further help, they were also able to see that they had the choice of showing that they cared through their quills or through their soft bellies – which they hesitated to even acknowledge they had because of the anticipation of being pierced by the quills of someone else in the family.

Looking deeper

THE GUEST HOUSE
This being human is a guest-house.
Every morning a new arrival.
A joy, a depression, a meanness,
some momentary awareness comes
as an unexpected visitor.
Welcome and entertain them all!
Even if they're a crowd of sorrows,
who violently sweep your house
empty of its furniture.
Still, treat each guest honorably.
He may be clearing you out
for some new delight.
The dark thought, the shame, the malice,
meet them at the door laughing,
and invite them in.
Be grateful for whoever comes,
because each has been sent
as a guide from beyond.
                                        - Jelaluddin Rumi

If you take a spiritual perspective, assuming that every experience in life is a potential healing lesson, an invitation from your higher self to learn and to grow, then challenges in your life may have a different "feel" to them. This is a major reframing!

If someone does something that disappoints or hurts you (if you can catch yourself before anger rises and derails you're your trains of thought and reasoning abilities, or after anger has abated), you might ask yourself, "What healing lessons am I being invited to learn?"

Focusing on the "other," you may come up with answers such as "compassion," "empathy," "understanding," "healing" or "gratitude" (for being in more fortunate circumstances yourself).

Focusing on yourself, you might explore such questions as, "What beliefs or attitudes in me could have raised my anger towards this person/ interaction/ situation?" or, "What old hurts could there be in my bucket that were stirred by this encounter?"

If you notice that you find yourself angry repeatedly in similar sorts of encounters, you might begin to ask, "What might there be in me that invites these angry interactions?" It could be that your unconscious mind is bringing you to behave in ways that elicit provocations to anger.

Case: When I was 8-15 years old, I was often left in charge of David, my younger brother (along with other household duties) because my single-parent mother had to work to support the family. There were periods when I resented the burden of baby-sitting, but couldn't allow myself to complain because everyone in our little family had to pull their weight to enable us to get by. I would do things to invite David to misbehave and would then vent my anger on him. By doing this, I developed situations where I could vent some of the resentments I was carrying – over having to be the man of the house in the absence of our father. I was totally unaware of doing this until my mother repeatedly pointed it out to me.

Lessons of this sort may also come "out of the blue," without any apparent ways in which we could possibly have invited them through our behaviors.

In my 35 years of practicing psychotherapy, I have often found my clients teaching me almost as much as I am teaching them. The issues they are struggling with are precisely the issues I am – or need to be – examining in myself. And if I don't get the lesson the first time, a second or third client appears within a very short period, with a similar problem. Clients often offer general reminders, such as to be more compassionate and considerate of others' feelings, but their lessons can be uncannily on target for more specific issues in my life. I share here just one of the uncountable examples of synchronicities I could muster:

Case: I was festering and fuming at work, furious with my new clinical administrator, who was forcing us to document clinical interventions in increasingly greater detail. This appeared to me to be totally unnecessary and an enormous waste of time that could be far better spent in direct clinical interventions. Within a few days of receiving the printed directives that detailed the new, tedious charting procedures, a child came for psychiatric evaluation. He had a serious post traumatic stress disorder (PTSD) following an automobile accident. His mother was obviously upset and harried. I thought her distress was due to her own PTSD and her son's problems, but discovered that she was upset just as much by job-related frustrations. She is a nurse and her employer had just instituted much stricter charting procedures on her hospital unit. As I counseled her on how to deal with her job-related issues through relaxation and imagery techniques, I could not but smile inside – as I listened to some part of myself saying, "And who else in this room could use this advice?"

The skeptic will say these apparent synchronicities are purely coincidental. I believe they are choreographed by our higher selves and by an unseen wisdom that far exceeds our own – to nudge or jar us into greater healing awarenesses.

These lessons from clients have come so often that I now regularly ask, in each therapy session, "Now, what has this client been sent to teach me?"

Group angers

In inter-racial or international angers, ingrained prejudices tend to be perpetuated. The targets of our angers are dehumanized as "others" – who are less than human, less than deserving of our understanding or compassion; ungrateful recipients of our aid who are draining our resources, sending criminals into our neighborhoods or terrorists into our country; unfortunate but necessary civilian casualties in our crusade for our own causes; and anyway, if they had stopped their leaders from being the nasty people they are, they wouldn't have to suffer these consequences.

If we look only at the surface manifestations of problems, it is easy to escalate to avenging the wrongs we feel have been perpetrated upon us by these "others." We fail, however, to solve the problem. We prosecute and jail perpetrators of crimes – but end up with criminals who are released from jail only to return to further crimes on the streets, more savvy for having spent lots of time behind bars with other, more experienced and vicious criminals. We attack Afghanistan and Iraq, and in fact increase the likelihood of further terrorist attacks.

We should be asking, "What has our nation done that may be feeding our angers – in the same way that we as individuals can ask what we may have done to provoke angers. Changing ourselves is so much easier than changing someone else!

Figure II-23

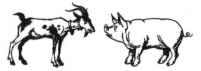

WHY AREN'T YOU
MORE GRATEFUL
WHEN I PROVE
HOW WRONG YOU'VE BEEN?

Choices: Revenge vs. forgiveness

> *There are two courses of action to follow when one is bitten by a rattlesnake. One may, in anger, fear or vengefulness, pursue the creature and kill it. Or one may make full haste to get the venom out of his system. If we pursue the latter course we will likely survive, but if we attempt to follow the former, we may not be around long enough to finish it.*
> – Brigham Young

There are countries where revenge is the accepted way of dealing with interpersonal hurts.[375] While I am not competent to judge whether this is any better a solution if it is culturally sanctioned, I am not inclined to believe it is.

In our own culture, on a personal level, revenge may be sweet but it tends to perpetuate and aggravate angry relationships. As mentioned above, this is much more so in revenge between clans and nations.

Forgiveness

Forgiveness is one of the best alternatives to anger. While this is seen by some to be the choice of a weakling or wimp, it is actually, in most cases, the choice of a deeply wise and spiritual person.

> *He who cannot forgive others destroys the bridge over which he himself must pass.*
> – George Herbert

Some outstanding examples of immediate forgiveness were seen after the events of 9-11. Phyllis and Orlando Rodriguez lost their son, Joe, in the World Trade Towers. When President Bush immediately began his campaign to attack the terrorists, they wrote a letter to the New York Times editor:

Saturday, Sep 15, 2001 8:35pm

Our son Greg is among the many missing from the World Trade Center attack. Since we first heard the news, we have shared moments of grief, comfort, hope, despair, fond memories with his wife, the two families, our friends and neighbors, his loving colleagues, and all the grieving families that daily meet at the Pierre Hotel.

We see our hurt and anger reflected among everybody we meet. We cannot pay attention to the daily flow of news about this disaster. But we read enough of the news to sense that our government is heading in the direction of violent revenge, with the prospect of sons, daughters, parents, friends in distant lands dying, suffering, and nursing further grievances against us. It is not the way to go. It will not avenge our son's death. Not in our son's name.

Our son died a victim of an inhuman ideology. Our actions should not serve the same purpose. Let us grieve. Let us reflect and pray. Let us think about a rational response that brings real peace and justice to our world. But let us not as a nation add to the inhumanity of our times.

Copy of letter to White House:

Dear President Bush:

Our son is one of the victims of Tuesday's attack on the World Trade Center. We read about your response in the last few days and about the resolutions from both Houses, giving you undefined power to respond to the terror attacks.

Your response to this attack does not make us feel better about our son's death. It makes us feel worse. It makes us feel that our government is using our son's memory as a justification to cause suffering for other sons and parents in other lands.

It is not the first time that a person in your position has been given unlimited power and came to regret it. This is not the time for empty gestures to make us feel better. It is not the time to act like bullies. We urge you to think about how our government can develop peaceful, rational solutions to terrorism, solutions that do not sink us to the inhuman level of terrorists.

Sincerely,

Phyllis and Orlando Rodriguez

Often, forgiveness follows a period of anger. This may come when tempers cool, immediately following an injury or altercation, or it may come only after years of bitter struggles and battles that leave the warring parties exhausted, bleeding and mourning their dead. It is helpful to have an outsider mediating between the aggrieved parties – to create a safe space in which to meet, to help explore differences in a gradual and reasoned (rather than heated) manner, to smooth ruffled feathers and calm prickly tempers, and to suggest alternatives to habitual patterns of perceptions, feelings, anticipations of being attacked, and other dysfunctional and counter-productive interactions.

The most important part of such mediation is getting the parties to sit down together and have some normalizing human interactions, breaking the pattern of perceiving the opposing parties as "other," as "enemy" or as "inhuman." In many cultures it is acknowledged that if you break bread together with another, then you are much less likely to be unkind to each other. So a an introductory period of getting acquainted and rubbing elbows with each other is important, prior to exploring differences.

> For it is in giving that we receive,
> It is in pardoning that we are pardoned...
> – St. Francis of Assisi

The most difficult parts of forgiveness may be forgiveness of self – for having let anger get out of control – and, even more difficult, examining the bucket of angers we carry from various personal experiences and from realizing we have dumped an undeserved load of buried emotional garbage on a convenient target. The last is so difficult that very few people manage this.

Love and compassion

> Man must evolve for all human conflict a method which rejects revenge,
> aggression and retaliation. The foundation of such a method is love.
> – Dr. Martin Luther King, Jr.

Addressing your life, including your problems, through your heart is a totally different experience from living your life through your head.

The heart knows the experiences of others directly. It resonates with their pains, their buckets of buried hurts, their wishes and aspirations and their fears of failure, their love of life and their yearning to receive love from others, and the shared experiences of being a part of something greater than any one individual.

The heart is more than a metaphor for these awarenesses. It is an actual organ of energetic and spiritual perception. Our heart chakra is the central energy center in the body. The lower charkas coordinate our physical being, the higher ones connect us with our higher, spiritual selves. At the same time, the heart chakra connects with the energetic heart centers of others.

The heart knows – within you and within every person you meet – your connection with the Infinite Source, that timeless kernel of core Truth which guides and inspires all life; the connection with the eternal soul that has chosen to come into this earthly existence to learn and to grow.

If we can hold an awareness that negative experiences are opportunities to choose – between dumping negativity from our inner bucket and finding ways to spread the balm of compassion and healing on the situation – then we may move from responding to negativity with care and love rather than with anger and revenge.

This is the deeper healing of life. To hold a connection with the inner knowing of the rightness of all being, so that every action and reaction comes from the heart.

> *It is a mistake to speak of a bad choice in love, since as soon as a choice exists, it can only be bad.*
>
> – Marcel Proust

No one who walks this earth is perfect. We will all make mistakes. The challenge is to learn compassionate lessons from our mistakes, deepening our love and acceptance of ourselves first of all, and then extending our unconditional acceptance to others.

When we can return to this place of love, after another and another and yet another forgetful lesson, we have reached a place of deep self-healing.

Changing patterns of behavior – individually and collectively

> *The Latin roots of 'resentment,' re and sentire, mean 'to feel again' – to feel over and over again the pain caused by the wrong that was done.   Letting go of that resentment is a lot of the 'personal work' done in forgiving, and is often what takes so long*
>
> – Andrew Knock

Once we establish individual and group behaviors for handling anger and revenge, they tend to persist. Blaming others and venting anger on them provides some relief from carrying around buckets full of hurts and angers. Not knowing any alternatives, this often feels like a successful way of handling frustrations.

Changing such patterns can be very difficult. First, we have to begin to feel there might be something wrong in the way we are handling our negative feelings. We might be confronted with pictures of "others" who are as human as we are. We might be inspired by healing responses of people who have been hurt in conflicts but did not respond with anger.

We might begin to see contradictions in the messages our leaders are putting out. The glaring self-interests of Bush and his supporters in promoting wars may come to roost in our awareness when we begin to pay the human and monetary costs of war, or when the media (if they are not censored) bring us information or images that sway us towards healing. Seeing our own soldiers wounded and dying, or seeing enemy civilian casualties of our attacks might just bring us to seek more healing approaches to problems.

We tend to think of healing as something one person does to another, but the most important healing is self-healing. This is as true on a group and national basis as it is with our individual selves.

Politicians take advantage of our tendencies to blame others. Politicians offer us convenient targets for our angers. By painting the "others" as despicable villains, deserving of punishment or death, they invite us to pour out our buckets of wrath. (This serves their interests well, crating a pool of soldiers who will sacrifice themselves for the politicians' gains.)

While we all feel better with this catharsis, we are still left with the real sources of our angers – the buried hurts we carry in our buckets – untouched. It is like throwing burning coals at an enemy from a fire in our home, giving us a sense that we have made good use of these embers of our misfortunes... but not dealing in any basic way with the flames that go on smoldering in our home.

Few people are asking, when we consider terrorist activities and other violence in the world, "What have we done that has contributed to or provoked the violence?" When we start to look in these directions, we find many things we can do to promote healing. Western arrogance in assuming that we have the best way of life, and Western promotion of ways of life that run contrary to traditional values in other cultures can be highly provocative to people who are not eager to give up their own values. While capitalism has improved material quality of life for those at the top of the social order, it has destroyed family ties and created a culture of competition and self-interest that easily degenerates to destructive selfishness and greed. America's growing poverty levels - witnessed by increasing numbers who find themselves unable to afford health care or even a home - are not good advertisements for our way of life. America's exploitation of material and human resources in other countries is increasingly perceived as a red flag in front of a bull. Fighting off the vengeful terrorists and adopting defensive lifestyles may prove less effective and more costly in terms of diminished quality of life for ourselves in the long run than dealing with some of the underlying problems that generate terrorism.

Healing our international conflicts should begin at home – on a personal level.

> *If there is light in the soul,*
> *There will be beauty in the person.*
> *If there is beauty in the person,*
> *There will be harmony in the house.*
> *If there is harmony in the house,*
> *There will be order in the nation.*
> *If there is order in the nation,*
> *There will be peace in the world.*
>
> – Chinese Proverb

Bioenergy protection and spiritual responses to anger from others

> *Your own mind is a sacred enclosure into which nothing harmful can enter except by your permission."*
> –Ralph Waldo Emerson

Some bioenergy practitioners recommend putting up a mirrored energy shield around ourselves, so that any angers directed at us will bounce right back to their source. While this may protect us from angers, it will also perpetuate the anger at the very least, and may spread it around to others who were not the original sources of anger.

My personal practice is to have a strong bioenergy shield that is coated with loving pink healing energies. The shield neutralizes any negative energies in the environment or negative thoughts that are directed at me.

Others have suggested inviting your guardian angels to coat the shield with healing light; praying for the light of Christ or God to surround you (Allah, Buddha, saints, or other protectors and guides may – literally – suit you better); or creating a slippery shield that directs any negativity deep into the earth, where Gaia can neutralize it. The latter was favored by a gardener in one of my workshops, who pointed out that the earth is a wonderful composter, and can transform all negativity to positive, nurturing energies.

Bioenergies "charge up" and strengthen physical realities. They are necessary for life and contribute to health and illness. We usually think of positive energies as building and creating and negative energies as destroying. While this can be the case, in a conflict situation we see that negative energies often add to the "charge," make the sparks fly, and fan the flames. Negative energies can give strength to and perpetuate negativity. If we enter into a conflict with those who are spoiling for a fight, our energies will fuel their energies.

If we can detach ourselves from angry responses, we will not fuel the fires. If we can bring ourselves to send loving, healing energies, we may be able to calm or even neutralize the negative energies.

Case: "Brenda," a 42 year-old mother of three young children, had been estranged from her family for more than two decades. Her father had abused her mother and her verbally and physically, during frequent alcoholic rages. Brenda had left home as soon as she could find a job as a waitress, and had cut all contact with her parents and her younger brother – who had been favored by her father and had not been abused.

While her children enjoyed the company of their grandparents on their father's side, contact with them was infrequent because they lived six hours away. Brenda wished her children could have the attention of her mother, who lived in the same city – but was afraid to contact her lest her father learn of her address and become abusive again.

After hearing a sermon on prayer for forgiveness, Brenda decided to work on her hatred of her father, to free herself of the searing angers she felt whenever she thought about him. Through meditation and prayer, she gradually came into a place of forgiveness, where she started to recall the stories she had heard about her father being severely beaten himself as a child by his father. Brenda added prayers of healing for her father, in addition to prayers for healing for herself; she added prayers for healing of her father's old wounds, and for her mother, who had sided with him out of fear of being abused even more.

She was utterly astounded to receive a phone call from her mother, two days later, telling her how much her mother missed her. She had had a dream about her and decided to track her down. She reported that Brenda's father had been attending Alcoholics Anonymous for several years, and was no longer violent or abusive.

Brenda was able to re-establish relationships with her parents, and her children enjoyed the love of the grandparents they had never before known.

Over the years, I have heard countless stories like this one. When a person who has been harboring resentments and angers against a relative can release them, moving into a space of forgiveness and healing, the universe responds with healings that are way beyond their expectations.

Neutralizing fears and anger

Carrying resentments is poisonous in many ways. When we have a potful of anger that is just waiting to spill, we often feel "prickly" to others. We are resentful, edgy, touchy, suspicious that others are going to hurt us, paranoid that we will be misunderstood, carry a frown or worse on our face, speak with an edgy or annoyed voice, and are likely to say and do things – minor and major – that we might later regret. Other around us will quickly sense they are dealing with a porcupine or a skunk. If their buckets aren't full, and they're not spoiling for a ruckus, they may steer clear of us till we calm down. If they're ready to dump some of their anger garbage they've stuffed away, they may use us as convenient sparring partners, as beating posts, or may provoke us to the point that we explode – expressing their angers for them while they don't have to take the consequences.

This works through subtle energies and intuition as well as on psychological and social levels. When we put out negative vibrations, negativity that is floating around is attracted to us. If we're seeking opportunities to discharge negativity, we will telepathically attract and be attracted to others who are seeking the same. Energetic like is attracted to like.

When we come from a space of love and healing, the universe resonates and responds in kind.

I have been exploring and practicing the use of love, acceptance, healing and forgiveness to neutralize every imaginable sort of negativity for several years, both with clients and for myself. I have yet to find a negativity that cannot be softened or eliminated using these positive energies that are born in a place of love. I am therefore certain that love is stronger than any negativity, so this works well for me and for my clients.

Case: "Merle" had been the victim of a brutal date rape at age 18. She had been too frightened to tell her parents, and had never disclosed this to anyone prior to coming for healing at age 33. She was suffering from menstrual cramps that were so severe she was considering having a hysterectomy – even though she dearly wanted to have children. This, too, had been a problem, as she was infertile and had not

If neutralizing approaches were taught to children in school, then people wouldn't grow up holding as many hurts in their buckets. There would be much more energy available for positive projects, for healing others, for building sweetening spirals - of loving acts for others that beget caring acts in return, that stimulate kindness in return.

Not only would this be helpful to them personally, it would reduce the collective angers that are manipulated by politicians to make war.

In summary
The bottom line is:

No one can make you angry

Anger is one of many choices you can elect in response to a life challenge.

VARIETIES OF HEALINGS FOR STRESS

Bioenergetic healing
Your energy body is another avenue for you to offer yourself healing. You can do this by placing your hands on or near the parts of your body where you have needs for healing, activating the energies with imagery/ visualization, and by intent/ meditation/ prayer.

Before starting bioenergy healing, always set your intention for safety, telling your higher self that you will accept only that which is for your highest good.[376]

Hand healing is something that most people can readily do. You hold your hands over the place needing healing and invite it to happen, allowing your higher self to guide the process. You may feel nothing or you may feel a variety of sensations in your hands and near them, including heat, tingling and vibrations. You can expect an easing of the symptoms as you do this – immediately and increasing over time. Pain responds particularly well, as do injuries (cuts, burns, abrasions, sprains, and fractures) and infections.

Case: I burned my hand in placing a pan in the oven. I thought it wasn't serious, but saw I was wrong when a blister developed. I held my other hand over the burn, asking for healing. The pain abated within minutes, and the next day I awoke with only a barely noticeable redness remaining.

Imagery of healing energies flowing through you can increase your self-healing. You can visualize these energies entering through your feet from the earth or through your head from the Infinite Source and flowing through your body to wherever they are needed, guided by your mind and your hands. Another way is to invite them in with your breath, reaching every part of your being – just as oxygen does.[377]

Intent, meditation and prayer can markedly enhance your self-healing with bioenergies. You may ask your higher self, your guides, angels or the Infinite Source to help you, bringing in more healing, taking it to where it needs to go, in the ways that it can be most helpful. Even though you, yourself, might not consciously know or understand how this will work best, your unconscious mind can manage this.[378]

These sorts of healing improve with practice. You will also gain confidence as you find success in doing this. You may also offer healing in such ways to others.

Intuitive and spiritual awareness

[S]pirituality deepens our notions of what success might be. It becomes inner peace instead of things. It becomes love rather than control. It becomes wealth of spirit rather than just bank account.

Spirit sees creatively into the essence of things, discovering the third way when the either/or is merely two ways of making a mistake.

But it only does that when we continue to stay awake, pay attention, take the humble responsibility that is needed where we are in the moment.

Spirituality is about having the strength to continue when things don't go well. If we quit when things go badly we don't give the numbers a chance to redeem us. If we keep going something good will happen.

Dr. Seuss had over twenty rejections before his first book was published. There is a spiritual energy in perseverance.

Letting go and letting God is what we do when we have done everything, walked the extra mile, paid our dues in full and then some. Then trust the result to the divine.

Spirituality is the bridge upon which dreams flow into reality.

Go ahead and be a human doing. Act out of spiritual consciousness.

Love flows when I do.

                                – John MacEnulty (4/10/2003)

Your higher self knows you are more than just a physical being with thoughts and feelings. It is that part of you which senses you are connected with the Infinite Source, with other people and with everything in nature.

You can call upon your higher self to help you deal with stresses and challenges in your life – through wishes, meditation and prayer.

While western society has tended to discount this aspect of our being, suggesting it is wishful or magical thinking, with no basis for expecting it could be effective, there are many studies showing these approaches can actually work.[379] They can help you deal with difficult situations and improve your life.

Skeptics suggest that we can't rely on such approaches when we don't know how they work. The fact is, they do work. So do aspirin and the force of gravity – and we rely on these regularly without being able to explain how they work.

What is true is that wishing and praying do not always produce the results we ask for, and sometimes seem to bring about unexpected responses from the universe, in ways we would never have anticipated nor even dreamed could happen.

CASE: I have been working on the four volumes of Healing Research for 23 years. There were many times when I wished and prayed the books would be published and out there for the public to enjoy and benefit from. There were times when I was incredibly frustrated at the countless problems which delayed publication. When the books have finally been published, I could see that there were important minor and major details and many significant segments which had been added to the manuscripts due to the delays. The books are better for my having had the leavening of greater time, experience and contemplation.

This process has been a lesson for me in going with the flow, in patience, and in accepting that my concept of the rightness and timing of events is very short-sighted compared to that of the collective consciousness and the Infinite Source which guide and inspire the unfolding of experience. Not only are the books better for my wishes not being answered, but I, myself, am better from these delays.

While there is no ordinary way to confirm reports that some of these responses to wishes and prayers come to us through the help of spirits, angels, Christ, other inspired beings, or of God, many people report that they feel they have these kinds of assistance when they pray for help. As fanciful as this may sound within our western ways of thinking, again there is a wealth of anecdotal reports and fascinating research suggesting that such reports may be based on realities we have just begun to appreciate.[380]

Protection

> *Your own mind is a sacred enclosure into which nothing harmful can enter except by your permission.*
>
> – Ralph Waldo Emerson

When we invite our higher selves to participate in our lives, several cautions are in order.

Our wishes and prayers are sometimes based on limited understanding of the situation, of its overall potentials for affecting us positively or negatively, and of the full potentials and consequences of our wishes for affecting our lives.

An apocryphal tale from China illustrates these points.

> The one horse a poor farmer owned, his prized possession, ran off one day and could not be found. This was a serious blow, as he depended on the horse for transportation, hauling heavy loads and plowing his small plot of land.
>
> The farmer's neighbors commiserated with him over his bad luck. All he would say was, "Well, we'll see."
>
> A week later, his horse returned, accompanied by a small herd of wild horses. His neighbors complimented him on his good fortune. All he would say was, "Well, we'll see."
>
> The farmer's son broke his leg when he was taming one of the wild horses. His neighbors again commiserated with him over his bad luck. Again, all he would say was, "We'll see."
>
> A week later, the local warlord sent his soldiers to conscript every able bodied young man to go to war. The farmer's son was spared, due to his broken leg. When his neighbors again marveled at his good fortune, all he would say, as usual, was, "Well, we'll see."

536 Vol. II Chapter 5 – Self-Healing Approaches and Exercises

Many people find that their wishes come true, and they are then sorry that they do. Wishes are often made in the throes of distress, anxieties and fears. At times like these, out of pain, fear or desperation, we may ask for things that at a later time we really do not need or want. Once set in motion, however, a wish may take on a life of its own. We may not be able to undo the energetics of the wish.

Unanswered prayers may thus be blessings in disguise.

> *There is no such thing as a problem without a gift for you in its hands. You seek problems because you need their gifts.*
> – Richard Bach (p. 57)

A safeguard against our making wishes that may not be in our best interests is to preface a petitionary prayer or any opening of our higher selves to the universe with a statement such as, "I accept only that which is for my highest good." or "If it be for my highest good, then please grant me this wish:" This allows our higher self and the healing powers beyond our ordinary reality to participate in choreographing our wishes into realities that are helpful and healing rather than negative or harmful.

People ask, "Why would God or the angels allow anything negative to come of a prayer?" I believe that what may feel painful and negative is often an invitation to healing lessons. It is like letting a child touch a hot cup of coffee in order to learn that when you say, "Hot!" or "Don't touch that!" you are warning the child away from something that might be unpleasant or painful. A lesson learned through experience is remembered and understood much better than a lesson told to us. And so it is with our prayers. We must sometimes suffer the consequences of our limited perceptions or understanding in order to learn deeper lessons of respect for the power of our wishes and prayers.[381]

Divination

> *Live the questions now. Perhaps then, someday far in the future, you will gradually, without even noticing it, live your way into the answer.*
> – Rainer Maria Rilke

Accessing your intuitive awareness may be a challenge. While all of us have varying degrees of intuitive abilities, western society discourages us from recognizing, acknowledging and using them. By letting them speak through externalized systems of projection, we can often find deeply meaningful and helpful suggestions to handle challenging issues in our lives.

Numerous systems have been developed in cultures around the world. A few are listed here.

Asking your inner self to answer Yes and No questions is the most direct approach.

You can do this through applied kinesiology[382] – letting your body speak through muscle testing; through imagery – inviting your unconscious mind to show you a mental image for *Yes* and another for *No*; looking within yourself for emotional feelings that distinguish *Yes* and *No*; or with the help of *divining rods* or a pendulum.[383]

Projected divination is another approach. You receive answers to your questions from a long list of possible responses, using what appears to be a random system of selection: you may pick a card from a deck; flip a coin, or use other such methods to select the statements that match your situation. It can be very helpful to have a written reference or live expert to help you interpret the answers you get.

The I Ching, or **Book of Changes** was developed over three thousand years ago, in the dawn of recorded Chinese culture. To read answers to your questions in the *I Ching,* you flip coins or throw yarrow stalks six times and record their patterns as a set of six full or broken lines called a *hexagram.* The sixty-four possible combinations of these hexagrams are then used as keys to select readings from the classic Chinese text, which speak to your questions.[384]

Figure II-24. Hexagrams of the I Ching

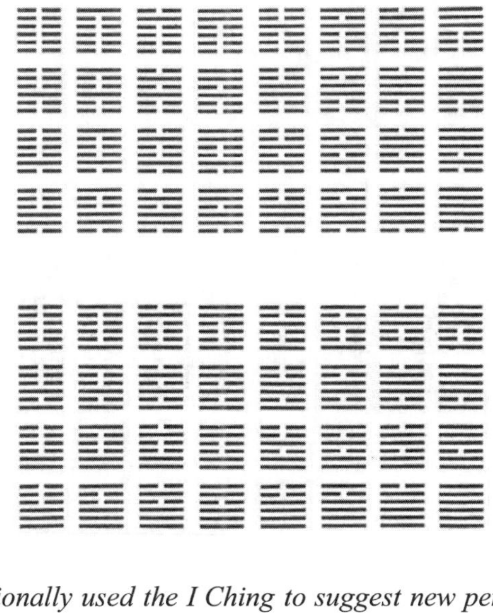

Case: I have occasionally used the I Ching to suggest new perspectives on a diffi-cult or unclear situation. The most striking experience I had was when I was applying for work and three openings were available. Two were at clinics within the same mental health system. I got the identical hexagram for these two and a completely different one when I threw the coins for the other. Since there are 64 possible combinations of lines in the hexagrams, it is highly unlikely to get the identical results twice.

Tarot cards offer a rich set of 78 images, each with a meaning that can relate to questions you are pondering. The 22 cards comprising the *Major Arcana* relate to the physical and spiritual forces of health, power, illness, relationships and religion. The 56 cards representing the *Minor Arcana* include four suits: pentacles, wands, cups and swords. These usually relate to work and to social positions.

While there are basic elements that are common denominators in tarot cards, there are distinct variations in the imagery in different decks of cards. The particular style and archetypal themes depicted on one deck or another may speak more clearly or resonate more deeply with your personality, cultural traditions and aesthetic preferences. A tarot reader will often bring out innumerable associations and help you to find your own meanings to the readings that you might otherwise miss.

Runes are a set of Norse letters, usually printed or carved into a set of stone tokens, each of which carries a detailed meaning. There is a different feel to picking a stone rune out of a pouch – compared to shuffling a deck of cards.[385] The meanings of the runes you choose are detailed in books (Blum) and may be accessed on the web.

Figure II-25. The Norse Runes

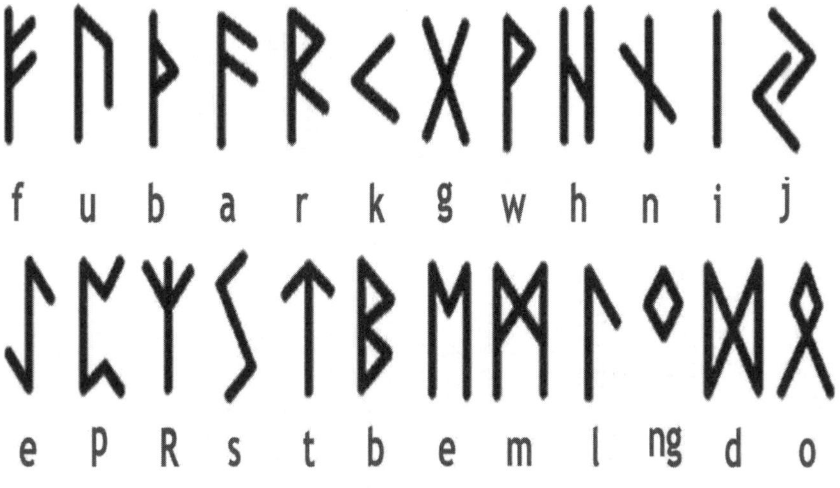

Medicine cards help you explore your issues through traditional Native American[386] or animal[387] symbols.

Pendulums and dowsing rods of many sorts are used to help people apply their intuition to questions that can be answered in simple terms. The most common is to ask, "What is my yes?" and then, "What is my no?" noting the direction of swing of the pendulum or rod in each case. You can then ask any yes/ no question and see what answer your unconscious mind produces through the pendulum or rod.[388]

Many other systems of divination are popular around the world. A common one is to hold a question in your mind and then crack open a large book, such as the

Bible or Qur'an, letting your index finger go intuitively to a line or paragraph that provides an answer. In Africa, shamans throw bones and interpret their patterns for guidance. Many fortune tellers from European backgrounds have used *scrying*, which involves gazing into a crystal ball, a bowl of water, or a mirror, allowing one's inner eyes to project images that relate to questions at hand.

In Native Americans and many other traditional societies, the behaviors of animals and any other occurrence that corresponds in time with your thoughts and actions are viewed as hints that you are thinking and/ or acting in propitious or inadvisable directions. For instance, if you're setting out to visit someone and your car is nearly hit by a careless driver, you might pause to reconsider whether this is the best time to make the journey. More subtle resonations of nature could be the appearance of a beautiful, powerful bird in the sky as you are contemplating an undertaking – which could be an encouraging hint from the collective consciousness that this is an endeavor worth pursuing.

How do these systems of divination work?
All of these approaches have the following common denominators:

1. Inviting you to hold a question in your mind while you are
2. Accessing an index of statements through what seems to be a random system, such as picking a card from a deck, tossing coins, or picking symbols in some other way;
3. Using the words or images indicated by (2) to access comments that relate to your question, as well as to your situation in life;
4. Finding the meanings in the readings that feel relevant to your question.

Though it appears that (2) is a random process, research has shown that mental intent can alter the random arrangements of elements in a system. If left on their own, these do distribute themselves randomly, but when influenced by the needs or intent of a living being they will tend to conform to the needs and expectations of that being.

For instance, an electronic random number generator (RNG) set to display either a number "1" or a "0" will produce very close to 50 percent of each when it is set to run automatically. If a person is asked to sit in front of the RNG and make it produce significantly more "1's" or more "0's."[389]

The devices used in divination allow the conscious mind to detach from responsibility for the outcome of the choice, while the unconscious mind can intuitively/ psychically/ spiritually select the symbol that is indexed to the answer that will be helpful.

On another level, the vagueness of the statements in (4) invites the seeker to bring up mental images and other associations that the unconscious mind is ready to raise on the screen of awareness in response to the questions that initiate the process.

While the skeptic may suggest that all of this is no more than wishful thinking, people through the ages have found these methods helpful in addressing challenging situations in their lives.

See also: Dowsing; Kinesiology

Groups

> *When spiders unite, they can tie down a lion.*
> – Ethiopian Proverb

Groups provide support when you are in need of information, understanding, acceptance, feedback, hope and nurturing. While it helps to have a professional therapist facilitating a group, this may not always be possible.

Self-help groups have been enormously helpful to addicts of every variety, to deal with dependence on alcohol, tobacco, street drugs, gambling, sex and more. Likewise, such groups have been enormously helpful to relatives of addicts who are often caught up in codependent relationships.

Support groups have been able to help some people with pain, cancer, cardio-vascular and other diseases to deal much more constructively and effectively with their physical as well as their psychological issues. In many cases this has brought about physical changes as well, such as reduced pain and lessening of other symptoms.[390]

Meditation, yoga and other self-healing practices are often more enjoyable as well as more effective in group settings. Participants provide instruction, encouragement and psychological support for each other.

Groups can be educational for caregivers – participants sharing new methods and approaches and support to deal with difficult cases.

Groups for healers have been helpful – to each other and to healees. Offering healing within a group, healers can more easily let go of any attachments to outcomes, as they are not totally responsible individually for responding to the healing needs of the healees. Combined efforts of healers have been reported at times to help, when prior individual healings were of limited success.

Imagery/ Visualization

> *We are what we think.*
> *All that we are arises with our thoughts.*
> *With our thoughts, we make our world.*
> – Gautama Buddha

In imagery we find the pictures (worth the thousands of words) that facilitate our thought processes and communications. Imagery helps us build analog maps in our minds that enable us orient ourselves and to navigate through the physical world, the worlds of relationships with other people, and our own inner worlds of thoughts and feelings.

We hold memory pictures in our minds of how the world is, inner maps that guide us through familiar territory. In some instances, these maps lead us to organize our perceptions in stereotyped ways; in other cases, they serve as starting points and more general guidelines for dealing with new situations.

Creativity and healing may be expressed and shaped through imagery. We may choreograph scenes in our minds, playing out imaginary roles in hypothetical situations, and rehearsing exploring in our minds various options and possibilities before acting upon them.

Healing energies may be activated and shaped by mental imagery. If I picture that I am projecting healing to another person, my hands and heart may warm to the task – quite literally. I often find that when I am opening myself to healing and wishing healing thoughts for someone, my hands get warm or even hot, as the healing energies are activated. The metaphor of "my heart warming to another person" is an accurate description of healing energies activated in the heart chakra, connecting my heart with that of the person I'm relating to in a healing way.

There are many wonderful applications of imagery in self-healing. The simplest use of imagery is for reducing emotional and physical tensions. You may find it relaxing to picture yourself on a holiday, enjoying fresh surroundings and pleasurable activities. You might image yourself on a beach or by a pool, savoring a cool drink after a refreshing swim. You'll find that your body will relax as you relax psychologically.

More complex imagery approaches may involve problem-solving exercises for issues that cause tension. You could allow yourself to imagine as many ways as possible of dealing with someone whom you find oppressive or abusive. Your visualizations could take the form of practicing being in control, or of healing interactions and problem resolution. You might bring up memories of pleasant and satisfying experiences with that person, to remind you during times of stress and distress that good things are still possible. Such imagery may introduce hope in situations where you feel despair, offer immediate emotional satisfaction, and suggest creative solutions that you might not have considered previously.

> *If you advance confidently*
> *in the direction of your dreams,*
> *and endeavor to live*
> *the life you have imagined,*
> *you will meet with a success*
> *unexpected in common hours.*
> *You will pass an invisible boundary:*
> *new, universal, and more liberal laws*
> *will begin to establish themselves*
> *around and within you*
> *and you will live*
> *with a higher order of beings.*
> *If you have built castles in the air,*
> *your work need not be lost;*
> *that is where they should be.*
> *Now put the foundation under them.*
>
> – Henry David Thoreau

Imagery can be used for healing in many situations, including meditation, relaxation, problem-solving, intuitive awareness, and self-healing for allergies, cancer, and other disorders.[391] As an example, here are some imagery exercises for pain.

Imagery for dealing with pain

As discussed in Chapter II-2, pain is a complex experience, composed of physical, neurological and psychological elements. On spiritual levels, pain is often an invitation to explore aspects of ourselves that we would otherwise rather ignore.

Much of our response to pain is a meta-reaction of anxiety about suffering from the pain. This sets up vicious circles like

> Pain → anxiety about suffering → tension → worsening of pain due to tension → more anxiety that the pain will never go away → etc.

There are many ways to stop these vicious circles, imagery being a potent one.

Imagery offers a series of potent vehicles that can take us into new spaces, where we can stop these vicious circles and reduce our pains.

Listening to your pain is a first step. As with any symptom, your should ask, "What is this pain telling me?" Picture to yourself that you are putting your pain on an empty chair and speak with it. (*See Gestalt Therapy*)

Once you have heard its messages and opened yourself to learning its lessons (which can be an ongoing, ever-deepening process), your pain may abate on its own, because your unconscious mind will no longer need to be calling your attention through the pain to the issues it wants you to deal with.

Pains may have physical components and habit components that are not cleared by just listening to them. Further exercises may then be helpful.

Picture a treatment or remedy for your pain. If you have a headache and you image that a compress of exactly the right temperature is being gently applied to the painful spot, the pain may diminish.

Picture your pain as a color. Close your eyes and invite your pain to dress itself in a color. Often, this will have intense, angry, hurt hues. Picture to yourself that you are shifting the color to lighter, more delicate shades of the same color, or ask your pain if it would like to have another color join it, to soothe it.

Case: "Evelyn" suffered from migraines, and medications barely took the edge off the headaches that frequently made her head feel like it was going to explode. She pictured her headaches as an angry red that filled her whole visual field, laced with black lightning symbols. Her headaches suggested that bringing in a white, healing light could help. As Evelyn pictured to herself that white light was coming from the Infinite Source to soothe her, she felt the painful red and black gradually shift to pink and gray. I encouraged her to practice this several times a day.

The next time she felt a migraine coming on, Evelyn repeated this imagery. Her pain was less than half as severe as it had been before, and the migraine attack lasted only half an hour, where previously it could have continued through the whole day, till she went to sleep at night.

Evelyn felt a major benefit of this exercise was that she had something to do about the terrible pain.

This is a good example of how any relaxation techniques can help in dealing with pain by reducing the meta-anxiety about the pain.

Colors may not speak to everyone's experience of pain. If colors don't speak to you, then invite your pain to suggest its own image. People have found their pains appearing as fire, a blowtorch, a knife, pincers, an angry monster, and so on. Work with whatever images come to you. Ask for suggestions from your inner wisdom, your higher self, from your guides or the Infinite Source for ways in which to soften the intensity of the pain imagery.

Case: "Gary," a musician, suffered from severe backaches. He had little success with color imagery. When he sought inner guidance, what came to him was an angry, loud synthesizer tone. When he adjusted the keyboard in his mind to make the tone softer and quieter, his pain lessened to almost nothing.

Stephen Levine (1986) observes that our natural tendency is to do our best to shut off or wall away the pain from our awareness. We tend to tighten ourselves against the pain. While the logic of walling off our awareness from the pain is obvious, if you thinks a bit further you will probably be able to see potential pitfalls in this approach. Pushing the pain away does not diminish the pain, and often leads to an internal struggle to overcome it that ends up creating more tension. This feeds into the vicious circles that worsen pain, rather than improve it.

Levine observes, from years of helping people who are suffering, that pains will lessen if you can soften the space around the pain. This imagery lowers tensions in the body and allows the pain to diminish.

The Sedona Method uses a visual analog scale to represent pain.[392] You assign a number to the pain – from "10" being the worst it could possibly be, to "0, " representing freedom from pain. You then simply ask whether you could release some of the pain, in essence giving yourself permission to do so, and check your pain level. It will often go down significantly with this simple approach.[393]

This is a key concept in my understanding of self-healing. In the Sedona Method the acceptance of your symptoms is the primary focus. By not running away from a problem and by not fighting it, by picturing that we are totally in touch with it, we lessen the mental focus and bioenergies attached to the problem. This may be a major component of placebo reactions and of the suggestion component that accompanies all therapies.[394]

Relaxation of any sort reduces the tension component that usually accompanies pain in its vicious circle. Picturing to yourself that you are in a comfortable, relaxing place can markedly reduce tensions and pain. My favorite is to retreat to a magical bubble that is under the water by a coral reef. I watch the colorful fish swimming by, and enjoy the patterns of the sun on the water surface above, making shadows on the sands below. (*See more under Relaxation*)

Meditation can help to not think about and dwell upon the pain, as well as increasing relaxation. Meditation may also open into insights about the origins of pains. (*See Meditation*)

Imagery for bowel problems

Visualizing your digestive system as a river has been helping people with Irritable Bowel Syndrome (IBS), at the hypnotherapy center in Withington Hospital, Manchester, England. IBS may include bloating, pains, constipation or diarrhea.

While symptoms are often mild, they can be debilitating and when severe can be incapacitating. Conventional treatments have had limited success.

Devised by Dr Peter Whorwell, a gastroenterologist, the aim is to make the river flow smoothly. If there is a blockage or a flood, they are asked to visualize ways that the problems can be solved. Therapy sessions are supplemented with practice at home.

For a person with constipation, they may visualize rocks that are blocking the river and needing removal, while someone with diarrhea might picture that they are shoring up the banks to slow the river from running so rapidly.

These imagery exercises have provide relief helped 71% of patients for up to five years after their course of treatment. While other doctors have been slow to pick up on these methods, patients have been very satisfied with the results (Ryan).

Imagery for other physical problems

Gerald Epstein, a psychiatrist in private practice, helps people to self-heal a wide range of illnesses and dis-eases with imagery exercises. His approaches are very direct and mechanistic. For instance, a person may have an enlarged prostate, which is the gland between the bladder and the penis that produces seminal fluid. This can swell and constrict the urethra, making it difficult to start and stop urinating, causing dribbling, etc. Epstein might prescribe practicing of mental imagery of the prostate encased in a net that the respant draws tight, constricting the swollen gland to encourage it to shrink. At the same time, the respant could visualize that he is massaging his prostate, encouraging the flow of urine and semen through the urethra. Though there is no known spontaneous mechanism whereby an enlarged prostate will shrink, Epstein's patients have had success with such exercises.

In another example, a pregnant woman whose baby was lying with its feet towards the cervix in the last days of pregnancy was in danger of delivering the baby feet-first. This can be dangerous because the umbilical cord is at risk of being squeezed shut by the head as it descends through the birth canal, constricting or obstructing the blood supply to the baby from the placenta. Because of this danger, caesarian delivery is often recommended. Epstein might suggest to the woman that she image herself entering her own body, going to the baby through the cervix and helping it to turn to the more common and safer head-down position. (Healers have reported success with the mother speaking mentally with her baby, explaining the need to turn head-down prior to the birth.)

Epstein does not emphasize exploration for psychological causes underlying physical conditions, although he does accept that emotional and social factors may become apparent in the course of treatment. He feels that if illness is present it should be addressed directly, and the rest will follow as required by the individual.

My own preference tends strongly toward exploring underlying psychological causes behind physical problems. Before assuming that a symptom, however troublesome, should be encouraged to diminish or disappear, I recommend to my respants that they ask their symptoms what lessons these problems might be offering. A neck pain may be a metaphor for someone in your life who is "a pain in the neck." A cough, stomach ache or indigestion may be the unconscious mind's way of bringing to your attention that you are having to "swallow down" feelings that you are uncomfortable with or fearful of expressing.[395] I believe that if underlying causes are not addressed then there is an increased likelihood that the same problem will return, or that other symptoms will develop in its place – until the unconscious feelings and issues gain a person's attention.

Imagery for dealing with cancer
Visualization is used in self-healing for cancer. Respants picture their bodies fighting off their disease in every way possible. Classical examples include: seeing their white cells as white knights attacking cancer cells; imaging the blood vessels that feed the cancer as pipes with spigots that the respant shuts off; and so on. Conversely, respants can picture themselves as being healthy (in particular organs and in general) and doing things they like (such as sports; visiting with family and friends; working). Each respant must find the specific images that work for her.

   Many find that self-generated imagery is the most potent, as it holds the structure and associations that are most suitable for the individual person's specific needs. Others find that imagery suggested by a therapist may be more helpful to them, as it can introduce new elements and variations on themes that have become habitual, or approaches that they may not have considered themselves. Even better, a therapist may suggest new approaches that people can then individualize to meet their own needs.

   Intensive practice has often produced improvement in quality of life and occasionally has brought about arrests or even complete remissions of cancer.[396]

Imagery for sports performance enhancement
If you practice your moves mentally, your game will improve. In part, this is a meditative focus, learning to focus your mind on the activity so that you are not distracted; in part, it is a preparation of your body for the physical motions required for the task – just as if your body had actually gone through the physical motions.

   See also: Fitness

Spiritual explorations with imagery

> *A man who works with his hands is a laborer; a man who works with his hands and his brain is a craftsman; but a man who works with his hands and his brain and his heart is an artist.*
> – Louis Nizer

Experiential exercise: a spiritual imagery stroll
Pick a time to do this when you feel confident that you are in a quiet psychological space. It should also be a time when you will not be interrupted for at least an hour or more. Find a comfortable chair that will support your back firmly, and settle yourself into the chair with your feet firmly planted on the floor. You might want to read the following instructions onto an audio tape so that you can have

their guidance as you move through the exercise, without having to interrupt yourself to find the steps of instruction on these pages.

Picture to yourself that you are on a holiday, with no obligations or cares. You start out from your country inn, taking a pleasant walk through a beautiful countryside on a clearly marked, winding path. See the bushes and flowers and trees along the path. Feel the crunch of the earth under your feet; the warm sun and pleasant breeze on your skin. Smell the smells of the earth and the fragrance of lush vegetation. Hear the rustle of the breeze through the leaves of the trees, and the twitter of birds.

As you round a turn in the path, you come upon a cottage, where a wise being dwells. He is sitting by his doorway, and welcomes you warmly. He invites you to sit down and enjoy a fresh drink, and offers to answer any questions you may have.

You ask him questions that you've pondered about your life and your relationship. You take as long as you need to pose all your unsolved problems, listening carefully to his answers.

Take some time to reflect on his observations, clarifying with this wise being any issues that remain unclear.

Feeling sated with his wise replies, you thank him, take your leave, and start back along the path.

You are surprised at how differently you feel on the path back, and how quickly you reach the inn.

Take whatever time you need to consider the answers you received to your questions. You might write them down for review at a later date. Were they helpful? Where did they come from?

Many people find such exercises incredibly enriching, stimulating inner resources which they never knew they had within them.[397]

Visualizations for insomnia

While insomnia can be tiring and draining, it is also an opportunity to practice various relaxation and imagery techniques that are wonderfully self-healing. Here is an exercise taught by Judith Landau, MD, a spiritual psychiatrist.

As you go to sleep, talk to your guardian angels and spirit guides and protectors, asking them to bring you messages only for your highest good. Remind them, "I want only those messages during the night that I absolutely need, because I need to sleep. You may bring me messages to help me waken and proceed through my day tomorrow, but only half an hour before I wake."

Take some deep, clearing breaths. Picture to yourself that you are inhaling light, exhaling gray impurities. Breathe at a normal rate, not pushing your breath, just watching how your body moves the air in and out, releasing any tensions or old "stuff" that you no longer want or need to hold onto out, bringing in healing and spiritual inspiration.

Gently tighten and relax the muscles of your toes and feet. Repeat with the muscles of your ankles; then your calves, thighs, and so on, right up your body to your face. (See muscle relaxation, above, for further details on progressive muscular relaxation.) Note any points of tension or pain in your body, but don't spend time focusing on them just yet.

When you are completely relaxed, visualize a colored crystal in the sky. Let the color come to you spontaneously. Direct the rays of the crystal at whatever points of anxiety or pain you sense in your body. Let the colored rays from the crystal spread from this spot, reaching every particle of your being.

Take your time in doing this exercise. If you fall asleep at any point along the way, that is just fine.

If you are still awake, picture to yourself that a piece of the crystal is now crystallized out of the light, residing in your body, and continuing to radiate its healing light – even when you are not paying attention to it.

See also: Cognitive Behavioral Therapy; Conditioning; Meditation; Neurolinguistic Programming; Psychoneuroimmunology (PNI) – especially the anchoring imagery exercise

Meditation

> *May we be guided through every experience along the direct path of love that leads from the human heart into the most sublime source of love.*
> – The Koran

Meditation is a mental discipline. It helps you to focus your mind as and when you want to.

You may not be aware how your mind tends to ruminate on frivolous, useless or, more annoyingly, on troublesome issues. For instance, have you ever thought of a purple camel? Well, now take a few moments to stop thinking of a purple camel.

What happens? Most of us find that we can't simply stop thinking about something by willing ourselves to stop. The mind does not accept negative orders. In fact, as we push against a thought, such as a purple camel, it tends to push back even stronger. In effect, by pushing it away we are actually giving it more energy and strengthening it.

So how can you get this purple camel to stop following you? Quite simply, actually – by focusing on something else.

The same is true of anxieties and worries. If you push them away, you are simply giving them more energy and they will pursue you even more persistently than your purple camel.

Meditation allows you to let go of anxieties, worries and problems, thereby slowing or even stopping the vicious circle. With meditation, you gain greater control over the focus of your mind.

With prolonged regular practice (usually over a period of years), meditation can also lead you into profound spiritual awarenesses.[398]

Practices:

Mindfulness meditation is an ancient classic, honed to a fine art in Zen and other traditions. You practice being aware of being aware. As you wake in the morning, you note every nuance of opening your eyes, stirring your body, the sensation of your feet touching the floor, your muscles moving your legs, and so on through the day. If your mind strays in the directions of what your legs are moving you towards, you have gone into your head and have to remind yourself to hold your focus strictly in the present moment, the ever-present *Now*.

Breathing meditations are as varied as cultures and traditions around the world can make them.

- Observe your breath coming in and going out. Simply watch your body being filled by the air and releasing it. This may not be as simple as it sounds, because there is a natural tendency to pull the air in or push it out, which interrupts its natural rhythm and flow.

- Silently say to yourself the word "in" as you breathe in, and "out" as you breathe out. Say this as the air is in mid-stream in each direction. You might watch for the precise turning point where the out-breath turns around and becomes the in-breath, saying "in" at this point, and "out" as it reverses to become the outgoing breath, or you might simply say, "now" at each of the turning points.

- Don't criticize, argue with yourself or get into mental discussions over thoughts, feelings or sensations that call for your attention. This simply locks you into the distractions.

- Picture to yourself that you breathe in *prana*, cosmic energy, along with the air that comes into your lungs. Like the oxygen, it spreads to every particle of your being. As you exhale, it carries away any tensions you're ready to release like an ocean tide.

- Count your breaths, starting with "and" on the in-breath and "one" on the out-breath. After a round of four, return to "one." If you get distracted, gently return to "one."

- There are many spiritual practices associated with breathing. One is to choose two inspirational words or brief phrases, such as, "I am" and "One with God." Silently say one phrase on the in-breath and the other on the out-breath. You might deepen this practice by deliberately saying, "I am" on the out-breath, picturing to yourself that you are emptying the vessel that is you, then filling your whole being with God's essence on the in-breath. Other common breath-pacing phrases: I am – love/ peace; Al – lah; Christ/ God/ Allah – heals / loves me/ is love; Explore how you feel with reversing the timing of the phrases, to match the opposite phase of breathing.

Meditations for chatty minds can help to deal with habits of distraction.

The bubble meditation can have surprisingly steadying effects on even the chattiest mind. Picture to yourself that you are in a big, magic bubble that you can adjust in any way you wish for your comfort. You can have it as large as a room or a house or a football field, as small as a space suit, or as small as a soap bubble you would blow as a child into the wind and yourself small and light enough to waft away on it. You can make the walls of your bubble transparent, opaque or mirrored on the outside for privacy; solid or windowed; static or flexible. You are perfectly safe and able to conjure up any comforts you wish within your private bubble. (I like to have mine about the size of a small room, underneath the waters of a coral lagoon where I can watch the fish swim by and enjoy the play of light on the water surface above, reflected as moving shadows on the sands below.)

Once you are settled into your bubble, observe any sensation, feeling or thought that comes along. Welcome it lovingly and put it into a bubble of its own, which you pop through the wall of your bubble. You may release it from your awareness immediately, or watch it float away till it disappears. Then, return to waiting for the next thing that comes along, welcoming it lovingly and releasing it into a bubble of its own. Continue to do this for as long as it feels helpful.

Variations on this theme: Picture that you are sitting by the side of a good sized stream after a heavy rain. There are lots of leaves, twigs, and even some good sized branches floating past you. Welcome lovingly any sensation, feeling or thought that comes along, placing it on a leaf or a branch that is floating by. You may release your awareness of it as you place it on its floating raft, or you may watch it float downstream till it is out of sight.

Another vehicle for carrying away your distractions could be an endless conveyor belt or train, if these feel more constructive to you.

Problem solving can be a meditative practice.
Here is a sample meditation for brainstorming creative solutions to problems: Picture to yourself that you are in the center of an enormous flower with many petals, such as a lotus or dahlia. Ask yourself, "What can I do about this problem?" Take any answer which pops into your mind and place it on a petal near you, without analyzing or criticizing it. Answers may be mundane, silly, foolish, or brilliant inspirations. Don't give in to temptations to abandon any one of them or to analyze them. Return and ask yourself the same question again and again, placing each answer on its own petal.

When you feel this process of inner exploration has run its course, stop asking your question. Sit back and examine each item on its own petal. I have often found this to be an extremely productive meditation.[399]

See also: Under imagery – The spiritual awareness stroll.

Meridian Based Therapies (MBTs)

We all make the mistake of letting a child program our lifetime computer. Meridian Based Therapies allow us to reprogram our hard drive.
– DB

Thought Field Therapy (TFT) was the original modern, western innovation of acupressure self-healing techniques. TFT assigns series of acupuncture points to tap or touch, each problem requiring its own specific cluster and order of points to tap for treatment. A therapist is therefore needed to direct your treatment.

Emotional Freedom Technique (EFT) and a whole alphabet soup of related therapies offer *generic series of points* to tap or touch for relief of your problems. Affirmations are recited as you tap, to focus your attention on the problem and to reprogram your cognitive and emotional response to it.[400]

Eye Movement Desensitization and Reprocessing (EMDR) by itself is a potent treatment for emotional traumas – even severe ones. While it is possible to do this on your own, it is essential with memories of serious emotional trauma to have a counselor or psychotherapist to assist you in sharpening your focus for this work, and in dealing with the memories and feelings that may be released – which sometimes can be intense.

To provide a safer, less traumatizing method for clients in my practice, I have added an affirmation to EMDR that eliminates the intense releases of emotions.[401]

The Wholistic Hybrid of EMDR and EFT (WHEE) is the briefest of these approaches, which I developed for use in my psychiatric psychotherapy.

You can easily experience for yourself how this process works.

Experiential exercise: When you feel comfortable and secure in releasing feelings, you can proceed with this exercise. (If you have any hesitations, I encourage you to find a therapist who can support you through this work.)

First focus your awareness on a mildly unpleasant anxiety, such as a fear of heights, spiders or snakes. Ask yourself, "On a scale of 0 - 10 (with 10 being the worst you could feel, and 0 being not bad at all), how bad do you feel when you recall this memory?" Write down the specific anxiety you want to deal with and your starting intensity number.

Then fold your arms and alternately pat the biceps under each hand for a period of 1-2 minutes. As you do this, recite the following generic affirmation (which you can adapt in any ways that feel best to you):

> *Even though I feel _____*
> *when I think about _____ ,*
> *I love and accept myself wholly and completely*
> *and God loves and accepts me wholly and completely and unconditionally.*[402]

Now reassess the intensity of your negative feeling, on the same scale of 0-10. Most people experience a distinct decrease in their negative feelings.

Alternatives to patting your biceps include: alternate tapping or gently touching the end of each eyebrow that is closest to your nose; alternate patting each of your thighs or knees, and tapping your feet on the floor. In "Silent WHEE" you alternate touching the teeth on the right and left sides of your mouth with your tongue; moving your eyes back and forth horizontally; or listening to sounds that stimulate your right and left ears [403]

Installing positive feelings/ beliefs to replace the negative ones you have released will strengthen your improvements. To do this, you formulate your positive statement (taking your time to select words and images that precisely fit and feel right to you), check your level of belief in the statement on a scale of 1 – 10, and then use your right-left sided stimulation as you recite the affirmation:

> *[POSITIVE AFFIRMATION e.g. I can succeed in _____]*
> *and I love and accept myself wholly and completely;*
> *and God loves and accepts me wholly and completely and unconditionally.*

There are varieties of further methods for dealing with blocks to progress and with more serious problems, for which you are strongly advised to obtain professional support.

These methods are helpful in treating physical as well as emotional pains, with poor self-esteem and negative self-image, with allergies, and with assorted other physical problems.[404]

Neurolinguistic Programming (NLP)

NLP alerts you to notice the modalities for conscious awareness available to you: visual, auditory and kinesthetic. One of these sensory channels may function more strongly and successfully for you. For example, I've discovered that my ears don't connect well to my memory hard drive. If I hear something, such as a name or a phone number, I can recall it for only a few minutes before I am likely to forget it. If I write it down, however, my eyes connect well to my hard drive and I will remember it much more readily.

Pay attention to your own sensory preferences, strengths and weaknesses. Using your stronger sense may make life a lot easier and less stressful for you.[405]

NLP is helpful for self-healing in other ways as well, taking advantage of the fact that your body is participating in your conscious and unconscious awarenesses and in your memories of experiences – particularly the traumatic ones. You can access and reprogram the feelings attached to negative and traumatic experiences with the help of your body. Here is a basic exercise that illustrates this:

Sit comfortably in a chair, and keep your hands in one position on your thighs throughout the exercise. Return to a memory of something that made you sad. When you feel the sadness, press your right thigh with one finger of your right hand, and hold the pressure for a few moments. Then release the pressure, without moving your hand from where it is resting. Now release the sad memory from your awareness, taking a few deep breaths to blow away all traces of the feelings it evoked in your mind and body. Next, turn to a happy memory. When you feel the joy of it, press on your left thigh with one finger of your left hand, and hold the pressure for a few moments. Then release the pressure without moving your hand from where it is resting. Now release your awareness from the happy memory, taking a few deep breaths to blow away all traces of the feelings it evoked in your body. Do not move your hands or fingers from the positions they are in on your thighs.

Now, simultaneously press both of the fingers that you used previously, holding the pressure for a few moments. Then return to the sad memory and observe the feelings that you experience. The following footnote will describe what many people find when performing this exercise. (The information is provided in a footnote so that you can be sure you did not read it subliminally and conform to a suggestion, rather than allowing yourself to have your own, unbiased experience.)[406]

Sometimes it is too large a step and too great a leap of faith for a person to go directly from their state of anxiety to a state of confidence. A therapist may insert several intermediate steps, anchoring each in a chain of spots from the original, problematic situation to the final, successful one.

CASE: If "George," who was fearful of speaking in public (described in Chapter 1) found it too much of a stretch to imagine himself feeling relaxed and competent while lecturing, the therapist might plant one or more intermediate anchors between the first that the final one. For instance, a second anchor might be "feeling confused about whether he might react differently to lecturing;" a third, "wondering whether he might someday feel differently about giving a lecture;" and a fourth, "feeling comfortable speaking to a small group of people he knew." After establishing this chain of five anchors, the therapist would then touch each one, in sequence. This would condition George to shift from his anxieties about lecturing, through each of the intermediate steps, and finally into the image of being comfortable as he made his presentation to a large audience. After repeating this chained release of anchors several times, George would find himself responding automatically with confident feelings to the thought of lecturing.

Anchoring can also be achieved through pairing of auditory, visual and visualized (imagined) stimuli. For instance, you might picture to yourself that your are holding (anchoring) the negative memory with its associated feelings in a bubble in your right hand, taking the time to connect with it deeply. You then picture a positive image and feelings in a bubble in your left hand. You collapse the two by bringing your two hands together. The effects are the same as when you touch two anchors simultaneously, as described above.

The Sedona Method

If we allow our pain to be felt and freed, our suffering does great work in softening our hearts. It is, in the words of Trungpa Rinpoche, "manure for the field of wisdom." In fact, it is important to know that any difficult mind state is welcome to arise at any moment just as the sky welcomes whatever arises in it without resistance. Our suffering, if we feel it deeply and allow its natural passing, makes us stronger and yet more tender. We are whole not only despite what we have suffered but often because of it.
                                                                                    – Catherine Ingram (p. 46)

You might not have to use the tapping techniques of the Meridian Based Therapies. Simply giving yourself permission to release your negative feelings and thoughts may work just as well. Similarly, when you have completely released the negatives, you may be able to install the positives by giving yourself permission to do so.

This approach has been formalized into a system of self-healing called The Sedona Method. Its originators are very protective of this simple but highly potent technique and discourage anyone not trained as a teacher from sharing its details.[407] My personal experience is that this works better for adults than for children.

Story telling

> *All human beings have an innate need to hear and tell stories and to have a story to live by...*
>
> – Harvey Cox

Whenever possible in the experiential healing workshops I lead, I invite participants to share their life stories. Telling your life story is an enormously healing experience. It allows you to share the images of your past in an accepting atmosphere, helping you bring healing to old hurts through the compassion of the listeners, as well as through realizing that you are not alone in your challenges and suffering.

Story: A rabbi was invited to visit a synagogue that was considering hiring him. He had heard that this was a particularly challenging community, in which many had suffered losses and were therefore bitter and angry. He announced prior to his visit that in his Sabbath discourse he would be picking several people to tell the stories of their lives, in order to help him get to know the congregation – just as they were seeking to know him. So he suggested that everyone write down the highlights of their lives and bring their lists of questions that they might ask God about why they had had particularly difficult or especially blessed experiences in their lives.

He was pleased to see that most of the congregation came to his discourse with papers ready in their hands. After hearing several of them read out their stories, and more of them to share their questions to God, he asked each one to picture the following to him- or herself: "Imagine that you have brought your life experiences here in a big sack, which you are holding now in front of you. Now, ask yourself, each one of you, who would you pick from this congregation to trade their sack for yours?" There was a long silence.

The rabbi continued, "I have asked this question of myself – not only once and not only twice in my life. I have come to accept that God knows what He is doing, because I certainly don't and I haven't found anyone else who does. So I have not come here today to tell you the answers, but to congratulate you on asking your questions."

People in today's society don't seem to have sufficient opportunities to tell their stories. This is particularly important when you are stressed, hurting or ill. In traditional societies, the shaman will listen carefully to every detail of the story of the person who is ill. Complementary therapists will often do the same. Careseekers feel heard, understood and accepted when they have had the opportunity to detail what is bothering and hurting them. One of the most frequent complaints against physicians is that they don't take any time to listen to their patients. This is one of the major factors leading people to seek out CAM therapists.

Stories also provide vehicles for healing in other ways. Many people come to caregivers hoping that they will tell them what their problems are and what they can do about them. However, when told what to do to make themselves better, many people ignore the advice or even rebel against being told what to do. Shamans, the wise women and men of their societies, will often tell healing stories and parables. In effect, they lay these remedies out on the ceremonial blanket in front of them, and leave it to the careseeker to choose which part of their healing offering they will take home with them.

Healing stories allow healees to match appropriate parts of this metaphoric story remedy to their situation, to how they have experienced it, and to how they understand it. Thus, one story may be a "fit" for many different people, with problems that differ in minor or even major ways from each other.

See also: Collective Consciousness; Journaling

Suggestions in various forms for self-healing

> *It is the nature of man to rise to greatness if greatness is expected of him.*
> – John Steinbeck

Affirmations are statements you repeat to yourself in order to program them into your memory. The classic is the affirmation of Emile Coué, "Every day, in every way, I am getting better and better." By reciting this or meditating on it regularly, you can imprint it on your hard drive and come to feel as you program yourself to feel.

Other helpful variations: I know I can --; I am a loved child of God/ Christ/ Nature/ The Infinite Source; I am love/ peace/ a healing presence; It moves me.[408]

Thinking positively creates a more positive feeling and attitude towards live. When you are feeling down, ask yourself whether your glass is half full or half empty. Are you remembering to count your blessings as well as to figure out how to deal with your challenges? By reminding yourself of the gifts you have been and are given; of the fact that you are more fortunate than a major portion of people living on this planet; of the healing that is inherent in your challenges, you can color your days in brighter colors.

Suggesting healing dreams as you retire to be at night can invite your unconscious mind to speak more clearly and loudly, to contribute from its enormous stores of creativity to your life.

Suggesting a greater openness to spiritual awareness can bring you into a clearer and firmer connection with your higher self, your guides, angels and the Infinite Source.

The best collection of affirmations I have seen comes from Asha Nahoma Clinton. Clinton has developed Seemorg Matrix Therapy, a chakra-focused energy psychology approach for dealing with limiting beliefs that can produce disease and may contribute to the development of physical, psychological, and spiritual problems. She has a manual with an incredibly helpful array of affirmations that can help you to focus your awareness on your troublesome issues and immediately identify affirmation antidotes to these. If you are uncertain about specific issues, you can use kinesiology muscle testing to identify any of these that are relevant to your problems and beliefs.

Here are some examples from among the 74 pages of affirmations covering 62 distinct issues (Clinton 2000).

MATRIX COVENANT[409]

I give permission for my soul to be healed.

a. I want my traumas to get much, much worse/I want to heal all my traumas.

b. I want to die/I want to live.

c. I have nothing to live for/I have my own healing and transformation to live for.

e. It's not safe to be healed/It's safe to be healed.

f. I don't deserve to be healed/I deserve to be healed.

v. I don't want to change/I want to change.

KEY CORE BELIEFS MATRIX

It is very important to clear this Matrix before you do any others, especially if the client suffers from significant pathology.

A. Pessimism

2. I can never heal myself/I can heal myself.

3. Something basic is missing in me/I have everything I need within me.

B. Self

2. I am unlovable/I am lovable.

13. I am fragile/I can become strong.

C. Others

2. People are unloving/Many people are loving.

ABANDONMENT MATRIX

A. General issues

4. No one loves me/Some people love me.

B. Bereavements and unresolved grief

I can't be the same ever again without my (parent/ partner/ job/ body part or organ or body function, job, possessions, etc.)/ I can and will learn to live a good life despite my loss of my (parent/ partner/ job/ body part or organ or body function, job, possessions, etc.)

ABUSE MATRIX

7. I deserve punishment/I deserve understanding, compassion, and acceptance.

BODY MATRIX

6. My body can't be healed/My body can be healed.

CONTROL MATRIX

A. For People Who Are Controlling

B. For People Who Don't Take Their Power

Using meridian therapies on the negative issues to reduce their intensity, and then installing and strengthening the positive affirmations offers a systematic way for reprogramming the hard drive of your unconscious mind.

See also: Imagery/ Visualization; Meditation; Meridian Based Therapies

Right and left brain preferences

> *There can be no knowledge without emotion. We may be aware of a truth,*
> *yet until we have felt its force, it is not ours. To the cognition of the brain*
> *must be added the experience of the soul.*
> — Arnold Bennett

As reviewed in Chapter II-1, there are distinct differences in the activities of the right and left brain hemispheres. In broad summary, the right brain hemisphere activity is intuitive, grasps concepts through imagery, and responds in feeling ways to situations. The left brain specializes in logic, linear reasoning, and other thinking functions.[410]

People tend to have distinct preferences for relating to the world more through right or left hemispheric approaches.[411] People may be stressed when challenged by situations that are better served by the modalities that they are not adept at or are uncomfortable in using. While left- and right-handedness are associated with right- and left- brain dominance, respectively, they do not necessarily indicate a person's preferences in approaching the world.

If you are stronger in left brain functions, you may need to consciously work on developing and maintaining sensitivity around feeling and emotional issues and relationships. If you are stronger in right brain functions, you may find yourself often asking for help with some of the mechanical or mathematical challenges in life.

Here are several interesting ways in which these brain function preferences may contribute to stress or help to relieve stresses

Fredric Schiffer, a psychiatrist at Harvard University, patented special eye-glasses with denser tinting on the right, shading to lighter on the left, and another pair with shading in the reverse direction. Wearing one of these pairs of glasses will stimulate the side of the brain opposite to the lighter tinting. These can stimulate the appropriate brain hemisphere to activate the more constructive personality, and promote its healing contribution to the patient's life. You can make a simpler version of these glasses with two pairs of safety goggles and some duct tape.

When you focus your mind on a problem while wearing one set of glasses you feel very differently about the issue than you do when wearing the opposite set of glasses. That is, when you thinking brain registers the problem it may be stuck in patterns of reasoning that find no solutions to your difficulties. Putting on the opposite pair of glasses, you may put your right brain in gear and find yourself feeling very differently about the problem.

Another fascinating bit of brain dominance activity can be found in the *ultradian rhythm*. This is a period shift of dominant activity from right to left brain hemisphere and back, which occurs about every 90 minutes. You can tell which side of your brain is active at any time by checking which of your nostrils is more open to the flow of air. If your right nostril is more open, then your left hemisphere is more active, and conversely.

You may find that you do better at certain tasks when the appropriate hemisphere is engaged. To check this out, you can simply wait till the shift occurs naturally – but if you want to catch yourself with the left nostril open, you had better set an alarm clock. If you don't, you are more likely than not to overlook this intention as your non-linear hemisphere gets into gear. As a more controlled alternative, it is often (but not always) possible to force the nostril of your choice to open more, by lying on your side on a pillow, so that the nostril you want to be open is not next to the pillow.

By choosing which hemisphere is active, or by timing your tasks to coincide with the rhythmic activation of your hemispheres, you may find yourself more in harmony with your work and play.

Experiential exercise with right and left brain hemisphere functions
Fredric ~Schiffer has explored simple ways in which to identify for yourself whether you have strongly divided functions between your left and right brain hemispheres. Think about a problem or memory that disturbs you (with feelings of hurt, anger, or remorse, etc.). Now, use your right palm to completely cover your right eye, and your left palm to cover all but a little of the ear-side of your left eye. This will allow a little light in from the left side of your left eye, which will stimulate and activate your right hemisphere. Spend a few moments exploring your feelings regarding the issue you have chosen to focus on. Then reverse the process and cover your left eye entirely, leaving only a little of the ear-side of your right eye uncovered, and spend a few minutes exploring how you feel about the same issue.

About 60 percent of people will notice a distinct difference, sometimes quite a strong one, between the responses of their right and left hemispheres to this type of stimulation while focusing on an emotionally distressing issue. For most, the left, thinking hemisphere is more rational and can sort out how to deal with the issue, while the right brain tends to be emotional, and when it is activated, they may feel quite upset about the issue.[412]

Schiffer finds that some people he sees in psychotherapy have distinct personalities that are evoked when the left and right brain hemispheres are stimulated. In some of his clients there is a very wounded, angry, immature, self-destructive personality that is more often evoked by stimulating the right brain, and a more mature, composed, rational, constructive personality, evoked in the left brain. This knowledge can allow the therapist to selectively access the wounded personality and thus facilitate releases of psychological traumas. The constructive personality is encouraged to provide support and control over the life of a person who may otherwise be dominated by the emotions of her wounded side, and may therefore be self-destructive. (See the case of Harriet, below.)

Schiffer patented special eyeglasses with shaded tinting from dark at the right to clear at the left and others with shaded tinting from left to right. (You can make a simpler version of these glasses with two pairs of safety goggles and some duct tape, to explore your own right/ left hemispheric awarenesses.) These can stimulate the appropriate brain hemisphere, by letting in more light to one side, to activate the more constructive personality, and promote its healing contribution to a person's life.

Case: "Harriet" was so emotional about her husband leaving her that she could not think straight. She was depressed, easily distracted, crying at the least stress, and barely able to function at her job as secretary in an elementary school. She was crying so much it was difficult for her to make constructive use of her time in therapy sessions.

A few minutes after putting on the taped glasses, Harriet was able to think and discuss her problems much more coherently.

In EMDR and WHEE people alternate stimulating the right and left hemispheres while focusing the mind on a problem, phobia, anxiety or other distressing feeling or memory. In EMDR there can be strong emotional releases while doing this. In WHEE, where an affirmation is recited that states the problem PLUS a positive affirmation immediately afterwards – while stimulating right and left hemispheres. This produces reductions in the emotional distress but prevents strong emotional releases.[413]

People have asked how such simple techniques could be so potently effective. Early brain studies are showing EMDR produces increased activity in the corpus callosum (the bridge of nerve pathways between the two brain hemispheres). My personal theory is that feeling memories appear to be stored in the right hemisphere. When the experiences producing the feelings are disturbing, the right brain, in effect, says to the left brain, "You don't want to suffer these negative feelings, do you?" The left brain, being the focus of conscious thought, is highly analytical and uncomfortable with negative feelings. It answers, "No, I'd rather not suffer through remembering these painful experiences." So the right brain locks the feelings away from conscious awareness and the left brain forgets about them and pretends they never happened. By stimulating the right and left sides of the body while focused on a distressing issue, the two hemispheres open communications again and can release the locks on the dark closets where the feelings were stored.

See also: Emotional intelligence

General healing and self-healing factors

Self-confidence may be an issue needing healing, but at the same time a lack of self-confidence may slow the progress of self-healing practices or even block them completely, especially through giving up too soon. In conventional psychotherapy a lack of self-confidence can be a serious impediment to progress, requiring extended efforts over months and years of treatment.

Using some of the techniques in this chapter it may be possible to overcome issues of self-confidence much more quickly. Helpful techniques include: WHEE and other meridian based therapies; cognitive behavioral techniques; NLP; affirmations; and imagery. Partializing and addressing individually each element you can identify that relates to self-confidence may lead to greater success.

Beliefs and disbeliefs about your ability to change and others' abilities to contribute to your self-healing may contribute to your greater or lesser success with self-healing techniques. Belief in the availability and willingness of others to help you gives you greater confidence to ask for the assistance you need.

Believing you can always change for the better opens you to greet each day with the anticipation of having new

If your beliefs include spirituality, then your illness and other life challenges may be experienced as a lesson that gives your life deeper meaning.

If your beliefs include an afterlife, then the worst that could happen is that you may shed your current physical garment sooner than you had hoped or planned, but you will have other opportunities to pursue the dreams and lessons your higher self knows will benefit you.

Hope helps you maintain your centeredness despite your problems, knowing that there will be resolutions to your issues in one way or another.

Acceptance

> I would like to beg of you, dear friend, as well as I can, to have patience with everything that remains unresolved in your heart. Try to love the QUESTIONS THEMSELVES... Do not look now for the answers. They cannot now be given to you because you could not live them. It is a question of experiencing everything. At present you need to LIVE the question. Perhaps you will gradually, without even noticing it, find yourself experiencing the answer, some distant day. Perhaps you are indeed carrying within yourself the potential to visualize, to design, and to create for yourself an utterly satisfying, joyful, and pure lifestyle. Discipline yourself to attain it, but accept that which comes to you with deep trust, and as long as it comes from your own will, from your own inner need, accept it, and do not hate anything.
>
> – Rainier Maria Rilke (1903)

Acceptance is the ability to maintain perspective on your problems, not ignoring or minimizing them but knowing that one way or another you will get through them and not worrying excessively about the outcome – over which you have no control in any case. Acceptance helps you to find an appropriate level of concern and to not slip into unnecessary and unproductive worrying. Acceptance allows you to make mistakes and learn from them, knowing that everyone makes mistakes and that some of your best lessons in life will come out of your mistakes and how you deal, learn and grow from them. Acceptance allows you to forget that you shouldn't worry, to catch yourself or be reminded of worrying, and to apply whatever self-healing remedies you need in order to transform your worry back into concern – without beating yourself up because this is the ninety-ninth time you've caught yourself doing this.[414]

Acceptance is going with the flow, trusting that if life doesn't unfold in the way you want it to, it will turn out even better in the end because of the unexpected turns your life has taken.

> *Happiness is like a cat. If you try to coax it or call it, it will avoid you. It will never come. But if you pay no attention to it and go about your business, you'll find it rubbing up against your legs and jumping into your lap.*
> – William Bennett

Determination

> *Try not.*
> *Do, or do not.*
> *There is no try.*
> – Yoda

Determination can make the whole difference between achieving significant changes in your life and remaining as you are today. Sometimes your physical and psychological problems change spontaneously, but many times they persist and may worsen with time. Even if your condition does not change, you can take steps to change how you relate to your state of being.

If you are determined to make changes in your life, you should not *try* to implement any of them. *Trying* is a cop-out. You are saying from the beginning that you don't believe you will succeed; your are stating that you will not be putting in your maximal effort.

By saying you will only try to do something, you are giving yourself an excuse for not following through to completion – even before you get started.

Experiential exercise: *Try to pick up a small, light object that is near you, such as a pen or a book. Did you actually pick it up? What is the difference between picking it up and trying to pick it up?*

You might think that with an unfamiliar or more difficult task, such as stopping a bad habit, you can't promise with any certainty that you will succeed, so *trying* is an honest statement of intent. Check out how it feels if you tell yourself instead, "I'm going to do the best I can to stop this bad habit." Doesn't this feel more positive than *trying* to stop the habit? By avoiding the word *try* and by using more affirming language, you will be setting a clearer and far more determined course towards succeeding.

Perseverance

Perseverance can get you to your goal, overcoming outer and inner obstacles. Too often, we give up on approaches that could be helpful if we just persisted with them. I find this is often a problem with parents who have willful or stubborn children. Parents apply one remedy after another for only a brief period and give up when the child does not change after only a few days with any one approach.

A lot of my work is simply to help parents agree on one way of dealing with their children and sticking with it. If it only works part way, then we go back to the drawing board and figure out where the blocks are and work to overcome them.

> *When Thomas Edison was asked, "Aren't you discouraged that you've tested more than 100 different materials and haven't found a single one that works for your light bulb?" He answered, "Not at all. Now I know more than 100 materials that don't work!"*

In my promotion of wholistic spiritual healing since 1980, I have found many skeptical people who believe I'm simply odd, weird or crazy. I have met scientists who are eager to study healing, in order to prove how it works – and when it doesn't work like a physical medicine, they abandon their studies. I continue to work with those who have the patience to study healing and simply observe it on its own terms, noting just how it does and doesn't work, and gradually building an understanding of what healing is and isn't.

Releasing attachments to outcomes can free up your energies to do your best.

> *If you keep your eyes on a distant mountain peak or star, you may stumble over the little rocks that are right in front of you.*
> – D.B.

When you keep your focus on what you are experiencing and doing at any given time, you are allowing yourself to be in the flow. You are engaging fully in the present moment. You are not allowing expectations, wishes or fears about the future to rob you of any of the energies you can give to this moment.

This overlaps with meditation, and may be a part of many meditations.

Rituals

> *Rituals allow us the means to come into the mystery realms of being. When ritual is done well, with great care, it becomes ceremony. Ritual per-formed with careless hands and a distracted heart is just a bunch of 'stuff.'*
> – Susan Chernak McElroy (2002, p. 71)

Rituals can provide considerable comfort in times of stress. They provide structure when there is chaos, offer prescribed manners of behaving and relating to others in difficult situations, and can help to control tensions.

Having a regular schedule (which is a form of ritual) for eating, exercising, and work can reduce stresses, particularly when a family of several generations is involved. If people all gather around a dinner table, there is a known time when issues can be raised and discussed, tensions shared, and problems addressed. A helpful ritual is a regular family "check-in," where each member of the family can tell the story of their day and hear how others in the family are faring. While this may not be possible every day of the week, a ritual of a family gathering at set times on the weekend can be the catalyst for many healings.

Rituals around holidays and times of life changes bring families and friends together. Celebrations of holidays, birth, baptism, birthday, confirmation, bar mitzvah, graduation, marriage, promotions, and support in times of illness, mourning and bereavements are healing occasions. Rituals remind you to affirm your caring for each other, and bring families and friends together for celebration and support.

Rituals can enhance your spiritual life, as in prayer and meditation. Having a special time of day when you connect with your higher self – to give thanks for the blessings in your life, to offer healing to others, and to ask for the support and help that will bring more healing into your life. Attending a house of worship, or participating in a meditation or prayer group can deepen your spiritual connections.

Rituals around set times are especially helpful to those who prefer life rhythms that are regular and evenly paced, as they affirm that way of being. Rituals may become too rigid or you may in other ways outgrow their usefulness. Rituals involving time may not appeal to those whose life rhythms are irregular.[415] When rituals chafe rather than nurture, it is time to review and discuss them with those who participate with you in these regular exchanges of energies and celebrations of life.

Generating and nurturing positive attitudes

> *In the calculus of the heart it is the ratio of positive to negative emotions that determines the sense of well-being.*
> – Daniel Goleman (1995, p. 57)

It is ever so much more pleasant to flash a smile to people around you than to frown. Positive thinking and feeling can become a way of relating to yourself and the world. You can practice this until it becomes your habit, your ordinary way of being.

Experiential exercise: Check out how it feels to you when you deliberately smile at everyone you pass and everyone you interact with.

Next day, check out how it feels to frown deliberately at everyone you pass and meet.

This is not to say your should ignore or shut away your negative emotions. Hurt, anger, depression, jealousy and other negative responses are a normal part of life. When they arise, don't run away from them. Feel them, process them for as long as you need to... but then let them go.

While you are down in the dumps, don't dump your feelings at random on others! Find those friends and counselors who can be there for you and understand you when you are feeling bad. Just as you don't throw a piece of clothing or food just anywhere when you're unhappy with it, find those compassionate human containers who can hold a space of compassion in which you can vent your feelings. If no one is around, you may find release and comfort in journaling your feelings.

Being human, it is virtually certain you will not come into the habit of positive thinking and feeling in one jump. Every misstep is an opportunity to practice kindness with yourself. While our natural tendencies may be to be critical of ourselves, we can equally choose to be supportive. If you catch yourself saying something like, "How could I be so dumb?!" or "#@*#!! There I go again, making the same old mistake!" You can turn it around. Let go of the negative feelings and say something supportive, like, "I'm doing well to catch myself before I really go off on a rampage or tear myself to shreds over silliness." or "I can do better than that next time!"

Prayers of thanks and gratitude can help in setting a positive tone to your day. If you are coming from a place of gratitude for whatever blessings are and have been in your life, then negativity or even misfortunes may not feel as overwhelming.

Starting from a positive space generated by prayer, problems may be turned into invitations to further prayer, or into challenges to find healing approaches for addressing them.

> ... The moment you shift from a mind state of negativity or judgment to one of appreciation, there are immediate effects at many levels of your being: brain function becomes more balanced, harmonized, and supple; your heart begins to pump in a much more coherent and harmoniously balanced rhythm; and biochemical changes trigger a host of healthful balancing reactions throughout your body. In the healing ways of indigenous people, the restorative power of gratitude was well understood.
>
> A heart filled with gratitude generates actions and prayers that complete the circle between the gift offered to us, the receiver of the gift, and the sacred source of the gift. To offer prayers of thanksgiving is a gesture of rejoicing in discovering the many gifts that life brings us.
>
> – Joel and Michelle Levey

Experiential exercise: Joel and Michelle Levey suggest a way to generate gratitude and thanksgiving: Start by quieting and centering yourself in meditation for a few minutes, perhaps by concentrating on your breathing. Focus your awareness on someone for whom have deep gratitude. With each in-breath, invite this person into your heart. With each out-breath, send your heartfelt gratitude to them. Allow the glow of love and gratitude with each breath to light up your whole being, knowing that the same light is warming their being with your love. Radiate love with each breath from the essence of your being to the essence of their being.

Nutrition

We are what we eat. Eating a balanced, nutritious diet is recommended by every therapist I know. Organically grown foods, including fish and meats, are also very highly recommended.

Some of the stresses we experience are from poor nutrition and from toxins that make their ways into our food – as additives, pesticides and pollutants.

Applied Kinesiology and other intuitive approaches to assessing your dietary needs and sensitivities may be helpful. If you hold a food in one hand and find that your muscle testing shows a weakness (compared to testing when you are not holding that food), you can assume that that food may not agree with your system. Of course, you might react in line with your expectations and beliefs rather than to the substance itself. A more objective way of testing is to have someone else do blinded surrogate testing for your sensitivity, particularly if they are experienced and gifted in kinesiology. That is, you would hold the substance you are testing, but they would do the kinesiology on themselves while being unaware of the substance you are holding. While this may sound pretty far out, the fact that it works suggests that we are all interconnected through intuitive and bioenergetic links.

Allergies and negative reactions to medications
Feeling stressed and tired may be a sign of allergies, particularly (but not exclusively) to food items. Again, Applied Kinesiology testing may be helpful – both in identifying allergies and in treating them.

Chronic tiredness may be a sign of chronic fatigue syndrome (CFS) or candidiasis, and when accompanied by muscle pains, of fibromyalgia.[416] Allergies are often major contributing factors in these disorders.

While avoiding the allergen is obviously the most direct way of dealing with such problems, this can become a challenge when multiple allergies are present or when the allergy is to a common food item such as wheat or dairy products.

Several stress reducing approaches discussed above can help treat allergies.

WHEE and the other meridian based therapies are particularly helpful. While following the routine of tapping on the appropriate points on your body, you can recite an affirmation such as: *Even though I get cramps and diarrhea when I eat ____, I still love and accept myself, wholly and completely, and God loves and accepts me wholly and completely and unconditionally.*[417]

Imagery of a protective field surrounding you can protect you from negative environmental allergens or toxins.

Case: When riding on the London underground (subway/ Metro), I found myself exhausted and irritable, particularly if I had to travel through the tube at the end of the day. This tiredness felt clearly disproportional to my exertions of the day. I realized I was picking up some of the tiredness, irritability and negativity of other passengers who were weary after their day at work. When I made it a point, prior to entering the underground, to invoke and periodically strengthen my image of a protective shield around myself, I found myself much less bothered by these negative vibrations.

Prayer and healing can lessen negative effects of toxic chemicals. If you pray or give healing to medications you are taking, you will have fewer side effects from these substances.

Case: A nurse on a chemotherapy unit was prohibited by her supervisor from giving healing to the people in her care, even though they were suffering from symptoms of their cancers (such as pain) that she could readily relieve with a brief touch of her hands.

Praying for inspiration for how to still be able to use her healing gifts with her patients, she was guided to give healing to the chemotherapy bottles. She was very pleased to find that her patients did not suffer from headaches, nausea, vomiting, diarrhea, or many of the other common annoying side effects of chemotherapy.

I have been suggesting this approach to people in my own practice of psychiatric psychotherapy for a decade, with excellent results. While this also gives people a positive attitude towards their medication, and could therefore be helpful through the mechanisms of suggestion, I am convinced that the effects are more powerful than I would expect from suggestion alone.

Finding centeredness, passion and meaning in your life

> *The minute you begin to do what you really want to do, it's really a different kind of life.*
> – Buckminster Fuller

When you are on a path that is harmonious with your being, when you have a sense that what you are doing is meaningful and satisfying, then you will be less likely to feel stressed – even in the face of serious challenges.

You don't have to be a millionaire, you don't have to have all sorts of degrees or other formal qualifications in order to find this special space. I have met a waitress, a nurse, several shopkeepers, and a number of healers who have a settledness and a warm glow about them that is obvious to all who interact with them. Each is totally present in the moment, totally focused on what they are doing. The most palpable aspect of their glow was their total attention when I spoke with them.

Case: Colleagues at a meeting of the American Holistic Medical Association, who knew of my interest in healers, suggested that I might like speaking with "Marla," a nurse who is a healer. I sat next to this quiet, unassuming woman at lunch and asked about her involvement with healing. She suggested she might be able to respond more fully to my questions after the meal. When the others left the table, she proposed that she could demonstrate her healing better than she could put it into words, if I was open to this. I assented, expecting she would do a laying-on of hands, meditation or prayer for healing.

She did none of these. All she did was to have me sit squarely opposite her as she looked quietly into my eyes. Her gaze was warm and steady, and her attention was completely and totally on me, and nowhere else. She said not a word. Within a few minutes, I found myself moved to tears – knowing I was in the presence of someone who was totally and unconditionally accepting of me. It mattered not that Marla knew nothing about me. I simply knew with an absolute certainty that she accepted me without reservation.

When I wanted to ask her about her healing, she shushed me, indicating that an important part of her healing is to accept it is – not questioning, analyzing or dissecting it. At the time, twenty-one years ago, I felt considerable frustration of my intellectual curiosity. Today, I understand better and am at peace with her brief healing – which I recall as though it were only yesterday.

While this degree of centeredness is rare, it is an inspiration to the rest of us to do our best to emulate. If we can be present in every moment, we are not going to stress ourselves with dissatisfactions over disparities between what IS in the present moment – in contrast with our memories of moments past or anticipations of what might be in moments future.

This is head "stuff."

Finding what our heart sings to do in the world, for which we jump out of bed – happy and eager to engage and be present with – is a tonic more powerful than any medicine we might swallow. It is best when our passion can also be our occupation that earns us a living – or when we can bring our passion in some significant manner to our workday job. Then our job is not a tedium. We are not watching the clock to see how many hours or minutes are left before we can leave. We are engaged with body, heart and head in giving of ourselves in every possible way to see that every moment is a healing moment.

For many (myself included), this can translate into efforts to move our work forward in the best ways possible. This can become a pitfall, as it involves expectations of how and of how fast our progress ought to be, which introduces unnecessary stress in our lives.

The most satisfying and least stressful path is to stay in the moment, being present in whatever our task is – knowing that as the ripeness of time unfolds, the products of our efforts will blossom and flourish. If we pull on the plant to make it grow faster, it will not help the plant and is likely to frustrate us from achieving our wishes and goals.

Are you puzzled that I mention goals and wishes? Are these not a contradiction to being in the moment? Well, yes and no! Having objectives and aspirations gives us directions for our work. The trick is not to become rigidly attached to these as absolutes; not to feel that we have to manifest them in particular manners and forms or within deadlines that we often set up arbitrarily and without true need or cause.

Michelle Small Wright (1997) writes beautifully about gardening projects. She suggests that we can invite nature (including nature spirits) to join us in our projects:

> In co-creative science, nature becomes a fully operational, functioning, conscious partner with the scientist. Together they create a team, with each member of the team providing specific and different information that is needed for understanding and solving a defined problem. (p. 1)

Everyone's class will be individually designed by and for that person.

When you are working directly in partnership with nature, you cannot simply announce, "Let's put in a garden!" and expect that you will get any information back from nature regarding the garden. You must supply the definition, direction and purpose of this garden. In other words, you must supply the evolution dynamic within the i/e balance, and you are the only one who can do that. Nature will not do your job for you. It will only supply the evolution dynamic for objects that fall within its "natural" domain: plants, rocks, deer, lightning, etc. (p. 17-18)

The average class takes 4 years.

You should decide how much time each week you will spend on this and set a time period as a study "term." 4-6 months is a comfortable time in which to see progress on a project.

Nature can sort out its lessons in a more structured and orderly way when you let them know the parameters for your availability. Your garden project does not have to be built around vegetables or flowers in a plot of land. Your growth project could be your business, your relationships, or your own personal development.

Here are some of Wright's suggestions for your garden:

1. Verbally state your intention to nature. Out loud is best. For instance, "I would like to open a co-creative science classroom with myself as the student and nature intelligence as my teacher. My intent is to be educated and trained as a co-creative scientist. I am ready to learn."

2. Select your classroom. This can be anything that provides structure for action. "Pick something that you can do alone, and remember that whatever you choose will become a classroom and you will need to hand over all the activity, timing and rhythms to your teacher. So, don't choose something you are not willing to release control of and don't pick something that is life-threatening either to yourself or anyone else. Your classroom has to remain personal for the amount of time you and nature are using it... "

3. Keep detailed notes, a log for each day. Be as complete as possible. Keep notes organized, so you can review them periodically.

This is an excellent self-help book, enriched by the author's sharing of her own path in opening to intuitive and spiritual awarenesses and learning to be a co-creative gardener.

Without turning your passion into a formal project, you can still seek and create joy in whatever you do.

Joy is increasingly obvious as a major factor that determines how people respond to challenges such as illness in their lives. People with cancer who have joy and purpose in their lives do better with their physical illness, as well as with their emotions and relationships.

While it may be difficult to hold onto a feeling of joy when faced with severe problems in life, sometimes these very challenges bring us into states where we do a healing through cost-benefits analyses of how we are investing the most valuable assets we have – our health and our time. You may be surprised to learn that people with cancer quite often state that they appreciate life much more since having this serious disease, and some even say they are grateful for getting cancer, because it forced them to reassess their lives and to make major changes are healing. Soul-destroying work situations, abrasive and abusive relationships, and other non-nurturing aspects of their lives are changed or abandoned after their soul-searching assessments of what is important in the time remaining to them on earth.

Meditation and spiritual practices may enhance the joy in one's life, initiated through major life challenges, as well as through regular disciplines. Conversely, difficult times may bring us into greater spiritual awareness and healing.

> *Joy is the most infallible sign of the presence of God.*
> – Teilhard de Chardin

COLLECTIVE CONSCIOUSNESS

> *Without... recognition and the direct experience of our interconnectedness on the emotional level, all cures are meaningless. The negative emotions of fear and anxiety which create the root energetic imbalances which lie beneath many illnesses are simply cultural imbalances manifesting locally in the individual.*
> – Michael Greenwood and Peter Nunn (p. 109)

Many shamans will address an illness in an individual as an opportunity to invoke healing for the entire community. The healing ritual dramas they create will activate the healing energies of the community, bringing psychological and spiritual awareness to all the participants.

This intuitive healing for the community acknowledges the interconnectedness of each individual within the society. Each of us is like a cell in the body of the whole group. In offering healing to one of the cells, a part of the whole society is healed and therefore the individual healing contributes to the healing of the whole.

The interconnectedness of each of us with the whole is not just as separate people living together in a larger social group that can be viewed as a collection of individuals. We are interconnected in many subtle ways: through telepathic and clairsentient awareness; through bioenergies that link us intimately with each other; through pre- and retrocognition, which connect us with our society across the boundaries of lifetimes; and through spiritual connections that exceed our limited comprehension from the vantage point of physical existence.

Each of us is thus a part of a vast collective consciousness. Perhaps each of us is more accurately described as a particle of awareness in the mind of the infinite All. Each of us thus participates in this all-encompassing consciousness. Through intuition, we can potentially access any and all knowledge that is presently in the minds of living beings, as well as that which exists in the past and future. We are also in intimate communications with nature spirits, angels and the Infinite Source.

This is how intuitive information can be obtained for identifying the roots of problems and finding cures; this is how bioenergies may be invited in to bring about unusual healings. Our unconscious mind and higher self are in touch with all knowledge, everywhere and everywhen.

By quieting your mind through meditation, by developing intuitive awareness, and by meditating or praying for guidance and help through your higher self, you can invite the more developed parts of the collective consciousness to advise and help you.[418]

YOU'RE ON YOUR WAY TO SELF-HEALING

Success is how high you bounce after you hit bottom.
                                        – General George Patton

Everyone is on a path of self-healing, whether they know it or not. Life gives us challenges in countless forms and we make our choices in dealing with them – learning lessons in the moment as well as in living with the later consequences of our decisions. As we advance in learning the many ways of healing, we continually improve our abilities to deal with physical, psychological and spiritual issues.

When you know a variety of ways to understand and deal with these challenges, you can live your life with greater joy and satisfaction. Problems become invitations to learn more about yourself and to grow.

I wish you good healings.

Conclusion

If a man will begin with certainties, he shall end in doubts; but if he will be content to begin with doubts, he shall end in certainties.
— Francis Bacon

Volume I of *Healing Research* presents rich anecdotal evidence that spiritual healing can accelerate recuperation from a variety of illnesses, and research evidence confirming many significant effects of healing on humans, animals, plants, bacteria, yeasts, cells in laboratory culture, enzymes, DNA and more.

It is therefore evident that through touch and mental intent we can influence the physical and psychological state of other people and of non-human organisms.

Volume II of *Healing Research* has explored a broader spectrum of healing phenomena. Here we have seen that there are a variety of ways in which we can both cause and heal ourselves of psychological and physical problems. Western medicine has assumed that such self-healings are brought about by the mind influencing the body – primarily through relaxation, with the concomitant harmonizing of functions of the nervous system and hormones. Recent research is beginning to add an appreciation of how the mind can also influence immune functions.

Complementary therapies are now being studied systematically, under rigorous research conditions. We are finding that many of the claims made over decades and centuries can be confirmed scientifically. Gradually, these therapies are being integrated into Western medical practice.

Studies of complementary therapies add to our understanding of how biological energy medicine works. The simplest explanation I have found is Einstein's Theory of Relativity, expressed in the equation $E = mc^2$. *Quantum physics* has confirmed that matter is interconvertible with energy. A living organism may be viewed as a physical object or as an energetic being. *Newtonian medicine* has barely begun to absorb the imports of this insight, while bioenergy practitioners have been saying for several millennia that the body can be understood and treated as energy.

The discipline of *biological energy medicine* is growing out of this understanding, shaped by health care practitioners with diverse beliefs and practices about bioenergies. We are in the earliest stages of exploring how these biological energies function. Various CAM therapies suggest that there are biological energy lines, energy centers, and energy fields that interact with the body, emotions, mind, relationships and spirit. There are many ways in which we can actively interact with these bioenergy systems in the interest of health management.

Excess flows or blocks to flows of energies in the meridians are identified by acupuncture and its derivatives (acupressure, applied kinesiology, reflexology, shiatsu), Therapeutic Touch, and other healing methods . Craniosacral therapists find bioenergy pulsations – especially around the head and spinal cord, but also around the rest of the body – which inform them about the state of the healee and the progress of the healing. Homeopathy and flower essences are given with the explanation that they convey a patterned biological essence in the water or in other vehicles that are used to administer these remedies. Spiritual healers report that they can sense (mostly through touch or visual perceptions) a bioenergy field around the body. Many people who are not healers can also sense these fields.[419]

Many bioenergy therapists believe that the biofield acts as a template for the physical body, and is also a reflection of the current condition of the body. Two lines of evidence support this assertion. First, the various treatments that influence the energy body can bring about changes in physical and psychological conditions. Second, some spiritual healers report that they can see abnormalities in the bioenergy field prior to the development of physical illness, often preceding the manifestation of physical evidence of disease by several weeks and months. The function of the biofield as a template also could explain how the physical body maintains its integrity during growth and during repairs following injuries.

Bioenergy therapists also suggest that the biofield is influenced by an individual's emotions, mind, relationships (with others and with the environment), and spirit.

At this stage in our explorations of bioenergy medicine, it is still difficult to be clear or certain regarding the patterns we are beginning to explore.

> *We are like flies crawling across the ceiling of the Sistine Chapel. We cannot see what angels lie underneath the threshold of our perceptions. We... live in our paradigms, our habituated perceptions... the illusions we share through culture we call reality, but the true... reality of our condition is invisible to us.*
>
> – William Irwin Thompson (p. 81)

Elements of spiritual healing appear to be common denominators in all of these complementary therapy frameworks (Benor 1995a).

Spiritual healing is practiced through an apparent exchange of bioenergies between healer and healee. These exchanges may promote healing by: 1. adding energies to a healee's depleted bioenergy system; 2. removing excesses of energies; 3. removing blocks to energy flows within the healee's bioenergy system; 4. converting bioenergy patterns of illness into patterns of health; 5. influencing the body directly, through interactions with the nervous, hormonal, and/or immune systems; or 6. through combinations of the above.

Some or all of the above mechanisms may include exchanges of information that accompany exchanges of bioenergies. In fact, we may come to understand bioenergies as combinations of information with energy.

Once we conceive of ourselves as energy organisms, we become more aware of vast, known and potential interactions with our environment. While our conventional instruments tell us that an electromagnetic field cannot have *material* influence beyond a measurable distance, the laws of physics tell us that EM fields extend to infinity. We may be influenced by vibrations of sound, of light, and of the entire electromagnetic spectrum that exists outside of our usual sensory awareness. As energy denizens of the cosmos, we are in constant energetic communication and interaction with all that is.

Homeopathy suggests even more profound resonations with our environment. Energetic patterns of various mineral and plant substances interact with the bioenergy patterns of humans and animals in ways that can harmonize physical and psychological functions and promote healing. The world – including plants, animals, minerals and universe around us are not just composed of non-human, inanimate or "dead" matter. Each and every element in the universe, including thoughts, words and metaphors, can have an influence on us – and we on them.

In summary, we see that there appear to be diverse biofields that can be accessed and manipulated through the practices of the various energy medicine specialties. The minds of healee and healer appear to be active elements in these bioenergy interactions with the body. Our beliefs and disbeliefs may influence our states of health and illness. Healing energy fields may enter into the processes of spiritual healing and self-healing through visualizations and through therapeutic ministrations of health professionals, even without the knowledge of the participants. Intentions of healers and healees may reshape disease processes through bioenergies and intentions.

We are just in the earliest stages of sorting out how biological energy approaches can be integrated with conventional medical care. The enormous complexities of both systems make this a monumental task.

Considering the sensitivity of bioenergy and consciousness interactions, the *how* of integrative medicine may be even more important than the *what*.

> *[B]ecause the whole is so much greater than the sum of the parts –*
> *the relationship between the parts becomes the biggest part of all.*
> – Stephen Covey (DiCarlo p. 220)

Our bioenergetic connections and interactions with our environment make us much more intimately a part of our environment than Western culture generally accepts. The evidence presented in Volumes I and II supports the evidence reviewed in this volume which suggests that all life on this planet is a part of the ecobiological entity *Gaia* and of the wider universe beyond.

Volume III extends the review of research in the fields of bioenergies and consciousness into the spiritual dimensions. It examines scientific evidence supporting reports from healers, mystics, and healees regarding the spirit and spiritual awareness. These are aspects of healing that are not yet included in much of mainstream energy medicine, but which are often reported as essential in spiritual healing.

Volume IV explores theories that may explain some elements of energy medicine and of healing processes, along with a detailed synthesis of our present-day understanding of healing. Some people object to the suggestion that there are biological energies that provide the substratum for spiritual healing and other complementary therapies. These skeptics demand that proof of such energies must be registered on some instrument in order to verify their existence. The best instrument for this purpose appears to be the human organism, which is an exquisitely delicate sensor and instrument for interventions with subtle energies. Volume IV reviews this and other theories that attempt to explain healing. Various reasons why healing has not been accepted by conventional, Newtonian, medicine are also discussed in detail. Volume IV also includes my personal experiences in learning to open myself to the infinite possibilities of spiritual awareness and healing.

> ... *It is we who, with our minds, determine the final shape of reality. Which is not to say that the world is "all in the mind." It would be more accurate to suggest that the mind is all in the world. That it is part of the world, in fact, because we are intimately involved.*
>
> – Lyall Watson (p. 40)

This book comes with user support and updates. I lecture and lead experiential workshops – posted as they unfold on www.WholisticHealingResearch.com; I am constantly updating the resources on that website; and I edit the International Journal of Healing and Caring – On line www.ijhc.org.

Our knowledge is but a speck in the cosmos awareness of how our personal and collective health and healing can unfold. By keeping our minds open to new possibilities, we will achieve the best healings possible.

Again, I wish you good healings!

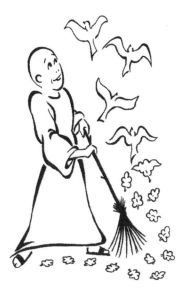

Image courtesy of Keith Chopping

Appendix A

VARIATIONS ON THE THEME OF PSYCHOTHERAPY

There are enormous variations in psychotherapy approaches from one school of practice to another. Here are just a few examples.

Bioenergy therapy Therapies that address the person as energy that interacts with the physical body, where the energies provide information about the body and offer avenues of access to shift the body towards greater harmony and health.[420]

Bodymind therapy Psychotherapy that invites awareness of what the body is saying about our past and present relationships with ourselves and each other.[421]

Cognitive therapy relies on clients' thinking functions to identify misperceptions and self-destructive behavior patterns. The therapist introduces new perspectives, and encourages clients to practice applying these in every day life.[422]

Cognitive behavior therapy combines elements of both the cognitive and behavioral approaches, which are symptom and goal oriented.[423]

Creative arts therapies Music, art, movement, dance, metaphor, poetry, journaling, psychodrama invite explorations that stage our issues and conflict in new and innovative ways, inviting us to explore and re-evaluate our relationships to ourselves, to others and to the cosmos.

Dream analysis Invites explorations of dramatic hints about our inner selves that are thrown up on the screen of our consciousness, inviting us to explore issues our unconscious minds consider important to our lives.[424]

Energy Psychology (See Meridian Based Therapies).

Eye Movement Desensitization and Reprocessing (*EMDR*) teaches clients to move their eyes back and forth laterally, or to alternate stimulating the right and left sides of their body as they focus on a problem.[425]

Gestalt Therapy invites clients to put words to aspects of their behaviors, the images in their dreams, their sub-personalities, and their anticipated reactions of others. Clients can then dialogue back and forth with their inner self to discover the sources of their discomforts.[426]

Hypnotherapy uses potent suggestions to explore the depths of clients' consciousness, and to introduce and strengthen new beliefs and behavior patterns.[427]

Imagery/ Visualization/ Metaphor Imaginary stages upon which we can explore old and new ways to deal with our lives creatively.[428]

Jungian analysis focuses mostly on dreams and archetypal imagery to sort out clients' belief systems. *Jungian analysis* can also extend into transpersonal realms, if the analyst is open to this. In my experience, psychoanalysis can help with existential issues, and is particularly useful for psychotherapists who wish to understand the workings of their own minds in order to be more helpful to their clients.[429]

Meditation Practice of mental discipline that allows one to not focus on stressful issues, promotes physical, psychogical and spiritual health in many ways.[430]

Meridian Based Therapies (also called *Energy Psychology*) invite clients to tap on acupressure points while mentally focused on a problem. Some of these therapies also have clients simultaneously recite an affirmation while tapping on these points.[431]

Metaphor See Imagery.

Mind-Body Therapy Therapy that addresses body issues through conscious and unconscious interventions. (See also Bodymind Therapy)

Neurolinguistic Programming or NLP (Bandler/ Grinder) introduces elements of hypnotic suggestion and conditioning to bring about focused, rapid changes in clients' beliefs, emotional responses, and behaviors.[432]

Primal Scream Therapy (Janov) encourages intense releases of emotions so clients will stop holding in negative feelings that could inhibit or even cripple them in their relationships.

Psychoanalysis is offered in several variations, all focused on uncovering inner psychological processes, and requiring sessions once (or preferably several times) weekly for many years. Deepening insight, rather than achieving behavioral change, is the goal of psychoanalysis. *Freudian analysis* (A. Freud; S. Freud) focuses on early childhood traumas, and uses the client's associations and dreams to guide therapists as they help clients to recognize the conflicts in their unconscious mind. The process of transference, or projection of beliefs and expectations onto the therapist, also reveals the inner workings of the clients's mind.[433]

Psychodrama invites clients to act out their conflicts with others who may have similar problems, but who may respond differently in the same situation. This allows clients to release buried feelings, acquire new insights about their responses to various situations, and explore new options for response.[434]

Psychoneuroimmunology Combination of relaxation, meditation, imagery and group support that enhances immune functions.

Psychosynthesis invites clients to find spiritual inspiration to help them deal with their problems. It combines a broad spectrum of techniques, including creative arts, gestalt therapy, and others.[435]

Relaxation Relaxing the body and mind individually and collectively promotes health.[436]

Rogerian therapy assumes that clients have all the tools they need to sort out their own problems, and requires only the listening ear and empathy of the therapist to bring these out. The principal agent for change is the therapist's unconditional acceptance.[437]

Transactional Analysis translates psychoanalytic terminology into everyday language that can alert clients to aspects of themselves and others that may be in conflict. For instance: your inner *parent* may plague you with injunctions about what you should and shouldn't be doing; your inner *child* may rebel against these injunctions; and your *adult* self may have a difficult time deciding how to resolve this inner conflict, and how to behave in this situation. TA combines insight, emotional clarity, and behavioral changes to help clients recognize and deal with their own self-defeating habits.[438]

Transpersonal psychotherapy introduces a variety of spiritual elements into psychotherapy, such as meditation, prayer, and discussions of spiritual issues.[439]

Visualization See imagery.

The ***Wholistic Hybrid of EMDR and EFT (WHEE)*** combines the Eye Movement Desensitization and Emotional Freedom Techniques, utilizing the alternating stimulation of both sides of the body while reciting an affirmation.

Stress levels associated with problems the clients focus on rapidly diminish with all of these approaches. Clients can then install positive affirmations to replace the negative feelings and beliefs they have relinquished.[440]

NOTES

Foreword
[1] C. Norman Shealy, MD, PhD is a neurosurgeon specializing in holistic therapies for pain and other problems. Dr. Shealy's research on healing for depression and clairvoyant diagnosis is reviewed in Healing Research, Volume I, Chapters 4, 5 (abbreviated as Chapters I-4; -5).

Notes: Introduction

[2] **Spiritual healing** is used here as a generic term for treatments using the laying-on of hands, intent, and/or prayer – such as Therapeutic Touch, Healing Touch, Reiki, external Qigong, and many others. These are extensively discussed, and 191 controlled studies of healing are reviewed in Chapters I-4, -5.

[3] More on **physicists and mystics** in Chapters III-10; IV-2, IV-3.

[4] The Professional Edition of this book focuses heavily on research that confirms CAM therapies and bioenergies provide valid and helpful ways for dealing with dis-ease and disease. *Healing Research, Volume II: Consciousness, Bioenergy and Healing: Self-Healing and Energy Medicine for the 21st Century*, Medford, NJ: Wholistic Healing Publications 2003.

[5] This is a composite clinical picture from several people who struggled with these problems.

[6] **Parapsychology** as related to healing is discussed in Chapter I-3.

[7] Genetically modified plants and animals could have characteristics that are harmful to the modified organism, to the environment, or to animals who consume them. It might take several generations to discover these damaging effects, by which time it might be impossible to stop the modified plants or animals from continuing their damaging effects.

[8] **Psi phenomena** are discussed in detail in Chapter I-3. See the **glossary** for explanations of terms.

[9] Healing has also been called *psi* healing, *faith* healing, *mental* healing, *paranormal* healing, etc. More on the many names for healing in I-Introduction.

Notes: Chapter 1 – Self-Healing

[10] **Spiritual issues** are discussed in Volume III.

[11] See more on sorting out **personality factor compatibilities and frictions** in Chapter II-5.

[12] The Jungian functions have been translated into the Myers-Briggs psychological test, and are quite useful in psychotherapy.

[13] See more on **Jungian polarities** and **shadow** under *reasons healing has not been accepted*, in Chapter IV-3.

[14] Healing is specifically helpful for chronic state anxiety. See **studies of healing for anxiety** summarized in Chapter I-4. See discussion of **healing for meta-anxiety** below and in Chapter IV-3

[15] Freud termed this *neurotic* anxiety.

[16] See a wide variety of **stress management techniques** is Chapter 5.

[17] See Chapter II-5 for a spectrum of **self-healing** approaches.

[18] See Appendix A for a brief **summary of a spectrum of therapies**.

[19] Eeman termed the presentation of physical symptoms that are based on emotional traumatic memories *myognosis*.

[20] Janov is a little hard to take when he touts his method as the only one that is worthwhile. His arrogant manner and readiness to make brash, poorly supported claims have left the vast majority of professionals resistant to what I see as quite penetrating observations regarding the process of intensive psychotherapy.

[21] I am not suggesting that conventional psychotherapists deliberately avoid intense emotional releases in order to keep their clients in therapy longer. However, there could be this unconscious reinforcement to keep these therapists in this groove.

[22] See discussion of **psi research** in Chapter I-3.

[23] Internal feedback loops are discussed under *Self-healing* and *Biofeedback*, later in this chapter.

[24] See Volume III of *Healing Research* for research and discussions of **spiritual** dimensions.

[25] A recent addition to the list is to cover the skin with duct tape for several days, finding that the warts come off when the tape is removed.

[26] James Randi and William Nolen do this with healing; Paris Flammonde does the same with radionics.

[27] It is paradoxical and distressing to find studies on *hope* which entail the killing of animals.

[28] Congenital ichthyosiform erythrodermia of Brocq, abbreviated as ichthyosis.

[29] Residues of past life trauma and related issues are discussed in Chapter III-3.

[30] See Chapter III-7 on **psychic surgery**.

[31] It is fascinating that **Hawaiian kahuna healings** described by M. Long in Chapter I-1 are also similar in many respects to hypnotherapy.

[32] Eye Movement Desensitization and Reprocessing (**EMDR**), discussed briefly later in this chapter and Chapter II-2, is also very helpful in treating multiple personality disorders.

[33] See discussion on super **ESP** in Chapter 1-3.

[34] See Newberg et al on brain imaging that shows particular areas of the brain that are active in meditative and spiritual experiences.

[35] More on **channeling** in Chapter III-5.

[36] For **possession as a part of the spectrum in multiple personality disorder** see Allison; Crabtree; Kenny and discussion in Chapter III-6..

[37] See the review of **allobiofeedback** in Chapter I-4.

[38] More on **ectoplasm** under **mediumistic experiences** in Chapter III-5.

[39] See Chapter II-2 for more on **meditation**; III-9 for more on **mystical** states.

[40] See Chapter IV-2 for more on **LeShan's "alternate" realities**.

[41] There is much more on **theories explaining healing** in Chapter IV-2.

[42] This average is obviously high, reflecting the enormous number of days lost by people with chronic pain problems – who are averaged in with ordinary people who have no major pain problems.

[43] More on **reincarnation** in Chapter III-3.

[44] WHEE is the Wholistic Hybrid of EMDR and EFT. More on this below, in the section on EMDR; Benor 2001.

[45] Discussed earlier in this chapter under **transpersonal psychotherapy**; also in Chapter III-8, III-12; IV-3.

[46] "Self" (spelled with capital "S" – The part of our self that is aware of a transpersonal, spiritual dimension, of which we are an integral part.

[47] Harlow; Spitz 1954.

[48] Qigong is a Chinese form of healing, discussed in Chapter II-2. See research on infrasonic healing devices in Chapter I-4.

[49] See discussion on **thoughtography** in Chapter IV-3.

[50] See discussions on **biological energy fields** in Chapter II-2; II-3; IV-2, 1V-3.

[51] About 30 percent of people note a strong difference with one eye or the other partly open; 30 percent note a mild difference; 40 percent note no difference. When the left outer quadrant of the left eye is stimulated by light, the right cerebral hemisphere is activated. This may shade the experience with emotional tones. When the right outer quadrant of the right eye is stimulated, the left hemisphere is activated. Your perception of the experience may be more analytical and less emotional from this perspective.

[52] As in dreams, or in the laboratory-induced ganzfeld state - discussed in Chapter I-3.

[53] Some might see in this a sinister (pun intended) plot for masculine domination in the world – the word, *sinister*, deriving from the Latin for "left."

[54] See II-Introduction; III-Iintroduction; III-12; IV-3.

[55] One out of every six people who are hospitalized is likely to acquire an infection in the hospital. Over 100,000 people die in US hospitals annually due to medications properly prescribed; another 100,000 annuallly due to **medical errors**. More on this in Chapter II-2.

[56] More on **surrender** in Eysenck, discussed below; under *acceptance,* earlier in this chapter; Chapters III-8; IV-3.

[57] Cardiac bypass surgery has been developed for people whose hearts are being starved of oxygen by hardened, narrowed arteries which are blocked by arteriosclerosis. Bypass surgery is a complicated procedure that carries considerable risk and discomfort for patients. Veins from the leg are transplanted to the heart to carry blood around the blocked portions of the diseased cardiac arteries. A significant percentage of patients develop further blocks following the surgery, and repeat operations may be necessary.

[58] The cardiac programs are called **psychoneurocardiology**, discussed in Chapter II-2.

⁵⁹ See Chapter II-2 on **auras**; Chapter II-3 on **biological energy templates for the body**.

⁶⁰ See discussion of **fear of death** in Chapters III-2, -8, -11; **fears of healing** in Chapters IV-3; Benor 1990.

⁶¹ Fascinating research is available on all of these pre-death and post-death experiences, reviewed and discussed in detail in Volume III of *Healing Research*.

⁶² I have sometimes wondered whether a psychologically-minded mathematician might develop equations for the various infinities of human experiences.

⁶³ CAT, PET and MRI scans

⁶⁴ In **out-of-body** (**OBE**) experiences, people perceive themselves to be located outside of their physical body. This may occur during sleep, surgery or life-threatening accidents. Some people can do this deliberately, in which case it is often called *remote viewing*. See Chapter III-1 on OBEs, and Chapter III-2 on similar reports during **near-death experiences,** and Chapters I-3 and IV-3 on **remote viewing**.

⁶⁵ While it is too complex to expand upon here, see discussions of **modern physics** in chapters III-10; IV-2; Capra; Jahn/ Dunne 1987; F. Wolf; Zukav 1979.

⁶⁶ All of science is built on basic assumptions that are ultimately unprovable. Some branches of science, however, are better supported than others by consistent bodies of observations and research.

⁶⁷ In Eastern terms, these stages are called *jhanas*. See H. Smith.

⁶⁸ See Wilber's personal experiences in meditation in Wilber 1999.

⁶⁹ Unity with the All is *Atman* in Buddhist terminology.

⁷⁰ An important theoretical side note: Freud, Rank, and others have postulated that the fear of death leads people to kill or sacrifice others. Symbolically, through the death of others, these killers attempt to deny their mortality and put off their own death.

⁷¹ Wilber's levels do not entirely conform to the levels described in the various conventional developmental theories. See also Chapter III-11 for discussions on developmental stages in transpersonal awareness (also Benor 2003) and in faith.

⁷² Pierrakos has an even broader perspective, and his methods are closer to healing per se than many others in this category.

⁷³ These rates of pulsation are similar to **craniosacral rhythms**, discussed in Chapter II-2. Perhaps they relate to the same biological energy field phenomena.

⁷⁴ 1974a; 19074b; 1995; 1998.

⁷⁵ More on this in Chapters III-3; -4; -5; -6; -8; -11; Benor 1994; 1996b;. Benor/ Mohr.

⁷⁶ See Chapter I-4 on **healing for anxiety**.

⁷⁷ **Many facets of healing** are discussed in greater detail in Chapter IV-3.

⁷⁸ **Karmic issues** are discussed in Chapters III-3; III-8; III-11.

⁷⁹ We have formed an International Association for Healing and Psychotherapy in England for mutual support and personal learning/growth, and are working on a similar organization in America. The International Journal of Healing and Caring – On line publishes articles on wholistic psychotherapy and healing www.ijhc.org.

[80] See description of Edwards in Chapter I-1.

[81] See Ruth Benor, Chapter I-1 on **healing unto death**; also Chapter III-8 on spirituality and death.

[82] **Psi powers** are discussed in chapter I-3. More on the collective unconscious in Chapters IV-2 and IV-3.

[83] More on **remote viewing** in Chapter I-3.

[84] Non-verbal communication can be as simple as gestures punctuating conversation, or may include unconscious psychological communications (Fast). If chronic tensions are communicated by the mind to the body, it may lead to physical changes in body morphology (Lowen).

[85] For **biological fields** see Chapters II-3; IV-3; Benor 1984; Brennan 1987; 1993; Gerber.

Notes: Chapter 2 – Wholistic Energy Medicine

[86] I use the term *wholistic medicine* to include nursing as an integral part of medical practice. Nurses have, in fact, made as many advances into wholistic care as doctors have, if not more.

[87] I pondered hard and long on whether to keep Chapters 1 and 2 as a single chapter – to emphasize the wholeness of self-healings and caregiver-assisted healings. The separation of these approaches in clinical practice is unfortunate. For ease of accessing discussions and references I have conceded to popular views and reluctantly separated these chapters.

[88] The code of conduct of the American Medical Association declares that it is unethical for medical doctors to use or abet in the use of a treatment that has no scientific basis, promotes false hope or delays "proper" care – as defined by medical doctors. This can lead to ethical conflicts between doctors and patients, particularly where children are involved. More on this at the end of this chapter.

[89] The ranking of causes of death varies with several forms of gathering statistics for each cause.

[90] This is not a new finding. In 1964, the Yale New Haven Medical Center reported in the Annals of Internal Medicine that deleterious effects of negligent medical care occurred in 20 percent of admissions, with major negative effects in 4.7 percent.

[91] See for instance discussion of adverse effects under Acupuncture; Kava and herb-medication interactions under nutritional and herbal therapies, below.

[92] See Mercola on statistics of iatrogenic deaths; Fonorow on mortuary statistics in Israel. Even more sobering are the ethical issues surrounding big business and government-led efforts to cover up such problems.

[93] On **treatments for back pain** see chiropractic, osteopathy, massage.

[94] On **treatment for cerebral palsy** see craniosacral therapy, later in this chapter.

[95] There is a pun here, as *consumption* was also used as a term for tuberculosis in Shakespeare's time.

[96] **Spiritual aspects of health and illness** are considered in great detail in Volume III.

[97] Figure from Swift, Gayle, A contextual model for holistic nursing practice, *Journal of Holistic Nursing* 1994 12 (3), 265-281, Copyright © 1994 by Gayle Swift, reprinted by permission of Sage Publications, Inc.

[98] Figure from Swift, Gayle, A contextual model for holistic nursing practice, *Journal of Holistic Nursing* 1994 12 (3), 265-281, Copyright © 1994 by Gayle Swift, reprinted by permission of Sage Publications, Inc.

[99] Several of these are listed in Chapter II-5.

[100] The American Board of Holistic Medicine has examinations in holistic medicine.

[101] The AHNA Holistic Nurse Certification Program (with examination) covers holistic caring/ healing nursing modalities over 18-24 months. Certification may be by examination without formal training.

[102] Much more on **dying and death** in *Healing Research Vol. III.*

[103] See particularly   Pietroni/ Pietroni and the following journals: *Alternative Therapies, Journal of Alternative and Complementary Medicine, Journal of Complementary and Alternative Medicine, Journal of Holistic Nursing.*

[104] The American Medical Student Association (AMSA) has put together a comprehensive listing of medical school courses, electives and interest groups relating to complementary, alternative and/ or integrative medicine www.amsa.orghumed.

[105] The numbers of people using CAM therapies is truly impressive. For instance, a review of cancer therapy patient surveys showed a rate of use ranging from 7% to 64% (mean 31%) worldwide.

[106] See Chapter I-5 for a brief discussion on **surveys of healee assessments of their treatments** in several countries. These show a very high rate of consumer satisfaction with healing.

[107] Acupuncture,   homeopathy, Ayurveda, naturopathy and Native American healing are good examples of **treatment systems with well developed philosophies**.

[108] There are extremists who even assert that there is no evidence for any benefits from CAM or wholistic approaches.

[109] http://www.nationalhealthfreedom.org/index.htm

[110] Because of these overlaps in effects of the various therapies, there are also overlaps in the discussions about them.

[111] Alternative English spellings: *Ki* or *Chi.*

[112] Sanskrit dates back 3,000 years in India, which shows that acupuncturists have been aware of the chakra energy centers for a very long time.

[113] More on **holograms and holographic organization of the body** in Chapter IV-2.

[114] See **healers' views and descriptions** of their work in Chapter 1-1.

[115] See description of Shubentsov and his healing work in Chapter I-1.

[116] **Iridology**, a system of diagnosis of body conditions through examination of the iris of the eye, represents another body hologram.

[117] The greatest part of this review is taken from the annotated bibliography of Birch/ Hammerschlag, in which studies are reported to have shown "significant" effects, with no statement about the criteria used in designating them as "significant."

[118] More on **holographic reality** and **cosmic awareness/ unity** in Volume III and Chapter IV-2 and IV-3.

[119] It is a sociological curiosity that in its early introductions into the West, acupuncture found a more ready acceptance in the US and healing was more readily accepted in Britain. This illustrates the processes of dissemination of information related to aspects of energy medicine. These treatments may be more or less available to individuals due to preferential allocations of research resources and input of prominent personalities in the sciences, government and media (through advertisement, politics and faddism), irrespective of the inherent benefits of the therapeutic modalities themselves.

[120] Bott 1984; 1996; Steiner/Wegman

[121] See under naturopathy; homeopathy.

[122] Eye Movement Desensitization and Reprocessings (EMDR, developed by Shapiro) and the Wholistic Hybrid of EMDR and EFT (WHEE, developed by Benor, 2001a) – the latter being one of the Meridian Based Therapies (MBTs) - are discussed below.

[123] On **intuitive assessment** see Chapter I-4; Benor 1992; 2001b.

[124] See Chapter I-3 on **parapsychological studies** and Chapters I-4 and IV-3 on **intuitive assessments**.

[125] See NLP anchoring exercise in Chapter II-5.

[126] See a spectrum of **breathing meditations** in Chapter II-5.

[127] Per the description in a research article

[128] The Upledger Institute identifies its work as CranioSacral Therapy[TM].

[129] **Energy cyst** is a term originated by Elmer Green (Upledger/ Vredevoogd). This theory was presaged many centuries ago in the yoga sutras of Patanjali, in the concept of *samskaras* or scars in the energy body that may impede proper body energy flows and physiological functions. On other origins of craniosacral therapy see Dove. More on energy cysts and their emotional components below and in Chapter II-5.

[130] These techniques have overlaps with Applied Kinesiology.

[131] This appears to be an example of psychic/ intuitive assessment.

[132] This is a further overlap of craniosacral therapy with spiritual healing. Very similar descriptions of spontaneous physical movements during spiritual healing are described in Chapter I-1.

[133] See Chapter I-4 for clinical studies of **infrasonic sound healing devices**.

[134] More on **mythic levels of awareness** in Chapter IV-2.

[135] *Mal ojo,* caused by staring, is often confused in common usage, as well as in translation, with *mal puesto,* as "the evil eye, which is the casting of a hex or curse."

[136] Much of this summary was taken from Harding.

[137] Quoted items have been extracted from a bulleted list in Oschman/ Pert. No references for these theories are cited in this fascinating book.

[138] In inner circles pronounced as in *batch*; elsewhere pronounced as for the composers of that name.

[139] See list of **flower essences**, posted at http://www.wholistichealingresearch.com/References/Genread.asp#fe.

[140] Bach remedy trade named **Rescue Remedy**, containing Rock Rose (to "bring about stabilization and calmness"), Clematis (to "draw one back into present time"), Clematis (to "balance and soothe away impulsiveness and irritability"), Cherry Plum (to "bring about inner peace and stillness which allows us to ease the contraction felt in the body") and Star of Bethlehem (to "help us regain our composure" and "for learning and mastery of our lives").

[141] **Yarrow Special Formula** includes Yarrow, Arnica and Echinacea.

[142] See chapter I-3 on **clairsentience**, or intuitive perception of the world that does not rely on our five outer senses.

[143] Case description courtesy of Judy Steele, MTP.

[144] Description of remedy spectrum of efficacy taken from R. Morrison

[145] Anonymous joke: "Did you hear about the homeopath who forgot to take his medicine? He died of an overdose."

[146] Scofield reviews numerous studies demonstrating this sinusoidal periodicity of clinical effects (periodic increases and decreases in potency) as the homeopathic remedies are diluted further and further. See also Davenas et al.

[147] Case related to me by a UK homeopath.

[148] More on **complexity theory, information as healing and chaos theory** in Chapter IV-3.

[149] See more about **Tiller and his theories** in Chapter II-4 under *radionics*; about healing in Chapter IV-2; and about the etheric body in Chapter II-3 under *auras*. Tiller 2003a; b also discusses how quantum physics can explain spiritual healing

[150] See more on **water as a vehicle for healing** in Chapters I-2 and I-4; **a summary of vehicles for healing energies** in Chapter IV-3.

[151] See **Applied Kinesiology** earlier in this chapter.

[152] See more on **metaphor and imagery in healing** in Chapter II-1; II-2; IV-3; and on **mythic dimensions of healing** in Chapters III-8; IV-2.

[153] On **state-specific consciousness** see LeShan; Tart, reviewed in Chapter IV-2.

[154] For more on **holographic realities** see Chapter IV-2.

[155] This holographic model is similar to perspectives in shamanic healings, where the individual is addressed as a part of the community and where influences of nature are also taken into consideration. It is also similar to the theory that our earth, *Gaia,* is a giant ecobiological unit in which every element is an integral part of the planet. Anything influencing the planet will impact everything on the planet.

[156] This sort of intuitive reading of an inanimate object is called **psychometry**, a form of extrasensory perception discussed in Chapter I-3.

[157] Other intuitives have developed such remedies, in the context of homeopathic and flower essence therapies. For instance, Madeline Evans has an excellent book on homeopathy, including essential, esoteric and chakra relevance.

[158] See discussion of **psi phenomena** in Chapter I-3.

[159] See Chapter I-2 on **IR and UV measurements of healing changes in water.**

[160] Overlaps with sacred geometry (Chapter II-4), vehicles for healing (IV-3) and healing rituals (IV-3) are suggested here as well. More on **healing through metaphor and imagery** in IV-2.

[161] See discussions of LeShan 1974a; 1976, reviewed in Chapter IV-2.

[162] It is of interest that these people (described by Shallis), who suffered from extreme allergies sometimes were also able to produce electrical effects, such as electric shocks given to other people and damage to electrical appliances. Many also have a variety of psi abilities.

[163] Governing bodies are: Arizona Board of Homeopathic Medical Examiners; Connecticut Dept. of Health Homeopathic Licensure; Nevada State Board of Homeopathic Medical Examiners.

[164] Warts may be treated with many forms of suggestions, including placebos, without full hypnosis.

[165] For further reading on **hypnotherapy** see Cheek 1994; Gilian; Rossi 1976; 1986a; H. Spiegel/ Spiegel.

[166] American Society for Clinical Hypnosis; Society for Clinical and Experimental Hypnosis; International Society for Hypnosis; American Boards of (Psychological, Medical, Dental) Hypnosis.

[167] See also discussion in Chapter I-1 for further applications and benefits of hypnotherapy.

[168] Massage is often termed *manipulation*, which is confusing because there are separate therapies that combine spinal manipulation with massage.

[169] Note also the impediment to including touch and massage in psychotherapy imposed by laws that are meant to prevent sexual malpractice within the therapeutic relationship.

[170] **Meridian Based Therapies (MBTs) include:** *Emotional Freedom Technique* (*EFT* – G. Craig), Thought Field Therapy (Callahan 1985; 1991; 1996; Durlacher; Gallo), *the Wholistic Hybrid of EMDR and EFT (WHEE*- Benor 2001a), *Touch and Breathing* (*TAB* – Diepold), Be Set Free Fast (*BSFF* – Nims), *Tapas Acupressure Technique* (*TAT* – Fleming) and numbers of other variations on this theme. More on MBTs in Gallo 1999; 2000; Gallo/ Furman; Gallo/ Vincenzi; M. Gordon 1998; 1999; Hartman-Kent; Lake/ Wells; Mountrose/ Mountrose; Pratt/ Lambrou; K. Zimmerman.

[171] I feel it is important to include these subtle energy interventions here, within the massage overview, despite the obvious redundancy. This is not only for the sake of thoroughness in discussing manual therapies. It is also to emphasize that many of the manual therapies may include elements of subtle energy healing – even without the awareness of the practitioners.

[172] A **proxy** is a person who receives the energy medicine intervention in place of the person for whom the treatment is intended. The proxy serves as an antenna or a form of living clairsentient *witness*, enabling the bioenergy therapist to connect with the person in need. More on the use of a witness to c onnect the healer with the healee for intuitive assessment and healing under *Radionics* in chapter II-4.

[173] See extensive review of **spiritual healing** in Volume I.

[174] **Radix** therapy, related to Reichian therapies such as Bioenergetics, Core Energetics and Hakomi, was developed by Charles Kelley and is described at http://www.radix.org .

[175] **Eutony** (G. Alexander); **Hakomi** (R. Kurtz); **Hawaiian massage** (Samet; Kahuna healing – S. King); **Metamorphic Technique** (R. St. John); **Thai massage**; **Zero balancing** (Hamwee/ Smith).

[176] The Psychological Corporation is a company that develops assessment tools.

[177] These have curricula of 500 hours or more covering anatomy, physiology and the theory, practice and ethics of massage. The US Massage Therapy Association (AMTA) is the most established of the professional massage associations, with over 20,000 members. It publishes the *Massage Therapy Journal*. The Federation of Therapeutic Massage and Bodywork Organizations is an umbrella group including the AMTA, the American Oriental Bodywork Therapy Association, the American Polarity Therapy Association, the Rolf Institute and the Trager Institute. For general discussions of **massage** see: Bentley (head); Cassar; Chia (bioenergetic self-massage); Downing; Hollis; Inkeles (for stress); Knaster; Lidell; Vickers (with aromatherapy).

[178] Benor 1992 (reviewed in Chapter I-4). See also brief mention of intuitive assessments using devices that read electromagnetic potentials at acupressure points, under Acupuncture.

[179] American Board of Scientific Medical Intuition www.absmi.com

[180] **Transpersonal psychology** is discussed later in this chapter and in Chapter II-1; III-11.

[181] Volume III reviews **research in spiritual dimensions of healing**. Of particular interest for intuitive assessments are the channeled perceptions that may provide suggestions to help identify the causes of illness and various cures that can help. In the basic sciences, Besant/ Leadbeater 1908 is particularly interesting – includes clairsentient perceptions of the elements in the periodic table before they were identified by conventional science.

[182] **Theories to explain healing** are discussed in Chapter IV-2.

[183] The American Board of Scientific Medical Intuition, founded by C. Norman Shealy, MD and Carolyn Myss - www.absmi.com.

[184] **Remote viewing** is discussed in Chapter I-3.

[185] See review of **LeShan's realities** in Chapter IV-2; also Table IV-2. LeShan (1974a) and Joyce Goodrich (1978) teach a method of spiritual healing that is based on achieving a focused, meditative state, described briefly earlier in this chapter.

[186] Murphy 1992b lists studies on meditative benefits for visual sensitivity, auditory acuity, other aspects of perception, reaction time and other motor skills, concentration, empathy, creativity, and more.

[187] See Chapter II-1 on **right and left brain functions**.

[188] See meditations for problem solving in Chapter II-5.

[189] See EmotionalBody Process in Benor et al 2001; 2002. See S. Levine 1986 for healing meditations with serious illness. The Sedona method at http://www.sedona.com.

[190] I have seen very penetrating insights arise from such meditations, in myself and in clients I have worked with.

[191] As examples of techniques for rapid release of problems see the Meridian Based Therapies (see endnote 170); EMDR; and the Sedona Method (http://www.sedona.com).

[192] See discussion on **mystical experiences** in Chapter III-8; LeShan 1974a on **alternative realities**, reviewed in Chapter IV-2.

[193] More on **meta-anxiety** in Chapter II-1.

[194] U. of Pennsylvania; U. of Massachusetts.

[195] R. Callahan; Hooke; Leonoff.

[196] See endnote 170.

[197] In addition, with the Tapas Acupressure Technique, roots of psychological problems in past lives may be discovered and released. Much more on past lives and past life therapy in Volume III.

[198] See discussion on applied kinesiology, below. No research literature is available as yet on TAT. See Chapter 5 for information on courses.

[199] EMDR, Eye Movement Desensitization and Reprocessing, is described under Bodymind therapies

[200] Naturopathic Physicians Licensing Examination (NPLEx).

[201] Alaska, Arizona, Connecticut, Hawaii, Maine, Montana, New Hampshire, Oregon, Puerto Rico, Utah, Vermont, Washington. Florida also has some naturopaths practicing under a sunsetted licensure law.

[202] Two years of basic medical sciences: anatomy, physiology, biochemistry, pharmacology, pathology, and microbiology/ immunology (total of 1025 hours) are blended with 2 years of naturopathic philosophy and therapeutics, plus 869 hours of clinical education and 1,500 hours of clinical training.

[203] I have always been amazed that medical schools offer next to no training in nutritional therapies.

[204] A tranquilizer, brand name Valium.

[205] More than half of physicians surveyed by the Association of American Medical Colleges complained that their education in nutrition and nutritional therapy was inadequate. Less than a third of medical schools have courses in nutrition, and there is rarely any extension of the course in clinical education. The Physicians' Committee for Responsible Medicine has designed a resource for medical students to fill this gap.

[206] Much of this discussion comes from Burton Goldberg Group 1997.

[207] Some of these studies are reviewed in Chapter I-4.

[208] Technically, a **medicine man** is defined as a traditional healer. **Shamans** are medicine **men**, but not all medicine men are shamans. Shamans serve in many other capacities within their culture, in addition to performing their duties as healers They may mediate disputes, provide counseling for emotional and relational problems, officiate at religious holidays and rites of passage, etc.

[209] Berman is especially cogent in arguing these points. In sociology and anthropology, these **polarities of attitudes towards other cultures** are termed:
Emic - Explanation which acknowledges that peoples from cultures other than our own, behaving in manners that are different from ours, usually have their own legitimate cultural explanations for their beliefs and behaviors. (Contrasted with *etic*)

Etic - Explanations based on Western convictions that modern science can provide "objective" explanations for every phenomenon - within the frameworks of Western scientific paradigms. (Contrasted with *emic*)

[210] Research confirms absent healing can influence people, animals, plants, bacteria, and yeasts – as reviewed in detail in Chapters I-4; I-5; and briefly in IV-3.

[211] See Chapter I-1 for over 100 pages of descriptions of **how healers around the world practice and how they explain their healing**.

[212] See **annotated healing research bibliography** in *Healing Research*, Vol. I.

[213] The Confederation of Healing Organisations in Britain includes 16 healer groups with around 6,000 members. Their Code of Conduct prescribes that they will not diagnose, and will suggest that healees see a doctor first for their problems. These have been strong labor unions, and effective in lobbying the government to accept healing. See Volume I, Chapter 5 for names of healing organizations.

[214] See reviews of spiritual healing studies in Chapter I-4.

[215] The Tibetan definition of chi differs from the Qi (same pronunciation) of Chinese medicine.

[216] Summary taken primarily from Badmaev.

[217] I see the colloquial use of the term **mystic** as a Western expression of our unfamiliarity and discomfort with the realms that these explorers of internal worlds are describing – immersed as we are in the materialistic, Cartesian dualism separates mind from matter. The research and theories reviewed in this book put mysticism in a different light, and make such reports of inner realms more easily comprehensible and acceptable. More on **mystical and transcendent experiences** in Chapter III-9.

[218] See Ferrer for an extraordinary (very philosophical and erudite) on the limitations of linear **ways of defining transpersonal realms**, and the suggestion that each of us co-creates these realms through our perceptions and participations when visiting them.

[219] See more on Estebany and Safonov in Chapter I-1.

[220] More on **psychic surgery in** Chapter III-7.

[221] The healing work and views of Edwards; Estebany; Ivanova in Mir/ Vilenskaya; Knowles; Lombardi; and Safonov are described in Chapter I-1.

[222] See **suggestion and hypnosis** in Chapter II-1; **metaphor in healing** under creative arts in this chapter; Chapter IV-2.

[223] See discussion on the **history of spiritual healing and paradigm shifts**, in I-Introduction.

[224] A clear example of this imprinting is seen James Peterson's study, where 20 percent of children were found to see auras – till they enter school, at which point the percent drops to close to zero.

[225] In **table rapping**, those sitting around the table hold a yes/ no question in their minds, with the anticipation that it will be answered by a spirit through psychokinetic raps that are heard from the table. Typically, one rap signals YES, and 2 raps mean NO. While skeptics suggest these raps are most likely produced by the participants in some covert physical manner, research suggests otherwise. The oscilloscope recordings of the sound of the raps show that these raps have a cres-

cendo profile, which is physically impossible. That is, the vibrations in the table start with a low intensity and build to a higher intensity. In contrast with this, ordinary raps start with a jar to the table and then have a decrescendo profile – as the vibrations from the initial physical tap on the table dissipate. See **research on mediumistic phenomena** in Chapter III-5.

[226] In similar ways, sightings of various **apparitions and nature devas** (van Gelder) or interactions with apparent **discarnate influences** (Eaton) may be projections of the perceivers, sometimes called "**Thought forms**." More on this in Chapter III-4, under Apparitions. Some reported sightings of UFOs and of the Loch Ness monster may also be thought forms of this sort.

[227] More on **mediumistic channeling** and **spirits** in Chapters III-4; III-5; and III-6.

[228] More on **OBEs** in Chapter III-1.

[229] More on these **spirit and spiritual aspects of healing** in Volume III. Edwards is described in Chapter I-l; Turner in I-1 and III-5.

[230] The Theosophical Society was formed by H.P. Blavatsky in India in 1871, "through which the West and the world in general would be instructed in 'true Spirituality.'" http://ts-adyar.org/history.html

[231] The very lack of a common term for the opposite of a "vicious circle" is an example of social resistance to altering reality. See more on self-perpetuating circles and spirals in Chapter II-1 under systems theory.

[232] See discussion on **rituals** above and in Chapter IV-3.

[233] I would expect other clusters of healers and healees to be found with strengths in different areas as well, which would similarly be reflected in the processes and/or results of their healings. Cooperstein has made a start at clarifying these points, as reviewed in Chapter I-5.

[234] **Numerous factors that may influence healing** are considered in Chapter IV-3.

[235] See Chapter IV-2 for a discussion of **morphogenetic fields.**

[236] See a more extensive discussion on **reasons that healing and psi have not been accepted** in Chapter IV-3; Benor 1990.

[237] In combination with relaxation, meditation, dietary and lifestyle changes, and group therapy

[238] **Healer effects on water** are reviewed in Chapter I-3; **water as a vehicle for healing** in Chapters I-4; IV-3.

[239] A few advanced practitioners of yoga have cooperated with Western scientists, allowing measurements of their bodily functions while they enter unusual meditative states or simply demonstrate exceptional control over their bodies. Some have exercised their egos along with their bodies, employing their unusual control over body functions to entertain or astound audiences.

[240] See Chapter III-3 on **reincarnation research** and **past life therapy.**

[241] All the Meridian Based Therapies can be used to treat allergies. See especially Nambudripad's Allergy Elimination Technique (NAET) http://www.naet.com/; List of MBTs at:

http://www.wholistichealingresearch.com/References/MBTs.htm

[242] It is estimated that close to 4 billion pounds are lost annually in the UK due to CFS (http://news.bbc.co.uk/2/hi/health/3014341.stm).

[243] See Chapters I-1; I-4; I-5.

[244] Many of the captions in this section were suggested in J. Stone; Stone/ Matthews.

[245] A sad example of persecution of CAM therapies is presented in E. Brown.

[246] See www.WholisticHealingResearch.com for a few companies that offer insurance coverage for CAM modalities and malpractice insurance for CAM practitioners. The numbers of such insurers is growing rapidly. See also discussion of Pelletier/ Astin.

[247] CME credits are required for the annual renewal of physicians' medical licenses. By discouraging the granting of credits for CAM courses, the AMA blocks doctors from learning about - and then recommending or using these therapies

[248] See Ernst 2000 for a study of **journal reviewer biases against CAM**; D. Haley for a more general discussion of **medical biases**; and Mahoney 2000 on medicine as a business rather than a helping profession.

[249] See Stratton et al. for a survey; www.mercola.com has a variety of discussions on suspected negative effects of immunizations. On legal rights to refuse immunizations see Mercola:
http://www.mercola.com/article/vaccines/legally_avoid_shots.htm

[250] Amazingly, this has been known for about 30 years and is very well accepted in Europe, but US physicians continue to prescribe antibiotics for children's ear infections.

[251] **Dying through negative suggestion** is discussed in Chapters II-1; III-8; IV-3.

[252] Canada, England, and Australia also have holistic conventional caregiver associations.

[253] Other helpful resources on **choosing complementary therapies**: Brewitt; Eisenberg 1997; R. Moss 1997; Sinclair; Woodham/ Peters.

[254] More on the **biological energy body** in Chapters II-3, II-4, Volumes III and IV.

[255] More on **spiritual templates** in Chapters III-8, 9, 10, 11; IV-2, 3 and on bio-energetic templates in II-3, 4.

[256] Some of the CAM modalities have professional associations, a number of which are listed in the Resource Guide of the Professional edition of this volume, in the CD-ROM version. To verify board certification of a physician, call the American Board of Medical Specialties at (800) 776-2378; for a surgeon or anesthesiologist call either the American Board of Surgery at (215) 568-4000 or the American Board of Anesthesiology at (919) 881-2570. Other resources: the Board Certification Directory, The American Medical Directory, and The Directory of Medical Specialists. For information on physicians who have a history of documented incompetence check the Questionable Doctors Directory, published by the Public Citizen's Health Research Group, Washington, D.C.

[257] See discussion of **transpersonal psychology** in Chapters II-1; III-11; Mystical experience in III-9.

[258] See extensive research **evidence for survival of the spirit and for reincarnation** in Volume III of *Healing Research*.

[259] See discussion on **holography** in Chapter IV-2; also Bohm 1957; 1980; Weber.

[260] See discussions on **the observer as part of the observed** in Chapters III-9; IV-2; also Bohm 1957; 1980; Capra; Jahn Danne; LeShan 1974a; Zukav.

[261] In effect, they are teaching their clients to be "**respants**" (Siegel 1986; 2002).

Notes: Chapter 3 – The Human Energy Field

[262] People experience a variety of **sensations in bioenergy field explorations**, ranging from feeling nothing to sensing a very light pressure (like a very soft bubble or like two magnets opposing each other), as well as heat, tingling, vibrations, prickliness, cold, and other sensations. Most people who report these perceptions find that they are distinctly different with different people and that they vary over time.

Rapidly opening and closing your hands may make them respond more strongly and sensitively.

You can explore further, by putting your hands over a broken green twig to get a sense of the sensations of injury, or over part of a person's body that has pain in order to sense what the bioenergy of pain feels like to you. Different people may report totally different sensations when they pass their hands over the same pain spot.

Going further yet, you may have someone mentally image that they are projecting energy through their hand as you hold your hand opposite theirs. Tell them to cease the projection at some point without letting you know when they do this. See if you can identify when they stop projecting.

These are some ways in which you can begin to develop your personal awareness and sensitivity to bioenergy and to healing.

Healers may have a natural gift that makes them more sensitive to these perceptions, or they may work diligently to develop them. Many healers find that one hand is more facile at sensing different energies and the other more open to projecting or channeling energies for healing. Some healers have no sensations when they engage in healing.

More on **sensations during spiritual healing** in Chapter IV-3.

[263] More on **research on spiritual dimensions** in Volume III.

[264] Clair*voyants* perceive psychic information as visual imagery – as I use this term. This term is often used generically, however, for direct perceptions of objects at a distance through any sensory modality.

[265] So-called inanimate objects also have auras. Sensitives report they also are sentient, with rocks being some of the wisest – as they connect through their collective conscious with elements that have been in existence for many eons.

[266] This does not mean that all clairvoyants see red bricks in the aura when a person is on insulin. That was Kunz's own personal visual code.

[267] The differences in perceptions between gifted aura seers are difficult to understand. It would be helpful to have gifted clairvoyants such as Kunz and Brennan observe the same people simultaneously and compare what they see. See Benor

1992, reviewed later in this chapter, on explorations of multiple aura sensors viewing the same subjects at the same time.

[268] See descriptions of **Philippine healers** in Chapter III-7.

[269] The following three research summaries are taken from Chapter I-4.

[270] While this study is strongly supportive of healers' claims of being able to sense the biofield, there were several weaknesses in the methodology. See full details of this study in Chapter I-4.

[271] See chapter I-4 for a discussion by the authors of the study for further improvements in the research design.

[272] See a detailed discussion of **reasons why healing and psi have not been accepted** in Chapter IV-3; earlier versions in Benor 1990; Dossey 1993.

[273] It is odd that the authors do not mention the actual number of subjects who made this complaint.

[274] p. 1007, column 1, para 3.

[275] See discussion on **sheep and goat effects** in Chapter I-3.

[276] This is a rather lengthy response to a very limited study. I feel it is warranted in view of the serious weight given to this study by the editor of the prestigious journal in which it appeared.

[277] **Dowsers** (people who can locate water and other materials underground and obtain information with the use of various hand-held devices) have been shown to respond to electromagnetic energy, discussed in Chapter II-4.

[278] **Bio-energy theories** are discussed in Chapter IV-2; **energies and fields** in IV-3.

[279] The evidence of **body storage of memories** from practitioners of Rolfing is similar to Upledger's results with craniosacral osteopathy (discussed in Chapter II-2); of Lowen and of Pierrakos with bioenergetics therapy; and of Bandler/Grinder with Neurolinguistic Programming, regarding storage in the body of tensions generated by emotional traumas (discussed in Chapter II-1).

[280] Formerly Jean Roberton.

[281] Personal communication 1990.

[282] My personal experience of intuitive perceptions is that it may take a while to learn to become more consciously aware of them, and even longer to learn to differentiate true perceptions from one's own imagined or projected images. See a brief description of a healee's varied sensory perceptions in Freed 1991.

[283] See Benor 1990, and further expansions in Chapter IV-3 for detailed discussions on **reasons why people reject psi and spiritual healing**.

[284] Complementary primary colors are red-green; orange-blue; and yellow-violet.

[285] Some even suggest that their tapes may be faked, but I have spoken personally with both of them and I would doubt that this is the case. In a demonstration of Oldfield's video camera (not performed by Oldfield himself) I was suspicious that the energies being picked up were either reflected light or heat, as the images appeared to vary with the angle of my body in front of the camera.

[286] See more on **OBEs** in Chapter III-1.

[287] The specific significance of the bubbles is not apparent.

[288] See Chapter II-2 on Chinese maps of the body represented in the hand and other body parts; Chapter IV-2 on **holographic aspects** of the body; and Monte

on Chinese and other Eastern cosmologies which view the body as an integrated energy system.

[289] Rupert Sheldrake 1981 makes a further observation that seems to support the hypothesis proposed by Burr and Ravitz that the L-Field has an organizing property: "... the spherical egg cells of the alga *Fucus* have no inherent electrical polarity and their development can begin only after they have been polarized by any one of a variety of directional stimuli including light, chemical gradients and electrical currents: in the absence of any such stimuli, a polarity is taken up at random, presumably owing to chance fluctuations."

This phenomenon may be due to polarization of an energy field, especially if it can be brought about by light.

An alternative explanation I see is that the findings with eggs and *Fucus* cells might involve chemical changes in these organisms that only secondarily are manifested as an electrical polarity.

[290] Becker/ Marino; Becker/ Selden

[291] These are taken from the reference, Workshop on Alternative Medicine.

[292] This might be related to the observation from acupuncture that the various meridians are active at different times of the day.

[293] See reviews of these studies in Chapter I-5.

[294] See studies by J. Smith; Edge; reviewed with **controlled studies of healing** in Chapter I-4.

[295] EM and other **effects of healers on the physical world** are reviewed in Chapter I-2.

[296] The **sheep/goat effect**, in which believers in psi (sheep) demonstrate psi effects at rates higher than chance, and disbelievers (goats) at rates poorer than chance, is discussed briefly on p. 397 and in greater detail in Chapter I-3.

[297] This parallels a similar hypothesis that homeopathic medicines may be effective due to energy patterning in the remedy solutions rather than to chemical substances in the remedies. Should such research be validated, this may open up new theoretical approaches to the investigation of effects of medications via their vibrational interactions with the physical and energy bodies. See Chapter II-2.

[298] This parallels the **energy cyst** discussed by Upledger in Chapter II-2.

[299] The US Food and Drug Administration continues to hound practitioners of radionics. **Radionics** is reviewed in Chapter II-4.

[300] Unlike electrons and electromagnetic fields, biofields can be explored directly by most people, as described earlier in this chapter.

[301] Also called *complexity theory*.

[302] See reviews and analyses of these studies in Chapter I-4.

[303] See discussions of other **theories to explain healing** in Chapters IV-2; IV-3.

[304] See for example the review of Goodrich in Chapter I-4; Turner in 1-5 regarding sensations perceived during distant healing.

[305] More on **quantum physics and spiritual healing** in Chapters III-9; -10; IV-2; IV-3. I am particularly impressed with the explorations of healing by William Tiller (2003a; 2003b), a physicist who is researching the imprinting of intent on electronic devices that are able to alter the acidity of water.

Notes: Chapter 4 – Geobiological Effects

[306] A few words about my choice of the term, **geobiological:** I've seen a variety of reports of apparent human interactions with forces attributed to Earth and other heavenly bodies. The term *geobiological* is intended to be as neutral as possible in designating these interactions, leaving us free to speculate on their nature. (I started out with *geomagnetic* but this implied that magnetic fields were the source of these effects, which is clearly a premature presumption.) *Dowsing* is included in this section rather than with fields and forces in the preceding chapter, because it may be more than or different from a mere sensitivity to fields, and perhaps even a special case of clairsentience (if this is not a field phenomenon too).

[307] *Feng-shui* means *wind and water*, referring to heaven and earth.

[308] See figure II-9, The Bagua, in Chapter II-2.

[309] See more on **electromagnetic pollution of buildings** in Chapter II-2 under Environmental Medicine.

[310] More on **negative spirit influences** in Chapter III-6.

[311] This is consistent with Mermet's observation that identification of water appeared to be more distinct the deeper the stream lay in the earth.

[312] **Linger effects with spiritual healing** have been reported in controlled studies of mice, reviewed in Chapter I-4.

[313] Not to be confused with Harvard's Herbert Benson.

[314] Operating in the 7-m and 5-cm bands, on 1.0 watt and 0.2 watts, respectively.

[315] In the range of .000001 gauss per second

[316] under 0.1 gauss per meter

[317] in the range of 0.3 to 0.5 milli-ohms/meter (approx. 0.0003 to 0.0005 gauss/m)

[318] 15 or 150 Cps.

[319] 0.1 to 10,000 Cps. with a field strength of 1 V/m.

[320] 1971a; b; 1972.

[321] About 10^{-6} Volts/m

[322] With a 70 mA (rectangular) current at 6 Cps., producing a magnetic field of 4×10^{-6}T (.04 G) at the center of the coil, 6 out of 30 trials had positive results. At 200 Cps., 6 out of 15 trials were positive. In one double-blind test a subject was able to identify the field at 59 Cps. with a 30 mA current (1.7×10^{-6}T, = .017 G). The intensities given were measured at the center of the coils, and decrease rapidly with distance. Dowsers walked past the coils at a distance of 0.5 - 0.75 meter, at which distance no more than 90 percent of the intensity is measurable.

[323] Gradients of 0.5 gamma per foot (0.000016 gauss/m)

[324] 0.1 amp

[325] Named after Dr. Manfred Curry, who studied these lines.

[326] Pope; von Pohl. See further von Pohl studies below on the geopathic sites.

[327] König et al. are the source for the next series of reports that I review, which extends to the end of this section.

[328] Sedimentation rate - blood test indicating a disturbance in health, often due to infection or an immune system problem.

[329] 21 cm. high-frequency radiation with 1.75 Cps. modulation, with a power density of 1 mW/cm^2

[330] A **witness** is a physical object belonging to the person who is being analyzed from a distance by a dowser.

[331] Westlake is comparing inner, intuitive perceptions with the flamboyant mediumistic séance rooms, where dramatic voices were heard and various objects, such as mediums' trumpets, were seen to levitate and move about the room. More on these phoenomena in Chapter III-5.

[332] See discussion on **LeShan's views** in Chapter IV-2.

[333] This suggests that **thoughtography** (producing pictures on film using PK) may have been the method of production for the pictures taken with the de la Warr camera. See further discussion on thoughtography in Chapter IV-3.

[334] More on **Backster's plant communication experiments** in Chapter I-4, the section on plant research.

[335] Similar mechanisms may unite colonial insects such as bees, ants, and termites (Marais; L. Thomas).

[336] More on Tiller's theories in Chapter IV-2; Tiller 2003a; b.

[337] **Remote viewing** is reviewed in Chapter I-3.

[338] See discussions on parapsychology in Chapter I-3; L. Rhine 1967. See also Chapter II-2 for a discussion on the differences between several aura perceivers who viewed the same subjects (Benor 1993).

[339] These and many related questions are considered in greater detail in Chapter IV-3.

[340] Lovelock is distinctly opposed to a hypothesis of cosmic guiding intelligence in the universe. Others have taken his theory further, considering that there may be a conscious, creative and guiding intelligence that has produced the universe.

[341] See Volume III for research on **spiritual dimensions of healing.**

[342] I have included astrology under geobiological effects because it appears to represent an influence of cosmic nature upon the organism; or, conversely, the interaction between the individual and the cosmos. The contiguity of astrology with dowsing may appear unusual, but it seems to me that both involve the elements of individual sensitivities to and interactions with the environment.

[343] There is great difficulty involved in conducting this sort of research in America because the 1974 Privacy Act prohibits the release of data from private records. The American CSICOP study which sought to replicate the Gauquelin findings could not obtain sufficient data on outstanding sports figures, and it included numerous athletes who were not of international class in the sample pool. For more criticisms of the CSICOP investigations see Curry 1982.

[344] The *synodic* cycle is the most familiar, measuring 29.53 days from one full moon to the next. The *anomalistic* cycle is 27.55 days, from apogee (greatest orbital distance from the Earth) to apogee; the *sidereal* cycle is 27.32 days (the period of a lunar orbit relative to a fixed-star background from a point on Earth); the *tropical* cycle is also 27.32 days (period of a lunar cycle relative to a given celestial longitude); and the *draconic* cycle of 27.21 days (period of a lunar cycle crossing the plane of the Earth/sun orbit).

[345] Including changes in positive and negative ions in the air.

[346] The work of Burr and Ravitz was discussed earlier, under EM effects on biological organisms.

[347] For brevity's sake and for easier reading I discuss these phenomena as though an influence of heavenly bodies upon earthly events is actually demonstrated, though I feel that in most cases this is far from solidly established. By "non-linear" I mean causalities such as are being explored in quantum physics, psi and healing research.

[348] See Chapter I-2 for more on healing effects in water.

Notes: Chapter 5 – Self-Healing

[349] More on anger management later in this chapter.

[350] See discussion on **personality development** – as a basis for understanding meditation – later in this chapter; more on personality development in Chapter II-1; **personality issues related to faith and transcendent awareness** in III-11.

[351] On **cognitive behavioral therapy** see: Greenberger; Sand.

[352] I am indebted to Wendy Hurwitz, MD for the term, "Cost-Benefit Analysis" in this context.

[353] See **Feng shui** and **environmental medicine** in Chapters II-2; II-4.

[354] See further discussions of **meta anxiety** in Chapter II-1.

[355] See also **Journaling**, later in this chapter.

[356] More on **massage** in Chapter II-2.

[357] See Table II-2 in Chapter II-1 for many more of these **body language metaphors** for stress.

[358] More on relaxation in Curtis; Rosen; J. Smith.

[359] More on the bioenergey body in Chapter II-3; II-2. I use the "All" as a global term to include your higher self, spirit, soul, and the unseen but very present worlds beyond ordinary consciousness, extending to and including the Infinite Source.

[360] See discussion of **bioenergy fields** in Chapter II-3.

[361] See **bodymind and self-healing**, in Chapter II-1; II-2; Barasch; Dethlefsen/Dahlke; J. Harrison; Hay; Roud.

[362] See Murphy/ White for a discussion of **peak experiences in sports**.

[363] See discussions of **yoga, t'ai chi and qigong** in Chapter II-2. See C. Jackson for a Christian adaptation of yoga.

[364] See discussion of **meta-anxiety**, above and in Chapters II-1; II-2.

[365] On **dealing constructively with emotions** see: Averill; Harmin; Hyde; Jonas; Keen; Kinder; Newberger; Preston; Sand; Viscott; Wegner; Wood

[366] See discussion of **psychotherapy** in Chapter II-1.

[367] More on **desensitization** in Rosen; E. Sutherland; Wenrich et al; Wolpe.

[368] See discussions of the **shadow** in Chapter II-1.

[369] **Psi** awareness is discussed in Chapter I-3.

[370] The *yes* is usually stronger. This is sometimes called the *bidigital O-ring test*, or *BDORT*.

[371] The *yes* often feels smoother; the *no* rougher or stickier.

[372] Sadness usually produces weakness, happiness strengthens the muscles. Occasionally an individual will have the reverse response. A woman I worked with once shared her experience: "I grew up in a tough neighborhood. I taught myself to be tough if I was sad and never to cry, because if I cried they made fun of me." Her arm was much stronger when she was sad.

[373] I conducted a pilot study with the help of Sushma Sharma, a physiotherapist/ acupuncturist in London. We found apparent differences between responses of people who are more sensitive to subtle energies and people who are less sensitive. The less sensitive people had less strong responses. I am impressed that qualitative reports on subjects and procedures must be included with quantitative assessments of energy medicine therapies. See Monti et al. for a study of AK for congruence of muscle strength with beliefs.

[374] More on this under **Protection**, in this chapter.

[375] In Iran, the relatives of murderers get to decide the punishment, which can include monetary compensation, precisely equal injury or even death. In many instances, injured parties or their relatives may physically participate in the exacting of the punishment – even to the extent of blinding the perpetrator of a blinding injury, or pulling the chair out from under a murderer to hang him. The rich have an obvious advantage of more alternatives in this system of justice, being able to buy their ways out of paying with an eye or other body part. Women are compensated at half the rate that men are; non-Muslims may have partial or no legitimate claims against Muslims. There are time limits on the acceptable exacting of vengeance (Blumenfeld, p. 91).

In Albania, personal revenge is the cultural norm, standardized in a *Canon*, compiled by a 15th-Century nobleman named Leke Dukagjini, which details injuries and compensation or the extent of revenge that is the accepted norm. This is the legal code for Albania, where revenge is a sacred duty – particularly now, in the chaotic social reality of a government that has collapsed and an economy that is disorganized and despairingly poor. However, revenge has been an essential element in the code of conduct of Albania for many hundreds of years (Blumenfeld, p. 75-76).

[376] See more on protection, above.

[377] See other **imagery approaches** in Chapter II-2; Benor et al 2001; 2002

[378] On the vast **powers of the unconscious mind for healing**, see Chapter II-1.

[379] See studies of **psychokinesis** (PK; mind over matter) in Chapter I-1; healing in Chapter I-4, I-5.

[380] See **research on spiritual dimensions** in Volume III.

[381] Much more on **prayer and spiritual issues** in Chapter III-8; III-11; III-12.

[382] **Applied kinesiology** is discussed above, in this chapter and in Chapter II-2.

[383] **Dowsing** with pendulums and divining rods is discussed in Chapter II-4.

[384] The hexagrams are composed of pairs of trigrams. There are eight different trigrams possible with full or broken lines. There are then 64 (eight times eight) possible pairs of trigrams that make up the set of hexagrams.

The classic reference is Wilhelm.

Gateway to internet *I Ching* resources: http://www.zhouyi.com; on-line readings http://users.lmi.net/~tlc/iching .

[385] Runes http://www.sunnyway.com/runes/origins.html; On-line brief readings http://www.ipcc.com/market/newage/runes.htm.

[386] Wa-Na-Nee-Che/ Harvey

[387] Sams et al

[388] See extensive discussion of **dowsing**, including research, in Chapter II-4.

[389] Mental influence on Random Number Generators (RNGs) is detailed in Chapter I-3. Animals have been shown to influence RNGs as well as humans.

[390] See **psychoneuroimmunology** and **psychonneurocaridiology** in Chapters II-1 and II-2.

[391] More on **imagery for healing** in Chapters II-1; II-2; IV-2; IV-3.

[392] This is identical to the subjective units of distress scale (SUDS) used in EMDR WHEE and other meridian and chakra based therapies.

[393] See more on the Sedona Technique at www.sedona.com,

[394] See more on **Suggestion and placebo responses** in Chapter II-2.

[395] Benor 2002b; Dethlefsen/ Dahlke; Hay; Harrison; Steadman.

[396] Achterberg; O. C. Simonton;/ Matthews-Simonton; Matthews-Simonton.

[397] Another such exercise is described in Benor et al 2001.

[398] More on meditation in Chapters II-1, II-2.

[399] More on meditation in Bloomfield; Forem; Kabat-Zinn; Kornfield; LeShan 1974; S. Levine 1986; 1991; Singh.

[400] See endnote 170 for more on MBTs.

[401] Benor 2001a
http://www.WholisticHealingResearch.com/Articles/Selfheal.htm

[402] This is a generic formula affirmation, pairing the negative experience and its feeling with a strong positive, commonly used in Emotional Freedom Technique (Craig). If you are not comfortable saying you love yourself, or that God loves you, then pick whatever positives suit you better. I've worked with children who chose to say, "My mother/ grandmother/ foster mother loves me," or "I know I'm safe now that my father is in jail." I've had adults say, "I know I'm going to get better soon," or "I trust [you/ my partner/ my relatives] to be there for me." If one affirmation doesn't work for you, explore others till you find the ones that do.

[403] More on **WHEE** at
http://www.WholisticHealingResearch.com/Articles/Selfheal.htm

[404] Gary Craig, originator of EFT, maintains an outstanding website with loads of observations by many clinicians on how MBTs can be helpful www.emofree.com

[405] These preferred avenues for awareness offer a variety of NLP healing approaches, that are potent but quite complex. You would do well to have the help of a skilled therapist to sort them out.

[406] Many people will notice that the feelings connected with the negative memory are markedly less intense.

[407] See www.Sedona.com.

[408] See **Autogenic Training** in Chapter II-2.

[409] Per Clinton's manual, "with thanks to Larry Nims and BSFF" (clinton's note).

[410] See Table II-4 for details of right and left hemispheric functions.

[411] Some of these preferences are reflected as well in the Jungian polarities, also discussed in Chapter Ii-1.

[412] About 30 percent of people note a strong difference with one eye or the other partly open; 30 percent note a mild difference; 40 percent note no difference. When the left outer quadrant of the left eye is stimulated by light, the right cerebral hemisphere is activated. This may shade the experience with emotional tones. When the right outer quadrant of the right eye is stimulated, the left hemisphere is activated. Your perception of the experience may be more analytical and less emotional from this perspective.

[413] More on EMDR and WHEE, above.

[414] Mason et al (reviewed in Chapter II-1) found that acceptance was associated with better responses to eye surgery.

[415] See discussion earlier in this chapter about personality traits that may impact preferences for rituals; endnote 349.

[416] These are discussed at the end of Chapter II-2.

[417] See the discussion of WHEE, above.

[418] Much more on **spiritual awareness and collective consciousness** in Healing Research, Volume III.

[419] See discussions of many different energy medicine approaches in Chapter 2.

Notes: Appendix A

[420] More on **bioenergy therapy** in Chapters II-1, II-2.

[421] More on **bodmind therapy** in Chapters II-1, II-2.

[422] More on **behavior therapy** in Chapter II-1.

[423] A. Ellis 1962; Ellis/ Grieger

[424] More on **dream analysis** in Chapter II-1.

[425] More on **EMDR** in Chapter II-2.

[426] Perls.

[427] More on **hypnotherapy** below and in Chapters II-1; II-2.

[428] More on **imagery/ visualization** in Chapters II-1, II-2.

[429] More on **Jungian explanatory systems** in Chapter II-1.

[430] More on **meditation** in Chapters II-1, II-2.

[431] More on **meridian based therapies** (MBTs) in Chapter II-2; Endnote 170.

[432] More on **NLP** in Chapter II-1 and II-2.

[433] More on **psychoanalysis** in Chapter II-1.

[434] Jung; Sharp; Von Franz. More on psychodrama in Chapter II-2.

[435] Assagioli

[436] More on **relaxation** in Chapters II-1.

[437] Rogers

[438] Stewart/ Joines

[439] More on **transpersonal therapy** in Chapters II-1; II-2; Volume III.

[440] See endnote 170.

References

A

Achterberg, Jeanne. *Imagery in Healing: Shamanism and Modem Medicine*, Boston/ London: New Science Library/ Shambala 1985.

Achterberg, Jeanne/ Dossey, Barbara/ Kolkmeier, Leslie. *Rituals of Healing: Using Imagery for Health and Wellnessi*, New York: Bantam 1994.

Achterberg, J/ Lawlis, GF. *Bridges of the Bodymind: Behavioral Approaches to Health Care*, Champaign, IL: Institute for Personality and Ability Testing 1980.

Achterberg, J/ Lawlis, GF. *Imagery and Disease: Diagnostic Tools?* Champaign, IL: Institute for Personality and Ability Testing 1984

Adamenko, Viktor. Living detectors, *J of Parametric* 1972, 6(l), 5-8.

Adamenko, Viktor. Give the 'green light' to red light!, Translator Larissa Vilenskaya) *Psi Research* 1982, 1(1), 97-106. (Orig. Russian, *Tekhnika molodezhi* 1981, No.6.)

Adams, K. *Journey to the Self: 22 Paths to Personal Growth*, New York: Warner 1990.

Adey W R/ Bawin SM. 1977 Brain interactions with weak electric and magnetic fields, *Neurosciences Research Program Bulletin* 15(1):1-29

Albright, P et al (eds). *Mind, Body and Spirit,* Findhorn: Thule 1981.

Alexander, Gerda. (Trans. From French) *Eutony: The Holistic Discovery of the Total Person*, Felix Morrow, Great Neck, New York 11021 - Distributed by The Talman Company 1985

Alexandersson, Olof, *Living Water: Viktor Schauberger and the Secrets of Natural Energy*, Bath, England: Gateway 1990.

Allison, Ralph/ Schwarz, Ted. *Minds in Many Pieces*, New York: Rawson Wade 1980.

Altaffer, Thomas. *Energetic Homeostasis*, http://home.att.net/~tom.altaffer/index.htm .

Alternative Link. www.alternativelink.com

American Academy of Family Practitioners for Physicians, *Curriculum in Clinical Nutrition*, Kansas City, MO: AACP.

Archimedes. Attributed.

Assagioli, Roberto. *Psychosynthesis*, London: Turnstone 1965.

Assisi, St. Francis of. Attributed.

B

Bach, Marcus. The religious experience in the healing process, *J of Holistic Health* 1977,

Bach, Richard. *Illusions: The Adventures of a Reluctant Messiah* Delacorte Press/ Eleanor Friede 1977.

Bacon, Francis. *The Advancement of Learning* 1605.

Badmaev, Vladimir. Tibetan medicine, In: Jonas/ Levin p. 252-274.

Baker, Julian. Personal communication 1996.

Bandler, Richard/ Grinder, John. *Frogs into Princes: Neurolinguistic Programming*, Moab, Utah: Real People 1979.

Barasch, Marc Ian, *The Healing Path: A Soul Approach to Illness*, New York/ London: Arkana/ Penguin 1993.

Barker, AT. (ed), *The Mahatma Letters to AP Sinnett, 2nd Ed.* (p. 455, Letter no. CXXVII, 13 August 1882), London: Rider 1948 (1st Ed. 1923).

Barnothy, Madeline F (ed). Biological *Effects of Magnetic Fields*, New York: Plenum Press 1964.

Batcheldor, K. J., Contribution to the theory of PK induction from sitter-group work, In: *Research in Parapsychology 1982*, Metuchen, NJ: Scarecrow *1983*, 45-61. *(Also in: J of the American Society for Psychical Research* 1984, 78(2), 105-132.)

Bateson, Gregory. *Steps to an Ecology of Mind*, New York: Ballantine Books 1972.

Beard, Paul. *Survival of Death: For and Against*, London: Hodder & Stoughton 1966.

Beard, Paul. *Living on*, London: Allen & Unwin 1980.

Beardall, AG. *Clinical Kinesiology, Volumes I, II, III, IV, V*, Lake Oswego, OR: Beardall, DC 1985.

Becker, Robert O. *Cross Currents: The Perils of Electropollution, The Promise of Electromedicine*, Los Angeles: Tarcher 1990.

Becker, Robert O/ Marino, Andrew A. *Electromagnetism and Life*, Albany: State University of New York 1982.
http://www.ortho.lsumc.edu/Faculty/Marino/EL/ELTOC.html

Beecher, HK. Surgery as placebo, *J of the American Medical Association* 1961, 176, 1102-1 107.

Beinfield, Harriet/ Korngold, Efrem, *Between Heaven and Earth: A Guide to Chinese Medicine,* New York: Ballantine 1991.

Beirnaent, Louis (Jesuit Father), Quoted from Meeting of Int'l Congress of Parapsychology, St. Paul, France, May 1945.

Bek, Lilla/ Pullar, Philippa. *The Seven Levels of Healing,* London: Century 1986.

Belsky, Marvin. Attributed.

Benor, Daniel J. Intuitive diagnosis, *Subtle Energies* 1992, 3(2), 37-59. http://wholistichealingresearchcom.readyhostin g.com/Articles/IntuitDx.htm

Benor, Daniel J. A psychiatrist examines fears of healing, *J of the Society for Psychical Research* 1990, 56, 287-299; excerpted in Dossey 1993.

Benor, Daniel J. Spiritual healing: a unifying influence in complementary therapies, *Complementary Therapies in Medicine* (UK) 1995, 3(4), 234-238. http://www.WholisticHealingResearch.com/Art icles/Unifying.htm

Benor, Daniel J. Self-Healing: Brief psychotherapy with WHEE (Wholistic Hybrid of EMDR & EFT) and other approaches 2001a. http://www.wholistichealingresearch.com/Articl es/Selfheal.htm

Benor, Daniel. *Healing Research, Volume I – Scientific Valiedation of a Healing Revolution,* Southfield, MI 2001b.

Benor, Daniel J. Intuitive Assessments: an overview 2001b Benor, Benor, Daniel J. *Healing Research: Volume I, Spiritual Healing: Scientific Validation of a Healing Revolution,* Southfield, MI: Vision Publications 2001c. http://wholistichealingresearchcom.readyhostin g.com/Articles/IntuitAssessOverv.htm

Benor, Daniel J. Choices in anger: Emotions, mind and spirit (Editorial), *International J Healing & Caring – On line* 2003, 3(1), 1-20.

Benor, Daniel/ von Stumpfeldt, Dorothea/ Benor, Ruth. EmotionalBodyProcess, Part I. Healing through Love, *International Journal of Heahng and Caring – On Line* www.ijhc.org 2001, 1(1). http://www.ijhc.org/Journal/0601articles/love-I-1.html

Benor, Daniel/ von Stumpfeldt, Dorothea/ Benor, Ruth. EmotionalBodyProcess, Part II: *International Journal of Heahng and Caring – On Line* www.ijhc.org 2002, 2(1), January,.

Benson, Herbert. *The Relaxation Response,* New York: Morrow 1975.

Bentley, Eilean, *Step-by-Step Head Massage,* London: Gaia 2000.

Benveniste, Jacques. Understanding digital biology http://www.digibio.com/cgi-bin/node.pl?nd=n3 1998. (accessed 5/3/03)

Berkowsky, Bruce, wwwl.samarabotane.com/Dr_BruceBerkowsky/index.htm .

Bernard, Claude. *An Introduction to the Study of Experimental Medicine* 1865.

Besant, Annie/ Leadbeater, CW. *Thought-Forms,* Wheaton, IL: Theosophical/ Quest 1971. (Orig. 1925, reprinted with permission of The Theosophical Publishing House, Adyar, Madras 600 020, India)

Bierce, Ambrose. Attributed.

Biffle, C. *A Journey Through Your Child-hood: A Write-in Guide for Reliving Your Past, Clarifying Your Present, and Charting Your Future,* Los angeles: Tarcher 1989.

Biffle, C. *The Castle of the Pearl* (rev ed), New York: Harper 1990.

Bigu, J. On the biophysical basis of the human 'aura,' *J of Research in Psi Phenomena* 1976, 1(2), 8-43.

Birch, Stephen/ Hammerschlag, Richard, *Acupuncture Efficacy: A Compendium of Controlled Clinical Studies,* Tarrytown, NY: National Academy of Acupuncture and Oriental Medicine, Inc. 1996.

Bird, Christopher. *The Divining Hand: The Five Hundred Year Old Mystery of Dowsing,* New York: EP Dutton 1979.

Black, Claudia. *It's Never Too Late to Have a Happy Childhood: Inspirations for Adult Children,* New York: Ballantine 1989.

Blake, William. Attributed.

Blake, William. *Auguries of Innocence* 1803.

Bloomfield, H.H.; Cain, D.T.; Jaffe, D.T. *TM: Discovering Inner Energy and Overcoming Stress,* New York: Delacorte, 1975.

Blum, Ralph H. *The Book of Runes,* New York: St. Martin's 1983.

Blumenfeld, Laura. *Revenge: A Story of Hope,* New York: Simon & Schuster 2002.

Blundell, Geoffrey. The wonderful brain, *Caduceus* (Summer) 1990, 17-21.

Bly, Robert/ Woodman, Marian, *The Divine Child,* Belleville, Ont. Canada: Applewood Centre 1991.

Bohm, David. *Causality and Chance in Modern Physics,* London: Routledge and Kegan Paul 1957.

Bohm, David. *Wholeness and the Implicate Order* London: Routledge and Kegan Paul 1980.

Bolen, Jean S. Meditation and psychotherapy in the treatment of cancer, *Psychic* 1973 (July-August), 19-22.

Bolen, Jean Shidona. *The Tau of Psychology: Synchronicity and the Self,* New York: Harper & Row 1979.

Borelli, Mariane D/ Heidt, Patricia (eds). *Therapeutic Touch: A Book of Readings,* New York: Springer 1981.

Borysenko, Joan, *Fire in the Soul: A New Psychology of Spiritual Optimism,* New York: Warner 1993.

Brecht, Bertholt. *Life of Gallileo* 1939.

Brennan, Barbara A. *Hands of Light*, New York: Bantam 1988.

Brennan, Barbara. *Light Emerging*, New York: Bantam 1993a.

Brennan, TA et al. Incidence of adverse events and negligence in hospitalized patients: results of the Harvard Medical Practice Study I, *New England J of Medicine* 1991, 324, 370-376.

Brewitt, B et al. Personality preferences of healthy and HIV+ people attracted to homeopathy, *Alternative Therapies* 1998, 4(2), 99; 102.

Brier, R et al. Tests of Silva mind control graduates, In: Roll, W.G et al. (eds), *Research in Parapsychology 1973*, 1974, 13-15.

Brilliant, Ashleigh. Quotes taken from a series of 8 books; cartoons with permission of the author.
http://ashleighbrilliant.com/

Brown, Ellen, *Forbidden Medicine*, Murrieta, CA: Third Millenium 1998.

Buddha, Gautama. Attributed.

Burr, Harold S. The meaning of bioelectric potentials, *Yale J of Biological Medicine* 1944, 16, 353.

Burr, Harold Saxton. *Blueprint for immortality,* London: Neville Spearman 1972.

Buscaglia, Leo, Love, New York: Fawcett Crest/Ballantine 1972.

Butler, Samuel. Attributed.

C

Cade, M/ Coxhead, N. *The Awakened Mind: Biofeedback and the Development of Higher States of Awareness,* New York: Delacorte Press/ Eleanor Friede 1978; *2nd ed.* Shaftesbury, UK: Element 1986.

Callahan, Roger J. *Five Minute Phobia Cure,* Wilmington, DE: Enterprise Publishing 1985.

Callahan, Roger J. *Why Do I Eat When I'm Not Hungry?* New York: Doubleday 1991.

Callahan, Roger J/ Trubo, Richard, *Tapping the Healer Within Using Thought Field Therapy to Instantly Conquer Your Fears,* Anxieties, and Emotional Distress, New York: Contemporary 2001

Campbell, Don, *Music Physician for Times to Come*, Wheaton, IL: Quest/ Theosophical 1991.

Campbell, Don (Compiler): *Music and Miracles,* Wheaton, 1L: Quest/ Theosophical 1992.

Campbell, Don. *The Mozart Effect: Tapping the Power of Music to Heal the Body, Strengthen the Mind, and Unlock the Creative Spirit,* Avon 1997.

Campbell, Joseph. *Myths to Live By,* New York: Bantam/ Viking Penguin 1972.

Capra, Fritjof. *The Tao of Physics,* Boulder, CO: Shambala 1975.

Carey, Ken. *Starseed, the Third Millenium: Living in the Posthistoric World,* HarperSanFrancisco 1991.

Carlson, Richard/ Shield, Benjamin. *Healers on Healing,* London: Rider 1988.

Carrington, Patricia: *Freedom in Meditation,* Garden City, NY: Anchor/ Doubleday 1978.

Cassar, Mario-Paul. *Massage Made Easy*, Toronto: Elan 1994.

Chardin, Teilhard de. Attributed.

Chaussée, Nivelle de la. Attributed.

Cheek, DB. *Hypnosis: The Application of Ideomotor Techniques*, New York: Allyn & Bacon 1994.

Chia, Mantak. *Chi Self-Massage: The Taoist Way of Rejuvenation,* Huntington, NY: Healing Tao 1986a.

Clinton, Nahoma Asha Matrix Work, Level 1 Manual, Princeton, NJ:
www.seemorgmatrix.org 2000.

Clough, Arthur Hugh. Attributed.

Cogprints.
http://cogprints.soton.ac.uk/documents/disk0/00/00/20/46/cog00002046-00/CompanionPlacebo.htm

Cohen, Kenneth S. *The Way of Qigong: The Art and Science of Chinese Energy Healing*, New York: Ballantine 1997.

Cohen, Ken "Bear Hawk." Native American medicine, in: Jonas/ Levin 1999, p. 233-251.

Cohen, Kenneth S. *Honoring the Medicine: Native American Healing*, New York: Ballantine 2003.

Colton, Charles Caleb. Attributed.

Connolly, Cyril. *The Unquiet Grave*, New York: Harper Collins 1944.

Cooper, Joan, *The Ancient Teaching of Yoga and the Spiritual Evolution of Man,* London: Research 1979.

Cortright, Brant, Psychotherapy and Spirit; Theory and Practice in *Transpersonal Psychotherapy*, State University of New York Press 1997.

Coué, Emile. *Self Mastery Through Conscious Auto-suggestion,* London: Allen & Unwin 1922.

Cousins, Norman. *Anatomy of an Illness*, New York: Bantam 1981, (Also in: *New England J of Medicine* 1976, 295, 1457-1462).

Cox, Harvey. Attributed.

Craig, Gary/ Fowlie, Adrienne, *Emotional Freedom Techniques: The Manual* (2nd ed), Gary H Craig, PO Box 398, The Sea Ranch, CA 95497, (707) 785-2848 Web site: http:/ / www.emofree.com 1997.

Cram, Jeffrey, Flower Essence Therapy - The Treatment of Major Depression: Preliminary Findings, *International J of Healing and Caring* 2001, 1(1), 1-8.

Curry, P. Research on the Mars effect, *Zetetic Scholar* 1982, Spring.

Curtis, J.D.; Detert, R.A. *How to Relax: A Holistic Approach to Stress Management*, Palo Alto, CA: Mayfield Publishing Co., 1981.

D

Darras, Jean-Claude/ de Vernejoul, P. Summary from World Research Foundation: Los Angeles, undated. (Very brief)

Dass, Ram. in Elliott 1996, 61-75.

Davenas, E et al. Effect on mouse peritoneal macrophages of orally administered very high dilutions of silica, *European J of Pharmacology* 1987 135, 313-319.

Davenas, E et al. Human basophil degranulation triggered by very dilute antiserum against IgE, *Nature* 1988, 333, 816-818.

David-Neel, Alexandra. *Magic and Mystery in Tibet,* New York: Viking/ Penguin 1956.

Del Guidice, E. Coherence in condensed and living matter, *Frontier Perspectives* 1993, 3, 16-20.

Dethlefsen, Thorwald/ Dahlke, Rudiger: *The Healing Power of Illness: The Meaning of Symptoms and How to Interpret Them,* Longmead, UK: Element 1990. (Orig. German 1983)

Diamond, John. *Your Body Doesn't Lie*, New York: Warner 1996.

Dicarlo, Russell E. Towards a New World View : Conversations at the Leading Edge, Las Vegas, NV: Epic 1996.

Diegh, Khigh Alex. Acupuncture: Origins, theory, history and evolution in practice, Quote from *Conference on Psychic- and Self-Healing (sponsored by the Association for Humanistic Psychology), San Francisco,* 1972 (May).

Dienstfrey, Harris. *Where the Mind Meets the Body*, New York: HarperPerennial 1991.

Diepold, John H Jr. Touch and Breathe (TAB): an alternative treatment approach with meridian based psychotherapies, *Paper presented at Innovative and Integrative Approaches to Psychotherapy Conference, Edison, NJ, November 1998.*

Dossey, Larry. *Space, Time and Medicine,* Boulder, CO: Shambala 1982.

Dossey, Larry. *Meaning and Medicine: Lessons from a Doctor's Tales of Breakthrough and Healing,* New York/ London: Bantam 1991.

Dossey, Larry. *Healing Words: The Power of Prayer and the Practice of Medicine*, New York: HarperSanFrancisco 1993.

Dossey, Larry. Cancelled funerals: a look at miracle cures, *Alternative Therapies* 1998a, 4(2), 10-18; 116-120 (34 refs).

Dossey, Larry. The right man syndrome: skepticism and alternative medicine, *Alternative Therapies* 1998b, 4(3), 12-19; 108-114 (91 refs).

Dossey, Larry, Maggots and leeches: when science and aesthetics collide, *Alternative Therapies* 2002, 8(4), 12-16; 106-107

Doust, Jenny / Del Mar, Chris. Editorial, *British Medical J,* 2004, 328, 474-475

Downing, George. *The Massage Book*, New York: Random House 1972; 1988.

Dressler, David. Light-touch manipulative technique, *J of Alternative and Comple-mentary Medicine* (UK) 1990 (April), 19-20.

Dubrov, AP. A new resonance-field interaction in biology, Translated by Vilenskaya, Larissa. *Psi Research* 1982, 1(2), 32-45.

Duggan, Robert. Does Russek and Schwartz's language serve future genera-tions? (Response to article by Russek/ Schwartz 1996), *Advances* 1996 12(4), 28-31.

Duggan, Sandra. *Edgar Cayce's Guide to Colon Care*, Virginia Beach, VA: Inner Vision 1995.

Dunn, Joseph (ed). *Humor and Health Letter*, PO Box 16814, Jackson, MS 39236.

Dunn, Tedi/ Williams, Marian. *Massage Therapy Guidelines for Hospital & Home Care: A Resource for Bodyworkers, Healthcare Administrators and Massage Educators*, Information for People, Inc, PO Box 1876, Olympia, WA 98507-1876 (800) 754-9790 info@info4people.com 5 p. Refs *Excellent resource*

Duplessis, Yvonne. *The Paranormal Perception of Colon, Trans*lated from French by Paul von Toal) New York: Parapsychology Foundation 1975.

Duplessis, Yvonne. Dermo-optical sensitivity and perception: its influence on human behavior, *International J of Biosocial Research* 1985, 7(2), 76-93.

Durlacher, James V. *Freedom From Fear Forever*, Arizona: Vaness 1995.

E

Eaton, Evelyn, *I Send a Voice*, London and Wheaton, IL:Quest/Theosophical 1978.

Eddy, David. *BMJ*, Oct. 5, 1991, 303, 798.

Edge, Hoyt L., et al, *Foundations of Parapsychology*, Boston & London: Routledge and Kegan Paul 1986.

Edlin, Gordon/ Golanty, Eric. *Health and Wellness*, Boston: Science Books International 982.

Edwards, Harry, *Thirty Years a Spiritual Healer*, London: Herbert Jenkins 1968.

Eeman, LE. *Co-Operative Healing: The Curative Properties of Human Radiations*, London: Frederick Muller 1947.

Einstein, Albert. Attributed.

Eisenberg, David M. Advising patients who seek alternative medical therapies, *Annals of Internal Medicine* 1997, 127(1), 61-19.

Eisenberg, David et al. Unconventional medicine in the United States: Prevalence, costs and patterns of use, *New England J of Medicine* 1993, 328, 246-252.

Eisenberg, David et al. Trends in alternative medicine use in the United States 1990-1997: results of a follow-up national survey, *J of the American Medical Association* 1998, 280(18), 1569-1575.

Eliade, Mircea. *Shamanism: Archaic Techniques of Ecstasy*, Translated by W. Trask, London: Routledge and Kegan Paul 1970.

Eliot, T.S. Attributed.

Ellerbrook, Wallace C. Language, thought and disease, *Co-Evolution Quarterly* 1978, No.l, 17, 38.

Ellis, Albert. *Reason and Emotion in Psychotherapy*, New York: lyle-Stuart 1962.

Ellis, A/ Grieger, R. *Handbook of Rational-Emotive Therapy*, new York: Springer 1977.

Epstein, Donald M. *The 12 Stages of Healing: A Network Approach to Wholeness*, San Rafael, CA: Amber-Allen/ New World 1994.

Epstein, Gerald. *Healing into Immortality: A New Spiritual Medicine of Healing Stories and Imagery*, New York/ London: Bantam 1994.

Ernst, Edzard. Are reviewers biased against unconventional therapies: a commentary, *The Scientist* 2000, 14(2), 6.

Ernst, Edzard/ Cassileth, Barrie R. The prevalence of complementary/ alternative medicine in cancer: a systematic review, *Cancer* 1998, 83(4), 777-82.

Evans, Madeline. *Meditative Provings*, Holgate, UK: Rose Press 2000.

Eysenck, Hans J. *Sense and Nonsense in Psychology*, New York: Penguin 1957.

Eysenck, HJ. Psychosocial factors, cancer, and ischaemic hearth disease, *British Medical J* 1992, 305,457-459.

Eysenck, HJ/ Nias, David. *Astrology: Science or Superstition?*, New York: Penguin/ London: Maurice Temple Smith 1982.

F

Fast, Julius. *Body Language*, New York: Pocket Books 1972,

Feinstein, David/ Krippner, Stanley. *Personal Mythology: The Psychology of Your Evolving Self*, Los angeles: Tarcher 1988.

Feldenkrais, Moshe. *Awareness through Movement*, New York: Harper & Row 1972.

Ferrer, Jorge N., *Revisioning Transpersonal Theory: A Participatory Vision of Human Spirituality*, Albany, New York: State University of New York Press, 2002

Flammonde, Paris, *The Mystic Healers*, New York: Stein and Day 1975.

Fleming, Tapas. *You Can Heal Now: The Tapas Acupressure Technique (TAT), 2ⁿᵈ Ed*, Redondo Beach, CA: TAT International 1999.

Floyd, Keith: Quote from: *ReVision* 1978, 3/4, 12.

Fonorow, Owen R. Doctors' strike in Israel good for health, *Townsend Letter* 2000 (Aug/Sep), 93-94 (letter).

France, Anatole. *The Crime of Sylvestre Bonnard,* 1881.

Frank, Jerome. *Persuasion and Healing,* New York: Schocken 1961.

Frankl, Viktor E. *Man's Search for Meaning,* London: Hodder Stoughton 1964.

Freud, Anna. The ego and mechanisms of defense, In: *Writings of Anna Freud, Vol.2,* New York: International Universities Press 1967. (Orig. 1953)

Freud, Sigmund. *Psychopathology of Every-day Life,* New York: Norton 1971.

Fuller, Buckmisnter. Attributed.

G

Gabirol, Ibn. Attributed.

Gallo, Fred. *Energy Psychology: Explora-tions at the Interface of Energy, Cognition,* Behavior and Health, CRC Press 1999

Gallo, Fred P. *Energy Diagnostic and Treatment Methods,* New York: Norton 2000.

Gallo, Fred/ Furman, Mark Evan. *The Neurophysics of Human Behavior: Explorations at the Interface of Brain, Mind, Behavior and Information,* CRC Press 2000.

Garcia, Raymond L. 'Witch doctor?' A hexing case of dermatitis, *Cutis* 1977, 19(1), 103-105.

Gauquelin, Michel. *The Scientific Basis of Astrology: Myth or Reality,* New York: Stein and Day 1969.

Gauquelin, Michel. *Dreams and Illusions of Astrology,* Buffalo: Prometheus 1979.

Gauquelin, Michel. *The Spheres of Destiny,* London: Dent 1980.

Gerber, Richard. *Vibrational Medicine for the 21st Century: The complete Guide to Energy Healing and Spiritual Transformation,* New York: Eagle Brook/ HarperCollins 2000.

Gibran, Khalil. *The Prophet,* Alfred A. Knopf 1995.

Gilian, S. *Therapeutic Trances: The Cooperation Principle in Ericksonian Hypnotherapy,* New York: Brunner/ Mazel 1987.

Goldberg, Burton Group, *Alternative Medicine: The definitive guide,* Fife, WA: Future Medicine Publishing 1997 (28 pp finely typed refs Outstanding reference book!)

Goleman, Dan. *The Varieties of Meditative Experience,* New York: Dutton 1977.

Goleman, Daniel. *The Meditative Mind,* Tarcher 1988.

Goleman, Daniel. *Emotional Intelligence,* New York: Bantam 1995 (28pp notes/ refs.).

Goleman, Daniel/ Gurin, Joel. *Mind/ Body Medicine: How to Use Your Mind for Better Health,* Fairfield, OH: Consumer Reports 1993.

Goodman, Felicitas D. *Where the Spirits Ride the Wind: Trance Journeys and Other Ecstatic Experiences,* Bloomington & Indianapolis: Indiana University 1990.

Goodrich, Joyce. The psychic healing training and research project, In: Fosshage, James L/ Olsen, Paul. *Healing: Implications for Psychotherapy,* New York: Human Sciences Press 1978, 84-110.

Gordon, James. Attributed.

Gordon, Marilyn. *Energy Therapy: Tapping The Next Dimension in Healing,*WiseWord Publishing 1998.

Gordon, Marilyn. *The New Manual for Transformational Healing with ypnotherapy and Energy Therapy,* WiseWord Publishing 1999.

Graham, Martha. *Blood Memory* Buschekbooks 2000.

Green, Elmer. Biofeedback training and yoga: Imagery and healing, *Presentation at Conference on Psychic Healing and Self Healing Sponsored by the Association for Humanistic Psychology,* 1972 (May).

Green, Elmer/ Green, Alyce. *Beyond Biofeedback,* New York: Delta/ Dell 1977.

Green, Elmer E et al. Anomalous electrostatic phenomena in exceptional subjects, *Subtle Energies* 1991, 2(3), 69-94

Greenberger, D.; Padesky, C.A. *Mind Over Mood: A Cognitive Therapy Treatment Manual for Clients,* New York: Guilford, 1995.

Greenwood, Michael. *Braving the Void: Journeys into Healing,* Victoria, BC Canada: Paradox 1998.

Greenwood, Michael/ Nunn, Peter. *Paradox & Healing: Medicine, Mythology & Transformation,* Victoria, BC Canada: Paradox 1994.

Griffiths, Colin. The Berlin Wall, a remedy proved by group meditation, *Promethius Unbound* 1995, Spring, 25-30.

Gurvits, BY/ Krylov, BA/ Korotkov, KG. A new concept in the early diagnosis of cancer http://www.kirlian.org/kirlian/korotov/korotkov.htm

H

Haley, Jay. *Uncommon Therapy: The Psychiatric Techniques of Milton H Erickson, MD* New York: Ballantine 1973. (Reprinted by permission of WW Norton & Company, Inc. Copyright 1973 Jay Haley.)

Hamwee, John/ Smith, Fritz. Zero Balancing: Touching the Energy of Bone North Atlantic Books 2000.

Hansen, GP. Dowsing: A review of experimental research, *J of the Society for Psychical Research* 1982, 51, 343-367.

Harburg, E. Y. Attributed.

Harding, Suzanne. Curanderas in the Americas, *Alternative & Complementary Therapies* (Oct) 1999, 5(5), 309-317.

Harlow, HF. Development of affectional patterns in infant monkeys, In: Foss, BM (ed). *Determinants of Infant Behavior* New York: John Wiley & Sons 1961, 75-88.

Harmin, M. *How to Get Rid of Emotions That Give You a Pain in the Neck*, Niles, IL: Argus, 1976.

Harner, Michael. The *Way of the Shaman*, New York: Bantam/ Harper& Row 1980.

Harrison, Eric. *How Meditation Heals*, London: Piatkus 2000.

Harrison, John. *Love Your Disease - It's Keeping You Healthy*, London: Angus & Robertson 1984.

Hartmann-Kent, Silvia. *Adventures in EFT*, DH Publications 1999.

Hay, Louise L. *You Can Heal Your Life*, Santa Monica, CA: Hay House 1984.

Heidegger, Martin. Attributed.

Hemingway, Tricia. Personal communica-tion 1997.

Herbert, Benson. Theory and practice of psychic healing, *Parapsychology Review* 1975, 6(6), 22-23 (excerpted in Benor 2001c).

Heron, John. *Confessions of a Janus-Brain: A Personal Account of Living in Two Worlds*, London: Endymion 1987, p. 55.

Hippocrates, *Law, Book I* .

Hirshberg, Caryl/ Barasch, Marc Ian. *Remarkable Recovery: What Extraordinary Healings Tell Us About Getting Well and Staying Well*, New York: Riverhead 1995.

Holden, Constance. Chiropractic: Healing or hokum? HEW is looking for answers, *Science* 1974, 185, 922-925.

Hollis, N. *Massage for Therapists*, Oxford: Blackswell 1987.

Holmes, Oliver Wendell. Attributed.

Hooke, Wayne. A review of Thought Field Therapy, *The International Electronic J in the Study of the Traumatization Process and Methods for Reducing or Eliminating Related Human Suffering* 1998, 3(2), article 2, www.fsu.edu/-trauma/v3i2art3.html

Horrigan, Bonnie/ Block, Bryna. News briefs, *Alternative Therapies* 2002, 8(4), p. 31

Hulke, Malcolm (ed). *The Encyclopedia of Alternative Medicine and Self-Help*, New York: Schocken 1979.

Hunt, Valerie. *A Study of Structural integration from Neuromuscular Energy Field, and Emotional Approaches*, Unpublished project report 1977.

Hunt, Valerie. Electromyographic high frequency recording of human informational fields, In: *Energy Fields in Medicine: A Study of Device Technology Based on Acupuncture Meridians and Chi Energy*, Kalamazoo, MI: Fetzer 1989,400-427.

Hunt, Valerie. *Lectures at* Healing Energy Medicine Conference, London 1992. (Taped, from Doctor-Healer Network)

Huxley, Aldous. *The Perennial Philosophy*, New York: Harper& Row 1944, p. 35-36.

Huxley, T. H. Attributed.

Hyde, M.; Forsyth, E.; *Know Your Feelings*, Watts, 1975.

Hyman, Ray. The mischief making of ideomotor action, *Scientific Review of Alternative Medicine* 1999, 3(2):34-43. (Psi skeptics' journal)

I

Inglis, Brian. *The Case for Unorthodox Medicine*, New York: GE Putnam's Sons 1965.

Ingram, Catherine, *Passionate Presence: Experiencing the Seven Qualities of Awakened Awareness*, New York: Gotham Books, 2003.

Inkeles, Gordon. *Unwinding: Super Massage for Stress Control*, New York: Weidenfeld and Nicolson 1988.

J

Jackson, Christina. Movement, breathing and Christian meditation: catalysts for spiritual growth, *International J of Healing and Caring* 2003, 3(2), 1-22.

Jaffe, Dennis T. *Healing from Within*, New York: Knopf 1980.

Jahn, Robert G/ Dunne, Brenda J. *The Margins of Reality,* San Diego, CA/ London: Harcourt, Brace Jovanovich 1987.

Jahnke, Roger. *The Healing Promise of Qi: Creating Extraordinary Wellness Through Qigong and Tai Chi,* New York: Contemporary/McGraw-Hill 2002.

James, William. *The Varieties of Religious Experience,* New York/ London: Collier/ Macmillan 1961.

Janov, Arthur. *The Primal Scream,* New York: Dell 1970.

Jeans, James. *The Mysterious Universe,* New York: Macmillan; Cambridge: University Press 1948.

Jeffrey, Francis. Working in isolation: States that alter consciousness, In: Wolman/ Ullman 1986, 249-285.

Johnson, Steve. *The Essence of Healing: A Guide to the Alaskan Flower, Gem, and Environmental Essences,* Homer, AK: Alaskan Flower Essence Project 1996.

Jonas, W/ Levin, J (eds). *Essentials of Complementary and Alternative,* Philadelphia: Lippincott Williams & Wilkins, 1999.

Joy, W Brugh. *Joy's Way: An Introduction to the Potentials for Healing with Body Energies,* Los Angeles: JP Tarcher 1979.

Joy, W Brugh. *Avalanche,* New York: Ballantine 1990.

Jung, Carl. Psychology and literature, in: *Modern Man in Search of a Soul,* New York: Harcourt, Brace, Jovanovich 1933.

Jung, Carl. *Memories, Dreams, Reflections,* New York: Vintage 1961.

Jung, Carl. *Man and His Symbols,* Garden City, NY: Windfall/ Doubleday 1964.

Jung, Carl. Psychology and alchemy, In: *Collected Works; Vol. 13.* Translated by RFC Hull, NJ: Princeton University 1967a.

Jung, Carl. The archetypes and the collective unconscious, In: *Collected Works; Vol. 13.* Translated by RFC Hull, NJ: Princeton University 1967b.

Jung, Carl.. On the relation of analytical psychology to poetry, in Campbell, J (ed), Hull, R.F., Trans, *The Portable Jung,* New York: Viking 1972 (orig. 1922).

Jung, Carl. *The Symbolic Life,* Taylor & Francis, (V. 18 of *Collected Works*) 1977.

Jung, Carl. *Collected Works,* Princeton Univ 2000.

K

Kabat-Zinn, John. *Full Catastrophe Living: Using the Wisdom of Your Body and Mind to Face Stress, Pain, and Illness,* New York: Delta 1990.

Kabat-Zinn, JL. Lipworth/ R. Burney. The clinical use of mindfulness meditation for the self-regulation of chronic pain, *J of Behavioral Medicine* 1985, 8, 163-190.

Kabat-Zinn, Myla. Attributed.

Kanary, John. Attributed,

Kaptchuk, Ted J. *The Web That Has No Weaver,* New York: Congdon and Weed 1984.

Karagulla, Shafica. Breakthrough to Creativity: Your Higher Sense Perception, Santa Monica, CA: De Vorss 1967.

Karagulla, Shafika/ Kunz, Dora van Glelder. *The Chakras and the Human Energy Fields,* Wheaton, IL: Quest/ Theosophical 1989.

Katz, Michael J. *Templates and the Explanation of Complex Patterns,* Cambridge, England: Cambridge University 1986.

Keller, Helen. Attributed.

Kelley, Charles http://www.radix.org

Kenny, MG. Multiple personality and spirit possession, *Psychiatry* 1981, 44, 337-352.

Khalsa, Dharma Singh. *Meditation as Medicine: Activate the Power of Your Natural Healing Force,* Atria Books 2002.

Khan, Hazrat Inayat. quoted in Welwood, John. *Journey of the Heart: Intimate Relationship and the Path of Love,* London: Mandala/ HarperCollins 1990.

Kiev, Ari (ed). Magic, Faith and Healing: Studies in Primitive Psychiatry Today, New York: Free Press/ Macmillan 1964.

Kiev, Ari. *Curanderismo: Mexican-American Folk Psychiatry,* New York: Free Press 1968.

King, Martin Luther Jr. Attributed.

King, Serge. Imagineering for Health: Self Healing Through the Use oft/ re Mind. Wheaton, IL: Quest/ Theosophical 1981.

King, Serge. Kahuna Healing: Holistic Health and Healing Practices of Polynesia, Wheaton, IL: Quest/ Theosophical 1983.

Klauser, H. *Writing on Both Sides of the Brain: Breakthrough Techniques for People Who Write,* New York: Harper & Row 1987.

Knaster, Mirka. *Discovering the Body's Wisdom,* New York: Bantam 1996 (15pp fine print refs).

Kofman, Fred/ Senge, Peter. Communities of commitment: the heart of learning organizations, *Organizational Dynamics*, Autumn 1993

König, HL et al. The divining rod phenomenon, Chapter 10 in *Biological Effects of Electromagnetism*, New York: Springer 1981 194-217.

Kornfield, Jack. *A Path with Heart: A Guide Through the Perils and Promises of Spiritual Life*, New York/ London: Bantam 1993.

Krebs, Charles/ Brown, Jenny. *A Revolutionary Way of Thinking: From a Near-Fatal Accident to a New Science of Healing*, Melbourne, Australia: Hill of Content 1998.

Krieger, Dolores. *The Therapeutic Touch: How to Use Your Hands to Help or Heal*, Englewood Cliffs, NJ: Prentice Hall 1979.

Krieger, Dolores. *Accepting Your Power to Heal: The Personal Practice of Therapeutic Touch*, Santa Fe, NM: Bear& Co.1993.

Krieger Dolores. *Therapeutic Touch as Transpersonal Healing*, New York: Lantern/Booklight 2002

Krippner, Stanley. *Song of the Siren: A Parapsychological Odyssey*, New York: Harper & Row 1975.

Krippner, Stanley/ Villoldo, Alberto, *The Realms of Healing*, Millbrae, CA: Celestial Arts 1976; *3rd.* Ed. Rev. 1986.

Krippner, Stanley/ Welch, Patrick. *Spiritual Dimensions of Healing: from Native Shamanism to Contemporary Health Care*, New York: Irvington 1992 (22 pp refs).

Krishnamurti. Attirbuted quote.

Kunz, Dora van Gelder. *The Personal Aura*, Wheaton, IL: Quest/ Theosophical 1991.

Kunzang, J/ Rechung, Rinpoche. *Tibetan Medicine*, Berkeley/ Los Angeles: University of California 1973.

Kurtz, Ron. *Body-Centered Psychotherapy: The Hakomi Method - The Integrated Use of Mindfulness, Nonviolence and the Body*, Mendocino, CA: LifeRhythm 1990.

Kurtz, Ron/ Prestera, H. *The Body Reveals: An Illustrated Guide to the Psychyology of the Body*, New York: Harper & Row 1976.

L

Laing, Ronald D. *Knots*, New York: Pantheon/ Random House 1970.

Lake, David/ Wells, Steve. *New Energy Therapies: Rapid Change Techniques for Emotional Healing*, 1999. Available through wells@iinet.net.au.

Lama, HH The Dalai, Thoughts on the millennium 2003.

Lawrence, D. H. Attributed.

Lawrence, Jerome/ Lee, Robert E. *Inherit the Wind*, English Theatre Guild 1961.

Leadbeater, CW. *Man Visible and Invisible*, Wheaton, IL: Quest 1969. (Orig. 1902)

Leadbeater, CW. *The Chakras*, Wheaton, IL: Quest 1977 (Orig. 1927)

Leonard, George. in DiCarlo, p.16.

Leonoff, G. The successful treatment of phobias and anxiety by telephone and radio: a replication of Callahan's 1987 study, TFT Newsletter 1995, 1(2).

LeShan, Lawrence. *The Medium, The Mystic and The Physicist: Toward a General Theory of the Paranormal*. New York Ballantine 1974a; (UK edition: *Clairvoyant Reality*).

LeShan, Lawrence. *The Medium, The Mystic and The Physicist: Toward a General Theory of the Paranormal*. New York Ballantine 1974a; (UK edition: *Clairvoyant Reality*).

LeShan, Lawrence. *How to Meditate: A Guide to Self-discovery*, New York: Bantam/ Little-Brown 1974b.

LeShan, Lawrence. *Alternate Realities*, New York: Ballantine 1976.

LeShan, Lawrence. *You Can Fight For Your Life: Emotional Factors in the Treatment of Cancer*, New York: M. Evans 1977.

LeShan, Lawrence. *Cancer as a Turning Point: A Handbook for People with Cancer; Their Families, and Health Professionals*, Bath: Gateway 1989.

Leskowitz, Eric D. Phantom limb pain: subtle energy perspectives, *Subtle Energies* 1997, 8(2), 125-154

Levey, Joel/ Levey, Michelle, *Simple Meditation & Relaxation*, Berkeley: Conari Press 1998.

Levey, Joel/ Levey, Michelle, *Wisdom at Work*, Berkeley: Conari Press 1999.

Levey, Michelle/ Levey, Joel. Internet quote.

Levine, Barbara Hoberman. *Your Body Believes Every Word You Say*, Lower Lake, CA: Aslan 1991.

Levine, Stephen. *Meetings at the Edge: Dialogues with the Grieving and the Dying the Healing and the Healed*, London/ New York: Anchor/ Doubleday 1984.

Levine, Stephen. Who Dies? An Investiga-tion of Conscious Living and Conscious Dying, Bath, England: Gateway 1986.

Levine, Stephen. *Healing into Life and Death,* Garden City, NY: Anchor/ Doubleday 1987.

Levine, Stephen. *Guided Meditations, Explorations and Healings,* London/ New York Anchor/ Doubleday 1991.

Levine, Stephen. *A Year to Live: How to Live This Year As If It Were Your Last,* New York: Bell Tower/ Harmony/ Crown 1997.

Liberman, J. The effect of syntonic colored light stimulation on certain visual and cognitive functions, *J of Optometric Vision Development* 1986, 17.

Liberman, Jacob. *Ligtht: Medicine of the Future,* Santa Fe, NM: Bear & Co. 1991.

Lidell, Lucinda. *The Book of Massage: The Complete Step-by-Step Guide to Eastern and Western Techniques,* New York: Simon & Schuster 1984.

Lipton, Bruce. The Evolving Science of Chiropractic Philosophy, Part I, *Today's Chiropractic* 1998 (Sept-Oct), 16-19. http://www.spiritcrossing.com/lipton/chiro1.shtm.

Locke, John. *An Essay Concerning Human Understanding* 1690.

Locke, Steven/ Colligan, Douglas. *The Healer Within,* New York: Mentor 1986.

Loehr, Franklin. *The Power of Prayer on Plants,* New York: Signet 1969.

Long, Max Freedom. *The Secret Science Behind Miracles,* Marina Del Rey, CA: De Vorss 1976. (Orig. 1948)

Long, Max Freedom. *Recovering the Ancient Magic,* Cape Girardeau, MO: Huna 1978. (Orig. 1936)

Lovelock, James. *The Ages of Gaia: A Biography of Our Living Earth,* New York: Oxford University 1988.

Lowen, Alexander. *The Language of the Body,* New York: Collier 1971. (Orig. 1958)

Luthe, Wolfgang/ Schultze, JH. *Autogenic Therapy, Vols. 1-6,* New York: Grune & Stratton 1969.

M

Macbeth, Jessica. *Moon Over Water: Meditation Made Clear with Techniques for Beginners and Initiates,* Bath: Gateway 1990.

MacEnulty, John *Eman8tions* 1/12/2002. http://Emanations.net

MacEnulty, John. St. Louis, MO 6/7/2003 http://Emanations.net

MacEnulty, John *Eman8tions* 4/10/2003 http://Emanations.net.

MacManaway, Bruce/ Turcan, Johanna. *Healing: The Energy That Can Restore Health,* Wellingborough, England: Thorsons 1983.

Mahony, Margaret A. *Business Masquerading as a Medical Care: Saving the Soul of Medicine,* San Francisco: Robert D. Reed Publishers 2000

Mann, W Edward. *Orgone, Reich and Eros: Wilhelm Reich's Theory of Life Energy,* New York: Touchstone/ Simon and Schuster 1973. (7pp refs)

Marais, Eugene. *The Soul of the White Ant,* West Drayton, Middlesex, England: Penguin 1973. (Orig. 1937)

Margenau, Henry. Attributed.

Martin, SJ/ Kelly, IW/ Saklofske, DH. Suicide and lunar cycles: a critical review over 28 years, *Psychological Reports* 1992, 71, 787-795.

Maslow, Abraham. *Religions, Values and Peak-Experiences,* Columbus, OH: Ohio State University 1964.

Mason, Keith. *Thoughts that Harm, Thoughts that Heal,* London: Piatkus 2000

Matthews-Simonton, Stephanie. *The Healing Family: The Simonton Approach for Families Facing Illness,* New York: Bantam 1984.

McDonald, Kathleen (Courtin, Robina, Ed). *How To Meditate: A Practical Guide,* London: Wisdom 1984.

McElroy, Susan Chernak. *Animals as Guides for the Soul,* New York: Ballantine/ Wellspring 1998.

McElroy, Susan Chernak, *Heart in the Wild,* New York: Ballatine Books, 2002, p. 71

McFadden, Steven. *Profiles in Wisdom: Native Elders Speak About the Earth,* Santa Fe, NM: Bear & Co. 1991.

McLaird, George. *Meditation/ Visualization: Transformation is an Inside Job,* Marina del Rey, CA: De Vorss 1982.

Medicine Eagle, Brooke. The circle of healing, in: Carlson/ Shield 1989, 58-62.

Mercola, John. http://www.mercola.com/2000/may/14/doctoraccidents.htm

Mesmer, Franz Anton. *Mesmerism: A Translation of the Original Medical and Scientific Writings of F.A. Mesmer, MD.,* Translated by Bloch, George J.) Los Altos, CA: William Kaufmann 1980.

Milton, John. Attributed..

Mison, Karel. Statistical processing of diagnostics done by subject and by physician, *Proceedings of the 6th International Conference on Psychotronic Research* 1986, 137-138.

Montagu, Ashley. *Touching: The Human Significance of the Skin*, New York: Perennial/ Harper & Row 1971.

Monte, Tom. Editors of EastWest Natural Health, *World Medicine: A Comperhensive View of Six Traditional Medical Systems* (Chinese, Ayur-Veda, Western Conventional Medicine, Homeopathy, Naturopathy, Greek), New York: Tarcher/ Putnam 1993.

Monti, Daniel A. et al. Muscle test comparisons of congruent and incongruent self-referential statements, *Perceptual Motor Skills* 1999, 88, 1019-1028.

Morrison, Roger. Desktop Guide To Keynotes and Confirmatory Symptoms, Calcutta: Hahnemann Clinic Pub 1993

Morse, Melvin with Perry, Paul. *Parting Visions: An Exploration of Pre-Death Psychic and Spiritual Experiences*, New York: Villard/ Random House 1995.

Moss, Ralph. *Alternative Medicine Online: A Guide to Natural Remedies on the Internet*, Brooklyn NY: Equinox 1997.

Moss, Richard. *How Shall I Live*, Berkeley, CA: Celestial Arts 1985.

Moss, Richard. *The Black Butterfly: An Invitation to Radical Aliveness*, Berkeley, CA: Celestial Arts 1986.

Motoyama, Hiroshi. *Theories of the Chakras: Bridge to Higher Consciousness*, Wheaton, IL: Theosophical 1981.

Mountrose, Phillip/ Mountrose, Jane. *Getting Through to Your Emotions with EFT*, Holistic Communications 2000.

Murphy, Michael. Scientific studies of contemplative experience, In: *The Future of the Body*, Los Angeles: Tarcher 1992a, 527-529.

Murphy, Michael. Appendix C, Scientific meditation studies, In: *The Future of the Body*, Los Angeles: Tarcher 1992b, 603 611.

Murphy, Michael/ Donovan, Steven. *The Physical and Psychological Effects of Meditation: A Review of Contemporary Meditation Research With a Comprehensive Bibliography*, 1931-1996. San Rafael.CA: Esalen Institute of Exceptional Functioning 1997.

Murphy, Michael/ White, Rhea A. *The Psychic Side of Sports*, Reading, MA: Addison-Wesley 1978.

Murray, JCC. Source of quote lost.

Myss, Caroline. *Anatomy of the Spirit: The Seven Stages of Power and Healing*, New York: Harmony 1996.

N

Nash, Carroll B.: *Science of Psi: ESP and PK*, Springfield, IL: C.C. Thomas 1978.

Nightingale, Florence. Attributed.

Nizer, Louis. Attributed.

Nolen, W. A, *Healing: A Doctor in Search of a Miracle*, New York: Random House 1974.

Nordenström, Björn. *Biologically Closed Electric Circuits: Clinical, Experimental, and Theoretical Evidence for an Additional Circulatory System*, self published. Nordic Medical Publications, Grev. Turegatan 2, S-11435 Stockholm, Sweden (Reviewed in Taubes).

Nordenström, Bjorn. Biologically Closed Electric Circuits: Clinical, Experimental, and Theoretical Evidence for an Additional Circulatory System, self published. (Rev. in Taubes.)

Norwood, Robin. *Why Me? Why This? Why Now?*, London: Century 1994, p. 205.

O

O'Donohue, John. *Anam Cara: A Book of Celtic Wisdom*, New York: Cliff Street/ HarperCollins 1998.

Oldfield, Harry/ Coghill, Roger. *The Dark Side of the Brain: Major Discoveries in the Use of Kirlian Photography and Electrocrystal Therapy*, Longmead, England: Element 1988.

O'Regan, Brendan/ Hirshberg, Caryl. *Spontaneous Remission: An Annotated Bibliography*, Sausalito, CA: Institute of Noetic Sciences 1993.

Ornish, Dean. *Reversing Heart Disease*, New York: Ballantine 1990.

Ornish, D. *Dr. Dean Ornish's Program for Reversing Heart Disease*, New York: Ivy/Ballantine 1996.

Ornish, Dean. *Love and Survival: The Scientific Basis for the Healing Power of Intimacy*, New York: HarperCollins 1998.

Oschman, James L. *Energy Medicine the Scientific Basis*, Harcourt Publishers Limited 2000.

Oschman, James L/ Oschman, Nora H. *Readings on the Scientific Basis of Bodywork, Energetic, and Movement Therapies*, Dover, NH: N.O.R.A. 1997 (PO Box 5101, Dover, NH 03821).

Oschman, James L/ Pert, Candace. *Energy Medicine: The Scientific Basis*, London: Churchill Livingstone 2000

Osis, Karlis/ Haraldsson, Erlendur. *At the Hour of Death*, New York: Discus/ Avon 1977.

Osler, Sir William. Attributed.

Oye, Robert K/ Shapiro, Martin E. Reporting results from chemotherapy trials, *J of the American Medical Association* 1984. 252, 2722-2725.

P

Palmer, DD. *The Science, Art, and Philosophy of Chiropractic*, Portland, OR: Portland Printing House 1910. (From Hastings et al; Lipton)

Parnell, Laurel. *Transforming Truama*, New York: Norton 1997.

Patanjali. Attributed. Circa 1st to 3rd century BC.

Patten, Leslie/ Patten, Terry. Biocircuits: *Amazing New Tools for Energy Health*, Tiburon, CA: H.J. Kramer 1988.

Patton, General George. Attributed.

Pearson, D. *The Gaia Natural House Book*, London: Gaia 1989.

Peat, F. *David: Synchronicity: The Bridge Between Matter and Mind*, New York/ London: Bantam 1987.

Pelletier, Kenneth R/ Astin, John A. Integration and reimbursement of complementary and alternative medicine by managed care and insurance providers: 2000 update and cohort analysis, *Alternative Therapies* 2002, 8(1), 38-48.

Perls, Frederick S. *Gestalt Therapy Verbatin*, New York: Bantam 1969.

Peterson, James W. *The Secret Life of Kids*, Wheaton, IL: Quest/ Theosophical 1987.

Phillips, Jan. *God Is at Eye Level: Photography as a Healing Art*, Wheaton, IL: Quest 2000.

Pierrakos, John C. *The Energy Field in Man and Nature*, New York: Institute for the New Age of Man 1971.

Pierrakos, John C. *The Core of Man*, New York; Institute for the New Age of Man 1974.

Pierrakos, John C. *The Core-Energetic Process in Group Therapy*, New York: Institute for the New Age of Man 1975.

Pierrakos, John C. *Human Energy Systems Theory: History and New Growth Perspectives*, New York: Institute for the New Age of Man 1976.

Pierrakos, John C. *Core Energetics: Developing the Capacity to Love and Heal*, Mendocino, CA: Life Rhythm 1987.

Pietroni, Patrick. *Holistic Living: A Guide to Self-Care*, London: J.M. Dent & Sons 1986.

Pietroni, Patrick/ Pietroni, Christopher. *Innovation in Community Care and Primary Health: The Marylebone Experiment*, London: Churchill Livingstone1996.

Pinchuck, Tony/ Clark, Richard. Attributed.

Pope, C/ Mays, N. Reaching the parts other methodologies cannot reach: an introduction to qaualitative methods in health and health services research, *British Medical J* 1995, 311, 42-45.

Pope, DH. Two reports on experiments with dowsing, *Parapsychology Bulletin* 1950,20, 1-3.

Pope, Ilse. A view of earth energies from Continental Europe, *J of the British Society of Dowsers* 1987,32, 130-139.

Popp, FA et al (eds). *Recent Advances in Biophoton Research and Its Applications*, Singapore/ New York: World Scientific Publishing 1992.

Potter, Dennis. Television interview with Melvyn Bragg, March 1994.

Progroff, I. *At a Journal Workshop*, New York: Dialogue House 1975.

Proust, Marcel. Attributed.

Prudden, Bonnie. *Myotherapy*, New York: Ballantine 1984.

Punch, 1855.

R

Radin, Dean I. Beyond belief: exploring interactions among mind, body and environment, *Subtle Energies* 1991, 2(3) 1-41.

Radin, Dean, *The Conscious Universe*, New York: HarperCollins 1997.

Radin, Dean I/ Rebman, Janine, Lunar correlates of normal, abnormal and anomalous human behavior, *Subtle Energies* 1994, 5(3), 209-238.

Raikov, Vladimir L. Artificial reincarnation through hypnosis, *Psychic* 1971 (June),

Rama, Swami. *A Practical Guide to Holistic Health*, Honesdale, PA: Himalayan 1980a.

Ramel, C/ Nordenstrom, B (eds). *Interaction Mechanisms of Low-Level Electromagnetic Fields With Living Systems*, London: Oxford University Press 1991.

Randi, James, *The Faith Healers*, Buffalo, NY: Promethius 1987.

Ravitz, Leonard J. History, measurement and applicability of periodic changes in the electromagnetic field in health and disease, *Annual of the New York Academy of Science,* 1962-98, 1144-1201.

Ravitz, Leonard J. Electromagnetic field monitoring of changing state functions, *J of the American Society for Psychosomatic Dentistry and Medicine* 1970, 17(4), 119-129.

Reich, Wilhelm. *Selected Writings,* New York: Farrar, Straus and Cudahy 1960.

Reich, W. *The Function of the Orgasm,* New York: Farrar, Straus, Giroux 1986.

Remen, Rachel Naomi. *Kitchen Table Wisdom: Stories that Heal,* New York: Riverhead 1997.

Retallack, Dorothy. *The Sound of Music and Plants,* Santa Monica, CA: de Vorss 1973.

Rhine, Louisa E, *ESP in Life and Lab: Tracing Hidden Channels,* New York: MacMillan 1967.

Richards, MC. *Centering,* Middletown, CT: Wesleyan University Press 1989.

Rilke Rainier Maria. *Letters* July 16, 1903.

Rinpoche, Sogyal.*The Tibetan Book of Living and Dying,* New York: HarperSanFrancisco 1992

Rindge, Jeane Pontius (ed). Quote from *Human Dimensions,* 1977, 5(1,2), 4.

Rogers, Carl. Attributed quote.

Rogers, Carl R. The necessary and sufficient conditions of therapeutic personality change, *J of Consulting Psychology* 1957, 21, 95-103.

Rogo, D Scott (ed). *Mind Beyond the Body: The Mystery of ESP Projection,* New York: Penguin 1978.

Roosevelt, Eleanor. Attributed.

Rolf, Ida. *Rolfing: The Integra-tion of Human Structures,* Santa Monica, CA: Dennis-Landman 1977.

Rosen, G.M. *Don't Be Afraid,* Englewood Cliffs, NJ: Prentice-Hall, 1976.

Rosen, G.M. *The Relaxation Book,* Englewood Cliffs, NJ: Prentice-Hall, 1977.

Rosenthal, Robert. Interpersonal expectations: Effects of the experimental hypothesis, In: Rosenthal, R/ Rosnow, RL. *Artifact in Behavioral Research,* New York: Academic 1969, 181-277.

Rossi, Ernest. *Hypnotic Realities: The Induction of Clinical Hypnosis and Forms of Indirect Suggestion,* New York: Irvington/ Halsted/Wiley 1976.

Rossi, Ernest. *The Psychobiology of Mind-Body Healing,* New York: WW Norton 1986.

Roth, Robert. *Transcendental Meditation,* New York: Donald I. Fine, Inc. 1988.

Rotton, J/ Kelly, IW. Much ado about the full moon: a meta-analysis of lunarlunacy research, *Psychological Bulletin* 1985, 97, 286-306.

Roud, Paul C. *Making Miracles: An Exploration into the Dynamics of Self-Healing,* Wellingborough, England Thorsons 1990.

Rozman, Deborah. *Meditation for Children,* San Francisco: Celestial Arts 1976.

Rubenfeld, Ilana. *The Listening Hand: Self-Healing Through the Rubenfeld Synergy Method of Talk and Touch,* New York: Banam 2000.

Rubin, Theodore. Attributed.

Rumi, Jelaluddin. Attributed.

Rush, Benjamin. Attributed.

Russell, Edward W. *Design for Destiny,* London: Neville Speannan 1971.

Russell, Edward W. *Report on Radionics,* London: Neville Spearman 1973.

Ryan, Caroline. Imagine your gut as a river... BBC News On line, January, 4 2004 http://news.bbc.co.uk/1/hi/health/3341093.stm

S

Sagan, Carl. UCLA Commencement Speech 1991, quoted in *Network* 1997 (Dec) 65, 33.

Saint-Exupéry, Antoine de. *The Little Prince,* New York: Harcourt 2000.

Sams, Jamie; Carson, David; Werneke, Angela C.; *Medicine Cards: The Discovery of Power Through the Ways of Animals,* New York: St. Martin's Press, 1999.

Samet, Rosalie Hawaiian Huna Massage (Kahuna Bodywork) The Wisdom of Paradise in Motion, *Positive Health* http://www.positivehealth.com/permit/Articles/Massage/samet20.htm

Sand, F. *The Life Wish,* New York: Hawthorne, 1974.

Sandoz, Bobbie. *Listening to Wild Dolphins: Learning Their Secrets for Living with Joy,* Hillsboro, OR: Beyond Words 1999.

Sarayadrian, H. *The Science of Meditation,* Agoura, CA: Aquarian Educational Group 1971.

Sargant, William. *The Mind Possessed,* New York: Penguin 1974.

Satchidananda, Swami. In: Elliott, William. *Tying Rocks to Clouds*, New York: Image/ Doubleday 1996, 223-235.

Satprem. *The Mind of the Cells, or Willed Mutation of Our Species*, Translated from French by Francine Mahak/ Luc Venet) NY: Institute for Evolutionary Research 1981.

Schauberger, Viktor (ed by Coats, Callum). *The Fertile Earth*, Bath, UK: Gateway 2000.

Schiffer, Fredric. *Of Two Minds: The Revolutionary Science of Dual-Brain Psychology*, New York: Free Press 1998

Schroeder-Sheker, Therese. Music for the dying, *Caduceus* 1994, No. 23, 24-26.

Schroeder-Sheker, Therese. Music thanat-ology and spiritual care for the dying, *Alternative Therapies* 2001, 7(1), 69-77.

Schulz, Mona Lisa. *Awakening Intuition*, New York: Harmony 1998.

Schumacher, EF. *Small is Beautiful: Economics as if People Mattered*, New York: Perennial 1989.

Schwartz, Gary E. Psychophysiology of imagery and healing: A systems perspective, In: Sheikh, Anees A,: *Imagination and Healing*, Farmingdale, NY: Baywood 1984.

Schwartz, Gary E et al. Interpersonal hand-energy registration: evidence for implicit performance and perception, *Subtle Energies* 1995, 6(3), 183-200.

Schwartz, Gary E et al. Electrostatic body-motion registration and the human antenna-receiver effect: a new method for investigating interpersonal dynamical energy system interactions, *Subtle Energy* 1996, 7(2), 149-184.

Schwarz, Berthold E. Ordeal by serpents, fire and strychnine, *Psychiatric Quarterly* 1970, 34, 405-429.

Schwarz, Jack. *Voluntary Controls: Exer-cises for Creative Meditation and for Activating the Potential of the Chakras*, New York: Dutton 1978.

Seard, M. Leon. Attributed.

Seattle, Chief. Taken from anonymously distributed pamphlet. See other versios at www.kyphilom.com/www/seattle.html

Selye, Hans. *The Stress of Life*, New York: McGraw-Hill 1956. (From CG Ellison 1994)

Seneca. Atributed.

Sermonti, G. The inadequacy of the molecular approach in biology, *Frontier Perspectives* 1995, 4, 31-34.

Seto, A et al. Detection of extraordinary large bio-magnetic fields strength from human hand, *Acupuncture and Electro-Therapeutics Research International J* 1992, 17, 75-94

Shallis, Michael. *The Electric Shock Book*, London: Souvenir 1988.

Shapira, Rabbi Kolonymus Kalman.*To Heal the Soul: The Spiritual Journal of a Chasidic Rebbe* (Trans. Starrett, Yehoshua), Northvale, NJ: Jason Aronson 1995.

Shapiro, Deanne H Jr/ Walsh, Roger N (eds). *Meditation. Classic and Contempor-ary Perspectives*, New York: Aldine 1984.

Shapiro, Francine. *Eye Movement Desens-itization and Reprocessing*, New York: Guildford 1995.

Shapiro, Francine/ Forrest, Margot Silk. *EMDR, The Breakthrough Therapy for Overcoming Anxiety, Stress, and Trauma*, New York: Basic 1998.

Sharp, Daryl. *Personality Types: Jung's Model of Typology*, Toronto: Inner City 1987.

Shattock, EH. *Mind Your Body: A Practical Method of Self-Healing*, Wellingborough, England: Turnstone 1979.

Shaw, George Bernard. *Back to Methuselah* 1921.

Shealy, Norman, The role of psychics in medical diagnosis, In: Carlson, Rick (ed), *Frontiers of Science and Medicine*, Chicago, IL: Contemporary 1975.

Shealy, C. Norman. The Nuprin pain report, *Holos' Practice Report* 1987, 3(3), 1.

Shealy, Norman, Clairvoyant diagnosis, In: Srinivasan, T. M, *Energy Medicine Around the World*, Phoenix, AZ: Gabriel 1988, 291-303.

Shealy, C Norman. *Miracles Do Happen: A Physician's Experience with Alternative Medicine*, Rockport, MA/ Shaftesbury, England 1995.

Shealy, C Norman et al. Non-pharmaceutical treatment of depression using a multimodal approach, *Subtle Energies* 1993, 4(2) 125-134.

Sheldrake, Rupert. *A New Science of Life: The Hypothesis of Formative Causation*, Los Angeles: Tarcher 1981; rev. ed. 1987.

Sheldrake, Rupert. How widely is blind assessment used in scientific research? *Alternative Therapies* 1999, 5(3), 88-91.

Sheldrake, Rupert. *Dogs that Know When Their Owners Are Coming Home: and Other Unexplained Powers of Animals*, New York: Three Rivers 1999.

Shubentsov, Yefim. Healing Seminar, Philadelphia 1982 (July); reviewed in Benor 2001b..

Siegel, Bernie S. *Love, Medicine & Miracles: Lessons Learned About Self-Healing from a Surgeon's Experience with Exceptional Patients*, New York: Harper & Row 1986.

Siegel, Bernie, Respants: Information, Inspiration and Expiration, *International J Healing and Caring* 2002, 2(1)

Siegelman, E. *Myths and Meaning in Psychotherapy*, New York: Guildford 1990.

Sills, Franklyn. *The Polarity Process: Energy as a Healing Art*, Shaftesbury, England: Element 1989.

Sills, Franklyn. *Craniosacral Biodynamics, Volume I: The Breath of Life, Biodynamics, and Fundamental Skills*, Berkeley, CA: North Atlantic/ Palm Beach Gardens, FL: UI Enterprises 2001.

Simonides. In Plutarch, *Moralia.*

Simonton, O. Carl/ Matthews-Simonton. Cancer and stress: counseling and the cancer patient, *Medical J of Australia* 1981, 1, 679-683.

Simonton, O. Carl/ Matthews-Simonton, Stephanie/ Creighton, IL. *Getting Well Again,* New York: Bantam 1980.

Sinclair, Brett Jason. *Alternative Health Care Resources: A Directory and Guide*, W. Nyack, NY: Parker 1992.

Singh, R. *Inner and Outer Peace Through Meditation*, Rockport, MA: Element, 1996.

Singh, Rajinder. *Empowering Your Soul Through Meditation*, Shaftesbury, England: Element 1999.

Sliker, Gretchen. *Multiple Mind: Healing the Split in Psyche and World*, Boston/ London: Shambhala 1992.

Smith, Cyril/ Best, Simon. *Electromagnetic Man*, London: J.M. Dent & Sons 1989.

Smith, Cyril W/ Choy, Roy/ Monro, Jean. Environmental, allergic and therapeutic effects of electromagnetic fields, *Paper at* 3rd Annual International Symposium on Man and His Environment in Health and Disease, Dallas, TX 1985.

Smith, Huston. *The Religions of Man,* New York: Harper/ Colophon 1965.

Smith, J.C. *Relaxation Dynamics*, Champaign, IL: Research Press, 1985.

Spear, Deena Zalkind, *Ears of the Angels*, Carlsbad, CA: Hay House 2002.

Spiegel, David. *Living Beyond Limits*, New York: Fawcett Columbine 1993.

Spiegel, David. Mind Matters: Group Therapy and Survival in Breast Cancer, *New England J of Medicine*, Volume 2001, 345, 1767-1768.

Spiegel, Herbert/ Spiegel, David. *Trance and Treatment: Clinical Uses of Hypnosis*, Wahsington, DC: American Psychiatric 1987.

Spitz, Renee. "Hospitalism," *The Psychoanalytic Study of the Child I*, International Universities Press, New York, 1954

Steadman, Alice. *Who's the Matter With Me?*, Marina del Rey; CA: De Vorss 1969.

Steinbeck, John. Attributed.

Steindl-Rast, Brother David. Attributed.

Steiner, Rudolf/ Wegman, Ita. *Fundamentals of Therapy*, Kessinger 2003.

Stelter, Alfred. *Psi-Healing,* New York: Bantam 1976.

Stevenson, Ian. *20 Cases Suggestive of Reincarnation*, Charlottesville, VA: University Press of Virginia 1974a.

Stevenson, Ian. *Xenoglossy: A Review and Report of a Case,* Charlottesville, VA: University Press of Virginia 1974b.

Stevenson, Ian. *Children Who Remember Previous Lives: A Question of Reincarnation*, Charlottesville, VA: Univ. of Virginia 1987.

Stevenson, Ian. *Reincarnation and Biology: A Contribution to the Etiology of Birthmarks and Birth Defrects, Vols. I and II*, Westport, CT: Greenwood 1995.

Stewart, Ian/ Joines, Vann, TA Today, Chapel Hill, NC: Lifespace 1991

Still, Andrew Taylor. *Osteopathy: Research and Practice*, Seattle, WA: Eastland 1992.

St. John, Robert. *The Metamorphic Technique: Principles and Practice,* Tisbury, Wilts, England: Element 1982.

Stoff, Jesse A/ Pellegrino, Charles R. *Chronic Fatigue Syndrome: The Hidden Epidemic*, New York: HarperPerennial 1992 (14 p. of refs).

Stone, Julie. Ethical issues in complementary and alternative medicine, *Complementary Therapies in Medicine* 2000, 8, 207-213.

Stone, J/ Matthews, J. *Complementary Medicine and the Law*, Oxford, UK: Oxford University 1996.

Stone, Randolph. *Polarity Therapy: The Complete Collected Works*, Sebastopol, CA: CRCS 1986.

Stone, Randolph. *Health Building: The Conscious Art of Living Well*, Sebastopol, CA: CRCS 1999.

Stoppard, Tom. Attributed.

Strand, Clark. *The Wooden Bowl: Simple Meditations for Everyday Life*, Newleaf 1988.

Stratton, KR et al (eds). *Adverse events associated with childhood vaccines; evidence bearing on causality*, Washington DC: Institute of Medicine, National Academy Press 1994, 211-236.

Studdert, David M/ Eisenberg, David M et al. Medical malpractice implications of alternative medicine, *J of the American Medical Association* 1998, 280(18), 1610-1615.

Sutherland, E.A.; Amit, Z.; Weiner, A. *Phobia Free*, New York: Jove, 1978.

Sutherland, WG. *Teachings in the Science of Osteopathy*, Wales, A. (ed), Cambridge, MA: Rudra 1990 .

Swift, Gayle. A contextual model for holistic nursing practice, *J of Holistic Nursing* 1994 12(3), 265-281.

Swift, Jonathan. *Polite Conversation,* 1738.

Szasz, Thomas. *The Myth of Mental Illness*, New York: Quill 1984.

Szymanski, Jan A. Application of electric field measurements in research of bioenergotherapeutic phenomena, *Proceedings of the 6th International Conference on Psychotronics 1986,* pp 68-71.

T

Tagore, Rabindranath. Attributed.

Talbot, Michael.*The Holographic Universe*, New York: Harper Collins 1991.

Tart, Charles.*Altered States of Conscious-ness,* NY: John Wiley & Sons, 1969.

Tart, Charles T. *Transpersonal Psychol-ogies,* New York: Harper & Row 1975a.

Tart, Charles. *Waking Up,* Boston: New Science/ Shambhala 1986b.

Taylor, J. Lionel. Quote from *The Stages of Human Life;* p 157, (From Montague 1921)

Taylor-Reilly, David/ Taylor, Morag Anne. Potent placebo or potency, *British Homeopathic J* 1985, 74(3),

Taylor-Reilly, David/ Taylor, Morag. *The Difficulty with Homeopathy,* Paper Presented at the British Pharmaceutical Conference, Manchester 1987.

Thomas, Alexander/ Chess, Stella/ Birch, Herbert G. *Temperament and Behavior Disorders of Children,* New York: New York University 1968.

Thomas, Lewis. *The Lives of a Cell: Notes of a Biology Watcher,* New York: Viking 1974.

Thoreau, Henry David. *Walden* 1854.

Tiller, William A. *Radionics, radiesthesia and physics, In: Varieties of Healing Experience:*

Exploring Psychic Phenomena in Healing, an Interdisciplinary Symposium, Los Altos, CA, Academy of Parapsychology and Medicine 1971 (October 30), 55-78.

Tiller, William A. *Science and Human Transformation: Subtle Energies, Intentionality and Consciousness,* 1997.

Tiller, William. Homeopathy: A laboratory for etheric science? *J of Holistic Medicine* 1983, 5(1), 25.

Tiller, William A. *Science and Human Transformation: Subtle Energies, Intentionality and Consciousness,* 1997.

Tiller, William A. Conscious Acts of Creation: The Emergence of a New Physics, *International Journal of Healing and Caring – On line* 2003a, 3(1).

Tiller, William A. Towards a quantitative model of both local and non-local energetic/ information healing, *Journal of Healing and Caring – On line* 2003b, 3(2).

Tiller, William A. Intention Imprinted Electrical Devices: Their effects upon both materials and space, *Presentation at Fifth Annual Energy Psychology Conference, Toronto* 2003c.

Tillotson, Alan K. Personal communications 1982.

Tolstoy, Leo. Attributed.

Tomatis, Alfred A. *The Conscious Ear: My Life of Transformation Through Listening*, Barrytown, NY: Station Hill 1991.

Tomatis, Alfred A. *The Ear and Language,* Stoddart 1997.

Tomatis, Alfred A et al. *The Conscious Ear: My Life Transformed Through Listening,* Station Hill Press 1992.

Tov, Baal Shem. Attibuted.

Tsu, Lao. *Tao Te Ching*

Turner, Gordon. *An Outline of Spiritual Healing,* London, Psychic Press 1970. (Orig. 1963)

Tweedie, Irina. *The Chasm of Fire: A Woman's Experience of Liberation through the Teachings of a Sufi Master,* Longmead, England: Element 1988.

Nitch, Grandmother Twylah. In McFadden, p. 109.

U

Uphoff, Walter/ Uphoff, Mary Jo. *New Psychic Frontiers: Your Key to New Worlds,*. Gerards Cross, Bucks, England: Colin Smythe 1980.

Upledger, John E. *Craniosacril Therapy II: Beyond the Dura,* Seattle, WA: Eastland 1986.

Upledger, John E. *Your Inner Physician and You: CranioSacral Therapy, Somato-Emotional Release,* Berkeley, CA: North Atlantic 1992.

Upledger, John E. CranioSacral Therapy part II: as it is today, *Subtle Energies* 1995a, 6(2), 135-166.

Upledger, John E. CranioSacral Therapy part III: in the future, *Subtle Energies* 1995b, 6(3), 201-216.

Upledger, John E/ Vrederoogd, Jon D. *Craniosacral Therapy,* Seattle, WA: Eastland 1983.

V

van der Post, Laurens, *Jung and the Story of Our Time,* New York: Hogarth/ Penguin 1976.

van der Post, Laurens. *The Voice of the Thunder,* New York/ London: Penguin 1994.

van Gelder, Dora (Kunz), *The Real World of Fairies,* Wheaton, IL: Quest/Theosophical 1978.

Vaughan, Frances. *The Inward Arc,* Nevada City, CA: Blue Dolphin 1995.

Vickers AJ. *Massage arid Aromatherapy: A Guide for Health Care Professionals,* London: Chapman and Hall 1996a.

Vilenskaya, Larissa. An eyewitness reports firewalking in Portland, Oregon, *Psi Research* 1983, 4(2), 89-109.

Vilenskaya, Larissa. *Firewalking,* Falls Village, CT: Bramble 1991.

Villoldo, Alberto/ Krippner, Stanley. *Healing States: A Journey into the World of Spiritual Healing and Shamanism,* New York: Fireside/ Simon & Schuster 1987.

Vinokurava, Svetlana. Life in a magnetic web, *J of Paraphysics* 1971, 5(4), 131-136.

Viscott, D. *The Language of Feelings,* New York: Arbor House, 1976.

Voll, R. Twenty years of electroacupuncture diagnosis in Germany, a progress report, *American J of Acupuncture,* 1975, 3(Special EAV issue), 7-17.

Voltaire. Attributed.

von Franz, Marie-Louise. *On Divination and Synchronicity: The Psychology of Meaningful Chance,* Toronto: Inner City 1980.

von Franz, Marie-Louise. *On Dreams and Death: A Jung-ian Interpretation, Trans.* by Emmanuel X. Kennedy and Vernon Brooks) Boston/ London: Shambhala 1987.

von Pohl, Gustav Freiherr. *Earth Currents: Causative Factor of Cancer and Other Diseases,* Diessen nr Munich: Jos C. Hubers Verlag 1932; Frech-Verlag GmbH 1987 (English, ISBN 3-7724-9402-1).

W

Walter, Katya, *Tao of Chaos: DNA & the I Ching - Unlocking the Code of the Universe,* Rockport, MA/ Shaftesbury, England: Element 1994.

Wardell, Diane Wind, *White Shadow: Walking with Janet Mentgen,* Lakewood, CO: Center for Healing Touch 2000.

Washburn, M. Observations relevant to a unified theory of meditation, *J of Transpersonal Psychology* 1978 10(1).

Watkins, Mary M. *Waking Dreams,* New York: Harper & Row 1977.

Watson, D/ Tharp, R. *Self-Directed Behavior: Self-modification for Personal Adjustment,* Monterey, CA: Brooks/Cole Oublsihing Co., 1978.

Watson, Lyall. *Neophilia: The Tradition of the New.* Sceptre/ Hoder & Stoughton 1989.

Watts, Alan. *Psychotherapy East and West,* New York: Ballantine 1961.

Wegner, D.; Pennebaker, J. *Handbook of Mental Control,* Englewood Cliffs, NJ: Prentice-Hall, 1993.

Wenrich, W.W.; Dawley, H.; General, D. *Self-directed Systematic Desensitization,* Kalamazoo, MI: Behaviordelia, 1976.

Westlake, Aubrey. *The Pattern of Health: A Search for a Greater Understanding of the Life Force in Health and Disease,* Berkeley, CA: Shambala 1973.

Whisenant, William F. *Psychologtical Kinesiology: Canging the Bdy's Beliefs,* HI: Monarch Butterfly Productions 1994.

Whitaker, Kay Cordell. *The Reluctant Shaman: A Woman's First Encounters with the Unseen Spirits of the Earth,* HarperSanFrancisco 1991, p. 42.

Whitman, Walt. *Leaves of Grass* 1855.

Whitmont, Edward C. *The Alchemy of Healing: Psyche and Soma,* Berkeley, CA: Homeopathic Education Services and North Atlantic Books 1993

Wilber, Ken. Eye to eye - science and transpersonal psychology, *ReVision* 1979, 2(1).

Wilber, Ken. *The Atman Project: A Transpersonal View of Human Develop-ment,* Wheaton, IL: Quest 1980.

Wilber, Ken. *No Boundary: Eastern and Western Approaches to Personal Growth*, Boulder, CO: Shambala 1981.

Wilber, Ken/ Engler Jack/ Brown, Daniel P. *Transformations of Consciousness: Conventional and Contemplative Perspectives on Development*, Boston: New Science Library/ Shambala 1986.

Wilhelm, Richard (Trans. Baynes, Cary F; Foreword Jung, Carl). *I Ching, or Book of Changes*, New York: Penguin/Arkana, 1989.

Wilson, Sheryl C/ Barber, Theodore X. The fantasy-prone personality: Implications for understanding imagery, hypnosis and parapsychological phenomena, *Psi Research* 1982,1(3), 94-116; also in: Sheikh, Anees A (ed). *Imagery: Current Theory REsearch and Application*, New York: John Wiley 1983.

Wolman, Benjamin B/ Ullman, Montague. *Handbook of Stales of Consciousness,* New York: Van Nostrand Reinhold 1986.

Wolpe, J. *Psychotherapy by Reciprocal Inhibition,* Palo Alto, CA: Stanford Univ. 1958.

Wolpe, J. *The Practice of Behavior Therapy*, New York: Pergamon Press, 1974.

Wood, T. *How Do You Feel? A Guide to Your Emotions*, Englewood Cliffs, NJ: Prentice-Hall, 1974.

Woodham, Anne/ Peters, David. *Encyclopedia of Healing Therapies: The Definitive guide to More than 90 Alternative therapies & the Best Complementary Treatment Options for Over 200 Health Problems*, London/ New York: Dorling Kindersley 1997.

Workshop on Alternative Medicine. *Alternative Medicine: Expanding Medical Horizons, A Report to the National Institutes of Health on Alternative Medical Systems and Practices in the United States*, NIH Publication No. 94-066, December 1994, US Govt. Printing Office, Mail Stop SSOP, Washington, DC 20402-9328 (Outstanding resource with many pages of refs on each subject, popularly called 'The Chantilly Report').

Wright, Machaelle. Small. *Flower Essences: Reordering Our Understanding and Approach to Illness and Health*, Jeffersonton, VA: Perelandra 1988.

Wright, Machaelle Small. *Co-Creative Science: A Revolution In Science Providing Real Solutions For Today's Health & Environment,* Warrenton, VA: Perelandra, Ltd 1997.

Wright, Susan Marie. *Development and Construct Validity of the Energy Field Assessment Form* (Dissertation), Rush University College of Nursing 1988.

Zzz

Zahourek, R ed. *Relaxation and Imagery*, Philadelphia: W.B. Saunders. 1988.

Zimmerman, B. et al. *is Marijuana the Right Medicine for You?* New Canaan, CT: Keats 1998.

Zimmerman, J. New technologies detect effects in healing hands, *Brain/Mind Bulletin* 1985, 10(2), 20-23.

Zimmerman, J. Laying-on-of-hands healing and therapeutic touch: a testable theory, *BEMI Currents: J of the Bioelectromagnetics Institute* 1990, 2, 8-17.

Zimmerman, Katherine. *Breakthrough: The Emotional Freedom Techniques*, 1999 (order at www.trancetime.com)

Zukav, Gary. *The Dancing Wu Li Masters*, New York William Morrow 1979

Glossary

Akashic Records - Records in spirit or psychic realms that contain all the information about everything that ever was or will be; in essence, a cosmic library.

The All – The totality of the universe in all its manifestations, from physical to spiritual, and extending beyond human awareness and comprehension.

Alternative State of Consciousness – A state of awareness that is different from everyday perceptions of the outer world through the five senses of sight, sound, smell, taste and touch, and linear analyses of these perceptions and associated linear thought processes and memories. (Alternative term: *Altered State of Consciousness*.)

Apophatic – Identifying that which *is not* Divine as a way of approaching some semblance of defining what *is* Divine.

ASC – See *Alternative State of Consciousness*.

Bioplasma – This is a suggested biological parallel with plasma from the world of physics. Plasma is a fourth state of matter (after solid, liquid, and gas). In physics, plasma is found only at very hot temperatures. In biology it is allegedly present at normal temperatures, and is hypothesized to be a basis for life

Channeling – See *Mediumship*

Clairsentience – Knowledge about an animate or inanimate object, without the use of sensory cues (sometimes called psychometry). This may appear in the mind of the perceiver as visual imagery (clairvoyance), auditory messages (clairandience), or other *internal* sensory awareness, such as taste, smell, or a mirroring of bodily sensations from another person.

Confidence - Belief based on experience of previous experiences, events and results

Control group –

Cps – Cycles per second (*Hertz* or *Hz*), a measure of alternating current and other repeating vibrational phenomena.

Cross-correspondences – Spirit communications through separate mediums, who did not know of each other, producing separate, fragmentary messages from two spirits. The fragments make sense only when combined later by investigators.

Cupping – A glass is inverted against the skin with burning cotton inside it (often placed on top of a coin that insulates the skin from the burning cotton). The fire uses up the oxygen and thereby creates a vacuum within the glass, which then acts like a suction cup to draw out blood from a superficial cut in the skin – along with negative energies that are associated with diseases. In some cases, no cuts are made, and the cupping is intended to draw out negative bioenergies alone.

Deductive reasoning - Logical thought leading from the general to the more specific

Double-blind study – Research study in which neither the patients nor the experimenters treating or assessing the patients know who is receiving the experimental treatment and who is in the control group.

Electrodermal activity – Measurement of skin resistance, as correlated with emotional and tension states; also the basis for the lie detector test.

Emic - Explanation that acknowledges that peoples from cultures other than our own, behaving in manners that are different from ours, usually have their own legitimate cultural explanations for their beliefs and behaviors. (Contrasted with *etic*)

Entheogen – Mind-altering drug used to awaken spiritual awareness.

Epistemology – The science dealing with origins and methods of knowledge, particularly relating to limits and validity of theories.

Etic - Explanations based on Western convictions that modern science can provide "objective"explanations for every phenomenon - within the frameworks of Western scientific paradigms. (Contrasted with *emic*)

ESP – See *Extrasensory Perception.*

Extrasensory Perception – Telepathy, clairvoyance, pre- and retro-cognition.

Faith - Belief without preliminary factual basis in the material world; also a meta-belief in the validity of another belief.

Gnosis – Direct, intuitive knowledge, which often carries with it an inner, numinous sense of certainty about its validity. To those who have experienced gnosis, it may feel even more real than physical reality, which, in comparison, is sometimes described as an illusion.

Hermeneutics – The science, methodology and art of interpreting scripture.

Hertz – See *cps/ cycles per second.*

Inductive reasoning - Logical thought leading from the specific to the more general

Ineffable – Beyond description in ordinary language.

Intercessory prayer – Prayer specifically for healing.

Intuition - Thought without underlying logical basis. The use of intuition alone does not imply that facts were gathered with other than the five usual senses. Intuition, of itself, is neutral… not necessarily spiritual. One can think intuitively about science or   mathematics, for example. Intuition can have several layers, including:

- pattern recognition based on pervious experiences with situations that are similar to the current one;
- psychic (psi) impressions deriving from telepathy, clairsentience, precognition and retrocognition
- bioenergy perceptions acquired through interactions of one person's biological energy field(s) with the field(s) of other living beings and non-living things.
- spiritual awareness, derived from transpersonal consciousness

IR – *Infrared* – Light waves that are slower than red and are invisible to the human eye.

Kundalini – Energies (described initially in Eastern traditions) originating at the base of the spine, which may rise up the spine as a part of a bioenergetic process of spiritual awakening.

Lucid dreaming – Dreams in which the dreamer feels awake and is in conscious control of the progress and unfolding of the dream experience.

Mediumship – Psychic perceptions of spirits and communications with them. (Alt. *Channeling*)

Metaphysical thought – Speculations on primary causes and ultimate significance of the world beyond its measurable and testable limits. Metaphysics addresses 'why' things are and makes value assessments of thought and actions. In some cases the reasoning is inductive, that is from personal experience which is positive, intuitive, or first person: *gnosis*. In most cases, the reasoning is deductive, usually based upon assumptions derived from cultural or religious traditions or another person's *gnosis*.

Morphogenetic field – Proposed by Rupert Sheldrake, this is an aggregate of individual experiences that resides in a field of consciousness related to a given species. Individuals contribute to this memory field and can draw from it, as for intuitive guidance.

Noetic – Awarenesses beyond description in linear words and concepts, derived from spiritual awareness, gnosis.

Obsession - See *Possession*

Ontology – Metaphysical study of the theories of basic reality or pure being.

Peritonitis – Infection in the abdominal cavity.

Physical phenomena – Ghostly figures that appear in mediumistic séances.

Possession (Obsession) – When a discarnate entity has taken over (*possessed* or *obsessed*) the mind and/ or body of an individual for its own purposes

Precognition – Knowledge of a future event prior to its occurrence.

PS-I - Manipulations by the psychic surgeon only in the aura or astral body, which is secondarily presumed to effect changes in the physical body

PS-II – Manipulation by the psychic surgeon of the healee's physical body.

Psi (Psychic or Extra Sensory Perception) - Thought or experience based on information or sensory inputs gathered without the use of the five usual senses, including telepathy, clairsentience, precognition and retrocognition. Once within the unconscious or conscious mind, this information may be processed in a logical way, or may be handled intuitively. Psi perceptions are not inherently good or bad any more than perceptions based on our physical senses. Psi may represent the most primitive or generalized form of knowing. Indications are that it is often an inherited capacity and can improve with use. It can also be a learned skill, as most people have some measure of psi ability. Examples: auric vision, telepathy, remote viewing, psychometry, psychokinesis (PK).

Psi healing – See *Spiritual healing.*

Psychometry – See *Clairvoyance.*

Reductionistic – Presuming that everything can ultimately be explained by dissecting it into ever more basic components and analyzing it into ever finer details.

Religion - Organized religion grows out of spiritual experience as a way of perpetuating and passing on *gnosis* to those who are not primary experiencers. It may or may not foster or encourage or welcome individuals other than the founders of the religion to themselves question basic assumptions, traditions or values. The more distant a religion is from a sense of personal experience with its basic truths, the more likely the religion will be to insist on absolute adherence to its fundamental doctrine(s) and tenets as a way to insure that its followers do not deviate or go astray from its central teachings – or from those who hold offices in the religious hierarchy.

Some religions require their adherents to demonstrate their faith by exhibiting prescribed behaviors (example: speaking in tongues, walking on burning coals, handling poisonous snakes without being harmed); passing tradition-based rituals or tests of knowledge or skill (catechism or Bar Mitzva); or being "born again." These are types of group-acknowledged and accepted *gnosis* and are usually rigidly adhered to within a particular group. For example, one would not usually speak in tongues in a Catholic Church service or be expected to sit in silent meditation for many hours in a Jewish synagogue observance.

Retrocognition – Knowledge of a past event, without use of sensory cues.

Scientistic (Science as a religion) - The scientific method can be elevated to the status of a religion when it is used to discount observations and theories that are not currently popular, such as psi abilities and transpersonal awarenesses.

Séance – A session in which a medium channels information from spirits.

Sedimentation rate – Non-specific blood test that can indicate presence of infections, some malignancies and heart attacks.

Soteriology.- Theology dealing with salvation, particularly relating to Jesus Christ

Shadow – Those parts of our unconscious mind that we would rather not be aware of, including major and minor traumatic experiences, feelings which we find uncomfortable, self-doubts and misgivings we would rather not perceive, and the like.

Soul – That part of a person which survives death integrates aspects of the person's most recent personality with their eternal Self. (Some prefer to call this part the *spirit*. See also *spirit* for my explanation of my preference for *soul* here and *spirit* there.)

Spirit – That part of a person which survives death and still retains aspects of the person's personality. (Some prefer to call this part the *soul*. I prefer *spirit* because of the popular use of this term to denote those who have passed on but return to communicate through channeled messages or as apparitions. See also *soul*.)

Spiritual gifts (Sitvas, Charisms) - Extraordinary abilities that may be acquired suddenly or as a result of spiritual practices, such as prolonged meditation or vision quests. For example: healing through touch or at a distance; prophesy; discernment of discarnate spirits; levitation; bilocation.

Spiritual healing – A systematic, purposeful intervention by one or more persons intending to help another living being (person, animal, plant, or other living system) by means of focused intention, hand contact, or movements of the hands around the body to improve their condition. Spiritual healing is brought about without the use of conventional energetic, mechanical, or chemical interventions. Some healers attribute spiritual healing occurrences to God, Christ, other "higher powers," spirits, universal or cosmic forces or energies, biological healing energies or forces residing in the healer, psychokinesis (mind over matter), or self-healing powers or energies latent in the healee. Psychological interventions are inevitably part of spiritual healing (as they are with every clinical intervention), but spiritual healing adds many dimensions to interpersonal healing factors.

Spirituality - The first is an individual's basic quest or alignment with ultimate meaning and value. Spirituality often results from primary experience, *gnosis*, which is often stimulated by traumatic or transformational life occurrences, such as dramatic loss and grief; kundalini phenomena; psychic or even psychotic episodes; and other encounters beyond ordinary experience. These may, but do not always, include healing crises.

Synchronicity – Meaningful conincidences that appear to suggest a hidden or guiding order of awareness in the world.

Teleology – The study of final causes; the study of actions as they relate to their utility or ends; activity leading towards achievement of goals.

Telepathy – The transfer of thoughts, images or commands from one living being to another, without use of sensory cues.

Transcendent – Relating to realities that are perceived as being outside of the physical world (but may include the physical), associated with a consciousness that is vastly higher and wiser than that of humanity.

Transpersonal – Awareness extending beyond people's physical boundaries.

UV – *Ultraviolet* – Wavelengths of light that are invisible to the human eye, beyond violet on the color spectrum.

Xenoglossy – Speaking in a language that has not been learned in the current lifetime.

Names Index

A

Achterberg, Jeanne, 124, 330
Adamenko, Viktor, 109–110, 425, 426, 435, 469
Ader, Robert, 50
Adey, 415, 417
Adler, Felix, 171, 501
Agpaoa, Tony, 333
Agricola, Georgius, 439
Allison, Ralph, 83
Altaffer, Thomas, 201
Alvarado, Carlos, 400, 402
Anderson, Sherwood, 35
Archimedes, 197
Aschoff, D., 451

B

Baal Shem Tov, 95
Bach, Edward, 247
Bach, Marcus, 291
Bach, Richard, 535
Bachler, Kaethe, 448
Backster, Cleve, 456
Bacon, Francis, 569
Baker, Julian, 281
Balanovski, Eduardo, 412, 446
Baldwin, H., 439
Ballentine, Rudolph, 163
Bandler, Richard, 49, 87
Barasch, Marc Ian, 131, 132, 178
Barber, Theodore X., 34, 77–78, 90
Barker, 418
Barnothy, M. F., 419
Barrow, John, 463
Barrows, C. M., 74, 78
Bassman, 377
Batcheldor, Kenneth, 336
Bateson, Gregory, 347
Bawin, 417
Beams, 414
Beard, Paul, 339
Bearden, 423
Becker, A. J., 469
Becker, Robert, 414, 419, 433–434, 464
Beecher, H. K., 65
Beinfield, Harriet, 279
Beirnaent, Louis, 163
Bek, Lilla, 229
Bellavita, Paolo, 257–258

Benford, 421
Bennett, Arnold, 555
Bennett, William, 559
Benor, Ruth, 278-279
Benson, Herbert, 93
Benveniste, Jacques, 253, 263, 266
Bergsmann, O., 448
Berkowsky, Bruce, 206
Berland, 125
Bernard, Claude, 364
Berne, Eric, 514
Besant, Annie, 339
Betz, Hans-Dieter, 442
Bierce, Ambrose, 134
Bigu, J., 415
Bird, Christopher, 334, 438, 452
Bishop, George, 60–61
Black, Claudia, 338
Blake, William, 247, 328, 372
Block, Keith, 387
Blundell, Geoffrey, 94, 118
Bohm, David, 423
Bolen, Jean Shinoda, 38–39, 122, 330
Borelli, Marianne, 291
Borysenko, Joan, 233
Bott, Victor, 199
Bouly, Alexis, 453
Bowen, Tom, 280
Brame, Edward, 473
Braud, William, 334
Brecht, Bertolt, 165
Brennan, Barbara, 209, 291, 390, 399, 403
Bresler, David, 404
Brier, Robert, 287
Brilliant, Ashleigh, 33, 34, 54, 104, 111, 169, 171, 243, 288, 442, 491
Brody, 171
Brown, Ellen, 365
Brown, Frank, 471, 472
Brüche, 450
Bruyere, Rosalind, 240, 398
Buchman, 349
Burbank, Luther, 334
Bürklin, F., 450
Burr, Harold Saxton, 192, 344, 412, 413, 433, 469, 472
Burton, Richard E., 105
Buscaglia, Leo, 274, 495
Butler, Lisa, 126
Butler, Samuel, 270

C

Cade, C. Maxwell, 94, 118
Cadoret, Remi, 443
Campbell, Joseph, 299
Canavor, 409
Carey, Ken, 150
Caroli, G., 468
Carrington, Patricia, 292–293
Casdorph, Richard, 82
Cayce, Edgar, 218, 219
Chadwick, Duane, 446
Chapman, J. B., 469
Chappell, L. T., 376
Cheek, D. B., 291
Chief Seattle, 13, 383
Chien, 397
Childre, 418
Chopping, Keith, 55
Chopra, Deepak, 50Chouhan, Ramesh
  Singh, 405–406
Chow, Effie, 202
Choy, Ray, 266, 420
Churchill, Winston, 438
Clark, 286
Clark, Richard, 170
Clinton, Asha Nahoma, 553–554
Clough, Arthur Hugh, 129
Cobb, 368
Cohen, Ken Bearhawk, 182, 303, 317, 511
Cohen, M., 171
Cohen, Nicholas, 50
Cole, Warren, 130
Colligan, Douglas, 64
Colton, Charles Caleb, 370
Comunetti, A. M., 442–443
Connolly, Cyril, 139
Cook, S. A., 446
Cooper, Joan, 350
Cortright, Brant, 505
Cousins, Norman, 118, 232
Covey, Stephen, 571
Cox, Harvey, 552
Cram, Jeffrey, 250
Creighton, James, 315

D

Dajo, Mirin, 96, 100
Dalai Lama, 487
Dale, L. A., 443
d'Alembert, Jean Le Rond, 22
Daquin, 469
Darras, Jean-Claude, 187
Daskalos, 156

David-Neel, Alexandra, 337–338
Day, Langston, 454–456
de Boer, Wilhelm, 444
de Chardin, Pierre Teilhard, 103, 567
de la Warr, George, 454–456
Del Mar, 379
DeMeo, 430
Desrosiers, 447
Devereaux, 447
Diamond, John, 200
DiCarlo, 571
Diegh, Khigh Alx, 185
Dienstfrey, Harris, 18
Disraeli, Benjamin, 181
Donovan, 349
Dossey, Larry, 100, 123, 131–132, 459
Douglas, Herbert, 449
Doust, Jenny, 379
Downer, S., 357, 377
Dressler, David, 218, 226
Dreyfus, 286
Drown, Ruth Beymer, 456
Dubrov, 423
Duggan, Robert, 400
Dumitrescu, 408
Dumoff, 387
Duplessis, Yvonne, 108, 400, 409, 427
Dykeman, Arthur, 293

E

Eagle, Brooke Medicine, 175
Eastwood, N. B., 443
Edge, Hoyt, 421
Edwards, Harry, 156, 339
Edwards, N., 177
Eeman, L. E., 430–432, 434
Einstein, Albert, 21, 169, 284, 412, 481
Eisenberg, David, 181, 363, 364, 366, 377
Eliade, Mircea, 146, 321
Eliot, T.S., 200
Ellenberger, 290
Ellerbroek, Wallace C., 154, 346
Ellison, Arthur, 397, 398
Emerson, Ralph Waldo, 464, 529, 534
Endler, P. C., 257
Engel, Hans G., 407
Epictectus, 106
Epstein, Donald, 218
Epstein, Gerald, 331, 543
Erickson, Milton, 268
Ernst, Edzard, 376
Eskinazi, Daniel, 259
Estebany, Oszkar, 332

Everson, Tilden, 130
Eysenck, Hans J., 126–127, 263, 465, 466–467

F
Fadini, 445
Fang, Lu Yan, 110, 422
Fawzy, F. I., 124
Feldenkrais, Moshe, 245–246
Feldman, 403
Finsen, Niels, 272
Floyd, Keith, 136
Fonorow, 172
Fontanarosa, Phil B., 395
Forrest, 447
Fosket, 171
Foulkes, R. A., 445
France, Anatole, 495
Francis of Assisi, Saint, 527
Frank, Jerome, 61–63
Frankl, Victor, 106, 516
Fraser-Harris, 401
Freud, Anna, 30
Freud, Sigmund, 81
Frey, 469
Friedman H., 469
Fuller, Buckminster, 278, 564

G
Galbraith, Jean, 398
Gallert, 429
Gallimore, 423
Gardener, 358
Gauquelin, Michel, 264, 464–466, 467, 469
Gautama Buddha, 539
Gawain, Shakti, 482
Geller, 469, 471
Gibran, Kahlil, 46
Gissurarson, Loftur, 397, 398
Glazewski, Andrew, 415, 433
Gleick, 433
Godman, Colin, 446
Golden, Joe, 274
Goleman, Daniel, 27, 114–115, 138, 161, 501, 561
Gonzalez, S, 69
Goodheart, George, Jr., 200
Goodman, Felicitas, 230
Goodrich, Joyce, 271
Gordon, James, 484
Gordon, Richard, 432
Graham, Martha, 232
Gralla, 357

Green, Alyce, 94, 210
Green, Elmer, 92, 94, 95, 210, 333, 418
Greenberg, Daniel, 119
Greenwell, 352
Greenwood, Michael, 11, 104, 105, 177, 476, 567
Griffiths, Colin, 261–262
Grigoriantz, Alexander, 436
Grinder, John, 49, 87
Grof, Stanislav, 213, 352
Gross, Henry, 447
Grunewald, Fritz, 422
Guibert, Herve, 129
Guiley, 469, 471
Guldager, B., 239
Gunnarsson, Asgeir, 398
Gurwitsch, A. G., 424–425

H
Hager, 448
Hahnemann, Samuel, 251
Halifax, Joan, 213, 352
Hall, Howard, 95
Hansen, G., 444
Haraldsson, 339
Harburg, E. Y., 228
Harner, Michael, 321, 322
Hartmann, E., 449–451
Harvalik, Zaboj V., 443–445
Hattersley, Joseph, 243
Haus, 379
Hay, Louise, 491
Hayman, 290
Hazrat Inayat Khan, 107
Heidegger, Martin, 379
Heller, Joseph, 278
Hemingway, Tricia, 198
Herbert, Benson, 332, 423, 443
Herbert, George, 525
Hieronymous, T. Galen, 456
Hill, Christopher, 352
Hillary, 357
Hippocrates, 246, 275, 378
Hirshberg, Caryl, 130–131, 131
Hoffman, E. J., 357
Holdstock, 469
Holmes, Oliver Wendell, 258
Honeysett, Martin, 181
Hoo Fang, 60
Hornig-Rohan, Mady, 124
Horowitz, Len, 172
Horrigan, 387

Hudson, Tori, 304
Hunt, Valerie, 240–241, 398, 402, 406
Huntley, 376
Hutchinson, 349
Huxley, Aldous, 169, 301
Hyman, Ray, 202

I
Ibn Gabirol, 285
Ingram, Catherine, 551
Inyushin, V. M., 425–427
Isaacs, Julian, 432

J
Jack, W. H., 446
Jackimczyk, 469
Jackson, Christina, 352
Jacobs, M., 357
Jacobson, Nils, 287
Jahn, Robert, 158
Jahnke, Roger, 186, 317
James, William, 126
Janov, Arthur, 44
Jean, James, 328
Jeffrey, Francis, 57, 316
Jensen, Larry, 446
Johannsen, 422
Johnson, Steve, 249
Joy, W. Brugh, 120, 300, 347
Joyeaux, Henri, 421
Jung, Carl, 157–158, 178, 189, 297, 502
Jurion, Jean, 453

K
Kabat-Zinn, Myla, 502
Kanary, John, 493
Kaptchuk, Ted, 136, 162, 189, 191, 321
Karagulla, Shafika, 389
Katz, Michael, 170
Kaune, 415
Kaye, Danny, 519
Kaznacheyev, Vlail, 427, 435, 472
Keller, 396
Keller, Helen, 276, 497
Keller, Jimmy, 365
Kelly, W., 469
Kennedy, Edward, 119
Kennedy, John F., 497
Kessler, 181
Khalsa, Dharma Singh, 352
Kiev, Ari, 235
King, M., 424

King, Martin Luther, Jr., 477, 527
King, Serge, 286
Kirlian, Semyon Davidovich, 404–405
Kiszkowski, P., 445
Kiyota, Masuaki, 110–111
Klinowska, M., 471
Knock, Andrew, 528
Knowles, F. W., 333
Kofman, Fred, 242
Kollerstrom, N., 472
König, Herbert, 445, 449
Konikiewicz, 409
Kornfield, Jack, 298–300
Korngold, Efrem, 279
Kraft, Dean, 333
Krebs, Charles, 202–203
Kreiger, Dolores, 183
Krieger, Dolores, 273, 325, 333, 390
Krippner, Stanley, 156, 182, 320, 321, 423, 426, 472
Kuhlman, Kathryn, 60, 82
Kunz, Dora van Gelder, 325, 389
Kuznetsov, Vladimir, 95

L
Laing, Ronald, 32
Landau, Judith, 545
Lao, Lixing, 195
Laurie, 423
Lawrence, Jerome, 83
Lawrence, Ron, 239
Lazarou, J., 171–172
Leadbeater, C. W., 339
LeCron, Leslie, 77
Lee, Robert E., 83
Lee, Si-Chen, 109
Leerner, M., 357
Lehman, G., 450
Leichtman, Robert, 342
Leonard, George, 230
LeShan, Lawrence, 98, 100, 121, 234, 271, 291–292, 333
Leskowitz, Eric, 106, 401
Leuchter, AF, 69
Levesque, 471
Levey, Joel, 213, 562
Levey, Michelle, 213, 562
Levine, Barbara Hoberman, 70
Levine, Stephen, 122, 149, 150, 542
Liberman, Jacob, 273, 409
Lieber, Arnold, 471–472
Lilly, 349
Linn, 125, 126

Lipinski, Boguslaw, 421
Lipton, Bruce, 215
Locke, John, 169, 380
Locke, Steven, 124
Loehr, Franklin, 341, 344
Lonegren, Sig, 457
Long, A., 376
Long, Max Freedom, 96
Lovelock, James, 462
Lowen, Alexander, 45
Luedtke, Dietrich, 427
Lukoff, 169
Lundberg, George D., 288, 395

M

Maanum, Armand, 277
Macbeth, Jessica, 37
MacEnulty, John, 2, 21, 498, 533
MacManaway, Bruce, 94, 218
Maddox, John, 263–264
Mallikarjun, 405
Mann, W. Edward, 427–428
Manning, Matthew, 334
Margenau, Henry, 136
Marino, Andrew A., 414
Markides, Kyriakos, 96, 156
Markova, Dawna, 24
Marsh, 414
Martin, S., 470
Mason, Keith, 373
Mason, Randall, 70
Masson, Alain, 411
Matthews-Simonton, Stephanie, 315, 357
McCraty, Rollin, 275, 418
McElroy, Susan Chernak, 560
McEnulty, John, 231
Mentgen, Janet, 250
Mercola, 172
Merker, Mordecai, 78–79
Mesmer, Franz Anton, 74, 239
Michaud, 419
Miller, M., 15
Miller, Robert, 421
Milton, John, 37, 339
Mison, Karel, 287
Monro, Jean, 266, 420
Montagu, Ashley, 276
Montaigne, Michel de, 64
Montgomery, 277
Moody, Raymond A., 339
Mootz, Robert, 214
Morenas, Jamshed, 522
Morrison, Van, 23

Morse, Melvin, 179
Mosely, 368
Moss, Ralph, 357, 368
Moss, Richard, 175, 382
Moss, Thelma, 406
Motoyama, Hiroshi, 187, 188
Muller, H. J., 265
Murphy, Michael, 96, 247, 328
Murray, A., 177
Murray, J. C., 463
Myss, Carolyn, 287

N

Neumann, Therese, 95
Newton, 357
Nias, D. K. B., 465–467
Nightingale, Florence, 172
Nin, Anais, 475
Nixon, Richard, 119
Nizer, Louis, 544
Nordenstrom, Bjorn, 240, 433
Norred, 377
Norwood, Robin, 153
Nuland, 368, 369
Nunn, Peter, 11, 476, 567

O

O'Donohue, John, 272
Oldfield, Harry, 402
Oliven, 469
O'Regan, Brendan, 130–131
Ornish, Dean, 50–51, 126, 274, 314
Orr, Leonard, 213, 352
Oschman, James, 239, 241, 393, 415,
   417–418
Osis, Karlis, 339, 443
Osler, William, 171
Owen, Iris, 335
Oye, Robert, 133

P

Padfield, Suzanne, 332
Palmer, D. D., 214, 215
Panser, Jan Joy, 472
Parnell, Laural, 116
Patanjali, 287
Patten, Leslie, 432
Patten, Terry, 432
Patton, George, 568
Pavek, Richard, 279, 322
Pearl, 420
Peat, F. David, 137
Pellegrino, Charles, 356

Pelletier, 376
Perls, 44
Perry, 420
Persinger, Michael, 419, 471, 472
Pert, Candace, 239, 241
Peterson, James, 402
Petschke, 449, 450
Phillips, Jan, 325
Picasso, Pablo, 403
Piccardi, Giorgio, 467–468
Pichotka, J., 468
Pierrakos, John, 45, 150–152, 282, 403
Pietroni, Patrick, 367, 377
Pinchuck, Tony, 170
Plume, Harold, 60
Pokorn, 469
Poock, 408
Pope, D. H., 443
Pope, Ilse, 447–448
Priore, 423
Proust, Marcel, 100, 389, 505

Q
Quinn, 396

R
Rabindranath Tagore, 205, 235
Radin, Dean, 469, 470
Rae, M., 441
Rahe, Richard H., 15
Rahn, Otto, 424–425, 435
Raikov, Vladimir L., 78
Raina, 312
Rajaram, 405–406
Ram Dass, 106, 134
Rambeau, Dr., 448
Ramirez, Amanda, 124
Randi, James, 263
Randolph, Theron, 242
Ravitz, Leonard, 192, 413, 469, 472
Ray, 213, 352
Rebman, Jannine, 469, 470
Reich, Wilhelm, 44–45, 428–430, 434
Reichmanis, 419
Rein, Glen, 275, 412, 422–423
Remen, Rachel Naomi, 199, 323
Retallach, Dorothy, 230
Rhine, J. B., 443
Rhine, Louisa, 510
Richards, M. C., 380
Richardson, J. L., 125
Richardson, M., 171
Richter, Curt, 73

Rilke, Rainer Maria, 535, 558
Rindge, Jeanne Pontius, 1
Ring, 339
Rinkel, Herbert, 242
Roberts, Kenneth, 447
Roberts, Oral, 60
Rocard, Yves, 445
Rodriguez, Orlando, 526
Rodriguez, Phyllis, 526
Rogers, Carl, 115
Rogo, D. Scott, 338
Romains, 399
Roosevelt, Eleanor, 507
Rosa, Emily, 393–397
Rosa, Linda, 288, 393–397
Rosch, Paul, 239
Rose, Louis, 59
Rosenthal, Robert, 62–63
Rossi, Ernest, 74, 268
Roszak, Theodore, 474
Rotton, 469, 471
Roy, Rustum, 96
Rubenfeld, Ilana, 45, 229
Rubin, Theodore, 384
Rumi, Maulana Jelaluddin, 228, 479, 524
Rush, Benjamin, 182
Russek, Linda, 397, 418
Russell, Edward W., 344, 388, 424, 456
Ryan, Carolyn, 544

S
Safonov, Vladimir, 332, 333
Sagan, Carl, 264
Saint-Exupery, Antoine de, 297, 501
Sancier, Kenneth, 202, 354
Sannella, 352
Sargant, William, 82
Satir, Virginia, 486
Satprem, 299
Sattilaro, Anthony J., 357
Schaefer, R. C., 214
Schauberg, Viktor, 349
Schaut, George B., 472
Schell, Jesse N., 22
Scheller, E. F., 449
Schiffer, Fredric, 111–112, 555–556
Schiowitz, 221
Schneck, G., 449
Schrock, Dean, 125
Schroeder-Sheker, Therese, 230
Schultz, J. H., 206–207
Schulz, Mona Lisa, 116
Schulze, N., 469

Schumacher, E. F., 244
Schwartz, Gary, 58–59, 287–288, 392, 397, 418, 434
Schwarz, Berthold, 96, 447
Schwarz, Jack, 95, 411
Scofield, Anthony, 456–457
Seard, M. Leon, 115
Seidel, S., 250
Selye, Hans, 222
Seneca, 286
Senge, Peter, 242
Sergeyev, Gennady, 427
Sermonti, 418
Servadio, Emilio, 63–64
Seto, A., 416–417
Setzer, Dr., 473
Seutemann, Sigrun, 265
Sewell, Ruth Benor, 162, 377
Shakespeare, William, 44, 63, 302
Shannon, 469, 471
Shapira, Kolonymus Kalman, 311
Shapiro, Francine, 115
Shapiro, Martin, 133
Shaw, George Bernard, 6, 102, 130
Shealy, C. Norman, 100–101, 235, 287, 420
Sheik Lex Hixon, 546
Sheldrake, Rupert, 158–159, 345
Shem, Samuel, 378
Sherin, 471
Sherman, Ronald, 275–276
Shubentsov, Yefim, 192
Siegel, Bernie, 12, 120–121, 274
Signorini, Andrea, 257–258
Sills, Franklyn, 220, 227, 432
Simonides, 232
Simonton, O. Carl, 121–122, 123, 315, 330
Sisken, B. F., 415
Skinner, S., 452
    dowsing as, 462
Sleep, Tony, 229, 277
Sliker, Gretchen, 83
Smith, Cyril, 266, 420, 435
Smith, Huston, 350
Smith, Justa, 421
Smith, Lendon, 243
Snoyman, 469
Solomon, Paul, 14, 127
Soomere, Dr., 472
Sparrow, Margaret, 335
Spear, Deena, 94, 482
Spencer, Paula Underwood, 515
Spiegel, David, 76, 124–126

Spiegel, Herbert, 76
St. Claire, Lindsay, 446
Steadman, Alice, 27
Steel, Rosemary, 407
Stein, Diane, 318
Steinbeck, John, 553
Steindl-Rast, David, 359
Steiner, Rudolf, 199
Stelter, Alfred, 95, 333
Stevenson, Ian, 152–153
Stewart, Walter, 263
Still, Andrew Taylor, 216
Stoff, Jesse, 356
Stone, Randolph, 279, 313
Stoppard, Tom, 234
Studdert, David, 364, 366
Sumrall, Joe, 292
Sutherland, William G., 220
Swami Rama, 136
Swami Satchidananda, 134
Swift, Jonathan, 314
Sykes, Bill, 66
Szasz, Thomas, 164
Szydlowski, H., 445
Szymanski, Jan, 416

T
Takata, Maki, 468
Talbot, Michael, 383
Tart, Charles, 335, 402
Taubes, 369
Taylor, 412
Taylor, Charles, 276
Taylor, George, 276
Taylor, J. G., 446
Taylor, J. Lionel, 107
Taylor-Reilly, David, 256, 258
Tenforde, 415
Tesla, Nikola, 423
Thomas, Alexander, 477
Thommen, 379
Thompson, William Irwin, 570
Thoreau, Henry David, 34, 383, 437, 463, 488, 540
Thrash, 349
Tiller, William, 187, 258, 432, 458–459
Tillotson, Alan K., 336
Tipler, Frank, 463
Tipton, 469
Tolstoy, Leo, 65, 298, 379
Tomatis, Alfred, 229
Tompkins, 334
Touitou, 379

Trager, Milton, 281
Tromp, Sol, 444, 446–447, 450
Turner, Gordon, 339, 390–391
Tweedie, Irina, 300

U

Uphoff, Mary Jo, 110–111
Uphoff, Walter, 110–111
Upledger, John E., 220, 222–225, 333, 498
Usui, Mikao, 318

V

van der Post, Laurens, 137, 503
Vasiliev, Leonid, 78, 90
Vaughan, Frances, 137, 149, 150, 189
Velkover, 469
Vernejoul, P. de, 187
Vilenskaya, Larissa, 98, 426
Villoldo, Alberto, 156
Vinokurava, Svetlana, 419, 420
Voll, R., 354
Voltaire, François, 378
von Franz, Marie-Louise, 148–149, 157
von Pohl, Freiherr, 447–448
Von Reichenbach, Karl, 427–428

W

Walker, J., 415
Walter, Katya, 118, 155
Wardell, Diane Wind, 250
Watson, Lyall, 73, 456, 572
Watts, Alan, 55
Wegman, Ita, 199
Weiskott, 469
Welch, Patrick, 320, 321
Westlake, Aubrey, 290, 432, 453–454
Wetzel, 376
Whitaker, Kay Cordell, 148
White, J., 352
White, Rhea, 96, 247, 328
Whitman, Walt, 414

Whitmont, Edward, 251, 255–256,
  260–261
Whitton, J. L., 446
Whorwell, Peter, 543
Wiesenfeld, 409
Wiklund, Nils, 287
Wilber, Ken, 140–146
Wilson, B., 419
Wilson, Sheryl, 78, 90, 334
Witt, J., 277
Wolinsky, Steven, 382
Wolpe, J., 48
Worrall, Olga, 402
Wright, Machaele Small, 334, 656–666
Wright, Susan Marie, 287, 391
Wüst, J., 450

Y

Yeats, W. B., 100
Yongje, 426
Young, Brigham, 525

Z

Zert, Vlastimil, 449
Zimmerman, John, 416–417, 421
Zingrone, Nancy, 400
Zlokazov, V. P., 333
Zuccarelli, H., 110

Subject Index

Page numbers in **bold** indicate a major discussion of a topic.

A

Abreactions, 42
Acceptance, **70-72**
  importance of, 70
  low, 71-72
  in self healing, 558-559
Access to treatment laws, 171
Acquired Immunodeficiency Syndrome (AIDS),
  self healing for, 127-128
Active listening, 487
Acupressure, 278
Acupuncture, **192-197**
  adverse effects, 194-195
  American Academy of Medical Acupuncture (AAMA), 197
  for arthritis, 355
  Eastern cosmologies and, 195-196
  healing and, 192
  mechanisms behind, 189-191
  meridians and, 185-186
  National Accreditation Commission for Schools & Colleges of Acupuncture & Oriental Medicine (NACSCAOM), 196
  for pain management, 105
  research evidence for, 192-194
  for strokes, 357
  training and licensing, 196-197
  triple warmer, 185
  Western study of, 186-189
  World Union of, 187
Adrenaline, production of, 36
Adverse drug reactions, 172, 563-564
Affirmations, **553-554**
Aggression, poor management of, 15, 18
  See also: Anger management
Akashic records, 342
Alexander Technique, 45, **197-199**, 355
  direction, 198
Allergies
  CAM therapies for, 354
  EM fields and, 420, 434
  environmental, 242
  food, 306
  homeopathic dilutions for, 266

  treating, **307-308**, 563-564
Allobiofeedback, 94
Allopathic medicine
  American Medical Association, 365
  acupuncture explored by, 186-189
  bioenergy medicine and, 4-5
  complementary therapy (CAM) advantages over, 375
  conditions useful for, 7, 367-371
  disadvantages, 371-372
  iatrogenocide, 172
  medical errors, 172, 371
  wholistic medicine, 162-164, 384-387
  See also: Wholistic Medicine; Integrative Medicine
Alternative Medicine (Burton Goldberg Group), 377
Alternative Medicine: Expanding Medical Horizons (NIH), 377
Alternative state of consciousness (ASC), 98-100, 291
  See also: Meditation; Reality, objective
American Academy of Medical Acupuncture (AAMA), 197
American Association of Naturopathic Physicians (AANP), 304
American Board of Holistic Medicine, 376
American College for Advancement in Medicine, 238
American Holistic Medical Association, 274, 287, 304, 376
American Holistic Nurses Association, 304, 376
American Medical Association, 365
American School of Osteopathy, 216
Anatomy of an Illness (book), 118
Anesthesia
  acupuncture for, 193
  hypnotic, 75
Anger management, **516-533**
  behavior changes, 529-530
  bioenergy protection, 530-532
  blame and, 520-523
  control issues, 517-518
  cost-benefit analysis, 520
  deeper meanings, 524-525
  expressing anger, 518-520
  forgiveness, 526-528
  group angers, 525-526
  neutralizing approaches, 532-533

Animal healings, **312-313**
Animal magnetism, 74
  See also: Hypnosis; Suggestion
Anthropomaximology
  alternative states of consciousness and,
    98-100
  defined, 95
Anthroposophic medicine, **199**, 354
Anxiety
  autogenic training for, 207
  defined, 29
  healing useful for, 153-154
  See also: Meta-anxiety
Applied Kinesiology (AK), **200-204**
  for allergies, 354
  case studies, 202-203
  cautions, 204
  dowsing and, 460
  mechanisms behind, 203-204
  muscle testing exercises, 511-513
Arahant, 139
Archetypes, 157
Aromatherapy, **205-206**, 278
Art therapy, **230**
Arthritis, 307, 354-355
Aston Patterning, 278
Astral bodies, 195
  See also: Auras
Astrology, 464-468
  See also: Cosmobiology
Athletics, alternative states of conscious-
  ness and, 98-100
  See also: Fitness
Attitudes, positive, 561-562
Auras, **389-404**.
  bioenergies and, 152
  health problems and, 389-390
  interaction of, 397-399
  research evidence for, 391-397
  sensing, 397
  tactile nature of, 390
  theories of, 401-404
  visualization of, 339-342
  See also: Kirlian photography
Autogenic Training (AT), **206-207**, 334-335
Autonomic nervous system (ANS), 35, 79
Autonomy, patient, 360
Awareness through movement, 246
  *See also: Dance therapy; Movement
    therapy*
Ayurvedic medicine, **207-209**, 354

B

Bacteria, therapeutic use of, 314
  See also: Probiotics
Bagua, 244-245
  *See also: Environmental medicine;
    Feng shui*
Behavior change, 528-529
Behavioral therapy. *See Cognitive
  behavioral therapy*
Bi-Digital O-Ring Test, 511
  See also: Applied Kinesiology
Bigu, 96
Bilberry extract, 309
Bioelectrography. *See Kirlian photography*
Bioelectromagnetics, 239
Bioenergetics, 45, **281-282**
Bioenergies
  auras and, 152
  electromagnetic. *See Electromagnetic
    (EM) fields*
  energy circuits, 430-432
  energy cysts, **222-223**, 333
  Energy Field Assessment (EFA) ques-
    tionnaire, 391
  healing contributions, 3-4
  interaction of, 397-399
  laboratory measurement of. *See Elec-
    tromagnetic (EM) fields*
  Pierrakos on, 150-152
  sensing, 397
  shielding, 529-531
  subtle, 160, 183-184, 203, 244, 439
  Western medicine and, 4-5
  yoga and, 351-352
Bioenergy therapy
  basic principles, 10
  Pierrakos on, 150-152
Biofeedback, **91-94**
  allobiofeedback, 94
  body control and, 93-94
  EEG, 94
  healing and, 94
  for pain management, 92-93
  research and applications, **210-211**
Biofeedback Certification Institute of
  America (BCIA), 210
Biofield levels. *See Bioenergies; Auras*
Biological rhythms, 272, 379-380
Bions, 428-429
  See also: Orgone
Bioplasm, 425
Bioresonators, 451
Black boxes. *See Radionics devices*

Blame, 519-522
Blended medicine, 8
    See also: Integrative medicine; Wholistic medicine
Body metaphors, 67-68
Bodymind therapy.
    case studies, 211-213
    in general, 159-160
    physical symptoms and, 46-47
    principles behind, 51-53
    See also: Mind-body therapy
Boggle threshold, 57
Book of Changes (*I Ching*), 536
Boundaries, maintaining, 361
Bowen technique, 47, **280**
Boxwood, 309
Brain hemispheres, **111-118**
    Applied Kinesiology and, 202-203
    exercises, 114, 556-557
    laterality, 116-118
    stress and, 555-556
    Western focus on left, 117
Brain, mind outside the, 134-136
Brainstorming, 494
Breathwork, **213-214**.
    See also: Yoga
Brennan, Barbara, healing, **209-210**
British Medical Association, 181

C
CAM (complementary/alternative medicine) therapies, 192
    in allopathic (conventional) medicine, 162, 162, 384-387
    versus allopathic medicine, 372, (table) 375
    for chronic illness, 172-173
    certification in, 361-363
    competence, establishing, 359
    complaint mechanisms, 361
    cost-effectiveness, 173, 374
    ethical, legal issues, 359-366
    general approaches, 372-374
    problems addressed, 354-358
    research evidence for, 169
    safety, 172
    selecting, 377-378
    spiritual healing and, 183-184
    weaknesses of, 173
    See also: individual therapies, integrative care
Cancer
    CAM therapies for, 357

    conventional treatments for, 119
    geopathic zones and, 448
    psychoneuroimmunology (PNI), 51, 127-128, 315, 357
    self healing with, **120-126**
    spontaneous remission, 130-133
    visual imagery for, 121-124, 330, 544
Candida yeast infections, **355-356**
Cardiovascular disease
    mind's influence on, 50-51
    Psychoneurocardiology, 51, 314
    self healing for, 126-127
Centauric Self, 146
Centeredness, 564-567
Certification in CAM, **359-363**
    competence and, 359
    professional development, 360
    standards for, 183
Chakras, **188-192**
    colors associated with, 272
    healer focus on, 191-192
    visually identified, 190, 389-390
    yoga and, 352
Chanda Maharosina Tantra, 336
Chaos theory, 433
Chelation therapy, **238**
Chemical sensitivity, 242
Chemotherapy, 119, 132-133, 368
Children
    auras sensed by, 402-403
    experiences of "inner child" in adulthood, Inner child, 338, 476, 514
    treating, 360-361
Chinese massage, 278
Chiropractic, **214-219**.
    adverse effects, 218-219
    Council for Chiropractic Education, 215
    development of, 214
    healing and, 218
    mechanisms behind, 214-215
    National Board of Chiropractic Examiners, 215
    subluxations, 214
    training and licensing, 215-216
    See also: Craniosacral therapy; Osteopathy
Chronic fatigue syndrome (CFS), 356
Chronic illness
    Ayurvedic medicine for, 209
    CAM useful for, 7, 172-173, 354, 373

Chronobiology, 379
Circadian rhythms, 272, 380
Clinical ecology. *See Environmental medicine*
Co-dependent relationships, 54
Code of Conduct, British healers, 184
Coenzyme Q10, 307
Cognitive behavioral therapy (CBT), 42, 48, 487-488
Cognitive development, 142-143
Collective consciousness, 157-159, 568-569
Colonic irrigation, **219-220**, 349
Color therapy, **272-273**, 333
Colors, dermal perception of, 108-109, 399-400, 427
Coma, 358
Commission on Massage Training Accreditation and Approval, 283
Committee for the Scientific Investigation of Claims of the Paranormal (CSICOP), 467
Committee for the Study of the Paranormal, 395
Committee Para, 467
Communication, exercises to increase, 484-487
Compassion, 527-528
    personhood of therapist, 380
Competence, establishing CAM, 359
Complaint mechanisms, CAM 361
Complementary therapies. *See CAM therapies*
Complexity theory, 258
Conditioning, psychological
    behavior therapy and, 48-49
    conditioned responses, 42
    immune responses and, 50-51
    Pavlov's study of, 47
    stress and, 505-507
Confederation of Healing Organisations, 184
Confidentiality, 361
Conjuring up Philip, 335-336
Consciousness
    alternative states of, 98-100, 291
    collective, 157-159, 567-568
    higher, 83
    matter shaped by, 136
    outward arc, 142
    split, 81-83
    transcendent, 7
    Wilber on, 140

Consejeras, 236
Consent, 360
Contracts, therapy, 359-360
Control groups, 165
Conventional medicine
    balancing with CAM, 384-387
    versus complementary therapy, 375
    conditions useful for, 367-371
    disadvantages, 371-372
Conversion reactions, 43, 81-83
Core-energetics therapy, 45, **282**
Cosmobiology, **464-474**
    versus astrology, 464
    Gauqelin's study of, 464-466
    lunar influences, 470-473
    solar effects, 467-469
    See also: Geobiological effects
Cosmologies, Eastern, **195-196**
Cost benefit analysis (CBA), 488-490, 519
Costs, healthcare, 371
Council for Chiropractic Education, 215
Council for Homeopathic Certification (CHC), 267
Council on Naturopathic Medical Education (CNME), 304
Cranfield Institute of Technology, 257
Craniosacral therapy, **220-227**
    conditions useful for, 221
    defined, 220-221
    facilitated segments, 222
    overlaps with healing, 224-225
    problems and questions, 225
    and spiritual awareness, 227
    Upledger theories, 222-225
Creative arts, **233-234**.
    See also: specific therapies: Art, Journaling, Movement and Dance, Music, Poetry
Crystals, **234-235**
Curanderismo, **235-237**
Curry net, 447, 456-457

D
Dance therapy, **230**
Death
    dealing with, 179-180, 371-372
    and music therapy, 230
    near-death experiences, 339
Deep-tissue massage, **277**
Defense mechanisms, 29-33
    armoring, body, 151, 281-282
Denial, 30

Depression
    CBT for, 50
    crystals for, 235
    herbal therapy for, 308-309
Dermal optics (vision), 108-109, 399-400, 427
Desensitization, 506-507
    See also: Conditioning
Determination, 559
Diagnosis
    approaches to, 384-385
    conventional emphasis on, 370
    varies in CAM, 372
Diet therapy, **305-307**
    Elimination diets, 306
Dietary supplements, **307-308**
Direction (Alexander Technique), 198
Displacement, 31
Dissociative disorders, 81-83
    Inner Self-Helper, 64, 83
Distant healing, 435-436
Divination, **535-538**
Doctors
    choosing, 381-382
    heavy responsibility of, 370-371
    stress management for, 386
Doshas, 208
Dowsing, **439-459**
    blocking, 459
    Curry net, 447, 456-457
    devices used in, 439-440, 537
    dragon paths, 447
    electrodermal responses during, 446-447
    of EM fields, 443-446
    history of, 439
    ley lines and, 448-451, 463-465
    map dowsing, 440
    medical, **289-290**, 354, 440-441, 452-454, **457-462**
    Pohl Scale, 447-448
    research evidence for, 442-446, 451-452
    theories of, 458-460
Dreams, analysis of, 39, 507-511
Drugs. *See Medications*
Duke University, 443

E
Echinacea, 309
École Normale, 445
Ecopsychology, 474
Ectoplasm, 97

EDTA Chelation, **238**
EEGs
    biofeedback with, 94
    brain cell activity and, 412-413
    during healing, 118
    Mind mirror, 94, 118
    muscle testing and, 204
Ego states, 514
Electrical skin resistance (ESR), 91-92
Electroacupuncture assessments, **187-188**
Electrocardiography (ECG/EKG), 413
Electrodermal activity (EDA), 446-447
Electroencephalograms. *See EEGs*
Electromagnetic (EM) fields
    dowsing of, 443-446
    effects of, 419-421
    healing and, 421-422
    near the body, 415-418
    non-Hertzian, 423
    organizing, 433
    research on, 412-418
    spirituial healing and, 420-422
    summary of, 433-434
EM pollution, 243, 419-420
EM therapy, **239-241**
    conditions useful for, 355, 240-241
    mechanisms behind, 241
    research evidence for, 241
Electromyography (EMG), 413
Emotional Freedom Technique (EFT), 116, 548
    See also: Meridian based therapies
Emotional intelligence, 27, 114-115, 501
Emotions
    expressing, 499-501
    handling in therapy, 56
    illness and, 14-15
    intense, 214
    meta-, 521
    trusting, 502
Enemas, **219-220**, 349
Energy fields. *See Auras; Bioenergies; Electromagnetic (EM) fields, unconventional fields*
Entelechy, 261
Environmental medicine, **242-245**
Eros, 141
Essential oils, **205-206**, 282
    See also: Aromatherapy
Etheric body, 404
Ethical issues, **359-361**

Etiquette, professional, 361
Evidence-based practice, 164
Evil eye, 64
Exercise, **246-247**, 497-499
Experimenter effects, *See Placebo effects*
Extroverts, 22
Eye Movement Desensitization and
    Reprocessing, 115-116, 212, 549

F
Faith healing. *See Spiritual healing*
Fasting, 306
    See also: Bigu
Fatigue, vitamins for, 308
Federation of State Medical Boards, 387
Feedback loops
    general, 53-54
    negative, 56-57
    self-validating, 55
    theories of, 58-59
Feelings. *See Emotions*
Feldenkrais method, 45, **245-246**
Feng shui, **244-245**, 438-439, 457
Fibromyalgia, **356-357**
Fight or flight response, 36
Firewalking, 96, 97-98
Fish-skin disease (ichthyosis), 75
Fitness, **246-247**, 497-499
Flexner Report, 253, 304
Flower essences, **247-250**
    Rescue Remedy, 248
Folk healing
    Ayurvedic medicine, **207-209**, 354
    curanderismo, **235-237**
    Italian, 63-64
    Native American, **303**, 538
    rituals and, 320
    shamans, 68, **320-322**
    Tibetan medicine, **326-327**
Food and Drug Administration (FDA), 166
Forgiveness, 525-527
Franklin Pierce College, 446
French Academy of Medicine, 464-465
Functional integration, 246

G
Gaia, 244, 321, 462-463
Galantamine, 307
Gardening projects, 656-666
Garlic, 309
Gastrointestinal illness, 542-543
General Council and Register of Naturo-
    paths (GCRN), 304

Genetic therapy, 369
Geobiological effects
    psi and, 473-474
    ecopsychology, 475
    See also Cosmobiology
Geomancy. *See Dowsing*
Geometry, sacred, 439
Geopathic zones, 441, 447, 450
Gestalt therapy, 38, 44, 56, **503-505**,
    541
Ginger, 309
Ginkgo biloba, 309
Glasses, brain-hemispheric influence,
    114
Goal-directedness, inherent, 83-86,
    261
Green tea, 309
Groups, self-help, 539
    *See also: Psychoneuroimmunology;
        Psychoneurocardiology*
Guidelines, practice, 387

H
Hair analysis, **250**
Hallucinations, under hypnosis, 76
Hand healing, 532
Handles, for intervention, 61-62
Harrogate Training College, 443
Healing. *See Spiritual healing*
Healing Touch (HT), 3, 250, 281
Heart, living life through, 527-528
Heavenly bodies.
    See Cosmobiology
Hedges, 58
Hellerwork method, 45, **278**
Hemophilia, self-hypnosis and, 75
Herbal medicine, **309-312**
    adverse effects, 311
    for cancer, 357
    in general, 308-309
    regulation of, 310
    training and licensing, 310
Hexes, 68, 73
Holistic medicine, 162.
    American Board of Holistic
        Medicine, 376
    American Holistic Medical
        Association, 274, 287, 304, 376
    American Holistic Nurses
        Association, 304, 376
    See also: Wholistic medicine
Holonomic therapy, **213**
Holophonic sound, 110

Homeopathy, **251-267**
  in 19th century, 171
  for allergies, 354
  approaches to, 252-253
  for arthritis, 355
  case studies, 254-255, 262-263
  conventional, 251-252
  Council for Homeopathic Certification
    (CHC), 267
  as energy medicine, 260
  Hahnemann, founder, 251
  healing and, 265-266
  intuitive, 252
  Low-dose responses, 259
  mechanisms behind, 257-263
  miasms, 259
  National Center for Homeopathy, 267
  nosodes, 254
  potency issues, 264-265
  remedy preparation, 253-254
  remedy symptom clusters, 251
  research evidence for, 256-257
  Royal Society of Homeopaths, 267
  sarcodes, 254
  self healing with, 256
  training and licensing, 267
Hookup principle, 281
Hope, promotion of, 374
Hormone replacement, 369
Hormones, 36
Humor, 232
Hydrotherapy, 349-350
Hypertension, hypnosis and, 75
Hypnosis
  for cancer, 357
  clinical applications, 80-82, **268-269**
  common features, 87-88
  conditions useful for, 75
  conversion reactions, 43-44, 81
  excellent candidates for, 78
  healing and, 90-91
  history of, 74-75
  ideomotor response, 202
  induction styles, 75-76
  mechanisms behind, **77-80**, 88
  nervous system and, 79
  plenary, 290
  psi abilities and, 90-91, 290
  regression during, 76
  self, 81-82
  self-image and, 86
  telepathic, 78-79
  training and licensing, 269

without formal induction, 83-86
  See also: Suggestion
Hysterical (conversion) reactions,
  43

I
I Ching (Book of Changes), 536
I messages, 484-487, 518
Iatrogenocide, 172
Illness, emotional factors of, 14-15
Imagery. See Visualization
Immune system
  conditioning and, 50-51
  electromagnetic fields and, 239
  stress and, 36, 89
Immunizations, 254, 369
Infections, 367
Inner child, 338, 514
Inner Self-Helper, 64, 83
Insomnia, visual imagery, 545-546
Institute of Medicine, 172
Insurance coverage for CAM, 363
Integrative medicine
  balancing CAM with conventional,
    367-378, 384-387
  in general, 8
  modes of, 180-181
  as whole-person care, 170-171
Intellectualization, 31
Intelligence, emotional, 501
Internal mammary artery ligation, 65
Introverts, 22
Intuition, 533-534
Intuitive assessment, **284-288**
  development of abilities, 284
  pattern recognition and, 286-287
  research evidence for, 287-288
  through palpation, 285
Ionizing radation, 241
Irritable bowel syndrome, 542-543
Isopathy, 254
Issues, facing personal, 482-484

J
Jin shin do, 278
Jin shin jyutsu, 278
Journal of the American Medical
  Association (JAMA), 395-397
Journal of the Centre for Cancer
  Research, 448
Journaling, 232, 502-503
Joy, 234, 566-567
Jungian personality types, 20

K
Kapha (dosha), 208
Kava, 172
Kinesiology
    applied.
    behavioral, **200-201**
    See also: Applied Kinesiology
Kirlian photography, 187, 207, 240, 265,
    404-411.
    See also: Auras
Kundalini, 352

L
Lachesis, 252-253
Laterality, brain and body, 116
Laws, health.
    access to treatment, 171
    CAM ban attempts, 182-183
    liability, 206-207, 364
    licensing, certification, 362-366
    See also: Legal status
Laying-on of hands. *See Touch healing*
Leeches, **270**
LeShan healing, **271**
Ley lines, 447-451, 456-457, 462
Liability, 206-207, 364
Licensing for CAM
    competence and, 359
    in general, 361-363
    professional development, 360
    standards for, 183
Life-Events Scale, 15, 16-17
Life fields, 344, 413, 424

Life force
    in Native American medicine, 303
    orgone energy, 44-45, 428-430
Light therapy, **272-273**, 355
Limpia, 236
Linear analyses, importance of, 7-8
Logical awareness, 144
Love, as therapy, **274-275**
Low energy emission therapy, **240**
Lowenwork, **282**
Lunar influences, **469-472**
Lymph drainage, 277

M
Maggots, **276**
Magnet therapy. *See Electromagnetic
    therapy*
Magnetic passes, 74
Maieutic Method, 231

Malpractice litigation, 371
Manual lymph drainage, 277
Manual therapy. *See Chiropractic;
    Craniosacral therapy; Osteopathy*
MariEl healing, 154
Marylebone Health Centre, 377
Massage, **277-283**
    aromatherapy with, 205
    Chinese, 278
    clinical applications, 283
    Commission on Massage Training
        Accreditation and Approval, 283
    effective components, 282
    exercises, 497
    history of, 276
    for stress, 45, 495
    training and licensing, 283
    types of, 277-279
Matrix Therapy, Seemorg, 554-555
Meaning, in life, 564-567
Medical dowsing.
    See Dowsing, medical
Medical errors, 172, 371
Medical intuition.
    See Intuitive assessment
Medications
    adverse effects, 172, 563-564
    conditions useful for, 367-368
    tranquilizers, 28
Medicine cards, 537
Medicine, conventional, *See Allopathic
    medicine;
    Integrative medicine*
Medicine men, 320.
    See also: Shamanism
Meditation, 143-146, **291-300**.
    adverse effects, 300
    approaches to, 291-293
    breathing, 547
    bypass, 299
    for chatty minds, 547-548
    concentrative, 138, 140
    effects and benefits, 295-300
    exercises, 546-548
    insight, 138
    lessons from, 294
    mantras, 292
    mindfulness, 138-139, 546
    Pranayama, 351
    receptive, 141-142
    research evidence for, 293
    samadhi, 352
    for stress relief, 46, 532

visualization and, 336-338
See also: Wilber, Ken; Yoga
Membership Self, 144
Meninger Institute, 418
Mentalin, 209, 309
Mentastics, 281
Meridian based therapies, **308-309**, 548-550
Meridians, **185-190**
scientific evidence of, 186-187
visually identified, 190
See also: Applied Kinesiology
Meta-anxiety
acceptance and, 70
defined, 300, 493
healing useful for, 153-154
reducing, 86
See also: Anxiety
Metaphors, body, 67-68
as basis for suggestion, 88-90
Miasms, 259
Microwave resonance therapy, **239-240**
Milk thistle, 309
Mind-body therapy
case studies, 211-212
in general, 46, 159-160
Pierrakos on, 150-152
principles behind, 51-53
psychotherapy with, 212-213
See also: Bodymind therapy; Metaphor;
Placebo; Self healing; Suggestion
Mind mirror, 94, 118
Mind, outside the brain, 134-136
Mitogenic radiation, 424-425
Mobius strips, 423
Morphogenetic fields, 159, 345, 424
Movement therapy, **230**
awareness through movement, 246
See also: Dance therapy
Multiple personality disorder (MPD), *See*
Dissociative disorder, 81-83
Multiple sclerosis, 358
Muscle relaxation exercises, 495-496
Muscle testing, **200-201**, 511-513.
See also: Applied Kinesiology
Music therapy, **228-230**
Musselman phenomenon, 73
Myotherapy, **277**
Myths, **233-234**

N

National Accreditation Commission for
Schools & Colleges of Acupuncture

& Oriental Medicine (NACSCAOM), 196
National Board of Chiropractic Examiners, 215
National Board of Osteopathic Medical Examiners, 219
National Cancer Act of 1971, 119
National Center for Complementary and Alternative Medicine (NCCAM), 387
National Center for Homeopathy, 267
National Electro-Acoustics Laboratory (China), 110
National Health Freedom Coalition, 182
Native American medicine, **303**, 538
Natural healing capacity, 378-380.
See also: Self healing
Nature (journal), 263
Naturopathic medicine, **304-305**
American Association of Naturopathic Physicians (AANP), 304
Council on Naturopathic Medical Education (CNME), 304
General Council and Register of Naturopaths (GCRN), 304
Near-death experiences, 339
Neckar Hospital (Paris), 187
Neo-Reichian therapy, **282**
Nervous system
autonomic, 35
studies of, 412-418
parasympathetic (PNS), 35, 36
sympathetic (SNS), 35-37
Network Spinal Analysis, 47, 216, 218
Neurolinguistic Programming (NLP), 49, 87, 212, 550-551
Neurological problems, 357-358
Neuromuscular massage, 277
Neuropeptides, 36, 50
Neuroses, 28-29
Newtonian medicine.
See Allopathic medicine
Nirvanic state, 139
Nocebo effects, 66
Non-steroidal-anti-inflammatory drugs (NSAIDs), 374
Normality, 33-34
Nuclear force, 412
Nuprin Pain Report, 100-101
Nurse Healers Professional Associates, Inc., 326

Nutritional therapies. **306-312**
    for allergies, 354
    for arthritis, 355
    for cancer, 357
    diets, **305-307**
    stress and, 562-563

O
Objective reality, 11
Observational studies, 167
Orgone energy, 44-45, 428-430
Ornish, Dean, psychoneurocardiology, 51, 314
Orthomolecular medicine, **307**
Osteoarthritis, 307, 354-355
Osteopathy, **216-219**.
    American School of Osteopathy, 216
    National Board of Osteopathic Medical
        Examiners, 219
    See also: Chiropractic; Craniosacral
        therapy
Out-of-body experiences (OBEs), 338, 404

P
Pain, **101-107**
    assessment of, 103-105
    incidence of, 101
    perception of, 101-103
    phantom limb pain, 357-358, 401
    psychological components, 107
Pain management
    acupuncture, 105, 193
    biofeedback, 92-93
    CAM useful, 106
    spiritual healing, 105-106
    visualization, 540-541
Parapsychology,
    See Psi phenomena
Parasympathetic nervous system (PNS), 35, 36
Parent Effectiveness Training, 484
Parmann Project, 95, 99
Partializing, 493-494
Past lives, 152-153, 382
Pattern recognition, intuition and, 286
Pendulums. See Dowsing
Perceptions, crossed-sensory (synesthe-sias), 108-109, 399-400
Perseverance, 559-560
Persona, 24, 29
Personal space, 491-492
Personality
    disorders, 26-28

shadow aspects, 23-24
stress and, 15, 18
traits, 19-20
types, 20-22
Type A, 15, 18
Pet therapy, **312-313**
Pharmaceutical companies, studies
    commissioned by, 166
Philip effects, 335-336
Phobias, 49, 86-87
Physical fitness, **246-247**, 497-499
Physical powers
    alternative states of consciousness
        and, 98-100
    defined, 95
    physical fitness, **246-247**, 497-499
Physicians
    choosing for yourself, 381-382
    heavy responsibility of, 370-371
    stress management for, 386
Physics, quantum.
    See Quantum physics
Phytotherapy. See Herbal medicine
Pineal gland, 36
Pitta (dosha), 208
Pituitary gland, 36
Placebo effects
    healing and, 1-2
    negative (nocebo), 66
    in RCTs, 165-166
    as response to suggestion, 64-65
    scorned by Western medicine, 60,
        164
Plenary trances, 77
Pleromatic Self, 143
Poetry, **232-233**
Polarity therapy, 279, **313-314**, 421
Positive thinking, 561-562
Post-traumatic stress disorder, EMDR
    for, 115
Practice Guidelines, 387
Pranayama, 351
Pranic Self, 143
Pressure point therapies, 278
Preventive medicine, 369-370
Primal scream therapy, 56
Probiotics, **314**
Professional development, CAM, 360
Projection, 31
Proving (homeopathy), 251, 257, 261-262
Pseudonirvana, 139

Psi phenomena, 7
  collective unconscious and, 158
  dreams and, 510
  geobiology and, 472-474
  healing and, 9
  hypnosis and, 90-91
  psychic readers, 153;
  right brain function and, 117
  thoughtography, 110-111
  See also: Medical intuition
Psychological conditioning
  behavior therapy and, 48-49
  immune responses and, 50-51
  Pavlov's study of, 47
Psychoneurocardiology, 51, **314**
Psychoneuroimmunology (PNI), 51, **127-128, 315-316,** 357
Psychoses, 26-28
Psychosomatic disorders, 34-35
Psychotherapy
  body-based, 44-45;
  clinical applications, **316-317**
  hypnosis and, 80-82
  meridian, 301-302
  relational, 37-40
  spectrum, Appendix A
  touch avoided during, 51-52
  training and licensing, 316
  transpersonal. *See Transpersonal psychotherapy*
  variation within, 133-134
  See also: Bodymind, Mind-body therapies
Psychotronic associations, 424
Pulsed electromagnetic fields (PEMFs), 239, 355

Q
Qi energy, 185-186
Qigong, 96, 196, **317-318**
Qualitative studies, 167, 169-170
Quantum physics
  bioenergy medicine and, 4
  and consciousness, 136
  homeopathy and, 258-259
  vs. Newtonian physics, 437, 569
  on observation, 383
  research, 11

R
Radiation
  ionizing, 241, 449
  mitogenic, 424-425

  ultraviolet, 426-427, 435
Radiation therapy, 368
Radiesthesia. *See Dowsing, medical*
Radionics devices
  homeopathy and, 265
  medical dowsing with, 289, 440
  research on, 455-456
  spiritual healing and, 458
  water healing and, 266-267
  See also: Dowsing
Radix, 282
Randomized controlled trials (RCTs)
  for CAM, 164-168
Rationalization, 31
Reaction formation, 31
Reality, objective, 11
  See also: Alternative States of Consciousness
Realms of being, 147
Rebirthing, 213, 352
Records, patient, 360
Red reflex, 223
Referrals, CAM 360
Reflexology, 279
Registration of CAM therapists, 361-363
Regression
  defined, 31
  hypnotic, 76
  in service of ego, 155
Regulating systems, 35-37
Reiki, 3, 154, 281, **319-320**
Reinforcement. *See Psychological conditioning*
Relaxation techniques, 44
Religion, psychology of, 136-137
Remission, spontaneous, 130-132
Repression, 26, 30
Rescue Remedy, 248
Research evidence in CAM.
  in general, 7-8
  methodological errors in, 166
  on selecting therapies, 376-377
  study types, 164-167
  See also: specific DAM therapies
Respant, 120
Rituals
  as self-healing, 561-562
  therapeutic nature of, **320**
  visualization and, 345
Rolfing, 45, **278,** 398
Rosenthal (experimenter) effect, 63
Royal Society of Homeopaths, 267

Rubenfeld Synergy Therapy, 45
Runes, 537

S
Sacred geometry, 439
Samadhi, 352
Scheller test, 449
Schizophrenia, 28
Schumann frequency, 419
Scrying, 538
Seasonal affective disorder (SAD), 272, 308
Secondary gain, 35, 55
Sedona Method, 542, 551
Self confidence, 557-558
Self, development of, 143-146
Self-healing, 118-119, **476-569**
    anger management, 515-532
    autonomy, patient, 360
    benefits of, 476-478
    and brain hemisphere functions, 557-558
    and the body, 496-500
    for cancer, 120-126, 357
    capacity for, 378-380
    for cardiovascular disease, 126-127
    collective consciousness, 568-569
    feeling your way through, 500-507
    head working with heart, 515-533
    finding meaning in life, 565-568
    meridian-based, 301-302
    natural healing, 378-380
    nutrition, 563-564
    objective research lacking, 128-129
    personal space, 492-493
    reasoning, and stress, 478-496
    respant (responsible participant), 120
    subtle energy and, 160
    sweetening spirals, 55, 481-482
    unconscious roots of stress, 506-514
    varieties of healing for, 533-568
    visualization in, 342-346
Self-healing exercises
    AK muscle testing, 512-514
    bioenergetic, 533-534
    brain hemisphere functions, 557-558
    building on successes, 482-484
        See also: Sweetening spirals
    cognitive behavioral therapy, 488-490
    communication, 485-488
    cost-benefit analysis, 489-491

desensitization, 506-507
divination, 536-539
dream analysis, 508-512
facing issues, 483-484
fitness, 497-499
gestalt therapy, 504-506
"gardening", 657-667
in groups, 540
journaling, 503-504
massage, 497
Matrix Therapy, Seemorg, 554-555
meditation, 547-549
meridian based therapies, 549-551
muscle relaxation, 496-497
neurolinguistic programming, 551-552
psychoneurocardiology, 51, 314-315
psychoneuroimmunology (PNI), 51, 127-128, 315, 357
rituals, 561-562
for stress, 477-479
Sedona method, 552
story telling, 553-554
suggestion in, 554-556
sweetening spirals, 481-482
Transactional Analysis, 56, 144, 515-516
for vicious circles, 479-481
visualization, 540-547
worry, turned into concern, 493-496
Self image, 86
    constructs of self, 29
Shadow aspects of personality, 23-24
Shamanism, 68, **321-323**.
    See also: Folk healing
Shen Tao, 195
SHEN healing, 106, 154, 279, **323**
Shiatsu, 278
Sick building syndrome, 243
Silva Mind Control, 287
Skepticism, 57-58
Skin
    diseases and hypnosis, 75
    special functions of, 107
Sobardoras, 236
Solar effects, 467-469
Somnambulism, 290
Sound, healing effects, 110-111
Space, personal, 491-492
Spiritual awareness, 533-534
Spiritual bypasses, 33
Spiritual Frontiers (journal), 472

Spiritual healing, **323-324**
   adverse effects, 324
   for anxiety, 153-154
   biofeedback and, 94
   in Britain, 184
   in CAM, 183-184
   for cancer, 357
   chakra focus, 191-192
   chiropractic and, 218
   conditioning and, 53
   for conversion reactions, 82-83
   craniosacral therapy and, 224-225
   defined, 1, 9, 323
   distant, 435-436
   electromagnetic fields and, 421-422
   energy fields and, 3
   homeopathy and, 265-266
   hypnosis and, 90-91
   infrasound and, 417, 422
   interpenetrating process, 177
   laterality and, 116
   for multiple sclerosis, 358
   for pain management, 105-106
   physical symptoms and, 46-47
   principles behind, 51-53
   self. *See Self healing*
   spontaneous remission, **130-132**
   touch. *See Touch healing*
   visualization and, 332-334
   See also: Brennan; Healing Touch;
      LeShan; Reiki; Shamanism; Shen
      Therapy; Therapeutic Touch;
      Touch healing
Spontaneous remission, **130-132**
Sports massage, 277
SQUID technology, 417
St. John's Wort, **308-309**
Statistical analyses, in RCTs, 165
Stigmata, 95
Storytelling, **231**, 552-553
Stress
   autogenic training for, 207
   brain hemispheres and, 555-556
   conditioning and, 505-507
   factors countering, 69-70
   in healthcare practitioners, 386
   immune disorders and, 36, 89
   personality factors, 15, 18, 477
   self healing exercises, 477-479
   touch for, 495
   unconscious roots, 506-515
Strokes, 193, 357
Structural Integration, 278

Subluxations, 214
Subtle energies, 160, 183-184, 203,
   244, 439
   See also: Bioenergies; Energy
      fields
Subtle realms, 147
Sudden infant death syndrome
   (SIDS), 243
Sufis, 95, 99
Sugar-pill reaction. *See Placebo*
   effects
Suggestion, **59-63**.
   for anxiety, 154
   Applied Kinesiology and, 203
   flower essences and, 249
   in general, 59-60
   legitimacy of, 61-63
   metaphor as basis for, 88-90
   negative, 376
   posthypnotic, 80
   in self healing, 553-555
   See also: Hypnosis
Superconducting quantum interfer-
   ence device (SQUID), 417
Surgery, **368-369**
Surveillance theory, 121-122
Surveys, as research method, 167
Swedish massage, 277
Swedish Mind Dynamics, 287
Sweetening spirals, 55, 481-482
Sympathetic nervous system (SNS),
   35-37
Synesthesias, 108-109, 399-400

T
T'ai Chi Ch'uan, 318, **325**
Talk therapy, 37-40
Tarot cards, 536-537
Tension, chronic, 34, 47, 89, 496
Tension circuit, 430-432
Thanatology, music, 230
Thanatos, 141
Theory of Relativity, 569
Theosophical Society, 339
Therapeutic Touch, 106, 281, 288,
   325-326, 390
Therapists
   choosing, 381-382
   contracts, 359-360
   importance of, 183
   personhood of, 380
   stress management for, 386
Third eye, 402

Thought Field Therapy, 301, 344, 548
Thoughtography, 110-111
Tibetan Book of the Dead, 339
Tibetan medicine, **326-328**
Touch healing, 3, 108
Touch, importance of, 107-108
Traditional Chinese Medicine (TCM)
    for arthritis, 355
    diagnosis in, 197
    health and illness viewed by, 189
    massage, 278
Trager psychophysical integration, 281
Training, issues of CAM, 178, 183-184.
    See also: specific therapies
Trances. *See Hypnosis, Alternative State
    of Consciousness*
Tranquilizers, for personality disorders, 28
Transactional Analysis, 56, 144, 514-515
Transcendent consciousness, 7
Transcranial electrostimulation (TCES),
    240, 241
Transcutaneous electrical nerve stimula-
    tion (TENS), 240
Transference, 315
Transformation process, 140, 145
Translation process, 140, 145
Transpersonal psychotherapy, **137-139**
    autogenic training and, 207
    bioenergies and, 152
    facets of, 137
    meditation as, 138-139
    in wholistic medicine, 382-384
Trial by fire, 96
Trigger points
    massage for, 277
    muscular, 282
Triple warmer, 185
Tsubo, 278
Tumo, 93
Type A personalities, 15, 18
Typhonic Self, 143

U
Ultradian rhythm, 111, 380, 555
Ultraviolet (UV) radiation, 426-427, 435
Unconventional Fields and radiations, 422-
    433
Unusual human abilities, 97
Uroboric Self, 143
Utah State University, 446

V
Valerian, 309

Vata (dosha), 208
Vegetarian diets, 306
Vibrations, atmospheric, 244, 491
Vicious circles, 480-482
Visual Analogue Scale (VAS), 104
Visualization, **328-349**
    applications, 328-329, 348
    for bowel problems, 542-543
    for cancer, 121-124, 544
    conditions treated with, 329-332
    exercises, 334, 539-546
    group, 335-336, 347
    for insomnia, 545-546
    mechanisms behind, 332
    meditative, 336-338
    muscle testing and, 512
    negative effects, 347-348
    of other realities, 338-339
    for pain management, 540-541
    with physical intervention, 346
    research evidence for, 334
    in self healing, 342-346
    spiritual exploration with, 544-545
    in spiritual healing, 332-334
    for stress relief, 532
    suggestion and, 88-90
    thought forms, 340-342
    transition and, 146
Vitamins, **307**
Voll instrument, 187

W
Water therapies, **349-350**
Western medicine. *See Allopathic
    medicine*
Wholistic Hybrid of EMDR and EFT
    (WHEE), 115, 302, **550-551**
Wholistic medicine, 162
    American Board of Holistic Medicine
        (ABHM), 376
    American Holistic Medical Association,
        274, 287, 304, 376
    American Holistic Nurses Association,
        304, 376
    CAM therapies and, 179-180
    popularity of, 177-178
    professional associations, 178
    self healing facilitated by, 163-164
    tenets of, 174-177
    transpersonal perspectives, 382-384
    and Western medicine, 164
Wholistic spiritual healing. *See Spiritual
    healing*

Wilber, Ken, meditation stages,143-146
    Centauric Self, 146
    Membership Self, 144
    Pleromatic Self, 143
    Pranic Self, 143
    Typhonic Self, 143
    Uroboric Self, 143
Will to live, 73
Worry, concern and, 492-493

Y
Yang, 190-191, 195-196
Yeast infections, **355-356**

Yerberas, 236
Yin, 190-191, 195-196
Yoga, **350-353**.
    approaches to, 350-351
    body control and, 93
    clinical applications, 353
    energy component, 351-352
    in integrative care, 352
    See also: Meditation
You messages, 484-487, 518

Z
Zone therapy, **279**

About the Author

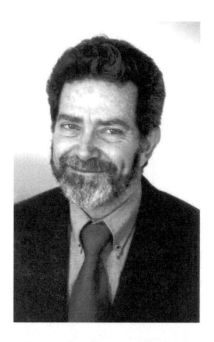

Daniel J. Benor, M.D. is a wholistic psychiatrist who includes bodymind approaches, spiritual awareness and healing in his practice. Dr. Benor is the author of Healing Research, Volumes I-IV and many articles on wholistic, spiritual healing. He appears internationally on radio and TV. He is a Founding Diplomate of the American Board of Holistic Medicine, Coordinator for the Council for Healing, a non-profit organization that promotes awareness of spiritual healing, and on the advisory boards of the journals, *Alternative Therapies in Health and Medicine, Subtle Energies* (ISSSEEM), *Frontier Sciences,* and the Advisory Council of the Association for Comprehensive Energy Psychotherapy (ACEP). He is editor and producer of the International Journal of Healing and Caring – On Line www.ijhc.org. See more by and about Dr. Benor at: www.WholisticHealingResearch.com